Inherited Metabolic Diseases

Georg F. Hoffmann
Johannes Zschocke
William L. Nyhan (Eds.)

Inherited Metabolic Diseases

A Clinical Approach

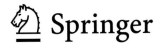 Springer

Prof. Dr. Georg F. Hoffmann
Ruprecht-Karls-University
University Children's Hospital
Im Neuenheimer Feld 430
69120 Heidelberg
Germany
Georg.Hoffmann@med.uni-heidelberg.de

William L. Nyhan, MD, PhD, Professor
University of California, San Diego
School of Medicine
Department of Pediatrics
9500 Gilman Drive
La Jolla, CA 92093
USA
wnyhan@ucsd.edu

Johannes Zschocke, Dr.med.habil., PhD,
Professor of Human Genetics
Divisions of Human Genetics
and Clinical Genetics
Medical University Innsbruck
Schöpfstr. 41
6020 Innsbruck
Austria
johannes.zschocke@i-med.ac.at

ISBN: 978-3-540-74722-2   e-ISBN: 978-3-540-74723-9

DOI: 10.1007/978-3-540-74723-9

Springer Heidelberg Dordrecht London New York

Library of Congress Control Number: 2009931335

Cover design: eStudio Calamar, Figueres/Berlin

Printed on acid-free paper

Springer is part of Springer Science+Business Media (www.springer.com)

Dedication

To our patients and their families

Preface

The field of inherited metabolic diseases has changed from a limited group of rare, untreatable, often fatal disorders to an important cause of acutely life-threatening but increasingly treatable illness. Unchanged is the orphan nature of these disorders with mostly relatively nonspecific initial clinical manifestations.

The patient does not come to the physician with the diagnosis; the patient comes with a history, symptoms, and signs. This book starts with those and proceeds logically through algorithms from questions to answers. Special emphasis is placed on acutely presenting disorders and emergency situations. The rationale of the approaches presented in this book are based on extensive, collective clinical experience. To utilize as broad an experience as possible, its concept has been extended from a pocket-size book written jointly by five colleagues to a textbook combining the experience of over 20 expert metabolic physicians. It is now imbedded in the environment of Springer Pediatric Metabolic Medicine in addition to the disease-based approach in Inborn Metabolic Diseases edited by John Fernandes and colleagues as well the series edited by Nenad Blau and colleagues on specific biochemical diagnostics, laboratory methods, and treatment.

A system and symptom-based approach to inherited metabolic diseases should help colleagues from different specialties to diagnose their patients and to come to an optimal program of therapy. For metabolic and genetic specialists, this book is designed as a quick reference for what may be (even for the specialist) infrequently encountered presentations.

Heidelberg, Germany   Georg F. Hoffmann
Innsbruck, Austria   Johannes Zschocke
San Diego, California, USA   William L. Nyhan

Contents

Contributors

Enrico Bertini Ospedale Pediatrico Bambino Gesù, Piazza S. Onofrio, 4, 00165 Rome, Italy, bertini@opbg.net

Alberto Burlina Department of Pediatrics, Division of Metabolic Disorders, University Hospital, Via Giustiniani 3, 35128 Padova, Italy burlina@pediatria.unipd.it

Alessandro P. Burlina Department of Neuroscience, Neurological Clinic, University of Padova, Via Giustiniani 5, 35128 Padova, Italy, alessandro.burlina@unipd.it

Ellen Crushell 26 Wainsfort Grove, Terenure, Dublin 6 W, Ireland, ellen.crushell@gmail.com

Joe T. R. Clarke Division of Clinical Genetics, Hospital for Sick Children, 555 University Avenue, Toronto, Ontario, M5G 1X8, Canada, jtrc@sickkids.ca

Carlo Dionisi-Vici Division of Metabolism, Bambino Gesu Hospital, Piazza S. Onofrio 4, 00165 Rome, Italy, dionisi@opbg.net

Guido Engelmann University Children's Hospital, Ruprecht-Karls-UniversityIm , Neuenheimer Feld 430, D-69120 Heidelberg, Germany, e-mail: guido.engelmann@med.uni-heidelberg.de

Angels García-Cazorla Servicio de Neurologia, Hospital Sant Joan de Deu, Passeig Sant Joan de Deu 2, 08950 Esplugues, Barcelona, Spain, agarcia@hsjdbcn.org

Kenneth M. Gibson Department of Biological Sciences, Michigan Technological University, Dow 740, ESE 1400, Townsend Drive, Houghton, MI 49931, USA kmgibson@mtu.edu

Hans H. Goebel Department of Neuropathology, Mainz University Medical Center, Langenbeckstraβe 1, 55131 Mainz, Germany, goebel@neuropatho.klinik.uni-mainz.de

Stephanie Grünewald Great Ormond Street Hospital, London WC1N 3JH United Kingdom, grune@gosh.nhs.uk

May El Hachem Ospedale Pediatrico Bambino Gesù, Piazza S. Onofrio, 4, 00165 Rome, Italy, elachem@opbg.net

Georg F. Hoffmann University Children's Hospital, Ruprecht-Karls-University, Im Neuenheimer Feld 430, 69120 Heidelberg, Germany, georg.hoffmann@med.uni-heidelberg.de

Cornelis Jakobs Department of Clinical Chemistry, Metabolic Unit, VU University Medical Center, De Boelelaan 1117, 1081 HV Amsterdam, The Netherlands C. Jakobs@vumc.nl

Stephen G. Kahler Department of Pediatrics, Division of Clinical Genetics, University of Arkansas for Medical Sciences, 4301 W. Markham Street, Little Rock, AR 72205, USA, KahlerStepheng@uams.edu

Division of Clinical Genetics, Slot 512–22, Arkansas Children's Hospital, 800 Marshall Street, Little Rock, AR 72202–3591, USA

Joachim Kreuder Department Pediatric Cardiology, University Children's Hospital, Feulgenstraße 12, 35385 Giessen, Germany, joachim.g.kreuder@paediat.med.uni-giessen.de

Dietrich Matern Biochemical Genetics Laboratory, Department of Laboratory Medicine and Pathology, Mayo Clinic, 200 First Street S. W., Rochester, MN 55905, USA, Dietrich.Matern@mayo.edu

Ertan Mayatepek Department of General Pediatrics, University Children's Hospital, Moorenstrasse 5, 40225 Düsseldorf, Germany mayatepek@uni-duesseldorf.de

Ute Moog Institute of Human Genetics, Ruprecht-Karls-University, Im Neuenheimer Feld 366, D-69120 Heidelberg, Germany, ute.moog@med.uni-heidelberg.de

William L. Nyhan Department of Pediatrics, University of California, UCSD School of Medicine, 9500 Gilman Drive, La Jolla, CA 92093, USA, wnyhan@ucsd.edu

Ben J. H. M. Poorthuis Department of Medical Biochemistry, K1–252, Academic Medical Centre, University of Amsterdam, Meibergdreef 9, 1105 AZ Amsterdam, The Netherlands, B. J. Poorthuis@amc.uva.nl

Piero Rinaldo Biochemical Genetics Laboratory, Mayo Clinic College of Medicine, 200 First Street S. W., Rochester, MN 55905, USA, rinaldo@mayo.edu

Richard J. T. Rodenburg Laboratory for Pediatrics and Neurology, University Medical Centre St Radboud, Nijmegen, The Netherlands, R. Rodenburg@cukz.umcn.nl

Ronald J. A. Wanders Laboratory of Genetic Metabolic Diseases, Academic Medical Center, University of Amsterdam, Meibergdreef 9, 1105 AZ Amsterdam, The Netherlands, r.j.wanders@amc.uva.nl

Nicole I. Wolf Department of Child Neurology, VU Medisch Centrum, 1007 MB Amsterdam, The Netherlands, n.wolf@vumc.nl

Johannes Zschocke Divisions of Human Genetics and Clinical Genetics, Medical University Innsbruck, Schöpfstr. 41,6020 Innsbruck, Austria, johannes.zschocke@i-med.ac.at

Introduction to Inborn Errors of Metabolism

Disorders of Intermediary Metabolism

A1

Johannes Zschocke

Key Facts

> The classical inborn errors of metabolism are defects in enzymes of the metabolism of amino acids, carbohydrates and fatty acids or in mitochondrial energy metabolism (Fig. A1.1).

> Disorders of intermediary metabolism are often dynamic, they fluctuate with changes in the metabolic state of the patient and frequently allow successful therapeutic intervention.

> Most disorders of intermediary metabolism are readily diagnosed through basic metabolic investigations which include blood gases, glucose, lactate, ammonia, plasma amino acids, urinary organic acids and an acylcarnitine profile.

The classical inborn errors of metabolism are defects in enzymes of the metabolism of amino acids, carbohydrates, and fatty acids or in mitochondrial energy metabolism (Fig. A1.1). These disorders are often dynamic; they fluctuate with changes in the metabolic state of the patient and frequently allow successful therapeutic intervention. Most of them are readily diagnosed through basic metabolic investigations, which include blood gases, glucose, lactate, ammonia, plasma amino acids, urinary organic acids, and an acylcarnitine profile.

A1.1 Disorders of Amino Acido Metabolism

Typical aminoacidopathies result from abnormalities in the breakdown of amino acids in the cytosol. In addition, several disorders involving mitochondrial enzymes such as branched-chain ketoacid dehydrogenase (maple syrup urine disease) or ornithine aminotransferase (gyrate atrophy of the choroidea) are classified as aminoacidopathies as they do not involve CoA-activated metabolites. This distinguishes aminoacidopathies from the organic acidurias, which are considered a separate group of disorders affecting mitochondrial enzymes, CoA-activated metabolites, and which have effects on other mitochondrial functions. Clinical symptoms of the aminoacidopathies may be thought of as caused by the accumulation of toxic intermediates that cause specific organ damage. Several defects of amino acid metabolism such as histidinemia are benign because

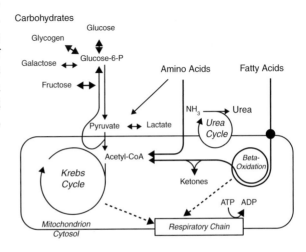

Fig. A1.1 Main pathways of intermediary metabolism

J. Zschocke
Divisions of Human Genetics and Clinical Genetics, Medical University Innsbruck, Schöpfstr. 41,6020 Innsbruck, Austria
e-mail: johannes.zschocke@i-med.ac.at

G. F. Hoffmann et al. (eds.), *Inherited Metabolic Diseases*,
DOI: 10.1007/978-3-540-74723-9_A1, © Springer-Verlag Berlin Heidelberg 2010

the metabolites that accumulate are not toxic. The pathogenetic relevance of an inborn error of amino acid metabolism is not always easy to ascertain as clinical symptoms observed in the child may be coincidental or the reason for performing the analysis in the first place. Aminoacidopathies are diagnosed through the analysis of plasma (or urinary) concentrations of amino acids and sometimes of urinary organic acids. A majority is treatable through dietary restriction of protein and of the amino acid involved in the defective pathway and by the avoidance or prompt treatment of catabolic states that lead to the breakdown of large amounts of protein. Another therapeutic strategy that has been successful in hepatorenal tyrosinemia is the inhibition of a biochemical step before the actual genetic deficiency, thereby changing a harmful disease into a more benign amino acid accumulation without the accumulation of the more damaging substances downstream.

A1.2 Organic Acidurias

The classical organic acidurias are deficiencies of enzymes in the mitochondrial metabolism of CoA-activated carboxylic acids, most of which are derived from amino acid breakdown. In this way, they are distinguished from disorders of fatty acid oxidation, which not only involve CoA esters but also present different diagnostic and therapeutic challenges. The term organic acidurias is preferred to the alternative term organic acidemias as they are most often detected by analysis of the urine. Biochemically, some of the reactions impaired in the organic acidurias are parallel to the dehydrogenase, hydratase, or ketothiolase reactions of the mitochondrial β-oxidation cycle. Clinical features are caused not only by the accumulation of toxic intermediates but also by a disturbance of mitochondrial energy metabolism and carnitine homeostasis; they may include encephalopathy and episodic metabolic acidosis. Organic acidurias are diagnosed through the analysis of organic acids in the urine or acylcarnitines in the blood. Treatment is similar to that of the aminoacidopathies and involves the dietary restriction of the relevant amino acid(s) and the avoidance of protein catabolism. However, as the defective enzymes are distant (more downstream) from the respective amino acids, restriction may not lead to a stoichiometric reduction of pathological metabolites, although it does in methylmalonic aciduria. Unexpected

fluctuations occur and complete return to normal intermediary metabolism is usually impossible. Supplementation with carnitine and sometimes other substances such as glycine (e.g., to form isovalerylglycine in isovaleric aciduria) are very useful adjuncts to the treatment.

Disorders of biotin metabolism are included among the organic acidurias. Biotin is a cofactor of the mitochondrial carboxylases and a deficiency of biotinidase or holocarboxylase synthetase leads to multiple carboxylase deficiency. It is also usually diagnosed through urinary organic acid analysis. Biotinidase enzyme analysis of dried blood spots has been included into programs of neonatal screening as it is well treated with biotin supplementation.

A1.3 Disorders of Ammonia Detoxification

The breakdown of protein produces large amounts of nitrogen in the form of ammonia that is highly neurotoxic but is normally converted to urea and excreted in the urine. Defects in enzymes of the urea cycle and other disorders of ammonia detoxification present clinically with encephalopathy and other symptoms of hyperammonemia. Metabolic investigations should include analysis of the amino acids in plasma and urine and urinary orotic acid. Treatment requires the reduction of protein intake in conjunction with the supplementation of essential amino acids, the avoidance of catabolic states and the administration of benzoate or phenylacetate/phenylbutyrate, which remove nitrogen in the form of alternative conjugates of amino acids such as glycine and glutamine.

A1.4 Disorders of Fatty Acid Oxidation and Ketogenesis

Mitochondrial fatty acid oxidation is required for the provision of energy during fasting, either through complete oxidation or through production of ketones in the liver that then serve as an alternative energy source for the brain. Disorders in this pathway typically present as hypoketotic hypoglycemia precipitated by fasting, leading to coma or convulsions. In addition, some disorders cause severe hepatopathy and (cardio-)myopathy, probably as results of the accumulation of toxic metabolites. The diagnosis is best reached in the acute situation through the analysis of free fatty acids and the ketone bodies 3-hydroxybutyrate and acetoacetate as well as the acylcarnitine profile and urinary organic acids. The diagnosis may be missed if samples are obtained in the normal interval between episodes or after the patient has been treated with intravenous glucose. Treatment consists of avoidance of fasting. Carnitine supplementation is mostly unessessary and must be carefully balanced in some defects, particularly those that cause cardiomyopathy or hepatopathy.

A1.5 Disorders of Carbohydrate Metabolism and Transport

The disorders in this group display a relatively wide range of clinical features and may cause clinical symptoms because of toxicity, deficiency of energy, hypoglycemia, or storage.

- *Disorders of Galactose and Fructose Metabolism*: Defects in the cytosolic metabolism of galactose and fructose for glycolysis cause disease through accumulation of pathogenic metabolites. Children with galactosemia and fructosemia typically develop evidence of severe damage to the liver and/or kidney after dietary intake of lactose (milk, milk products) or fructose (fruit, sucrose), respectively. Treatment requires the elimination of the intake of galactose or fructose.
- *Disorders of Gluconeogenesis and Glycogen Storage*: Typical metabolic features are hypoglycemia after relatively short periods of fasting and lactic acidemia. There may be variable organ dysfunction, most frequently hepatopathy. Glycogen storage leads to hepatic enlargement, which in infancy may be massive. In some disorders such as glycogenosis type III there are elevations of the transaminases and creatine phosphate kinase, and there may be clinical myopathy. Treatment includes frequent meals, cornstarch supplementation, or continuous overnight tube feeding to avoid hypoglycemia.
- *Disorders of Carbohydrate Transport*: There are a number of different glucose and other carbohydrate carriers, and clinical symptoms differ greatly

depending on the tissue localization of the individual defect. Symptoms are frequently gastrointestinal or renal but also include the central nervous system (deficient glucose transport across the blood/brain barrier).

A1.6 Mitochondrial Disorders

Disorders of energy metabolism (usually summarized as mitochondrial disorders although enzymes deficient, e.g., in organic acidurias or fatty acid oxidation defects are also located in the mitochondrion) include genetic defects of the pyruvate dehydrogenase complex, the Krebs cycle and the respiratory electron transport chain, comprising the final pathways of substrate breakdown and the production of ATP. Mitochondrial disorders manifest clinically with symptoms and signs of energy deficiency and a highly variable pattern of organ dysfunctions. In many cases, there are lactic acidemia and progressive neurodegenerative disease. Periods of metabolic stress such as intercurrent infections may trigger a deterioration of the patient's condition. The diagnostic work-up may be difficult and should include frequent measurements of blood lactate levels, CSF lactate, plasma amino acids and alanine, and often a search for mutations in mitochondrial DNA. Repeated, careful examinations of organ functions as well as imaging are essential. Treatment options are limited but usually include various vitamins and cofactors such as riboflavin, coenzyme Q, or thiamine. Heterozygous mutations in the genes of some Krebs cycle enzymes (e.g., fumarase) cause inherited cancer predisposition syndromes.

A1.7 Disorders of Cobalamine and Folate Metabolism

Genetically determined or nutritional deficiencies of vitamin cofactors may affect various metabolic pathways and cause a wide range of clinical symptoms. They can frequently be satisfactorily treated by supplementation of the deficient substance. Of particular importance in intermediary metabolism are cobalamin (vitamin B_{12}) and folate which are essential for cytosolic methyl group transfer. The cellular methylation reactions require methyl group transfer from serine to *S*-adenosylmethionine involving the folate cycle, cobalamin (vitamin B_{12}) and the methionine–homocysteine cycle. A disturbance in this pathway may be caused by methylcobalamin deficiency, a disturbance of the folate cycle, or by deficient remethylation of homocysteine to methionine. Most disorders of cobalamin metabolism as well as nutritional deficiency of vitamin B_{12} cause methylmalonic aciduria. Clinically, disorders of cytosolic methyl group transfer cause an encephaloneuropathy, often with additional hematological problems such as megaloblastic anemia and thrombembolic complications of hyperhomocysteinemia. The diagnosis involves the analysis of urinary organic acids, plasma amino acids (homocysteine), and levels of folate and cobalamin. Treatment includes supplementation of cobalamin and folate, in some situations with addition of betain and methionine.

A1.8 Disorders of Amino Acid Transport

Deficiencies in the intestinal and/or renal transport of amino acids may be nonsymptomatic or cause symptoms because of deficient absorption of essential amino acids (e.g., tryptophan in Hartnup disease) or because of increased urinary concentration of unsoluble amino acids which causes nephrolithiasis (e.g., cystein in cystinuria). These disorders are diagnosed by the quantitative analysis of amino acids in plasma and urine. Treatment depends on the clinical picture. Deficiency of essential amino acids is treated by supplementation with large amounts of these compounds, or in the case of tryptophan deficiency, supply of the cofactor nicotinic acid that is normally synthesized from tryptophan. Renal calculi in cystinuria can be prevented by treatment with a chelating agent such as penicillamine, which forms mixed disulfides with cysteine, and calculi once formed can be resorbed if they have not incorporated too much calcium.

A1.9 Disorders of Peptide Metabolism

- The tripeptide *glutathione* and the *gammaglutamyl cycle* have multiple functions in cellular metabolism, ranging from amino acid transport across membranes

to detoxification of peroxides. Deficiencies may cause neurological and hematological as well as metabolic problems. Investigations should include the determination of organic acids in the urine and glutathione in various body fluids. Treatment is largely symptomatic; certain drugs should be avoided.

- Defective breakdown of *dipeptides* of histidine such as homocarnosine or carnosine may be found in patients with mental retardation, although the causative relationship is not always proven. Ulcers of the skin, particularly of the legs are seen in prolidase deficiency. Investigations should include amino acid and peptide analysis of the urine. Treatment is symptomatic; some individuals with disorders of dipeptide metabolism are asymptomatic and do not require treatment.

A1.10 Disorders of the Transport or Utilization of Copper, Iron, and Zinc

- *Disorders of copper metabolism*: Wilson disease causes a chronic hepatopathy and symptoms of central nervous dysfunction, while patients with Menke disease suffer from neurological problems in conjunction with abnormalities of hair, connective tissue, and bones. Diagnosis involves the analysis of copper and coeruloplasmin in serum, urine, and liver tissue. Treatment in Wilson disease is aimed at reducing copper load, while copper should be parenterally substituted in Menke disease.
- *Disorders of iron metabolism*: Patients affected with such disorders may present with iron-deficient anemia, e.g., due to insufficient intestinal absorption of iron, or with iron overload and liver dysfunction as in hemochromatosis. Secondary iron overload may be observed in some hemolytic anemias. Treatment is directed at substitution or removal of iron.
- *Disorders of zinc metabolism*: Acrodermatitis enteropathica is characterized by chronic skin problems, alopecia, and central nervous symptoms. It is diagnosed through reduced levels of zinc and alkaline phosphatase and is treated with supplementation of zinc.

Disorders of the Biosynthesis and Breakdown of Complex Molecules

A2

Johannes Zschocke

Key Facts

> Disorders of the biosynthesis and breakdown of complex molecules typically show slowly progressive clinical symptoms and are less likely to cause acute metabolic crises.

> Disorders in this group are not usually recognised by basic metabolic analyses but require specific investigations for their diagnosis.

Disorders in this group typically show slowly progressive clinical symptoms and are less likely to cause acute metabolic crises. They are not usually recognized by basic metabolic analyses but require specific investigations for their diagnosis.

A2.1 Disorders of Purine and Pyrimidine Metabolism

Deficiencies in enzymes required for the biosynthesis or breakdown of purines and pyrimidines cause neuromuscular abnormalities, nephrolithiasis, gouty arthritis, or anemia and immune dysfunction. They may be recognized through increased or reduced urinary urea in relation to creatinine, urine microscopy, or specifically through the analysis of urinary purines and pyrimidines. Some metabolites of pyrimidine breakdown are only recognized by urinary organic acid analysis. Nephrolithiasis may be treated or prevented by allopurinol. A high fluid intake is helpful. Some disorders of pyrimidine metabolism, notably orotic aciduria and overactivity of 5' nucleotidase (nucleotide depletion syndrome), are treatable with uridine or triacetyluridine. There is no effective treatment for most of the primarily neurological manifestations of disorders of purine metabolism.

A2.2 Lysosomal Storage Disorders

Lysosomes contain a number of hydrolases required for the intracellular breakdown of large lipid and mucopolysaccharide molecules. If one of these enzymes is deficient, its substrate accumulates and causes enlargement and/or functional impairment of the organ system. Clinical features include progressive neurological deterioration, dysmorphic features, and organomegaly. There is usually no metabolic decompensation, although acute symptoms (e.g., severe pain) is a major feature in some conditions. Investigations include careful roentgenographic examination of the skeleton for dysostosis multiplex, analysis of leukocytes and other cells for vacuoles, and assessment of parenchymatous organs. The urine may be investigated for abnormal glycosaminoglycans and oligosaccharides; specific enzyme studies are usually required to make the exact diagnosis. For most disorders there is no specific therapy yet, although enzyme replacement therapy or bone marrow transplantation has been shown beneficial in several disorders.

J. Zschocke
Divisions of Human Genetics and Clinical Genetics, Medical University Innsbruck, Schöpfstr. 41,6020 Innsbruck, Austria
e-mail: johannes.zschocke@i-med.ac.at

G. F. Hoffmann et al. (eds.), *Inherited Metabolic Diseases*,
DOI: 10.1007/978-3-540-74723-9_A2, © Springer-Verlag Berlin Heidelberg 2010

- *Mucopolysaccharidoses (MPS)*, affected children typically develop progressive dysmorphic features, hepatomegaly and psychomotor retardation or regression. They are usually recognized through the analysis of urine for glycosaminoglycans.
- *Oligosaccharidoses* may resemble the MPS, but many show more severe neurological symptoms and are more frequently symptomatic at birth (nonimmune hydrops fetalis). The diagnosis is made through the demonstration of abnormal oligosaccharide patterns in the urine or enzyme analyses.
- *Sphingolipidoses* and *lipid storage disorders* usually present with progressive neurological deterioration. Hepatomegaly may be present, skeletal deformities and dysmorphic features are rare. Other presentation patterns are found particularly in Fabry disease (pain and paresthesias) and nonneuronopathic Gaucher disease (hematoma, anemia, massive splenomegaly, and abdominal/bone pain). The specific diagnosis usually requires enzyme analysis. The neuronal ceroid lipofuscinoses are usually suspected by electron microscopy and confirmed by mutation analysis. *Mucolipidoses* combine clinical features of the mucopolysaccharidoses and sphingolipidoses and may reflect the deficiency of several lysosomal enzymes as a consequence of defective enzyme processing.
- *Lysosomal transport defects:* Cystinosis causes nephropathy and dysfunction of other organs including the thyroid gland and the eyes; it is diagnosed on the basis of increased cystine content of leucocytes. Sialic acid storage disease causes progressive encephaloneuropathy; it is recognized through elevated free sialic acid in the urine. Both of these disorders result from defective transport out of lysosomes. Cystinosis is treated with oral cysteamine, cysteamine eye drops, and renal transplantation.

A2.3 Peroxisomal Disorders

The biochemical roles of peroxisomes are very diverse. Peroxisomal defects usually cause severe, progressive multisystem disorders.

- Defects of *peroxisome biogenesis* or the *activation and β-oxidation of long-chain fatty acids* cause progressive neurological disease, structural abnormalities as in Zellweger syndrome, and abnormalities in hepatic, intestinal, or adrenal function. They are usually recognized through the analysis of very long-chain fatty acids in blood or cultured fibroblasts. There is no effective treatment.
- Refsum disease is a defect in the metabolism of exogenous *phytanic acid*. It causes slowly progressive neurological, visual, and auditory abnormalities, and often does not present until adulthood. It is diagnosed through the quantification of serum phytanic acid and is treatable by a diet restricted of phytanic acid.
- Defects of *ether-phospholipid biosynthesis* cause rhizomelic chondrodysplasia punctata characterized by proximal shortening of the limbs in addition to neurological and other manifestations. It is diagnosed through quantification of plasmalogens in erythrocytes. There is no effective treatment.
- Catalase deficiency is the only known defect of the *detoxification of oxygen radicals*. It causes chronic ulcers in the oral mucosal membranes.
- Primary hyperoxaluria type I is the only known defect of *glyoxylate metabolism*; it causes nephrolithiasis and nephrocalcinosis. It is recognizable by organic acid or HPLC analysis for oxalate and glyoxylate. It has been treated by transplantation of liver and kidney.

A2.4 Disorders of the Metabolism of Isoprenoids and Sterols

Isoprenoids and sterols are essential in many cellular and developmental processes. Most defects of their synthesis are caused by enzyme deficiencies in the postsqualene portion of the pathway. Only mevalonic aciduria and hyperimmunoglobulinemia D syndrome, both due to mevalonate kinase deficiency, are found in the proximal part of the pathway.

- Mevalonate kinase deficiency is the only known defect of *isoprenoid biosynthesis*. It causes dysmorphic features, failure to thrive, mental retardation, and recurrent febrile crises. An attenuated variant causes hyper-IgD syndrome. Treatment is symptomatic.
- Defects of *sterol biosynthesis* cause various structural abnormalities including the dysmorphic features of the Smith–Lemli–Opitz syndrome and mental retardation. Diagnosis involves plasma sterol analysis. In Smith–Lemli–Opitz syndrome, specific treatment by cholesterol supplementation has been of limited success.

A2.5 Disorders of Bile Acid and Bilirubine Metabolism, Inherited Cholestasis and Porphyrias

- Genetic defects of *bile acid biosynthesis* cause symptoms either through bile acid deficiency or through deposition of precursors. The former causes progressive cholestasis and malabsorption, while the precursors can lead to progressive neurological dysfunction and xanthomas. The bile acid biosynthetic pathway is located partly in the peroxisomes and is affected by peroxisomal disorders. Diagnosis involves the analysis of urinary bile acids. Treatment with bile acids is effective in the bile acid deficiency states and to down-regulate bile acid biosynthesis.
- Hem is metabolized to bilirubin and excreted together with bile acids in the urine. Genetic defects may involve specific enzymes or mechanisms of transport into the bile ducts. They cause indirect or direct hyperbilirubinemia. Specific treatment strategies have been developed for some disorders.
- Porphyrias are disorders of hem biosynthesis, frequently inherited as autosomal dominant traits. Neurotoxic metabolites accumulate in deficiencies affecting the first few steps of the pathway and typically cause intermittent acute symptoms such as abdominal pain triggered by various factors, in particular induction of hem-containing enzymes. Porphyrins accumulating in more distal enzyme deficiencies are associated with photosensitivity and dermatologial symptoms. The diagnosis involves analysis of porphyrins and porphyrin precursors in urine, feces, or erythrocytes. Management entails the avoidance of precipitating factors.

A2.6 Congenital Disorders of Glycosylation (CDG)

Many proteins including enzymes, transport and membrane proteins, as well as hormones require glycosylation in the Golgi apparatus or endoplasmatic reticulum to render them functional glycoproteins. A deficiency of one of the more than 40 different enzymes involved in glycosylation leads to a wide range of structural abnormalities and disturbances of physiological functions. A disorder from the CDG group should be considered in all patients with unclear multisystem or neurological disorder. The diagnosis in *N*-glycosylation disorders is usually made by isoelectric focussing of transferrin in serum. There is no effective treatment for most disorders of this group.

A2.7 Disorders of Lipoprotein Metabolism

Many disorders of lipoprotein metabolism cause clinical symptoms through the deposition of lipid in tissues and premature atherosclerosis. Others cause gastrointestinal or peripheral neurological problems. They are recognized by quantification of cholesterol and triglycerides and through lipoprotein electrophoresis. Many disorders are open to dietary or pharmacological therapy.

- Elevated blood cholesterol levels in *hypercholesterolemias and mixed hyperlipidemias* cause lipid deposition in the form of xanthomas and xanthelasma. They lead to complications of premature atherosclerosis, especially myocardial infarction and cerebrovascular disease. Therapeutic options include diet, drugs, and lipid apharesis.
- *Hypertriglyceridemia* may be caused by genetic disorders that affect the utilization of chylomicrons and very low-density lipoproteins. They may cause failure to thrive and abdominal symptoms, and sometimes severe pancreatitis. These disorders require stringent restriction of dietary fat.
- Genetic disorders affecting *HDL metabolism* cause a variety of clinical manifestations including premature atherosclerosis, neuropathy, nephropathy, and corneal clouding. Therapy is symptomatic.
- Genetic disorders in which there are *reduced LDL cholesterol and triglycerides* lead to symptoms of fat malabsorption. They are treated by restriction of fat and supplementation with fat soluble vitamins.

Neurotransmitter Defects and Related Disorders

Georg F. Hoffmann

Genetic disorders of neurotransmitter metabolism are increasingly recognised as causes of severe metabolic encephalopathy often starting before birth or soon thereafter. Diagnosis usually requires investigations of the CSF. This group should be considered in children with neurological problems when basic metabolic investigations are normal.

A3.1 Disorders of Glycine and Serine Metabolism

Nonketotic hyperglycinemia is one of the best known causes of early-onset epileptic encephalopathy. It is recognised via concomitant amino acid analysis of plasma and CSF. Glycine levels in both are elevated, and the CSF to plasma ratio is increased. Treatment with dextrometorphan, benzoate or folate is of limited success. Disorders of serine biosynthesis cause neurological symptoms. They have been treated with serine and glycine supplementation.

A3.2 Disorders of the Metabolism of Pterins and Biogenic Amines

Affected children suffer from progressive developmental retardation and epileptic encephalopathy. There may be specific symptoms of dopamine and/ or serotonine deficiency, such as infantile parkinsonism, dopa-responsive dystonia, oculogyric crises or disturbed temperature regulation. These diseases are sometimes recognised by hyperphenylalaninemias but many exclusively through the analyis of biogenic amines and pterins in CSF.

Disorders of tetrahydrobiopterin biosynthesis and recycling affect the hydroxylation of phenylalanine and have been called atypical or malignant phenylketonuria. The hydroxylations of tyrosine and tryptophan are also affected, leading to deficiency of both, dopamine and serotonine. Investigations should include the analysis of biogenic amines, pterins and amino acids in the CSF as well as amino acids in plasma and pterins in urine. The disorders are treated with L-dopa along with carbidopa and 5-hydroxytryptophan and/or tetrahydrobiopterin and/or tetrahydrobiopterin substitution.

Disorders of the biosynthesis of biogenic amines present similarly with progressive extrapyramidal symptoms and encephalopathy. The deficiency of biogenic amines is treated with of L-dopa along with carbidopa and 5-hydroxytryptophan and/or dopamine agonists.

A3.3 Disorders of Gamma-Aminobutyrate Metabolism

These disorders cause central nervous dysfunction, often including seizures and encephalopathy. They are diagnosed through CSF analysis of amino acids and gamma-aminobutyrate (GABA). Urinary organic acid analysis may reveal 4-hydroxybutyric acid indicative of succinate semialdehyde dehydrogenase deficiency. Vigabatrin has been used in the treatment of SSADH deficiency.

G. F. Hoffmann
University Children's Hospital, Ruprecht-Karls-University,
Im Neuenheimer Feld 430, D-69120 Heidelberg, Germany
e-mail: georg.hoffmann@med.uni-heidelberg.de

G. F. Hoffmann et al. (eds.), *Inherited Metabolic Diseases*,
DOI: 10.1007/978-3-540-74723-9_A3, © Springer-Verlag Berlin Heidelberg 2010

A3.4 Disorders of Vitamin B$_6$ Metabolism

Pyridoxal phosphate (PLP, vitamin B$_6$) is a cofactor of all the transamination reactions and some decarboxylation and deamination reactions of amino acids, and as such is also required for the biosynthesis of several neurotransmitters including dopamine and GABA. Intracellular deficiency may be caused by primary or secondary disorders in the biosynthetic pathway and leads to a neonatal epileptic encephalopathy. In the well-known entity of vitamin B$_6$-dependent seizures, PLP is inactivated by delta 1-piperideine-6-carboxylate, which accumulates because of an enzyme deficiency in a different pathway. Disorders of vitamin B$_6$ metabolism are generally treatable with pyridoxine or PLP.

A3.5 Disorders of Creatine Metabolism

Creatine is the central compound in cytosolic energy metabolism, and deficiencies in the biosynthesis or transport of creatine manifest as neurometabolic disorders with progressive central nervous dysfunction.

They are usually diagnosed through the analysis of creatine and guanidinoacetate in urine and serum; treatment centers on creatine supplementation.

A3.6 Other Neurometabolic Disorders

- *Sulphite oxidase deficiency* is a cause of severe infantile seizures and encephalopathy. It is recognised through a sulphite stix test of the urine. Amino acid analysis of plasma and urine may be diagnostic but is less reliable. When it is caused by molybdenum cofactor deficiency there is also xanthine oxidase deficiency, which may be detected by purine analysis of the urine. There is no specific treatment.
- Various *cerebral organic acidurias* including Canavan disease, L-2- and D-2-hydroxyglutaric aciduria, 2-ketoglutaric aciduria, fumaric aciduria and malonic aciduria present with central nervous dysfunction, which is usually progressive. General metabolic abnormalities are absent, but the specific metabolites are found on organic acid analyis of the urine. The molecular basis of most of the conditions has now been established. There is no specific treatment.

Part **B**

Approach to the Patient with Metabolic Disease

When to Suspect Metabolic Disease

B1

William L. Nyhan

B1.1 History

B1.1.1 Family History

A careful family history may reveal important clues that point towards the diagnosis of an inborn error of metabolism. Most metabolic disorders are inherited as autosomal recessive traits, which may be suspected if the parents are consanguineous or the family has a confined ethnic or geographic background. Carriers for particular disorders, and as a consequence affected children, may be more frequent in remote villages, close-knit communities (such as the Amish in Pennsylvania), certain ethnic groups (such as Ashkenazi Jews), or countries that have seen little immigration over many centuries (such as Finland).

Quite often specialist investigations are started only after a second affected child is born into a family. Older siblings may be found to suffer from a similar disorder as the index patient or may have died from an acute unexplained disease classified as "sepsis with unidentified pathogen," "encephalopathy" or "sudden infant

W. L. Nyhan
Department of Pediatrics, University of California, UCSD
School of Medicine, 9500 Gilman Drive, La Jolla, CA 92093,
USA
e-mail: wnyhan@ucsd.edu

G. F. Hoffmann et al. (eds.), *Inherited Metabolic Diseases*,
DOI: 10.1007/978-3-540-74723-9_B1, © Springer-Verlag Berlin Heidelberg 2010

death syndrome." The latter is a frequent feature in disorders of intermediary metabolism that may have acute lethal presentations such as disorders of ammonia detoxification, organic acidurias, or fatty acid oxidation disorders.

In assessing medical records of previously affected but undiagnosed family members, it should be taken into account that the written clinical descriptions of complex conditions can be inconsistent and even misleading. Depending on the presumptive diagnosis at that time, important clinical clues may be missing. Parents are sometimes more reliable sources of information. On the other hand, the clinical expression of the same inborn error of metabolism may be variable even within families. Some more common Mendelian disorders are caused by a wide range of different mutations with different degrees of disease severity. Disease manifestations are especially variable in females with X-linked traits because of differences in the lyonization of the X chromosome in carrier females, e.g., ornithine transcarbamylase deficiency. Similarly, dominant disorders with variable penetrance may cause variable clinical problems in different members and generations even of one family, such as Segawa syndrome due to GTP cyclohydrolase deficiency.

As a result of the successful treatment of disorders of intermediary metabolism in which toxic small molecules accumulate, an increasing number of relatively healthy affected women are reaching the reproductive age. If they become pregnant, there is a risk for their fetuses to be harmed by pathological amounts of toxic metabolites from the mother, although the children are themselves not affected but heterozygous. Especially important is maternal phenylketonuria (PKU), which is likely to become a major health problem. Some women at risk may not even know that they are affected with PKU, if they come from countries where newborn screening did not exist or if they have discontinued dietary treatment and medical follow-up in late childhood. The latter will however remember that they had followed a special diet, which should be specifically asked for. Several mothers have been found to suffer from mild PKU only after maternal PKU was diagnosed in one of her children. Other maternal conditions may cause "metabolic" disease in the neonate or infant postnatally, e.g., methylmalonic aciduria and hyperhomocystinemia in fully breastfed children of mothers ingesting a vegan diet, which causes nutritional vitamin B_{12} deficiency.

B1.1.2 Prenatal Development and Complications of Pregnancy

Toxic small molecules that accumulate in many disorders of intermediary metabolism do not harm the fetus because they are removed via the placenta and metabolized by the mother. Children affected with such disorders usually have a completely normal intrauterine development and are born with normal birth measurements at term. In contrast, disorders that interfere with cellular energy metabolism, e.g., mitochondrial disorders, may impair fetal organ development and prenatal growth, causing structural (in particular cerebral) abnormalities, dysmorphic features, and dystrophy. Structural abnormalities and dysmorphic features may be even more pronounced in disorders of the biosynthesis of complex molecules that are necessary for developmental pathways and networks. Notable examples are the defects of sterol biosynthesis that interfere with cholesterol-dependent signaling pathways of development and cause, for example, the Smith–Lemli–Opitz syndrome. Disorders affecting the breakdown of complex molecules such as lysosomal storage disorders cause specific dysmorphic characteristics as in the Hurler disease, and when severe, may already present at birth. An unusual prenatal disease manifestation is found in mothers carrying a fetus affected with long-chain hydroxyacyl-CoA dehydrogenase (LCHAD) deficiency or carnitine palmitoyltransferase II deficiency, defects of fatty acid β-oxidation. These mothers have an increased risk of developing acute fatty liver of pregnancy, preeclampsia, or hemolysis, elevated liver enzymes, and low platelets (the HELLP syndrome). Systematic studies in mothers showed that fetal LCHAD deficiency is present in a significant number of women with acute fatty liver of pregnancy, but only in a very small proportion of the far more common HELLP syndrome. The neonates of such mothers should be screened for fatty acid oxidation disorders by acylcarnitine analysis in a dried blood spot.

B1.1.3 Age of Presentation and Precipitating Factors

The "typical" ages of manifestation of different groups of metabolic disorders in the first year of life are depicted

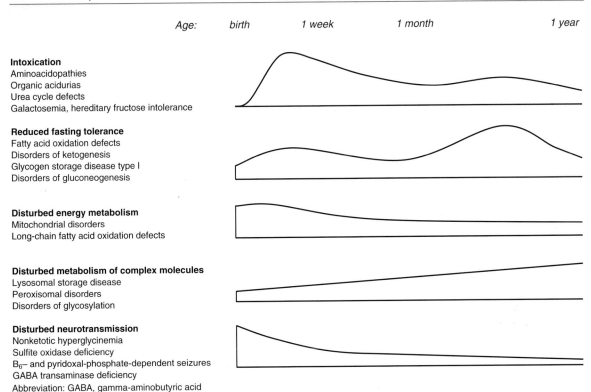

Fig. B1.1 Typical ages of manifestation of metabolic disorders in the first year of life

in Fig. B1.1. Disorders of intermediary metabolism that cause symptoms through the accumulation of toxic molecules ("*intoxication*") are usually asymptomatic in the first hours of life. They present after exposure to the respective substrate derived from catabolism or diet. Postnatal protein breakdown requires amino acid catabolism and nitrogen detoxification. Patients with acute aminoacidopathies (e.g., maple syrup urine disease (MSUD)), classical organic acidurias, or urea cycle defects most frequently develop progressive symptoms between days 2 and 5 of life. Subsequent risk periods include the second half of the first year of life (in particular, age 6–8 months) when solid meals with higher protein content are introduced and the children start to fast overnight, and late puberty when hormonal changes and a reduced growth rate change the metabolic state. Important precipitating factors throughout life are catabolic states caused by infections, fever, vaccinations, high-dose steroid therapy, surgery and accidents, as well as prolonged fasting.

Of the disorders of carbohydrate metabolism, galactosemia usually presents after the introduction of milk (which contains the galactose–glucose disaccharide

lactose) in the first week of life, while children with hereditary fructose intolerance develop symptoms after the introduction of fruits, vegetables, and particularly table sugar (the fructose–glucose disaccharide sucrose) to the diet, often between 4 and 8 months of age.

Disorders with a *reduced fasting tolerance* include genetic defects of fatty acid oxidation and ketogenesis, as well as deficiencies in the production and release of glucose. They typically present during periods of reduced food intake and/or increased energy requirement such as prolonged fasting or metabolic stress, and the age of presentation thus overlaps with the "intoxication" disorders. However, the disorders with reduced fasting tolerance are less frequently or less severely symptomatic in the postnatal period and more frequently present in association with infections in the second half of infancy.

Disorders of *energy metabolism* are frequently symptomatic at birth, but may essentially present at any time of life, depending on the severity of the genetic defect and the organs involved. Acute decompensation in mitochondrial disorders may specifically be triggered by major alterations in carbohydrate intake or the ingestion of large amounts of rapidly absorbed carbo-hydrates, while long-chain fatty acids that interfere with energy metabolism in some β-oxidation defects cause clinical features of a mitochondrial disorder dur-ing fasting periods. Another characteristic feature of mitochondrial disorders is a marked and frequently irreversible deterioration of the clinical condition with intercurrent illnesses.

Disorders in the *metabolism of complex molecules* rarely show acute metabolic crises but present with variable and often progressive organ dysfunction throughout childhood. There are usually no precipitat-ing factors. The clinical presentation of *neurotransmit-ter defects and related disorders* depends on the ontogenetic expression of neurotransmitter systems and receptors. Affected children are often symptom-atic immediately after birth, and there may even be symptoms of intrauterine epilepsy as evidence of pre-natal disease manifestations. There are usually no pre-cipitating factors.

B1.2 Physical Examination

Every child who is suspected of suffering from an inborn error of metabolism requires a thorough physi-cal examination and a careful evaluation of organ func-tions aided by routine laboratory and imaging investigations. In addition, hearing and vision should be examined at specialist appointments. Depending on the presenting symptoms and the clinical course, a reevaluation, especially a detailed physical examina-tion, should be repeated every 6 months. The detection of additional manifestations is of great importance even if the patient does not complain of them, particu-larly if the final diagnosis is still unknown.

The involvement of multiple organ systems is one of the strongest arguments in favor of an inherited metabolic disease. This is especially true for defects of organelle metabolism such as mitochondrial or per-oxisomal disorders or the quickly enlarging group of glycosylation defects or CDG syndromes. Structural abnormalities such as dysmorphic features or malfor-mations may be caused by disorders in the metabolism of complex molecules as well as disorders affecting mitochondrial energy metabolism, but are not usually observed in other disorders of intermediary metabolism.

Generalized organomegaly is often indicative of a (lys-osomal) storage disorder, while isolated hepatomegaly is observed in a great variety of enzyme defects. Urine color and body odor can provide diagnostic clues, as discussed later. A list of differential diagnoses of char-acteristic symptoms and signs is given in the appendix.

B1.2.1 Unusual Odor

Unaccustomed odors can serve as alerting signals for several metabolic diseases (Table B1.1). The most commonly encountered is the sweet smell of acetone found in the acute ketoacidosis of diabetes mellitus and the organic acidemias. Other characteristic odors are that of *MSUD*, the acrid smell of *isovaleric aci-demia* and *glutaric aciduria type II*, and the odor of phenylacetic acid in *PKU*. The phenylacetic acid odor is much more prominent in patients with urea cycle defects, treated with sodium phenylacetate, or phenyl-butyrate. Very prominent unpleasant odors are found in *trimethylaminuria* and *dimethylglycinuria*. Odors can be very useful in suggesting a diagnosis or an appropriate test. It is also important not to discard a potential diagnosis because of the absence of the odor. Some people are simply unable to detect some odors. Many physicians have never really been able to smell the ketotic patient. In other conditions, the acute meta-bolic crisis leads to a cessation of oral intake and vig-orous parental fluid therapy, so that by the time the

Table B1.1 Diagnostic utility of unusual odors

Odor	Substance	Disorder
Animal like	Phenylacetate	PKU
Maple syrup	Sotolone	Maple syrup urine disease
Acrid, short-chain acid	Isovaleric acid	Isovaleric aciduria, glutaric aciduria type II
Cabbage	2-Hydroxy-butyric acid	Tyrosinemia type I, Methionine malabsorption
Rancid butter	2-Keto-4-methiolbu-tyric acid	Tyrosinemia type I
Rotten fish	Trimethylamine, dimethylgly-cine	Trimethlaminuria, dimethylglycinuria

patient reaches the referral hospital the odor has long since disappeared.

The odor of maple syrup led to the recognition and original description of *MSUD*, before it was known that this was a disorder in the metabolism of the branched-chain amino acids. A keen sense of smell can still be useful in the detection of this disease, but the seriousness of the presentation of metabolic imbalance and a readiness to carry out an analysis of amino acids in plasma are such that most patients diagnosed today do not trigger the smell test. This is also true of acute exacerbation in established patients. Testing for urinary ketones with DNPH and organic acid analysis of the urine are also useful in the diagnosis of this disease. The odor of the patient with isovaleric acidemia has been described as like that of sweaty feet, but it does not smell anything like a locker room. The smell is penetrating, pervasive, and readily recognized. It is the odor of a short-chain volatile acid, and the same smell may be appreciated in patients with *multiple acyl-CoA dehydrogenase deficiency* (*glutaric aciduria type II*) during times of acute illness.

Now that screening of newborns for *PKU* is universal in developed countries, patients with this disease are not likely to be diagnosed because of the characteristic odor, but some of us have made the diagnosis in this way in patients born prior to the development of screening. The odor has variously been described as musty, barny, animal-like or wolf-like. It is actually the odor of phenylacetic acid. Now that patients with defects in the urea cycle are treated with phenylacetic acid or its precursor phenylbutyric acid, specialists in inherited metabolic disease are quite as accustomed to this odor.

Patients with *hepatorenal tyrosinemia* and other nonmetabolic patients with hepatic cirrhosis may have a very unpleasant odor that results from the accumulation of methionine.

The classic unpleasant odor is that of patients with *trimethylaminuria*. Trimethylamine is the odor of fish that is not fresh. The compound is a major end product of nitrogen metabolism of teleost fishes, which convert it to the oxide and employ the resulting compound to balance their osmotic pressure with surrounding sea water. In man, trimethylamine is formed from dietary trimethylamine oxide in fish and from choline absorbed from the intestine and transported to the liver, where the trimethylamine oxide is formed and ultimately excreted in the urine. Patients with trimethylaminuria have an inborn error in the metabolism of the oxide, defective activity of hepatic trimethyamine N-oxide synthetase. The metabolic abnormality does not *appear to* produce a disease as we usually know one; its consequences are nevertheless terrible. An odor so unpleasant leads to social ostracism, poor performance in school, depression, and loss of employment. Suicide is a possibility. Diagnosis is important because a diet low in fish, liver, and egg yolks is usually sufficient to eliminate the odor. The diagnosis is made by identifying the compound by gas chromatography, gas chromatography–mass spectroscopy (GC–MS), FAB-MS, or nuclear magnetic resonance (NMR) spectroscopy. Its excretion is increased by loading with choline, and this may be necessary for the diagnosis in patients who have found dietary ways of minimizing their odor. Following a morning specimen of urine, a 5 g oral supply of choline bitartrate in 3 doses over 24 h led to a 44-fold increase in trimethylamine excretion to 1.098 μmol/mg creatinine. Normal individuals excreted 0.0042–0.405 μmol/mg creatinine. The activity of the enzyme has been measured in biopsied liver. It is a flavin-containing monooxidase, designated FMO_3. Several mutations in the gene have been identified.

Patients have been described in whom the odor of trimethylamine is mild or intermittent. Mutations have been identified in the FMO_3 gene on chromosome 1q23–25. For instance, the P153L mutation has been identified in patients with severe trimethylaminuria and no enzyme activity in vitro. The patients with the mild phenotype have had an allele with two common polymorphisms, E158K in which a 472G→A mutation coded for a lysine instead of a glutamate, and E3086 in which a 923A→G mutation coded for glycine instead of glutamate. Patients have generally been heterozygous for this allele and a disease-producing mutation, but one patient has been homozygous for the variant allele. The variant allele is common in Caucasian populations; allele frequency was found to be 20% in Germans.

Dimethylglycinuria is a newly recognised inborn error of metabolism that causes a fishy odor. The defective enzyme is the dimethylglycine dehydrogenase, which catalyzes the conversion of this compound to sarcosine. A missense mutation in the gene has been identified in an affected patient. Trimethylamine was absent from the patient's urine. He also complained of muscle fatigue and had elevated levels of creatine kinase in the serum. Dimethylglycine is most readily detected by ^{1}H-NMR spectroscopy. Its presence was confirmed by ^{13}C-NMR spectroscopy and by GC–MS of nonextracted urine, but the compound could not be detected by GC–MS after the usual ethylacetate extraction.

B1.2.2 Color of the Urine or Diaper

Physicians since at least the time of Hippocrates have recognized that the color of the urine may be the clue that leads to the diagnosis. It was Garrod's recognition of the significance of the dark urine of patients and families with alkaptonuria that led to the conceptualization of the inborn errors of metabolism.

Alkaptonuria is recognized surprisingly infrequently in this way, and many patients reach adulthood and clinical arthritis before the diagnosis is made. This is the result of many factors, among them that the black pigment forms with time and oxygen, and that flushing does away with both. In a patient in whom one seeks to make this visual diagnosis, it is best to alkalinize and shake the urine and look with excellent light for the fine black precipitate. In times past when infants wore cloth diapers, which were laundered with strong alkaline soap, the conditions were perfect, and the diagnosis could be made by the appearance of black pigment in the diaper. Now they wear plastic disposable diapers, many of which turn pink on contact with alkaptonuric urine. So, we can still make the diagnosis early by examining the diaper.

Alkaptonuric urine also gives a positive test for reducing substance and is glucose-negative, and this may be an alerting signal for the diagnosis. Homogentisic acid also reduces the silver in photographic emulsion, and alkaptonuric urine has been used to develop a photograph, an interesting qualitative test for the diagnosis.

The diagnosis is confirmed by quantitative analysis of homogentisic acid in the urine.

Remember

The diagnostic black pigment of alkaptonuria is often missed. A red color may be seen in plastic diaper, or a positive test for reducing substance may be alerting (See Table B1.2).

B1.2.2.1 Examination of the Urine for the Significance of Color

Urine has a normal amber color that is the color of the pigment urochrome. Pale, dilute, or watery urine results from a plentiful fluid intake or diuresis as in diabetes mellitus or diabetes insipidus, or in the recovery phase of a tubular necrosis. Very dark urine or concentrated urine results from dehydration. Pale urine with a high specific gravity suggests diabetes mellitus. Dark urine with a low specific gravity suggests the presence of urobilin or bilirubin and is best checked by analysis of the blood for bilirubin. Very bright yellow urine may be seen in infants who ingest large amounts of carotene, but the skin of such infants is usually carotenemic. Urine may, of course, be red because of hematuria, but this is readily recognized by microscopic analysis, and such a specimen is not the subject of differential diagnosis by color. Free hemoglobin in the urine appears brown or black as methemoglobin is formed. The most famous example of this is the black water fever of malaria.

B1.2.2.2 Dark Brown or Black Urines

In addition to alkaptonuria, *hemoglobinuria* and *myoglobinuria* both produce brown or dark urine and both are detected by the dipstix for hemoglobin or by the benzidine test. Hemoglobin in the urine is often accompanied by hematuria. Hemoglobinuria in the absence of red cells in the urine is accompanied by evidence of hemolysis, such as anemia, reticulocytosis, or hyperbilirubinemia, while myoglobinuria is often accompanied by muscle pains or cramps and elevation of creatine phosphokinase and uric acid. An

Table B1.2 Syndromes of abnormally colored urine or diapers

	Conditions	Confirmation
Dark brown or black urine or diapers		
Alkaptonuria (Pampers become red)	Standing, alkaline	Homogentisic aciduria Clinitest positive
Melaninuria		Disseminated melanotic sarcoma
Red urine or diapers		
Hematuria		Microscopic
Hemoglobinuria		Guaiac, benzidine History
Beets (anthrocyanins)		
Congenital erythropoietic porphyria		Blood, urine, stool, uroporphyrin, uroporphyrin-III cosynthase (CEP) activity
Red dyes (Monday morning disorder, rhodamine B)		History
Red diaper syndrome (Serratia marcescens)	24–36 h of oxidation after passage	Culture Neomycin Rx
Phenolphthalein		History pH sensitive
Green-blue urine		
Blue diaper syndrome (indigotin)		Tryptophan malabsorption
		Indicanuria Indole-acetic aciduria
Biliverdin (obstructive jaundice)		Serum bilirubin
Methylene blue (ingestion, Rx)		History
Orange sand		
Urate overproduction (urates may stain diaper red in neonatal period)		Chemical assay for uric acid, blood and urine Hypoxanthine-guanine phosphoribosyl transferase (HPRT)

attack of myoglobinuria should signal a work-up for a disorder of fatty acid oxidation (Chap. C6). It is also seen in enzyme defects localized to muscle, such as myophosphorylase deficiency (McArdle disease) and myodenylate deaminase deficiency. *Melaninuria* is seen in disseminated melanotic sarcoma.

B1.2.2.3 Red Urine

Porphyrias are the major metabolic cause of red urine. Congenital erythropoietic porphyria is an autosomal recessive disease caused by mutations in the gene for uroporphyrinogen synthase. Uroporphyria and coproporphyria are found in the urine. It manifests a variable phenotype from nonimmune hydrops fetalis to a mild adult-onset form with only photosensitive cutaneous lesions. The disease is often first recognized because of a pink, red, or brown stain in the diapers. These patients also develop erythrodontia in which a red fluorescence of the teeth is visible with ultraviolet illumination.

Red urine may also be seen following the ingestion of large quantities of colored foods. The anthrocyaninuria of beet ingestion is quite common. Blackberries have also been associated with red urine. Red dyes, such as rhodamine B, used to color foods and cold drinks have led to red urine of so many children after a weekend party that the condition was termed the Monday morning disorder of children. Phenolphthalein in laxatives may also cause red urine. In the neonatal period, distinct red spots in the diaper were seen where crystals of ammonium urate dried out. In previous days when cloth diapers were used and accumulated for a while before laundering, a red diaper syndrome was recognized in which the color developed after 24 h of incubation and came from the growth of the chromobacterium, *Seratia marcescens*, which does not produce pigment in the infant's intestine, but only after aerobic growth at 25–30°C. Red stools may also be seen after the ingestion of red crayons, and in some patients receiving cefdinir, in most but not all of whom receive oral iron.

B1.2.2.4 Green or Blue Urines

Blue pigment in urine containing urochrome usually leads to a green color. Blue color was seen in the blue diaper syndrome. This disorder of the intestinal absorption of tryptophan was described in two siblings who also had hypercalcemia and nephrocalcinosis.

When tryptophan is not efficiently absorbed, intestinal bacteria convert it to indole metabolites that are absorbed and excreted in the urine. The blue color comes from the oxidative conjugation of two molecules of indican to indigotin, or indigo blue, a water insoluble dye. The excretion of indole products is increased by an oral tryptophan load. The condition must be very rare because further patients have not been reported since the initial report in 1964. Indoles including indican are also found in the urine of patients with Hartnup disease, in which there is defective renal tubular reabsorption, as well as intestinal absorption of a number of amino acids including tryptophan, but blue diapers or urine have not been observed.

Biliverdin, the oxidation product of bilirubin, is excreted in the urine, and so green urine may be seen in jaundiced patients, particularly those with chronic obstructive jaundice.

Benign pigments such as methylene blue, found in some tablets, are excreted in urine, and if a sufficient quantity is taken, will color the urine. Indigo-carmine is another blue dye that may find its way into food stuffs.

B1.3 Routine Laboratory Investigations

Unexpected findings in the "routine" laboratory require critical evaluation. Particularly in patients with unusual and unexplained symptoms they may be indicative of an inborn error of metabolism and can help to direct specific diagnostic investigations. Table B1.3 gives a noncomprehensive collection of such sometimes unexpectedly obtained laboratory abnormalities that may be suggestive of certain metabolic disorders.

B1.4 When Not to Suspect a Metabolic Disease

Inborn errors of metabolism may be considered in the differential diagnosis of a great variety of clinical problems, and at times it can be difficult to decide that specialist metabolic investigations are not warranted. Whether or not certain specialist investigations are indicated quite obviously also depends on secondary factors such as local or national availability, costs of the

Table B1.3 Routine laboratory investigations

Finding	Indicative of
Anemia (macrocytic)	Disturbances in cobalamin or folic acid metabolism or transport
Reticulocytosis	Glycolysis defects, disorders of the γ-glutamyl cycle
Vacuolized lymphocytes	Lysosomal storage disorders
↑ Alkaline phosphatase	Hypoparathyreoidism, bile acid synthesis defects
↓ Cholesterol	A-, hypobetalipoproteinemia, sterol synthesis defects, peroxisomal disorders
↑ Triglycerides	Glycogen storage disorders, lipoprotein disorders, e.g., lipoprotein lipase deficiency
↑ CK	Mitochondrial disorders, fatty acid oxidation defects, glycogen storage disease types II, III, and IV, glycolysis defects, muscle-AMP-deaminase deficiency, dystrophinopathies
↑ α-Fetoprotein	Ataxia telangiectasia, hepatorenal tyrosinemia
↓ Glucose in CSF	Mitochondrial disorders, glucose transport protein deficiency
↑ Uric acid	Glycogen storage disorders, disorders of purine metabolism, fatty acid oxidation defects, mitochondrial disorders
↓ Uric acid	Disorders of purine metabolism, molybdenum cofactor deficiency
↓ Creatinine	Creatine synthesis defect
↑ Iron, transferrin	Hemochromatosis, peroxisomal disorders
↓ Copper (in plasma)	Wilson disease, Menkes disease
↑ Copper (in plasma)	Peroxisomal disorders
↑ Copper (in urine and liver)	Wilson disease, peroxisomal disorders
↓ Ceruloplasmin	Wilson disease, Menkes disease, aceruloplasminemia
Hypothyroidism, hypoparathyreoidism	Mitochondrial disorders, CDG syndromes

AMP adenosine monophosphate; *CDG* congenital disorders of glycosylation; *CK* creatine kinase

test, the likelihood of litigation, and the personal experience of the clinician. It is imperative to exclude disorders for which effective treatments are available, while in cases of slowly progressive, and by experience often incurable disorders diagnostic procedures should be performed stepwise depending on the results of the first investigations and the appearance and development of signs and symptoms with time. The diagnosis of some metabolic disorders involves procedures that are stressful, such as sedation or lumbar puncture, or potentially dangerous for the child (e.g., fasting or loading studies), and that are often also stressful for the parents. Psychosocial factors should be taken into consideration when the diagnostic work-up is planned. The families need to be guided and supported. In the worst case, a specific diagnosis with a doomed prognosis that shatters the expectations of the parents can even damage the parent–child relationship. On the other hand, in almost all families a specific diagnosis no matter how negative will be one of the most important supports for coping, and of course is critical for timely genetic diagnosis in young families and appropriate counseling.

Specialist metabolic investigations are not usually indicated in children with moderate developmental delay, isolated delay in speech development in early childhood, moderate failure to thrive, frequent infections, occasional seizures, e.g., during fever, or defined epileptic syndromes. An inborn error of metabolism is also unlikely in the healthy sibling of an infant who died of SIDS, provided that this child had been previously asymptomatic. Key factors in the evaluation of symptoms are their isolated appearance vs. the presence of additional pathology, however subtle, i.e., the lack or presence of additional neurological and/or systemic abnormalities, and a static vs. a progressive clinical course. Multisystem or progressive disorders are much more likely to be caused by inborn errors of metabolism.

Key References

Moolenaar SH, Poggi-Bach J, Engelke UFH, Corstaensen JMB, Heerschap A, De Jong JGN, Binzak BA, Vockley J, Wevers RA (1999) Defect in dimethylglycine dehydrogenase, a new inborn error of metabolism: NMR spectroscopy study. Clin Chem 45:459–464

Nyhan WL, Barshop BA, Ozand PT (2005) Atlas of metabolic diseases, 2nd edn. Hodder Arnold, London

Saudubray JM, Charpentier C (2001) Clinical phenotypes: diagnosis/algorithms. In: Scriver CR, Beaudet AL, Valle D, Sly WL (eds) The metabolic and molecular bases of inherited disease, 7th edn, Vol 1 . McGraw-Hill, New York, pp 1327–1403

Zschocke J, Kohlmueller D, Quak E, Meissner T, Hoffmann GF, Mayatepek E (1999) Mild trimethylaminuria caused by common variants in FMO3 gene. Lancet 354:834–835

Metabolic Emergencies

B2

William L. Nyhan

Key Facts

> The classic presentation of inborn errors of metabolism is with a free period of apparent health that may last days or even years, but it is followed by overwhelming life threatening disease.

> The episode usually follows catabolism introduced usually by acute infection; sometimes after surgery.

> Initial laboratory evaluation needs only the routine clinical laboratory to establish acidosis or alkaoisis, hyperammonemia, ketosis, hypoclycimia, or latic acidemia.

B2.1 General Considerations

The most demanding cases in the field of genetic disease that pose problems for rapid diagnosis and rapid initiation of effective treatment are patients who present with episodes of acute life-threatening illness. This is the mode of presentation of a considerable number of inherited metabolic diseases (Table B2.1.1). It is particularly characteristic of the organic acidurias, the disorders of the urea cycle, maple syrup urine disease, nonketotic hyperglycinemia, and the disorders of fatty acid oxidation. The lactic acidemias may present in

this way, but usually the presentation is more indolent. Disorders which present with potentially lethal metabolic emergencies usually do so first in the neonatal period or early infancy. In fact, we have felt that prior to the advent of programs of expanded neonatal screening a large number of such infants probably die(d) without the benefit of diagnosis.

Episodes of acute illness and metabolic decompensation are often precipitated by acute infection and its attendant catabolism. Catabolism may also be induced by surgery or injury. The duress of birth may be sufficiently catabolic to induce an early neonatal attack. The diseases in which the fundamental defect is in an enzyme involved in the catabolism of a component of food, such as protein, are often characterized by a period of build-up of body stores of toxic intermediates until the levels are great enough to produce metabolic imbalance. Such a patient may have cycles of acute illness precipitating admission to the hospital, cessation of feedings and administration of parenteral fluids and electrolytes with recovery and discharge only to repeat the cycle until the diagnosis is made and appropriate therapy initiated, or the patient dies in such an episode. In the disorders of fatty acid oxidation, episodes of metabolic emergency are brought on by fasting. This can be when the infant begins to sleep longer, or more commonly, when intercurrent infection leads to vomiting or failure to feed.

The *classic presentation* of the diseases that produce metabolic emergencies is, for the initial acute presentation in infancy, often in the neonatal period, followed by recurrent episodes of metabolic decompensation usually with infection. Nevertheless, some patients with these diseases, usually those with variant enzymes in which there is some residual activity, may present first in childhood or even in adulthood. The diseases of fatty acid oxidation typically require fasting for 16–24 h

W. L. Nyhan
Department of Pediatrics, University of California, UCSD
School of Medicine, 9500 Gilman Drive, La Jolla, CA 92093,
USA
e-mail: wnyhan@ucsd.edu

G. F. Hoffmann et al. (eds.), *Inherited Metabolic Diseases*,
DOI: 10.1007/978-3-540-74723-9_B2, © Springer-Verlag Berlin Heidelberg 2010

Table B2.1.1 Metabolic diseases presenting as acute overwhelming disease

Disorder	Detect	Definitive diagnosis
Maple syrup urine disease	Urinary 2,4-DNP, plasma amino acids	Branched-chain amino academia, branched chain ketoacid decarboxylase
Organic acidurias, e.g., isovaleric aciduria	Smell	Isovaleric acid in blood, isovalerylglycinuria
methylmalonic aciduria	Methymalonic acid in urine	Methylmalonic acid in blood and urine, methyl-malonyl-CoA mutase, complementation assay
propionic aciduria	Hyperglycinemia, urinary organic acid pattern	Propionic acidemia, propionyl-CoA carboxylase
multiple carboxylase deficiency	Urinary organic acid pattern	Biotinidase, holocarboxylase synthetase
d-2-hydroxyglutaric aciduria	Urinary organic acid pattern	Isomer differentiation of 2-hydroxyglutaric acid
Urea cycle defects	Blood NH_3, plasma amino acids, urinary orotic acid	Ornithine transcarbamylase, c carbamoyl phosphate synthetase, N-acetylglutamate synthetase, argininosuccinate synthetase, argininosuccinate lyase, HHH syndrome
Disorders of fatty acid oxidation	Hypoketotic hypoglycemia	Acylcarnitine profile, enzyme assay, MCAD DNA
Lactic acidemias	Lactate, alanine	Enzyme assay; mitochondrial DNA
Hyperglycinemia, nonketotic	Glycinemia, CSF glycine	Glycine cleavage enzyme in liver
Methylenetetrahydrofolate reductase deficiency	Homocysteinemia, hypomethioninemia	Enzyme assay
Sulfite oxidase deficiency	Sulfite test, amino acid pattern	Sulfite oxidase
Adenylosuccinate lyase deficiency	Succinyladenosine, SAICA riboside	Enzyme assay
Lysosomal acid phosphatase deficiency	Lysosomal acid phosphatase	Enzyme assay
Adrenogenital syndrome	17 – ketosteroids	Pregnanetriol, testosterone
Fructose intolerance	Fructosuria	Hepatic fructose -1-P-aldolase
Galactosemia	Urinary reducing substance	Galactose-1-phosphate-uridyl transferase

CSF cerebrospinal fluid; *2,4-DNP* 2,4-dinitrophenol; *HHH* hyperammonemia, hyperornithinemia, homocitrullinuria; *MCAD* medium-chain acyl-CoA dehydrogenase; *SAICA* succinylaminoimadazole carboxamide

before metabolic imbalance ensues. Some people reach adulthood without ever fasting that long. Nevertheless, the first episode may be lethal, regardless of age.

The *initial clinical manifestations* of metabolic emergency are often vomiting and anorexia, or failure to take feedings. This may be followed by rapid deep breathing in the acidotic infant. A characteristically ketotic odor may be observed. There may be rapid progression through lethargy to coma, or there may be convulsions. Hypothermia can be the only manifestation besides failure to feed and lethargy. Further progression is to apnea and, in the absence of intubation and assisted ventilation, death.

The *initial laboratory evaluation* (Table B2.1.2) involves tests that are readily available in most hospital laboratories, particularly clinical chemistry. Most important in early discrimination are the electrolytes and the ammonia. Blood gases are listed because they are often the first data available in a very sick infant. They give some of the same information as the electrolytes on the presence or absence of metabolic acidosis. In general, it is advisable to get everything on the list on admission of the patient suspected of having a

metabolic emergency. Acidosis and hyperammonemia are indicative of an organic acidemia. Hyperammonemia and alkalosis are characteristic of urea cycle defects. Hypoglycemia along with elevation of uric acid and creatine kinase (CK) is seen in disorders of fatty acid oxidation. If ketones are absent from the urine, this is almost certainly the diagnostic category. The presence of ketones in the urine does not rule it out; the blood level of 3-hydroxybutyrate is a better indicator of the adequacy of ketogenesis. Hypocalcemia may be a nonspecific harbinger of metabolic disease.

Elevated levels of lactate in the absence of cardiac disease, shock, or hypoxemia are significant, and seen in organic acidemias and even hyperammonemias, as well as in the lactic acidemias of mitochondrial disease (Chap. B.2.3). A normal pH in the blood does not rule out lactic acidemia; the pH usually remains neutral until lactic acid concentrations reach 5 mM. The blood count is useful in indicating the presence or absence of infection. More importantly, neutropenia with or without thrombocytopenia or even with pancytopenia is characteristic of organic acidemia, while patients with mitochondrial disease often develop thrombocytosis.

The dinitrophenylhydrazine (DNPH) test is positive in any disorder in which there are large amounts of ketones in the urine. It is particularly useful as a spot indicator of the presence of maple syrup urine disease. A positive urine reducing substance may be the first indicator of galactosemia. Today in most developed countries this disorder is discovered through routine neonatal screening for the defective enzyme. Chemical testing for blood in the urine is also useful in detecting hemoglobinuria and myoglobinuria, the latter indicating a crisis in a disorder of fatty acid oxidation. The test for sulfite indicates the presence of sulfite oxidase deficiency, either isolated or as a result of molybdenum cofactor deficiency, which may present with intractable seizures shortly after birth.

It is advisable in a seriously ill infant to save some blood and urine (Table B2.1.2) while this initial testing is taking place. Then if the initial indicators point to an area of metabolic disease, these samples can be processed appropriately, obviating such problems as a later lack of availability of urine in an infant in whom dehydration and shock lead to a renal tubular necrosis. Further testing requires a biochemical genetics laboratory expert in these procedures. Programs of proficiency testing indicate that not all laboratories that undertake these specialized procedures do them properly.

Table B2.1.2 Initial laboratory investigations

Blood
Electrolytes: bicarbonate, anion gap
Blood gases: pH, pCO_2, HCO_3, pO_2
Ammonia
Glucose
Lactate, pyruvate
Calcium
3-Hydroxybutyrate
Uric acid
Creatine kinase
Complete blood count
Urine
Ketones
Reducing substance
Dinitrophenyl hydrazine
Sulfites (sulfite test)
Benzidine, guaiac
Store at −20°C (−4°F)
Urine
Heparinized plasma
CSF
Store at 4°C (39°F)
Heparinized whole blood

In the presence of acidosis suggesting organic aciduria the assay of choice is organic acid analysis of the urine. A positive DNPH in the absence of acidosis or with mild acidosis indicates amino acid analysis of the plasma for maple syrup urine disease. Hyperammonemia without acidosis indicates that a urea cycle defect should be followed up by amino acid analysis of the plasma and analysis of the urine for orotic acid. This can be done by organic acid analysis or better by a specific assay for orotic acid. In an infant found to have an elevated plasma concentration of glycine, the availability of simultaneously obtained CSF permits a definitive diagnosis of nonketotic hyperglycinemia. Following initial testing indicating a disorder of fatty acid oxidation, definitive testing requires organic acid analysis of the urine, an acylcarnitine pattern of the blood, and a medium-chain acyl-CoA dehydrogenase (MCAD) assay of the DNA. In most of these patients, quantification of concentrations of carnitine in blood and urine is useful.

Precise molecular diagnosis is made by enzyme assay, usually of lymphocytes or cultured fibroblasts, or by determination of the mutation in the DNA. DNA analysis is particularly useful in those situations in which there is a common mutation, such as the A 985G mutation in the MCAD gene in Caucasians.

B2.1.1 Neonates

The classic presentation of the metabolic disorders that lead to medical emergencies is with life-threatening illness in the newborn period. These infants are usually born healthy, and there is classically a hiatus, or period of apparent well-being, before the onset of symptoms. This free period can be as short as 12 h, or even less; it is usually at least 48 h; it can be as long as 6–8 months (Fig. B1.1). Nevertheless, within 24 h of the first symptom the infant is usually admitted to the intensive care unit with artificial ventilation begun.

Remember

Acute life-threatening neonatal illness following a hiatus in which the infant appears well is a strong indicator of the presence of inherited metabolic disease.

The most important key to the diagnosis of a metabolic disease in such an infant is a high index of suspicion.

Table B2.1.3 Clinical features suggesting the presence of metabolic disease in an infant

Overwhelming illness in the neonatal period
Vomiting, pyloric stenosis
Acute acidosis, anion gap
Massive ketosis
Hypoglycemia
Coagulopathy
Deep coma
Seizures, especially myoclonic
Hiccups, chronic
Unusual odor
Extensive dermatosis, especially monilial
Family history of siblings dying early

There are some alerting signals (Table B2.1.3). The picture of overwhelming illness in a neonate most often calls to mind a diagnosis of sepsis. Some alert physicians have initiated a metabolic work-up in such an infant once the blood culture is negative. In general, awareness toward metabolic disorders still needs to be increased. In a full-term newborn with an uncomplicated delivery, septicemia is also not as common as it is pursued, and a metabolic emergency should be considered and investigated in parallel. This approach may well provide an earlier diagnosis than is unfortunately the standard outcome in the diagnosis of most neonates with metabolic disease. However, it should be kept in mind that some patients with metabolic disease may actually present in the newborn period with septicemia. Prior to the advent of newborn screening for galactosemia, the earliest diagnoses of this disease were often made by physicians who recognized that these patients present with neonatal *Escherichia coli* sepsis. We have also encountered positive blood cultures and clinical sepsis in citrullinemia, propionic aciduria, and other disorders. Cerebral hemorrhage and pulmonary hemorrhage may complicate the initial episode of metabolic imbalance. Coagulopathy may be the first sign of the presence of hepatorenal tyrosinemia.

Many metabolic diseases and particularly the organic acidurias and the hyperammonemias present first with vomiting. This has led frequently to a diagnosis of pyloric stenosis or duodenal obstruction, and a number of pyloromyotomies or other explorations have been carried out. The organic acidurias should not be missed this way by the alert physician, because for all such patients results of electrolyte analysis are available, and pyloric stenosis causes alkalosis. A patient who appears to have pyloric stenosis and has acidosis has an organic aciduria even if someone can feel an olive.

Remember

An infant who is thought to have pyloric stenosis, but is acidotic, must be worked up for metabolic disease.

Electrolyte analysis also serves to indicate the presence of adrenal insufficiency or the adrenogenital syndrome, especially in the male, which may present in this way. Some patients present with poor sucking or a complete inability to feed. An odd smell may be very helpful in the diagnosis of metabolic disease (Table B1.1 in Chap. B1), especially isovaleric acidemia and maple syrup urine disease.

The critically ill infant is often first seen in coma in an intensive care unit. An algorithmic approach to the infant in coma is shown in Fig. B2.1.1. Initial evaluation of NH_3, pH, and electrolytes permits early separation into those with elevated ammonia and no acidosis, most of whom have urea cycle defects (Chap. B2.6). Similarly, those in whom the ammonia is elevated or normal, but there is metabolic acidosis and usually massive ketosis, commonly have organic aciduria. Patients with lactic acidemia and pyroglutaric aciduria may present with neonatal acidosis, but not usually with coma. The patient with maple syrup urine disease may be convulsant or opisthotonic as well as comatose, but there is usually little or no acidosis, and the DNPH test is positive.

Comatose patients without hyperammonemia or acidosis and a negative DNPH most commonly have nonketotic hyperglycinemia. The identical presentation can be seen in babies suffering from the treatable disorders of pyridoxine metabolism or from sulfite oxidase deficiency, molybdenum cofactor deficiency, adenylosuccinase lyase deficiency, methylenetetrahydrofolate reductase deficiency, or leukotriene C_4-synthesis deficiency (see Chap. C5). A urinary sulfite test must therefore be done in every child presenting with catastrophic encephalopathy, and specific tests for homocysteine in blood as well as urinary purine analysis should be ordered. Leukotrienes are best analyzed in CSF, which must be stored at $-70°C$ or, as an intermediate measure, in dry ice or under liquid nitrogen. If intractable seizures dominate the clinical picture, folinic acid responsive seizures should be considered, and so should pyridoxine- (B_6-) as well as pyridoxal-phosphate-responsive seizures. A therapeutic trial pyridoxine and pyridoxal-phosphate is followed, if negative, by the administration of folinic acid with 5 mg/kg/day in three doses intravenously or orally (see Chap. C5).

Fig. B2.1.1 The metabolic diagnosis of a newborn infant in coma

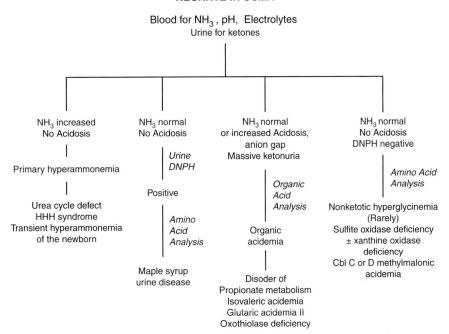

Severe neonatal/infantile epileptic encephalopathy is one indication for specialized CSF analyses testing metabolic pathways of brain metabolism, especially neurotransmitters (see Chap. C2 – Epilepsy – Neonatal Period, page 11). Defects in the metabolism of biogenic monoamines are diagnosed this way and so is GABA transaminase deficiency. An electroencephalographic finding of a burst suppression pattern is characteristic of nonketotic hyperglycinemia, but it is also found in other metabolic disorders such as disorders of pyridoxine metabolism, propionic aciduria or molybdenum cofactor deficiency causing sulfite oxidase deficiency.

The occurrence of ketosis and acidosis in the neonatal period is an almost certain indicator of metabolic disease. Ketosis is rare in newborns. Even the neonatal diabetic is not ketotic; so testing of the urine at this time is often not performed. However, this is a mistake because infants with organic acidemia have massive ketosis. A reasonable position might be that any infant admitted to a neonatal intensive care unit with life-threatening non-surgical illness should be tested for blood pH, NH_3, electrolytes, glucose, and for ketonuria. One could argue that valuable time would be saved by testing at the outset for lactate and amino acids in the blood, organic acids in the urine, and acylcarnitines in blood spots.

> **Remember**
>
> The urine of the ill newborn should always be tested for ketones. Massive ketonuria indicates an organic acidemia, while an absence of ketosis in a hypoglycemic infant leads to a diagnosis of a fatty acid oxidation defect.

B2.1.2 Infancy

The infant with a metabolic emergency that presents after the neonatal period may have a period of some months of failure to thrive. Such an infant may feed poorly and vomit frequently, but the metabolic crisis is avoided until the advent of an intercurrent infection or a switch from human to cow's milk. Such an infant may then promptly develop the picture of life-threatening illness just like that of the newborn. The etiologies are often the same, organic acidurias, hyperammonemias, hepatorenal tyrosinosis, and fructose intolerance.

The disorders of fatty acid oxidation (Chap. B2.5) present classically at 7–12 months of age, consistent with the time infants begin to sleep longer or the timing of the first intercurrent infection that leads to prolonged fasting because of anorexia or vomiting. They can of course present first at any age in which these conditions are met. The infantile presentation of these diseases is with hypoketotic hypoglycemia. Clinically, there may be convulsions or coma. Cardiac arrhythmias are common. It is important to assess the level of glucose in the blood, and the adequacy of ketogenesis. A urine negative for ketones in the presence of hypoglycemia is very helpful, but if there are ketones in the urine, examination of blood concentrations of free fatty acids and 3-hydroxybutyrate is necessary to evaluate ketogenesis. Roentgenographic examination of the chest, electrocardiography, and echocardiography should be carried out.

Muscle tone is affected in a variety of infants with metabolic diseases. These include the organic acidurias and the disorders of fatty acid oxidation, which are classically complicated by metabolic emergencies. Thus, inclusion of a work-up for metabolic disease in the hypotonic or floppy infant may bring to light the more important need to treat an infant prior to the onset of that first episode of metabolic decompensation that so often leads to death or mental retardation.

Neutropenia, thrombocytopenia, and even pancytopenia are concomitants of a number of metabolic diseases, notably the organic acidurias and the cobalamin-related disorders. Recognition of this association in infancy may lead to an early diagnosis and forestall what is usually the most life-threatening crisis, the first.

The infant thought to have *Reye syndrome* is an excellent candidate for a diagnosis of an inborn error of metabolism. Single episode Reye syndrome was once relatively common, but it is not any longer, presumably related to the sparing use of salicylates in acute viral illness. Today, most infants with the typical Reye presentation of hypoglycemia, hyperammonemia, and elevated transaminases have inherited metabolic disease. Most of them have MCAD deficiency (Chap. B2.5) or ornithine transcarbamylase (OTC) deficiency (Chap. B2.6), but any disorder of fatty acid oxidation or of the urea cycle may produce this picture. We have diagnosed the hyperammonemia, hyperornithinemia, homocitrullinuria syndrome (Chap. B2.6) in an infant thought to have Reye syndrome. The liver biopsy in this infant had the typical Reye picture of microvesicular steatosis, and so have

infants with the other metabolic diseases. So a positive liver biopsy will not make the diagnosis. A metabolic work-up is required.

Remember

An infant thought to have Reye syndrome has a metabolic disease until proven otherwise.

The differential diagnosis of primary *metabolic coma* in infancy overlaps with that of the neonatal period as shown in Fig. B2.1.1 and described earlier. In later infancy patients with defective B_{12} metabolism, including cobalamin C disease, transcobalamin II deficiency, and the breast fed infant of a mother on a vegan diet or a mother suffering from sometimes unrecognized pernicious anemia may also present in this way. A patient in coma may also have hypoglycemia (Chap. B2.4). A very specific cause of hypoglucorrachia is due to the defects of the glucose transporter 1 protein, the facilitative glucose transporter of the brain. This diagnosis, also termed De Vivo syndrome, can be anticipated from a pathologically decreased CSF/blood glucose ratio <0.45, normal mean 0.8 ± 0.1, in the absence of pleocytosis or elevated CSF lactate. Care must be taken to perform the lumbar puncture and determinations of blood sugar at least 4 h postprandially. Recurrent exaggerations of neurological and psychiatric symptoms often leading to metabolic coma are a major presenting feature of several late-onset inborn errors of metabolism in older children and adults. Clinical and laboratory presentations are especially variable and require a high index of suspicion on the part of the physician. These constellations and the most important diagnostic approaches are discussed in Chaps. B2. 7 and C5.

B2.1.3 Older Children and Adults

Any of the disorders, which present in early infancy, may develop repeated attacks of metabolic emergency at any age, despite generally successful therapy. Late-onset forms are also seen, albeit uncommonly, in many of the diseases that present classically in infancy. They are more common for the urea cycle defects and determination of ammonia should be tested in every patient with fluctuating consciousness or unexplained coma.

The lateness of onset is usually a function of the fact that the variant enzyme resulting from the mutation has greater residual activity than that of the patient with the early neonatal presentation. Nevertheless, the dangerous nature of these diseases is clearly indicated by the fact that episodes of metabolic imbalance occurring in childhood, adulthood, or even old age may be quickly fatal. This is particularly true of urea cycle defects, and OTC deficiency is notoriously unpredictable. A series of readily manageable hyperammonemic episodes may be followed by one that leads promptly to cerebral edema, herniation, and death. We have also observed carbamoyl phosphate synthetase deficiency leading to edema in a first episode in adults up to the age of 50. Branched-chain ketoaciduria has been reported in a small number of late-presentation patients. Again, as in the case of urea cycle defects, a late-onset patient is still in danger of dying from the first or a subsequent episode of metabolic imbalance.

The defects in fatty acid oxidation may present late, simply because the patient has never before fasted long enough to exhaust liver glycogen and call upon oxidation of fats. In this way, a MCAD deficiency can present first as a fatal episode of hypoketotic hypoglycemia in an adult. Other diseases of fatty acid oxidation may present later with acute rhabdomyolysis and cardiac arrhythmias. These patients usually have elevated levels of CK and uric acid at the time of the crisis. Others may present with acute cardiac failure, a consequence of year after year accumulated cardiomyopathy and the depletion of body stores of carnitine.

Mitochondrial diseases (Chaps. B2.3 and D1) may present at any age, but they more commonly present first in childhood or even adulthood. The first episode could be of coma with lactic acidosis and ketoacidosis. More commonly, particularly in the MELAS disease (Chap. B2.3), there is a stroke or stroke-like episode. Such episodes have also been seen in propionic aciduria, methylmalonic aciduria, OTC deficiency, and congenital disorders of glycosylation (CDG). Patients with mitochondrial disease often have abnormal neuroimaging studies. In addition to CT or MRI evidence of stroke, there are areas of increased signal in the basal ganglia and elsewhere. Many have the radiological appearance of Leigh syndrome. We have diagnosed NARP mutation in a patient who carried a radiological diagnosis of acute demyelinating encephalomyelitis. Basal ganglia lesions are also characteristic of propionic acidemia and methylmalonic acidemia.

B2.2 Work-up of the Patient with Metabolic Acidosis and Massive Ketosis

William L. Nyhan

Key Facts

> Massive ketosis in a neonate or young infant is a key to the diagnosis of an organic aciduria. Testing of the urine for ketones is a must in all ill infants.

> The most frequent organic acidurias are propionic aciduria, methylmalonic aciduria, multiple carboxylase deficiency, isovaleric aciduria, and 3-oxothiolase deficiency.

> Routine clinical chemistry reveals low pH, low bicarbonate, and an increased anion gap. The urine pH is low. Hyperchloremic acidosis and a normal anion gap mean intestinal losses or a renal tubular acidosis, the former with acidic urine and the latter with alkaline urine.

> Quantitative organic acid analysis by gas-chromatography mass-spectrometry is essential in differential diagnosis.

> Acylcarnitine (MS/MS) profile may be a quicker route to diagnosis.

There are a number of metabolic diseases that present with acidosis (Table B2.2.1), most of them for the first time in the neonatal period. Metabolic acidosis may be caused by the accumulation of the carboxylic acid itself, as in the case of lactic acidemia (Chap. B2.3) or pyroglutamic aciduria, or hawkinsinuria in infancy. However, in most of the severe acidoses, the acidosis is caused by a massive ketoacidosis, in which acetoacetic

W. L. Nyhan
Department of Pediatrics, University of California, UCSD
School of Medicine, 9500 Gilman Drive, La Jolla, CA 92093, USA
e-mail: wnyhan@ucsd.edu

acid and 3-hydroxybutyric acid accumulate in the blood, and the urine tests strongly for ketones. These are classic metabolic emergencies. It is critical to make the diagnosis as soon as possible, and to get therapy started, even before the precise diagnosis is known (Chap. B2.8). It is important that testing of the urine for ketones be incorporated into the work-up of a severely ill infant. Until the recognition of the organic acidurias, it was thought that ketonuria did not occur in the neonatal period, and testing for ketones early in life is often neglected. Its presence can signify an underlying metabolic diagnosis.

Remember

Testing for ketones in the urine is essential in any profoundly ill neonate. Massive ketosis is the hallmark feature of the organic acidosis.

Ketosis can be readily quantified by measuring the concentration of 3-hydroxybutyrate in the blood. Normally this is <1.0 mM in the nonfasting state, and <0.1 mM in children and adults. After a 24-h fast, levels of 2–3.5 mM are achieved. Infants and children with ketoacidosis may have levels over 7 mM.

Massive ketosis and metabolic acidosis are the hallmark features of the organic acidurias. Those most frequently encountered are propionic aciduria, methylmalonic aciduria, multiple carboxylase deficiency, isovaleric aciduria, and 3-oxothiolase deficiency (Table B2.2.1). 3-Hydroxyisobutyric aciduria causes episodic ketoacidosis and may otherwise mimic lactic acidemia. 3-Hydroxyisobutyryl-CoA deacylase deficiency, methacrylic aciduria, may also present with ketoacidosis and 3-hydroxyisobutyric aciduria.

The initial episode may begin with vomiting, anorexia, and lethargy, but progresses rapidly to life-threatening acidosis, dehydration, coma, and apnea. In the absence of intubation and assisted ventilation, the infant dies.

Table B2.2.1 Metabolic diseases which may present with acute metabolic acidosis

Disorder	Detect or suspect	Definitive diagnosis
Propionic aciduria, Ketotic hyperglycinemia	Massive ketosis, propionic acidemia, hyperglycinemia	Methylcitraturia, Propionic acidemia, Propionyl-CoA carboxylase
Methylmalonic aciduria	Massive ketosis, methylmalonic acid in urine	Methylmalonic acid in blood and urine, methylmalonyl-CoA mutase, Complementation analysis
Isovaleric aciduria	Acrid smell	Isovalerylglycinuria, isovaleric acid in blood, hydroxyisovaleric aciduria
Multiple carboxylase deficiency	Hydroxyisovaleric aciduria, 3-methylcrotonylg-lycinuria, methylcitrate	Biotinidase, holocarboxylase synthetase
Oxothiolase deficiency	Massive ketosis, tiglylglycinuria	3-Oxothiolase
Methylcrotonyl-CoA carboxylase deficiency	3-methylcrotonylglycinuria	3-Methylcrotonyl-CoA carboxylase
Maple syrup urine disease	Urinary 2,4-DNP	Branched-chain amino acidemia, branched-chain keto acid dehydrogenase
Lactic acidemia	Growth retardation, ataxia, stroke, hyperalaninemia, lactic acid in blood, CSF	Defective fructose-1,6- diphosphatase or pyruvate dehydrogenase, mitochondrial DNA, electron transport chain enzymes
Lysosomal acid phosphatase deficiency		Lysosomal acid phosphatase
Pyroglutamic aciduria		Pyroglutamic acid in blood or urine
Hawkinsinuria	Iodoplatinate	Cysteinyl-dihydrocyclohexyl acetic acid
Ketolysis defects	Ketosis	Cytosolic or mitochondrial acetoacetyl-CoA thiolase, succinyl-CoA 3-oxoacid CoA transferase
LCHAD deficiency	(Cardio)-Myopathy, hypoglycemia, lactic acidemia	Acylcarnitine profile, LCHAD
SCHAD deficiency	Hypoglycemia	Acylcarnitine profile, SCHAD

2,4-DNP 2,4-dinitrophenylhydrazones; *LCHAD* long-chain hydroxyacyl-CoA dehydrogenase; *SCHAD* short-chain hydroxyacyl-CoA dehydrogenase

A clinical clue to the diagnosis is acidosis with vomiting. Some infants with organic aciduria have been thought to have pyloric stenosis and some have been treated surgically; however, pyloric stenosis and its attendant vomiting lead to alkalosis. A patient who seems to have pyloric stenosis and has paradoxical acidosis has an organic aciduria.

These infants are often thought to have sepsis and some even have positive blood cultures. Septic infants can certainly be acidotic, but they are not ketotic, at least in the neonatal period. So an infant with real or apparent sepsis and massive ketonuria should be investigated and treated for an organic aciduria.

Patients with these disorders go on to have recurrent episodes of acidosis, always heralded by ketonuria. This is in response to the intake of the usual amounts of protein in patients prior to a specific diagnosis and the introduction of dietary therapies, and in response to infection in patients with an established diagnosis and receiving an appropriate therapeutic regimen.

The results from the clinical chemistry laboratory indicate severe acidosis. The arterial pH may be 6.9–7.2. The serum concentration of bicarbonate is low, and may be as low as 5 mEq/L or less. The anion gap is increased. The pH of the urine is <5.5. An acidosis with a high urinary pH signifies a renal tubular acidosis, but these disorders are usually chronic problems, not acute metabolic emergencies and the anion gap is not increased. Hyperchloremia and a normal anion gap in an acidotic infant indicate renal tubular acidosis or intestinal losses of electrolyte. In the acute crisis of the organic acidurias, levels of lactic acid in the blood are also elevated, and this may contribute to the acidosis. There may also be hypoglycemia (Chap. B2.4), hypocalcemia, and, at least in the neonatal period, hyperammonemia (Chap. B2.6), and each of these may be symptomatic. Hyperammonemia leads to respiratory alkalosis. An elevated ammonia in a patient with acidosis indicates that the diagnosis is an organic aciduria. Routine clinical hematology may also indicate the presence of an organic aciduria, especially in a very young infant. These disorders lead regularly to neutropenia, often to thrombocytopenia, and sometimes to anemia. Pancytopenia and acidosis are seen in infants with sepsis; they are also seen in infants with organic aciduria. If there are also large amounts of ketones in the urine, it is an organic aciduria. Chronic moniliasis may also indicate the presence of an organic aciduria. In a known patient with organic aciduria, abnormal hematological findings and moniliasis indicate a lack of metabolic control.

The definitive diagnosis of an organic aciduria is made by gas-chromatography mass-spectrometry (GCMS). In this way, the presence of isovalerylglycine indicates the diagnosis is isovaleric acidemia; methylmalonate, methylmalonic aciduria; methylcitrate, 3-hydroxypropionate and tiglylglycine, propionic aciduria; tiglylglycine and 2-methyl-3-hydroxybutyrate, 3-oxothialase deficiency; and 3-hydroxyisovalerate, 3-methylcrotonylglycine, 3-hydroxypropionate and methylcitrate, multiple carboxylase deficiency.

> **Remember**
>
> If you suspect organic aciduria, order GCMS, organic acid analysis of the urine and acylcarnitine profiling.

Among the organic acidurias, 3-oxothiolase deficiency is the most likely to be cryptic. For reasons that are not clear the key metabolites may not be found in the urine at the time of the acute crisis, as they may be masked somehow by the massive quantities of acetoacetate and 3-hydroxybutyrate. On the other hand, when the patient is well, the tiglylglycine and 2-methyl-3-hydroxybutyrate may be missing from the urine. In such a situation, an isoleucine loading test will reveal the characteristic presence of these organic acid products of isoleucine.

Quantification may also be important in diagnosis. For instance, the presence of 3-hydroxyisovalerate, 3-hydroxypropionate, and methylcitrate may suggest a diagnosis of multiple carboxylase deficiency, but these compounds are also found in propionic aciduria, because 3-hydroxyisovalerate increases in any patient with ketosis. The two are readily distinguished by quantification. In multiple carboxylase deficiency, the amounts of 3-hydroxyisovalerate are large and those of the other compounds small, while in propionic aciduria, the reverse is found. The distinction is important, because to send a patient home with biotin and no restriction of protein intake, thinking that the diagnosis was multiple carboxylase, could be lethal in propionic aciduria.

Most of the organic acidurias may be detected by analysis of the blood or urine for acylcarnitines by tandem mass spectrometry. Today, an elevated plasma C3-carnitine is often the first indication that the diagnosis is propionic acidemia or methylmalonic aciduria.

Once this biochemical genetic diagnosis is made, definitive molecular diagnosis may be undertaken at the level of the enzyme or the gene. Enzyme analysis can often be made by analysis of freshly isolated leukocytes, but for precision in diagnosis, especially at a distant laboratory, it is usually preferable to establish a fibroblast culture, send a confluent culture, and ensure enzymatic analysis of viable cells.

Most of the other disorders listed in Table B2.2.1, while causing acidosis, do not usually present as a metabolic emergency. Pyroglutamic aciduria may rarely present with severe acidosis without ketonuria, but more commonly the acidosis is mild or absent. Maple syrup urine disease (MSUD), on the other hand, presents as a metabolic emergency (Chap. B.2.1), but the acidosis is usually absent or minor. In MSUD, the DNPH test is very useful in detecting the presence of the large quantities of the keto acid derivatives of the branched-chain amino acids. GCMS analysis of the organic acids of the urine will identify these keto acids and also their hydroxy acids. The specific pattern is diagnostic of MSUD; as of course is the analysis of the amino acids of the plasma.

Ketoacidosis occurs, of course, in diabetes mellitus. This diagnosis is readily made clinically. A diabetic infant or child is not likely to be missed if routine clinical chemistry is employed. On the other hand, an occasional organic aciduria has been mistaken for diabetes when an isolated elevation of glucose occurred at the time of presentation in ketoacidosis. In these patients, there may be elevated ammonia or lactic acid in the blood, providing keys to the diagnosis. The hyperglycemia is also transient and responds exaggeratedly quickly to a small amount of insulin. Disorders of carbohydrate metabolism, especially von Gierke glucose-6-phosphatase deficiency, but also fructose-1,6-diphosphatase deficiency and glycogen synthase deficiency, can have impressive levels of ketones in the blood. However, these disorders seldom present with an acute metabolic acidotic emergency. They present rather with hypoglycemia (Chap. B2.4). Ketosis is seldom considered in the lactic acidoses (Chap. B2.3). However, we have repeatedly observed crises of ketoacidosis in patients with episodic illness in electron transport abnormalities, such as the NARP mutation. These episodes respond to the administration of parenteral glucose and water (Chap. B2.8).

The disorders of ketolysis may present with a more or less pure ketoacidosis in which there is no hypoglycemia, hyperglycemia, organic aciduria, lactic acidemia, or hyperammonemia. It is thought that they have defective peripheral utilization of acetoacetate and 3-hydroxybutyrate. The prototype condition is cytosolic acetoacetyl-CoA thiolase deficiency. Actually, at least one patient with this disorder was reported to have moderate hypoglycemia; and others had elevated concentrations of lactate and pyruvate and a normal lactate to pyruvate ratio. Other ketolytic defects include the mitochondrial acetoacetyl-CoA thiolase deficiency and succinyl-CoA:3-oxoacid CoA transferase deficiency. This last enzyme catalyzes the conversion of acetoacetate to acetyl-CoA. Patients with this disorder are ketotic in the fed condition.

Key References

Nyhan WL, Barshop BA, Ozand PA (2005) Atlas of metabolic disease, 2nd edn. Hodder Arnold, London, pp 3–56

Wendel U, Ogier de Baulny H (2006) Branched-chain organic acidurias/acidemias. In: Fernandes J, Saudubray JM, van den Berghe G, Walter JH (eds) Inborn metabolic diseases, 4th edn. Springer, Berlin, pp 245–72

B2.3 Workup of the Patient with Lactic Acidemia – Mitochondrial Disease

William L. Nyhan

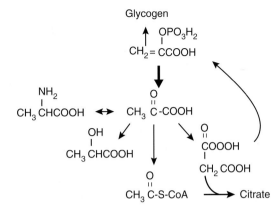

Fig. B2.3. 1 Pathway of pyruvate metabolism with pyruvate in the center and lactate and alanine sinks to the left

Key Facts

> Inborn errors characterized by lactic acidemia fall into two categories: abnormalities in gluconeogenesis and defects of oxidation. Distinction is important because management and prognosis are different.

> As a first step exclude factitious and secondary elevations of levels of lactic acid in order to focus on specifics of work-up.

> Ratios of lactate to pyruvate and 3-hydroxybutyrate to acetoacetate are useful in elucidating the area of metabolic defect.

> Postprandial rise or fall in lactate gives important information.

> A monitored fast may be required to distinguish oxidative defects from those of gluconeogenesis. Molecular methods have decreased the necessity for this.

The lactic acidemias represent a family of disorders of pyruvate metabolism. Under these circumstances large elevations of pyruvate concentration might be expected, but are seldom seen. Accumulating pyruvate does not lead to large elevations of pyruvate concentration; but rather to conversion to its two sinks, lactate and alanine (Fig. B2.3.1).

Genetically determined causes of lactic acidemia fall into two categories, defects in gluconeogenesis and defects in oxidation (Fig. B2.3.2). It is important in the work-up to distinguish clearly into which of the two categories each patient falls. The distinction is useful in determining optimal therapy, even in those

W. L. Nyhan
Department of Pediatrics, University of California, UCSD
School of Medicine, 9500 Gilman Drive, La Jolla, CA 92093,
USA
e-mail: wnyhan@ucsd.edu

patients in whom a molecular diagnosis remains elusive. Definitive diagnosis documents deficiencies in activity of a growing group of enzymes and mutations in DNA, first in mitochondrial and lately also in nuclear DNA (See also Chap. E1).

The first step in investigation of a patient with lactic acidemia is the documentation that the level of lactic acid in the blood or cerebrospinal fluid (CSF) is truly elevated. The most common situation in which the concentration of lactic acid in blood is elevated is factitious, the result of improper technique, the use of a tourniquet, or difficulty in drawing the blood. It is also true that levels are variable; even in patients with known mitochondrial disease the concentration of lactic acid is not always increased. Lactic and pyruvic acids are located distant from many of the enzymatic steps that are defective, especially those of the electron transport chain.

For the evaluation of energy metabolism, lactate should be determined repeatedly throughout the day (especially before and after meals). It is useful to also determine levels of pyruvic acid and alanine in the blood, as well as lactic acid. Alanine is not falsely raised by problems of technique. It is important to be rigorous about methods of sampling and to obtain blood flowing freely without a tourniquet. The concentration of lactate and alanine in the CSF should also be determined, particularly in those who appear to have mitochondrial disease with neurological symptoms despite normal levels of lactate in the blood. Many have elevated concentrations of lactate in the CSF, while the plasma level is normal, slightly, or intermittently elevated. Lactate to creatinine ratios in urine are less sensitive. Raised urinary lactate does,

ALGORITHMIC WORK UP OF PATIENT WITH LACTIC ACIDMIA

Document elevated Lactic Acid
and/or Pyruvic Acid and/or Alanine in Blood and/or CSF and Urine

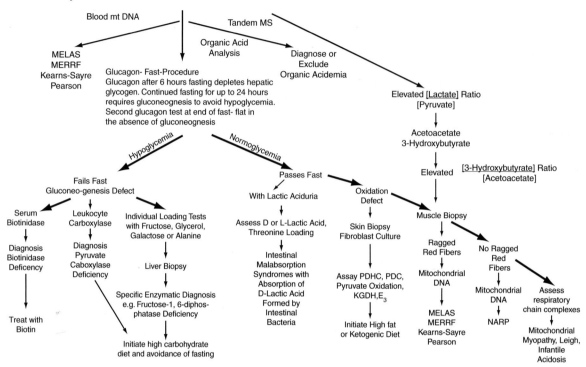

Fig. B2.3.2 An approach to the stepwise evaluation of a patient with lactic acidemia. E_3 estriol; *MELAS* Mitochondrial encephalomyelopathy, lactic acidemia and stroke-like episodes; *MERRF* Myoclonus epilepsy with ragged red fibres; *MS* mass spectroscopy; *mt* mitochondrial; *NARP* Neuropathy, ataxia, and retinitis pigmentosa; *PDHC* pyruvate dehydrogenase complex

however, support the significance of questionable increased lactate levels in blood. If urinary lactate is found more consistently elevated than blood lactate, predominant or even isolated disease of the kidney is to be considered. At first seemingly unrelated to the underlying mitochondrial disorders, patients often show a constant thrombocytosis and hypertrichosis.

Before embarking on a specific investigation for lactic acidemia it is important to exclude conditions that cause secondary lactic acidemia. Patients with hypoxemia, hypoventilation, shock, or hypoperfusion are generally readily recognized as patients with sepsis, cardiac, or pulmonary disease. Anaerobic exercise also produces lactic acidemia, but this is seldom clinically relevant except in the convulsing patient. A variety of inherited metabolic diseases produce secondary lactic acidemia including propionic aciduria, methylmalonic aciduria, isovaleric aciduria, 3-hydroxy-3-methylglutaric aciduria, and pyroglutamic aciduria. Each of these conditions can be excluded by organic acid analysis.

An uncommon cause of lactic acidosis is D-lactic acidemia, resulting from absorption of D-lactic acid produced by intestinal bacteria (see also Chap. C3). Most such patients have obvious malabsorption or short-gut syndromes, metabolic acidosis, and massive lactic aciduria, found by colorimetric test or by urinary organic acid analysis. Testing for lactate in routine clinical chemistry is now usually done in an enzymatic assay, which is specific for L-lactate, so this situation is often not even recognized. The discrepancy between urine and blood lactate levels, plus the history, is the key to diagnosis. A short course of treatment with oral neomycin or metronidazole will cause a dramatic fall in D-lactate production, and the lactic acidemia will disappear.

Remember

Before embarking on a work-up for lactic acidemia exclude functions or secondary lactic acidemias, which are even more common, and even D-lactic acidemia.

B2.3.1 Workup of a Patient with Lactic Acidemia (Congenital or Late-Onset)

Once it has been decided that a patient has lactic acidemia the redox status and the response to a carbohydrate load may be evaluated first. Lactate should be determined preprandially and postprandially together with pyruvate, 3-hydroxybutyrate and acetoacetate preferably from the same samples collected in tubes prefilled with perchloric acid. Plasma glucose must be determined as well. Elevated ratios of the cytosolic (lactate:pyruvate >20) as well as of the mitochondrial redox status (3-hydroxybutyrate:acetoacetate >3) point to a disturbance of oxidative phosphorylation. An elevated ratio of lactate:pyruvate without elevation of the 3-hydroxybutyrate:acetoacetate ratio is indicative of severe pyruvate carboxylase deficiency. In these patients, elevations of the amino acids citrulline and lysine may also be found, as well as hyperammonemia.

A postprandial rise of lactate ($\geq$ twofold) occurs in pyruvate dehydrogenase deficiency and also in glycogen storage diseases types 0, III, and VI/IX. In primary defects of the respiratory chain, the redox state may become more abnormal; in addition, and there may even be a rise of total ketone bodies (paradoxical ketonemia). A postprandial fall of lactate occurs in glycogen storage disease type I and defects of gluconeogenesis.

The differentiation between problems in gluconeogenesis or in oxidation (Fig. B2.3.2) can be achieved by evaluating the response to a prolonged fast. Fasting studies are not appropriate in the diagnosis of a child with a defect in fatty acid oxidation. An intravenous catheter is inserted to facilitate the drawing of samples. Prior to the initiation of fasting, blood is obtained for glucose, lactate, pyruvate, and alanine. In this method, 0.5 mg of glucagon is given intramuscularly at 6 h in order to deplete the liver of glycogen made from glucose, and the glucose response is determined at 15, 30, 45, 60, and 90 min. The response to glucagon should be a sizeable increase in glucose (>20%) except in glycogenosis type I. As the fast is continued for 18–24 h, or until the development of hypoglycemia, the body is dependent on gluconeogenesis for the maintenance of normal levels of glucose in the blood. Hypoglycemia

Table B2.3.1 Twenty-four hour fast for lactic acidemia

Protocol and specimens

Begin fast at time T = 0° at 4 p.m. The first 16 h are the least hazardous; so should happen overnight

T(ime) = 0° (4 p.m.): end of last meal with documented intake

T = 1° (5 p.m.): serum glucose, electrolytes, phosphate, uric acid, (transaminases, creatine kinase). Lactate, pyruvate, 3-hydroxybutyrate, acetoacetate from perchloric acid tube. Plasma alanine. Plasma for acylcarnitines. Can be spotted on Guthrie card. Blood spot sample should be collected as backup

T = 6° (10 p.m.): blood glucose

T = 6° (10 p.m.): 1 mg glucagon is given i.m. or i.v. after flushing the line with 5 mL 5% albumin

T = 6°15′: blood glucose

T = 6°30′: blood glucose

T = 6°45′: blood glucose

T = 6°90′: blood glucose

T = 9° (1 a.m.): blood glucose

If any glucose level from the 9° and after blood draws is

>85 mg/dL (4.7 mM), collect glucose levels q3 h

>65 but <85 mg/dL (3.6–4.7 mM), collect glucose levels q2 h

>50 but <65 mg/dL (2.8–3.6 mM), collect glucose levels q1 h

> 40 but <50 mg/dL (2.2–2.8 mM), collect glucose levels q1/2 h

T = 15° (7 a.m.): serum glucose, electrolytes, phosphate, uric acid. Lactate, pyruvate, 3-hydroxybutyrate. Plasma alanine

T = 24° (4 p.m.) or at the time of development of hypoglycemia: serum glucose, electrolytes, phosphate, uric acid, creatine kinase, (transaminases). Blood gases. Lactate, pyruvate, 3-hydroxybutyrate, acetoacetate collected in perchloric acid tube. Plasma alanine, free fatty acids. Plasma acylcarnitines. Collect urine for quantitative analysis of organic acids

If blood sugar is <40 mg/dL (2.3 mM) draw samples as above and in addition for insulin, growth hormone, and glucagon. Give 1 mg glucagon i.m. or i.v. and collect blood glucose at 15 min. If glucose rises, collect at 30 and 45 min followed by 3–5 mL 10% glucose/kg b.w./h. In the presence of any symptoms or if glucose does not rise, give 2 mL of 20% or 4 mL of 10% glucose/kg b.w. intravenously as a bolus, followed by 3–5 mL 10% glucose/kg b.w./h until normoglycemia is restored, and the patient is able to resume adequate oral intake (blood glucose <45 mg/dL = 2.6 mM) at any time signals the conclusion of the fast. If the patient is asymptomatic, glucagon is given again. During this time if there is no rise in glucose, the defect is in gluconeogenesis. Glucose is given intravenously to restore normoglycemia without waiting for the usual interval of a glucagon test, and in the presence of any symptoms is given immediately without testing glucagon responsiveness. Concentrations of lactic and pyruvic acids, alanine, acylcarnitines, free fatty acids, and ketone bodies are determined at the end of the fast. In a hypoglycemic patient concentrations of insulin, growth hormone and glucagon are also obtained at the time the fast is terminated. It must be remembered that lactate will be raised in a struggling child, and as a result of a convulsion, as might occur with severe hypoglycemia. Errors in sample acquisition, technique, and sample handling all raise the lactate level measured by the laboratory.

Fed and fasted responses to glucagon can provide a discrimination between glycogenosis type I and glycogenosis type III. In suspected glycogen storage diseases, it is useful to test the response to glucagon in the fed as well as in the fasted state. After a fast of 24-h or fasting to mild hypoglycemia, if a fast of 24-h is too long, administration of glucagon yields a flat response in glycogen storage diseases type I and type III, while blood glucose rises normally in glycogenosis type VI/IX. On the other hand, when glucagon is given 2, 3, or 6 h after a meal, the blood glucose rises in type III glycogen storage disease, reflecting glucose molecules on the outer branches released by phosphorylase. In type I glycogen storage disease, there is minimal production of glucose in response to glucagon, whereas lactate will increase markedly.

In the further work-up of a patient with a defect in gluconeogenesis who fails the fasting test it is convenient to assay biotinidase in serum or blood spot, and carboxylase activity in leukocytes or fibroblasts; in this way a definitive diagnosis of multiple carboxylase deficiency (due to holocarboxylase synthetase or biotinidase deficiency) or pyruvate carboxylase deficiency can be made. Patients with disorders of gluconeogenesis in whom these are not the diagnoses, such as those with fructose-1,6-diphosphatase deficiency, require liver biopsy for definitive enzyme assay, but the diagnosis

will be suspected and effective treatment can be instituted on the basis of fasting and loading data. Information as to the area of the defect may be obtained by loading tests, with fructose (Chap. D8), alanine, or glycerol. Each compound is given by mouth as a 20% solution 6–12 h postprandially in a dose of 1 g/kg.

Most patients who pass the fasting test have defects in oxidation of pyruvate, reflecting mitochondrial dysfunction (see also Chap. D6). The elucidation of oxidation defects may be initiated by obtaining a skin biopsy for fibroblast culture. A diet high in fat and low in carbohydrate, with vitamin supplementation can be begun while waiting for sufficient quantities of cells for analysis. Fibroblasts may be assayed for defects in the pyruvate dehydrogenase complex. Defects in the first enzyme of the complex, pyruvate decarboxylase or E1α, can also be tested for by mutational analysis. Measuring respiratory chain complex activities, and identifying the cause of the dysfunction, may require lengthy laboratory investigations. A more immediate answer may be obtained by the analysis of blood for abnormalities in mitochondrial DNA (Chaps. D4 and D6). Among the newly recognised mitochondrial diseases of electronic transport are the mitochondrial DNA depletion syndromes. Among the causes of mitochondrial/DNA depletion is mutation in the gene for the mitochondrial DNA polymerase γ. Other patients with this syndrome have had defects in deoxyguanosine kinase and in thymidine kinase. The syndrome is now known also to be the result of mutation in the gene (SUCLA$_2$) for succinyl CoA ligase.

Key References

Munnich A (2006) Defects of the respiratory chain. In: Fernandes J, Saudubray JM, van den Berghe G, Walter JH (eds) Inborn metabolic diseases, 4th edn. Springer, Berlin, pp 197–209

Nyhan WL, Barshop BA, Ozand PA (2005) Atlas of metabolic disease, 2nd edn. Hodder Arnold, London, pp 303–369

Smeitink J, van den Heuvel L, DiMauro S (2001) The genetics and pathology of oxidative phosphorylation. Nat Rev Genet 2:342–352

B2.4 Work-Up of the Patient with Hypoglycemia

William L. Nyhan

Key Facts

> Timely determination of blood concentrations of insulin, growth hormone, and cortisol at the time of hypoglycemia can elucidate endocrinologic causes of hypoglycemia. The endocrinologist may be the first consultant to see the patient, and if these determinations have not been made, often orders a control LED fast. It is important to educate these colleagues of the importance of obtaining metabolic testing (Fig. B2.4.1) under these circumstances.

> Liver disease is a common cause of hypoglycemia even in pediatric patients.

> The important distinction of ketotic vs. hypoketotic hypoglycemia is best made by determination of free-fatty acids, acetoacetate, and 3-hydroxybutyrate at the time of hypoglycemia.

> Hypoglycemia after a short fast is the hallmark of a disorder of carbohydrate metabolism; after a long fast, it signifies a disorder of fatty acid oxidation.

Hypoglycemia must be recognized promptly and treated effectively, if permanent damage to the brain is to be prevented. Treatment means bringing the blood glucose to a normal concentration and maintaining it there. Rational treatment demands a specific diagnosis of the disease causing the hypoglycemia. Determination of the blood concentrations of insulin, growth hormone, and cortisol at the time of hypoglycemia leads to the definition of the classic forms of hypoglycemia. Liver disease must be excluded as a cause. The metabolic causes of hypoglycemia may be elucidated by the response to fasting and determination of the levels of free-fatty acids, acetoacetate, and 3-hydroxybutyrate in

the blood. This permits the distinction of ketotic hypoglycemia, which includes the disorders of carbohydrate metabolism and the transient disorder termed ketotic hypoglycemia, from hypoketotic hypoglycemia, which, in the absence of hyperinsulinemia, includes most of the disorders of fatty acid oxidation.

Acute hypoglycemia is a manifestation of a variety of different disorders. Its prompt recognition and reversal are critical because this absence of substrate for cerebral metabolism can lead to permanent damage of brain just as surely as can lack of oxygen. The acute episode can also be fatal. Its management requires the provision of enough glucose to bring the blood concentration of glucose to normal and enough on a continuing basis to keep it there. Hypoglycemia is defined as a serum concentration under 50 mg/dL (3 mmol/L) or a concentration in whole blood under 45 mg/dL. Low concentrations of glucose are so common in the neonatal period that neonatologists (used to) define hypoglycemia as a concentration under 30–35 mg/dL and in preterm infants <25 mg/dL. However, there is little evidence that the brain of the very young is any more tolerant of hypoglycemia, and we prefer to maintain concentrations of glucose >45 mg/dL in any age group.

The classic symptoms of hypoglycemia are sweating, pallor, irritability, and tremulousness, but there may be considerable variability even in the same individual, and convulsions or coma may be the initial manifestation, particularly in the neonate. There may be vomiting, but this may be the result of an intercurrent illness that induces the acute hypoglycemic episode. Headache, lethargy, altered behavior, or psychosis may be seen in older children and adults, while apnea, tachypnea, cyanosis, or hypothermia may occur in the newborn. Some individuals for whom very low levels of glucose are a chronic occurrence, for example, patients with von Gierke disease or glycogen synthase deficiency tolerate surprisingly low levels without symptomatology. Also, sudden drops in glucose levels are more apt to induce symptoms than those achieved slowly.

B2.4.1 Algorithmic Approach to Diagnosis

Definitive diagnosis is the elucidation of the cause of the hypoglycemia. This is an essential feature of the design of therapy. It also permits prognostication of a transitory or a potentially recurrent nature.

W. L. Nyhan
Department of Pediatrics, University of California, UCSD
School of Medicine, 9500 Gilman Drive, La Jolla, CA 92093, USA
e-mail: wnyhan@ucsd.edu

Fig. B2.4.1 An algorithmic approach to the definitive diagnosis of the cause of hypoglycemia

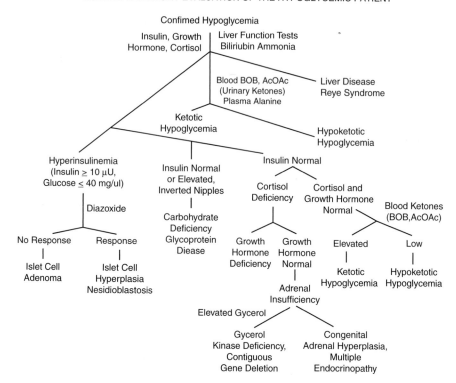

The diagnostic work-up is ideally initiated when the patient is seen at the time of the acute attack of hypoglycemia at which time blood can be obtained for insulin, growth hormone and cortisol to elucidate the common endocrine causes of hypoglycemia, tests of hepatic function to elucidate disease of the liver, a very common cause of hypoglycemia, as well as specialized tests, such as the blood concentrations of free-fatty acids, acetoacetate, and 3-hydroxybutyrate and plasma alanine to elucidate whether hypoglycemia is ketotic or hypoketotic (Fig. B2.4.1). More often, we are called upon to evaluate the patient after treatment of the acute attack when euglycemia has been restored. In this situation, a controlled monitored fast may be required to reproduce the hypoglycemic state and initiate the work-up.

The clinical history may guide the differential diagnosis. The age of the patient may help in certain types of hypoglycemia that are commonly encountered at different ages. Transient neonatal hypoglycemia is a condition of the first days of life and is seen particularly in preterm and small for gestational age (SGA) babies. Ketotic hypoglycemia is a common transient disease with onset usually between 1 and 2 years of age and disappearing by 6–8 years of age. Endocrine and metabolic causes may present first of any age, including the stressful first days of life, but there is a tendency to onset after 7 months of life when infants sleep longer and are more likely to acquire infectious illnesses that lead to anorexia or vomiting and hence fasting.

Patients with disorders of carbohydrate metabolism become hypoglycemic after short periods of fasting; 6–8 h leads to hypoglycemia in a patient with glycogenosis type I or glycogen synthase deficiency. On the other hand, even an infant may have to fast 16–24 h before stores of glycogen are exhausted, and fatty acid oxidation must be carried out to avoid hypoglycemia. Hypoglycemia resulting from the ingestion of a toxin, such as salicylate or ethanol is usually evident from the history, but covert administration of insulin in the Munchausen-by-proxy-syndrome is more difficult to suspect. Hyperinsulinemia with a normal C-peptide gives this situation away.

> **Remember**
>
> Hypoglycemia after a short fast signifies a disorder of carbohydrate metabolizing, and after a long fast, a disorder of fatty acid oxidation.

The physical examination is useful in leading to the diagnosis of specific syndromes, in which hypoglycemia is common. Macrosomia in an infant with full rounded cheeks and a plethoric, edematous appearance is the alerting picture for the danger of hypoglycemia in the infant of the diabetic mother. These infants also have a behavioral phenotype of drowsiness, hypotonia, a long latency for response and only brief periods of alertness. Macrosomia and hypoglycemia are also seen in the *Beckwith–Wiedemann syndrome* along with macroglossia, omphalocele and hepatomegaly. In both the syndromes, hypoglycemia is transitory, lasting 1–3 days; other syndromes associated with hyperinsulinism are congential disorders of glycosylation (CDG) and Pearlman, Simpson–Golabi–Behmel, Sotos, and Usher syndromes. A micropenis may be the only external clue to the presence of *panhypopituitarism*. Some such infants have midline defects, such as clefts of the lip and palate. Hepatomegaly is characteristic of even very young infants with glycogen storage disease. In the older child, it can sometimes be differentiated from the hepatomegaly of acute liver disease by its lack of tenderness.

The initial laboratory evaluation of the hypoglycemic patient (Fig. B2.4.1) rests on tests readily available in the clinical laboratory. Hyperinsulinemia is present when the insulin value is 10 U/mL or more in the presence of a plasma glucose concentration of 40 mg/dL or less. Another level of definition is >3 U/L of insulin, while glucose is <3 mmol/L (54 mg/dL) along with a positive response to injected glucagon (increase > 2 mmol/L after 1.0 mg). Many of the infants labeled as having idiopathic hypoglycemia, the infants of diabetic mothers, and those with leucine sensitive hypoglycemia have hyperinsulinism. *Persistent or recurrent hyperinsulinemic hypoglycemia* results from hyperplasia of the β-cells of the pancreatic islets, referred to as nesidioblastosis, or less commonly in older children an islet cell adenoma. In both the conditions, there is a relative absence of ketosis and a substantial risk of damage to the brain. Some patients without adenomas respond to diazoxide with a lessening of hypoglycemia.

Most of either group with persistent hyperinsulinemia require surgical removal of most of the pancreas. In children, many with diffuse hyperinsulinism can be managed medically, while those with focal lesions require surgery as do adults with true adenomas. Distinction between focal and diffuse lesions of the pancreas has been difficult short of surgery; the use of [¹⁸F] fluoro-L-dopa positron emission tomography (PET) appears to be useful in making that distinction. Hypoglycemia is also seen in patients with a variety of tumors that secrete insulin-like material. An interesting cause of hyperinsulinemic hypoglycemia is known as the *Hyperinsulism-Hyperammonemia Syndrome* and is caused by mutations in the gene (*GLUD1*) for glutamate dehydrogenase (GDH). Mutations in this gene impair sensitivity to its allosteric inhibitor GTP, leading to gain of function enzyme activity and increased sensitivity to its activator leucine. Concentrations of ammonia in these patients, while clearly elevated are not very high and patients have not had symptoms attributable to hyperammonemia. Changes in protein intake do not change the hyperammonemia – some of these patients have epilepsy without hypoglycemia. Persistent hyperinsulinemic hypoglycemia of infants is also caused by mutation in the pancreatic β-cell sulfonylurea receptor gene (SUR1) and in the inward rectifier potassium channels gene (KIR6.2), as well as in the glucokinase gene (*GK*).

SUR1 and KIR6.2 are channelopathy genes. Channels are composed of four KIR6.2 subunits and four SUR1 subunits. Dominant mutations may lead to haploinsufficiency in which the channel may be unable to stay open enough to maintain depolarization of the membrane, or dominant negative mutation may lead to destruction of channel structure. Mutations in the same gene may lead to diabetes or hyperinsulinism. Some patients with the same mutations have hyperinsulinism in infancy and diabetes later.

Patients with hypoglycemia and normal levels of insulin may have deficiency of cortisol with or without growth hormone deficiency and may be diagnosed as having one of the classic endocrine disorders (Fig. B2.4.1).

Patients in whom endocrine evaluations are normal may have ketotic or hypoketotic hypoglycemia (Chap. B2.5). This distinction can sometimes be made on the basis of the presence or absence of ketonuria at the time of hypoglycemia. However, the presence of ketones in the urine may be misleading. Many patients with documented disorders of fatty acid oxidation have been missed because of the presence of positive tests for ketones in the urine. Quantitative assays of acetoacetate and 3-hydroxybutyrate in the blood along with the levels of free-fatty acids clearly show that such a patient is hypoketotic at the time of hypoglycemia.

B2.4.2 Ketotic Hypoglycemia

Ketotic hypoglycemia is the name given to a very common disorder of late infancy and childhood which seldom begins before 18 months and disappears by 4–9 years of age. Actually there are a number of disorders in which abundant amounts of ketones accompany hypoglycemia. Massive ketosis is the hallmark of the organic acidurias (Chap. B2.2) in which hypoglycemia sometimes accompanies the acute attack of ketoacidosis. The other molecularly defined conditions in which ketosis accompanies hypoglycemia are disorders of carbohydrate metabolism, notably von Gierke disease (see also Chap. B2.3).

The syndrome known as ketotic hypoglycemia presents classically with symptomatic hypoglycemia in the morning after a long fast, often precipitated by an intercurrent illness that causes the child to miss dinner. At the time of the hypoglycemia tests of the urine for ketones are positive, and concentrations of acetoacetate and 3-hydroxybutyrate in the blood are elevated. Analysis of amino acids indicates the concentration of alanine to be low. This is often a hallmark of a problem with gluconeogenesis.

Physical examination is often unremarkable, but the patient may be short and have diminished subcutaneous fat, and there may be a history of low birth weight. Glucagon administered at the time of hypoglycemia is followed by little or no increase in glucose concentration.

In patients seen after recovery from hypoglycemia, the syndrome may be reproduced by fasting (see Sect. D8.2.1), but in some patients, this test may be negative. In these patients, a test of a ketogenic diet containing 67% of the calories as fat initiated after an overnight fast may reproduce the syndrome, and again there is no response to glucagon. Although in more severe or familial cases a definitive inborn error of energy homeostasis is suspected this can rarely be

ascertained. Two true inborn errors of metabolism that present with this constellation are the deficiency of glycogen synthase (see later) or of succinyl-CoA:3-oxoacid CoA-transferase (SCOT). In the latter, there is usually constant ketonuria even in the fed state.

B2.4.3 Disorders of Carbohydrate Metabolism

Patients with *glycogenosis type III*, a consequence of deficiency of the debrancher enzyme, also have low blood concentrations of alanine consistent with their very active gluconeogenesis. They are distinguished on examination from those with ketotic hypoglycemia because they have quite large livers. They do not respond to glucagon after fasting, but they do respond to the fed glucagon test.

Patients with *glycogenosis type I* or von Gierke disease, by contrast, have very high concentrations of alanine. Hypoglycemia occurs early in life and is recurrent. Concentrations of lactate are high, as are those of acetoacetate and 3-hydroxybutyrate, and ketonuria is frequent. Hypercholesterolemia and hypertriglyceridemia lead ultimately to cutaneous xanthomata. Hyperuricemia may lead to gouty arthritis or renal disease. The liver is quite large, stature is short, and there may be a cherubic facial appearance. In these patients, the glucagon test is flat under all conditions. The enzyme deficiency is in glucose-6-phosphatase. Patients with disorders of gluconeogenesis, such as glycerol kinase deficiency, pyruvate carboxylase deficiency, pyruvate carboxykinase deficiency, or fructose 1,6-diphosphosphatase deficiency, also tend to have high concentrations of alanine and lactate in the blood. Definitive diagnosis is by enzyme assay in leukocytes or fibroblasts in the case of fructose-1,6-diphosphatase deficiency of biopsied liver. They may be elucidated by the occurrence of hypoglycemia during a monitored fast (see Sect. D8.5.2) especially if glucagon is given after 6 h to deplete the liver of glycogen. The glycemic response to glucagon is normal at 6 h. Loading tests with fructose, glycerol, or alanine may clarify what enzyme to assay. Patients with glycerol kinase deficiency may have adrenal insufficiency as part of a X-chromosomal contiguous gene deletion syndrome. Some may also have ornithine transcarbamylase deficiency and Duchene muscular dystrophy.

B2.4.3.1 Glycogen Synthase Deficiency

Deficiency of glycogen synthase is a rare, unique cause of hypoglycemia in which there is a distinctive pattern of biochemical abnormality. Patients have fasting hypoglycemia, usually without acidosis but with high concentrations of acetoacetate and 3-hydroxybutyrate along with ketonuria. Thus, this is a ketotic hypoglycemia. Concentrations of alanine and lactate are low at times of hypoglycemia, but feeding or a glucose tolerance test (see Sect. D8.3.2) leads to hyperglycemia and elevated concentrations of lactate in the blood. Glucagon during fasting has no effect on blood concentrations of glucose, lactate, or alanine, while the fed glucagon test yields a glycemic response (see Sect. D8.5.1). Molecular diagnosis by enzyme assay requires biopsied liver, but mutational analysis can define the defect in the gene.

Key References

Cornblath M, Schwartz R (1976) Disorders of carbohydrate metabolism in infancy. W.R. Saunders, Philadelphia

De Lonlay P, Giuregea I, Sempoux C et al (2005) Dominantly inherited hyperinsulinaemic hypoglycaemia. J Inherit Metab Dis 28:267–276

Nyhan WL, Barshop BA, Ozand PT (2005) Atlas of metabolic diseases, 2nd edn. Hodder Arnold, London, pp 241–245;303–311

Orho M, Bosshard NW, Buist NRM et al (1998) Mutations in the liver glycogen synthase gene in children with hypoglycemia due to glycogen storage disease type 0. J Clin Invest 102:507–515

B2.5 Approach to the Child Suspected of Having a Disorder of Fatty Acid Oxidation

William L. Nyhan

> **Key Facts**
>
> - Hypoketotic hypoglycemia signifies a disorder of fatty acid oxidation. An absence of ketones in urine at the time of hypoglycemia is an important clue; but the presence of ketonuria may be misleading. Blood levels of free fatty acids and 3-hydroxybutyrate may be required to differentiate.
> - The acylcarnitine (MS/MS) profile is a very helpful clue to the diagnosis.
> - Medium-chain acyl-CoA dehydrogenase (MCAD) deficiency resulting from the A985G mutation is so common that this test should be added to the initial work up of a patient with hypoketotic hypoglycemia.

Initial presentation of disorders of fatty acid oxidation is usually with hypoketotic hypoglycemia. Hyperammonemia may suggest Reye syndrome. Sudden infant death syndrome (SIDS) is another acute presentation. Some patients present more chronically with myopathy or cardiomyopathy. Medium-chain acyl-CoA dehydrogenase (MCAD) deficiency is the only common disorder, and most patients have the same mutation. So a modern work-up may begin with assay of the DNA for the A-985G mutation. Those not revealed in this way are now assayed by tandem mass spectrometry for the acylcarnitine profile, and this may indicate the diagnosis and the appropriate enzymatic assay. Organic acid analysis should reveal the diagnosis in those with

W. L. Nyhan
Department of Pediatrics, University of California, UCSD
School of Medicine, 9500 Gilman Drive, La Jolla, CA 92093, USA
e-mail: wnyhan@ucsd.edu

3-hydroxy-3-methylglutaryl-CoA lyase deficiency. Those not elucidated by these measures are subjected to an algorithmic investigation, central to which is a prolonged monitored fast (Chap. D8) followed up by loading tests with specific lipids.

Most patients with disorders of fatty acid oxidation present with hypoglycemia (Chap. B2.4). The classic initial presentation is with hypoketotic hypoglycemia, usually at 6–12 months of age following a period of fasting of more than 12 h induced by vomiting or anorexia of an intercurrent respiratory or gastrointestinal infection. The hypoglycemia may be manifest as lethargy or a seizure. It may progress rapidly to coma. There may be hyperammonemia, and this may lead to diagnosis of Reye syndrome. Liver biopsy in such a patient may reveal microvesicular fat, and this may seem to confirm the diagnosis of Reye syndrome. Actually most patients, we see these days, in whom a diagnosis of Reye syndrome has been made have a disorder of fatty acid oxidation. A few have a urea cycle defect. Orotic aciduria, a hallmark of ornithine transcarbamylase deficiency has been seen acutely in disordered fatty acid oxidation.

The other major presentation is myopathic (see also Chap. C6). This may be acute with muscle pains and rhabdomyolysis, with or without hypoglycemia. It may be chronic with weakness and hypotonia. A major common presentation is with cardiomyopathy. The first manifestations in some patients are those of congestive failure. Arrhythmias are also common, especially in the acute episode of metabolic imbalance.

A third presentation is with the SIDS. One scenario has been to make a diagnosis of a disorder of fatty acid oxidation, most commonly MCAD deficiency, in an infant and to obtain a history of a previous infant dying of SIDS. We have obtained blood samples saved from neonatal screening programs representing the previous infant and made a diagnosis of MCAD deficiency by DNA analysis. This type of posthumous diagnosis has also been made by assay for octanoylcarnitine. Disorders of fatty acid oxidation have also been detected in studies of sudden infant death by assay of postmortem liver for deficiency of carnitine and the presence of key organic acids by gas-chromatography mass-spectrometry (GCMS).

In the patient presenting with hypoglycemia, it is really helpful in suggesting the diagnosis if the test for ketones in the urine is negative. In this situation, hypoglycemia is cleary hypoketotic. However, these patients may be treated with parenteral glucose in the emergency room and the first urine analysis done hours or days after the hypoglycemia has resolved, and so this clue to the diagnosis is not available. More commonly the diagnosis may be missed because ketones are found in the urine at the time of acute illness. These patients can readily be shown to be hypoketotic by analysing the blood, but that does not exclude the possibility that the urine test for ketones may be positive. Documentation that hypoglycemia is hypoketotic is best done by quantification of the concentrations of free fatty acids, acetoacetate and 3-hydroxybutyrate in the blood. This is most commonly done in the context of a controlled or monitored fast, because the stability of acetoacetate requires planning ahead for its analysis and is seldom considered at the time of the initial acute episode. Nevertheless a good idea of the presence of hypoketosis can be obtained simply by the assay of 3-hydroxybutyrate and free fatty acids in the blood at the time of the acute hypoglycemic illness.

> **Remember**
>
> Do not be led away from a diagnosis of a disorder of fatty acid oxidation by the presence of ketones in the urine. Absence of ketones in a hypoglycemic patient is useful; their presence may be misleading.

Clues from the routine clinical chemistry laboratory that suggest the presence of a disorder of fatty acid oxidation are elevated levels of uric acid and creatine kinase (CK). Uric acid determinations are not regularly included in metabolic panels for pediatric patients; so it may have to be ordered separately and so may be the CK; levels over a 1000 U/L are commonly encountered on presentation. Transaminase levels may also be elevated. Analysis of organic acids in the urine may reveal dicarboxylic aciduria, and its pattern may provide direction as to the site of the enzymatic defect. During intervals between episodes of illness, these patients usually appear completely well. Furthermore abnormalities such as the dicarboxylic aciduria and elevations of uric acid and CK usually disappear completely. The patient is most often seen first in consultation after the initial hypoglycemia has been treated, and none of the abnormalities seen in the acute situation are present. Therefore is has become important to develop a systematic algorithmic approach to the work-up (Fig. B2.5.1). In a patient suspected of having a disorder of fatty acid oxidation the algorithm starts with an assay of the DNA from a blood sample for the common mutation in

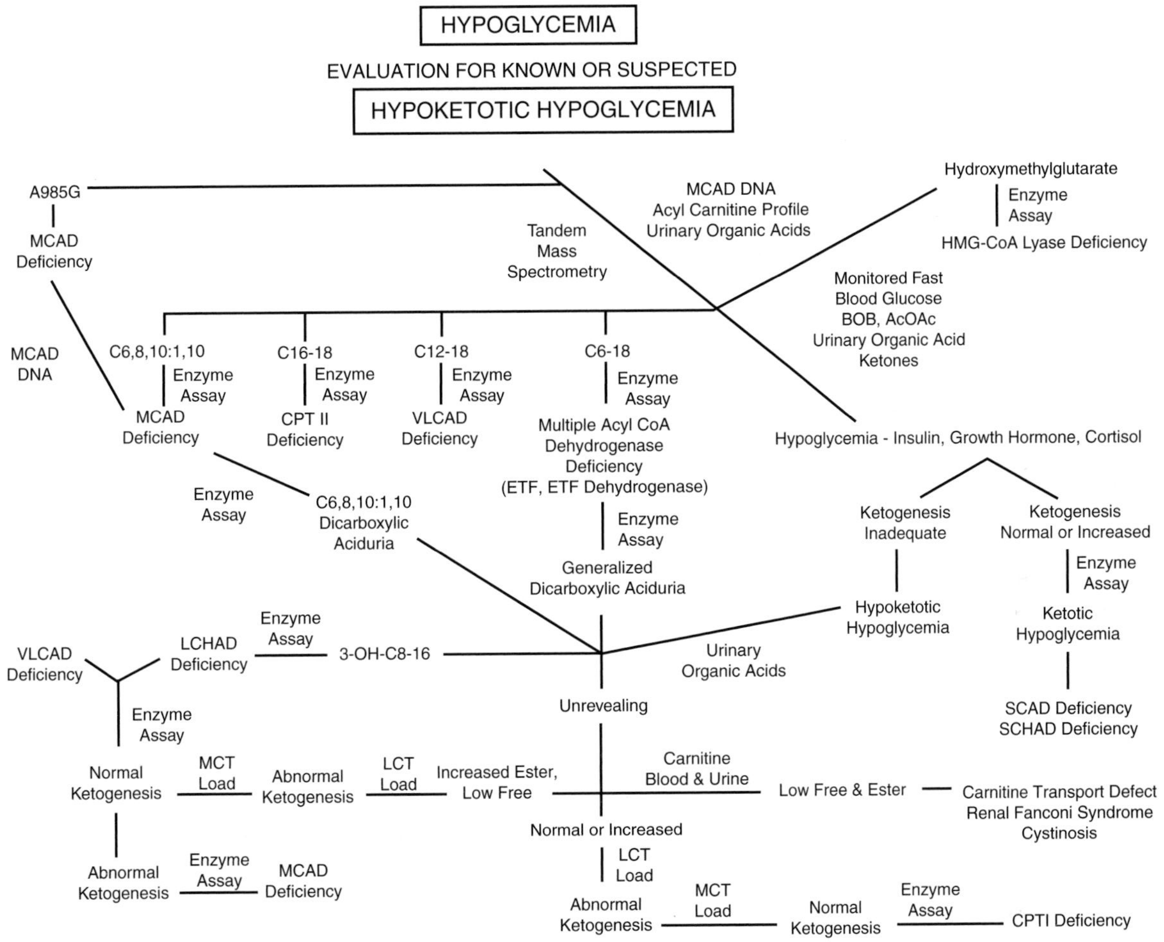

Fig. B2.5.1 An algorithmic approach to the work up of a child with a possible disorder of fatty acid oxidation. *MCAD* medium-chain acyl-CoA dehydrogenase; *DNA* deoxynucleic acid; *CPT* carnitine palmitoyltransferase; *VLCAD* very long-chain acyl-CoA dehydrogenase; *ETF* electron transfer flavoprotein; *BOB* 3-hydroxybutyric acid; *AcOAc* acetoacetic acid; *HMG* 3-hydroxy-3-methylglutaric acid; *SCAD* short-chain acyl-CoA dehydrogenase; *SCHAD* short-chain hydroxyacyl-CoA dehydrogenase; *MCT* medium-chain triglycerides; *LCT* long-chain triglycerides; *LCHAD* long-chain hydroxyacyl-CoA dehydrogenase

MCAD deficiency, assay of the blood for an acylcarnitine profile and assay of the organic acids of the urine.

MCAD deficiency is the only common disorder of fatty acid oxidation. Its frequency has been estimated at 1 in 6–10,000 caucasians. Most patients have the same mutation, an A985G change which makes for a protein containing glutamic acid where a lysine is found in the normal enzyme. So this simple DNA-diagnostic approach can be expected to yield a rapid diagnosis in a large number of the patients with this group of disorders. The acylcarnitine profile obtained by tandem mass spectrometry can also detect MCAD deficiency; in this instance octanoylcarnitine is the key compound; hexanoylcarnitine may be present as well. In a patient negative for the A986G mutation and positive in the acylcarnitine assay enzyme analysis will document MCAD deficiency. In that case it might be useful to test for the 4 bp deletion, for which there is a rapid test, as there is for A985G and which with A985G accounts for 93% of the MCAD mutations seen in patients representing illness.

Patients detected by newborn screening have another common mutation T199C and these patients seldom develop clinical symptomatology.

Acylcarnitine assay may also point to enzyme assay for carnitine palmitoyltransferase (CPT) deficiency, very long-chain acyl-CoA dehydrogenase (VLCAD) deficiency or multiple acyl-CoA dehydrogenase (MAD) deficiency. Acylcarnitine profiles are obtained by tandem mass spectrometry, which can be done on as little as a drop of dry blood.

Organic acid analysis can be expected to reveal the presence of 3-hydroxy-3-methylglutarate (HMG) in the presence of HMG-CoA lyase deficiency. This compound is abundant in the urine of affected patients even after recovery from the acute hypoglycemic episode. It has already been indicated that in most of the other disorders organic acid analysis is more often normal than abnormal in intervals between episodes of acute illness.

In some patients, essentially all of those not elucidated by the tests of the last three paragraphs, a controlled prolonged fast is necessary to document that the hypoglycemia really is hypoketotic and to elucidate the nature of the defect. As fasting is not only unpleasant but can be very dangerous in disorders of fatty acid oxidation, it is mandatory that carnitine status and acylcarnitine profile is reliably negative before planning a fasting study. In response to this long fast the body's first step is lipolysis which releases free fatty acids. In patients with disorders of fatty acid oxidation, concentrations of free fatty acids are higher than those of 3-hydroxybutyrate in the blood when hypoglycemia develops. In addition fatty acids that accumulate in the presence of defective oxidation undergo Ω-oxidation to dicarboxylic acids giving an elevated ratio of dicarboxylic acids to 3-hydroxybutyrate in the analysis of organic acids of the urine. The nature of the dicarboxylic aciduria at the time the hypoglycemia develops may indicate the site of the defect. Thus C8 to C10 dicarboxylic aciduria is seen in MCAD deficiency and 3-hydroxy long-chain acids in LCHAD deficiency.

Patients during the long fast must be monitored closely so that symptomatic hypoglycemia is avoided. Testing is best done in units where the staff has experience with the protocol. An intravenous line is placed to ensure access for therapeutic glucose, and bedside monitoring of blood concentrations of glucose is done at regular intervals. In abnormalities of fatty acid oxidation, fasting must be long enough to exhaust stores of glycogen and require the mobilization of fat and its oxidation.

Study of the concentrations of carnitine in the plasma and the urine and its esterification may point to the answer, particularly if a low level of free carnitine is documented in the blood and large amounts of esters are being excreted in the urine. Transport of long-chain fatty acid into the mitochondria, where β-oxidation takes place, requires carnitine, and the entry of carnitine into cells such as muscle requires a specific transporter which may be deficient as a cause of hypoketotic hypoglycemia. Assay of carnitine in the blood and urine reveals very low levels of free and esterified carnitine in these patients.

In patients in whom the blood and urine carnitine is normal or increased a long-chain triglycerides (LCT) load may reveal abnormal ketogenesis, and MCT load normal ketogenesis. In such patients MCT administration may even reverse fasting-induced hypoglycemia. In such patients enzyme assay reveals the deficiency of carnitine palmitoyl transferase (CPT I). Esterification of carnitine with fatty acyl-CoA esters is catalyzed by acyltransferases, such as CPT I. The transport of acylcarnitines across the mitochondrial membrane is catalyzed by carnitine translocase; and then hydrolysis, releasing free carnitine and the fatty acid acyl-CoA, is catalyzed by a second acyltransferase, CPT II. Inborn errors are known for each of these three enzymatic steps.

When the carnitine ester level of the urine is high and the free carnitine level of the blood is low, the basic problem is one in which the metabolic block causes the accumulation of acyl-CoA compounds which are esterified with carnitine and excreted in the urine, particularly in disorders of β-oxidation.

In β-oxidation the fatty acid is successively shortened by two carbons, releasing acetyl-CoA. Specific dehydro-

> **Remember**
>
> Low plasma free carnitine may be seen in defective carnitine transporter, or may be secondary to any condition in which acyl-CoA esters accumulate. These include the disorders of fatty acid oxidation and the organic acidurias (see Chap. B2.2) Elevation in the level of urinary esterifed carnitine are also seen in both latter sets of conditions.

genases with overlapping specificities for chain length include: short-chain acyl-CoA dehydrogenase (SCAD), MCAD, and VLCAD. Recently, defects of an additional acyl-CoA dehydrogenase, ACAD9, specialized for the oxidation of unsaturated long chain acyl-CoAs was proven to also result in clinical pathology. In addition, a tri-functional enzyme catalyzes longchain 3-hydroxyacyl-CoA dehydrogenation (LCHAD), 2-enoyl-CoA hydration, and 3-oxoacyl-CoA thiolysis. Diseases involving defects in each of these steps have been defined. The last two known defects leading to hypoketotic hypoglycemia are HMG-CoA synthetase and HMG-CoA lyase deficiencies, the enzymes producing ketone bodies from acetyl-CoA. Whereas the latter usually constantly shows a characteristic organic aciduria, the first one is very difficult to spot as organic acid analysis is unspecific and acylcarnitines normal. In this constellation enzyme analysis of the liver or direct mutation analysis will provide the diagnosis. All of these patients would be expected to have abnormal ketogenesis following an LCT load. When these patients are tested with MCT, MCAD patients display abnormal ketogenesis, while those with LCAD, LCHAD and VLCAD deficiency have normal ketogenesis. The follow-up of this testing is via assay for the specific enzyme or enzymes as suggested in Fig. B2.5.1.

The specific enzyme assays for specific disorders are technically demanding and not generally available. A reasonable step following the fast, if a specific disease is not identified, is to pursue a more general study of metabolism in cultured cells in which oxidation of fatty acids of varying chain length is studied in vitro and carnitine esters are separated and identified after incubation with ^{14}C- or ^{13}C-labeled long-chain fatty acids such as hexadecanoate. Impaired oxidation of long-chain fatty acids such as palmitate in vitro may also be seen in patients with mitochondrial disorders (see Chap. B2.3). Such patients may also have hypoketotic hypoglycemia with increased levels of 3-hydroxydicarboxylic acids because of failure to oxidise the NADH produced in the 3-hydroxyacyl-CoA dehydrogenase step via the electron transport chain. Such patients usually display lactic acidemia.

Key References

Aledo R, Zschocke J, Pié J et al (2001) Genetic basis of mitochondrial HMG-CoA synthase deficiency. Hum Genet 109:19–23

Saudubray JM, Martin D, de Lonlay P et al (1999) Recognition and management of fatty acid oxidation defects: a series of 107 patients. J Inherit Metab Dis 22:488–502

Vreken P, van Lint AEM, Bootsma Ah et al (1999) Rapid diagnosis of organic acidemias and fatty acid oxidation defects by quantitative electrospray tandem-MS acyl-carnitine analysis in plasma. In: Quant PA, Eaton S (eds) Current views of fatty acid oxidation of ketogenesis. From organelles to point mutations. Kluwer Academic/Plenum Publishers, New York, pp 327–337

B2.6 Work-up of the Patient with Hyperammonemia

William L. Nyhan

Key Facts

> Routine clinical chemistry is very helpful in pointing the direction of the work-up of a patient with hyperammonemia. Patients with urea cycle defects are alkalotic or normal; those with organic acidemias or disorders of fatty acid oxidation are acidotic. Presence or absence of ketosis distinguishes the latter two.

> Urea cycle defects are elucidated by analysis of the amino acids of the plasma (citrullinemia and argininemia) and urine (argininosuccinic aciduria).

> Urinary orotic aciduria distinguishes ornithine transcarbamylase deficiency from carbamoylphosphate synthetase and N-acetylglutamate synthetase deficiencies.

Elevated concentrations of ammonia occur episodically in a variety of inherited diseases of metabolism. These include not only the disorders of the urea cycle but also organic acidurias and disorders of fatty acid oxidation. Effective management is predicated on a precise diagnosis and understanding of the nature of the pathophysiology. A systematic progression from routine clinical chemistry to more specific analyses of amino acids, organic acids, and acylcarnitines will lead the clinician to the diagnosis. Liver biopsy has been required for enzymatic diagnosis of carbamyl phosphate synthetase deficiency and ornithine transcarbamylase (OTC) deficiency, as well as N-acetylglutamate

W. L. Nyhan
Department of Pediatrics, University of California, UCSD
School of Medicine, 9500 Gilman Drive, La Jolla, CA 92093, USA
e-mail: wnyhan@ucsd.edu

synthetase deficiency. Mutational analysis may obviate this invasive approach.

Deficiencies of enzymes of the urea cycle and some other disorders, such as the organic acidemias and the disorders of fatty acid oxidation present with hyperammonemia. Normally, values of NH_3 are $<110\,\mu mol/L$ ($190\,\mu g/dL$) in newborns and below $80\,\mu mol/L$ ($140\,\mu g/dL$) in older infants to adults. In the newborn period, a diagnostic work-up for hyperammonemia is warranted at values $>150\,\mu mol/L$ ($260\,\mu g/dL$) and in older infants to adults at values $>100\,\mu mol/L$ ($175\,\mu g/dL$). The classic onset of urea cycle defects is with sudden potentially lethal neonatal coma. The male with OTC exemplifies the classic presentation, but distinct disorders result from deficient activity of each of the enzymes of the urea cycle (Fig. B2.6.1).

The work-up of an infant in hyperammonemic coma is shown (Fig. B2.6.2). The differential diagnosis is very important because different disorders require different treatments. It must proceed with dispatch if the correct diagnosis is to be made and appropriate therapy instituted to prevent death or permanent damage to the brain be done. The initial steps in the algorithm are available in the routine clinical chemistry laboratory. Definitive diagnosis requires the services of a biochemical genetics laboratory.

The first step in the evaluation of a patient, especially an infant in coma, is the measurement of the concentration of ammonia in the blood. The next step is the quantification of serum concentrations of bicarbonate, sodium, chloride, and the anion gap and testing of the urine for ketones. Acidosis and/or an anion gap indicate against the disorders of the urea cycle, which tend to present with respiratory alkalosis. The acidotic patient with massive ketosis has an organic aciduria, such as propionic aciduria, methylmalonic aciduria, isovaleric aciduria, or multiple carboxylase deficiency (see Chap. B2.2). A specific diagnosis is made by quantitative analysis of the organic acids of the urine or of the acylcarnitines from dried blood spots. The disorders of fatty acid oxidation, which may present with hyperammonemia, are characteristically hypoketotic (see Chap. B2.5). However, testing of the urine for ketones may be misleading. We have observed impressively positive urinary ketostix tests in patients with disorders of fatty acid oxidation. Quantification of concentrations of free fatty acids together with acetoacetic and 3-hydroxybutyric acid in the blood of such patients reliably indicate them to have defective ketogenesis. The acute crises in these patients often display hypoglycemia, and diagnoses of Reye syndrome have been made. We have reported an acute hyperammonemic episode in a teenage girl with medium-chain acyl-CoA dehydrogenase deficiency that met all the criteria for a diagnosis of OTC deficiency including orotic aciduria; however, when biopsied liver was tested for OTC activity, it was normal. A patient

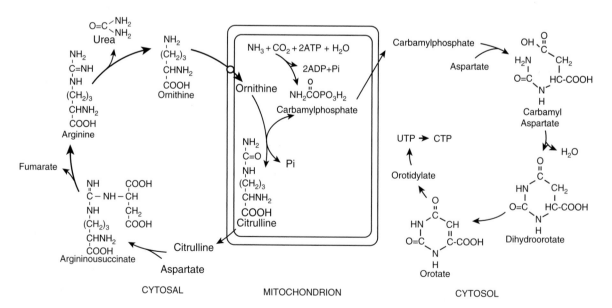

Fig. B2.6.1 Urea cycle

Fig. B2.6. 2 An approach to the stepwise evaluation of a patient with hyperammonemia

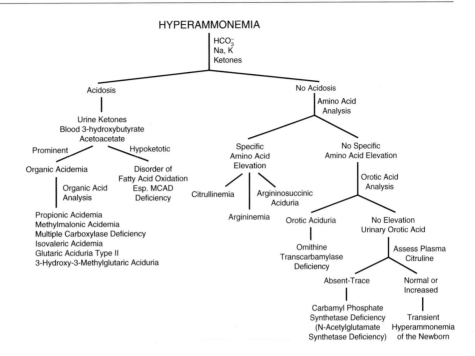

with hyperammonemic coma resulting from a urea cycle defect may develop hypoxia, leading to lactic acidosis. Adequate oxygenation and perfusion should be assured before a urea cycle defect is conceptually excluded and a diagnosis of organic acidemia pursued.

Remember

Hyperammonemia occurs not only in disorders of the urea cycle but also in organic acidemias and disorders of fatty acid oxidation. Testing for organic acids in urine and acylcarnitine profiles lead to the correct diagnosis.

The definitive diagnosis of a urea cycle abnormality is initiated by the quantitative assay of the concentrations of amino acids in blood and urine. The plasma concentrations of amino acids provide the diagnosis in patients with argininemia and citrullinemia. Study of the urine is required in argininosuccinic aciduria.

If hyperammonemic patients are found not to have a diagnostic abnormality in the concentration of an amino acid, the urine should be tested for the excretion of orotic acid. This is not reliably performed as a part of organic acid analysis by GCMS and a specific assay for the compound should be employed. Orotic aciduria

is found in patients with OTC. It is also found in citrullinemia and in argininemia. In a patient without an elevation of a specific amino acid and without orotic aciduria, the usual diagnosis is carbamylphosphate synthetase (CPS) deficiency. *N*-acetylglutamate synthetase deficiency will present with an indistinguishable clinical and biochemical constellation, but is much rarer. Transient hyperammonemia of the newborn may also present this picture, but for reasons that are not clear this disorder is nowhere near as commonly encountered as it was 20 years ago. Failure of immediate closure of the ductus Avenosus after birth is thought to result in (transient) hyperammonemia of the newborn because portal blood bypasses the liver. The definitive diagnoses of CPS, OTC, and *N*-acetylglutamate synthetase deficiencies are made by assay of enzyme activity in biopsied liver or determination of the mutation. If transient hyperammonemia of the newborn is suspected, it is well to wait before performing liver biopsy because the elevated ammonia in this disorder could resolve within 5 days. Too, this gives time to bring the patient into control of the blood concentration of ammonia. The level of citrulline in the blood may be helpful in distinguishing CPS deficiency from transient hyperammonemia of the newborn, in which it is usually normal or elevated. In neonatal CPS, OTC or *N*-acetylglutamate synthetase deficiencies, citrulline is barely detectable. In citrullinemia, concentrations of citrulline in plasma usually exceed 1,000 μmol/L. They are elevated to levels of 150–250 μmol/L in argininosuccinic aciduria, and to 54 ± 22 μmol/L in transient hyperammonemia in the newborn. The normal range is 6–20 μmol/L. Persistent hypocitrullinemia can, in general, be viewed as a marker for disorders of mitochondrial urea cycle enzymes (*N*-acetylglutamate synthetase, CPS I, and ornithine carbamoyltransferase) as well as for deficient pyrroline-5-carboxylate synthetase. Citrulline synthesis is directly coupled to ATP concentration. Consequently, hypocitrullinemia can also be observed in patients with respiratory chain disorders, especially as caused by NARP mutation.

Amino acid analysis also reveals concentrations of glutamine to be regularly elevated in patients with hyperammonemia. Concentrations of alanine are usually elevated, while concentrations of aspartic acid are elevated in some patients. These are nonspecific findings. They are not helpful in the differentiation of the different causes of hyperammonemia. They are potentially helpful in diagnosis, as sometimes an elevated level of glutamine is found in a patient that had not been expected to have hyperammonemia, and while concentrations of ammonia may vary from hour to hour, the elevated concentration of glutamine signifies a state in which there has been more chronic overabundance of ammonia. The transamination of pyruvic acid to alanine and oxaloacetic acid to aspartic acid, as well as 2-oxoglutaric acid to glutamic acid and its subsequent amidation to glutamine are detoxification responses to the presence of excessive quantities of ammonia.

Amino acid analysis may also reveal elevations of tyrosine, phenylalanine, and the branched-chain amino acids. If these are substantial, a primary liver disease should be carefully sought.

Some patients with defects of urea cycle and residual enzyme activity, especially many females with OTC deficiency, display completely unremarkable values of NH_3, amino acids, and orotate in between the crises. It is indispensable that the cause of an unexplained symptomatic episode of hyperammonemia should always be investigated in detail even after the patient recovers, even in adults or aged adults. In those instances, in which the amino acids are normal, an allopurinol loading test may reveal the diagnostic direction.

The differential diagnosis of hyperammonemia also includes the HHH syndrome, which results from deficiency of the ornithine transporter in the mitochondrial membrane, and lysinuric protein intolerance. HHH signifies hyperammonemia, hyperornithinemia, and homocitrullinuria. It is usually suspected first by the identification of large amounts of homocitrulline in the urine. The diagnosis of lysinuric protein intolerance is best made by finding very low levels of lysine in the blood. These patients fail to thrive, and when body stores of lysine are much depleted, the characteristic amino aciduria may not be present; it returns when the diagnosis is made, and blood amino acid concentrations are brought to normal. The metabolic abnormalities become more obvious by calculating the fractional clearances of lysine and other dibasic amino acids. The concentration of citrulline in the blood may be high. Symptomatic hyperammonemia may also finally result from a urinary tract infection in which the infecting *Proteus mirabilis* has urease activity, which produces ammonia from urea.

Key References

Ballard RA, Vinocur B, Reynolds JW Wennberg RP, Merritt A, Sweetman L, Nyhan WL (1978) Transient hyperammonemia of the preterm infant. N Engl J Med 299:920–925

Batshaw ML, Bachmann C, Tuchmann M (eds) (1998) Advances in inherited urea cycle disorders. J Inher Metab Dis 1(21):1–159

Batshaw ML, Brusilow S, Waber L, et al Treatment of inborn errors of urea synthesis: activation of alternative pathways of waste nitrogen synthesis and excretion. N Engl J Med 1982:306:1387

Nyhan WL, Barshop BA, Ozand PA (2005) Ornithine transcarbamylase deficiency. In: Atlas of metabolic diseases, 2nd edn. Hodder Arnold, London, pp 199–205

Thoene JG (1999) Treatment of urea cycle disorders. J Pediatr 134:255–256

B2.7 Work-Up of the Patient with Acute Neurological or Psychiatric Manifestations

Georg F. Hoffmann

Acute or recurrent attacks of neurological or psychiatric features such as coma, ataxia, or abnormal behavior are major presenting features especially of several late-onset, inborn errors of metabolism. The initial diagnostic approach to these disorders is based on a few metabolic screening tests. It is important that the biologic fluids are collected during the acute attack, and at the same time it is also useful to take specimens both before and after treatment. Some of the most significant metabolic manifestations, such as acidosis and ketosis, may be moderate or transient, dependant on symptomatic treatment. On the other hand, at an advanced state of organ dysfunction, many laboratory abnormalities such as metabolic acidosis, hyperlactic acidemia, hyperammonemia, and signs of liver failure may be secondary consequences of hemodynamic shock and multisystem failure. Flow charts for the differential diagnosis and diagnostic approach to acute neurological manifestations such as ataxia and psychiatric aberrations are presented in Figs. B2.7.1–B2.7.3.

Acute attacks of neurological or psychiatric manifestations, such as coma, intractable seizures, stroke, ataxia, or abnormal behavior, resulting from inherited metabolic diseases require prompt and appropriate diagnostic and therapeutic measures (see also Chap. C5). Acute metabolic cerebral edema must be especially quickly recognized and treated in order to prevent herniation and death. All too often, only a diagnosis of encephalitis is initially pursued. Cerebral edema is observed particularly in the acute hyperammonemias (most frequently ornithine transcarbamylase (OTC) deficiency) and maple syrup urine disease (MSUD). In contrast to respiratory chain defects or organic acidurias that involve the mitochondrial metabolism of CoA-activated compounds, the metabolic blocks in urea cycle defects and MSUD do not directly interfere with mitochondrial energy production, and the typical signs of acute mitochondrial decompensation such as lactic acidosis may be lacking. They may develop later as the condition of the patient deteriorates. Acute hemiplegia may be a presenting symptom; it has also been reported in patients with organic acidurias, in particular propionic aciduria and methylmalonic aciduria as well as phosphoglycerate kinase deficiency and mitochondriopthies.

An acute onset of extrapyramidal signs during the

> **Remember**
>
> Acute or recurrent attacks of neurological or psychiatric symptoms such as coma, ataxia, or abnormal behavior are major presenting features of several late-onset, inborn errors of metabolism. The initial diagnostic approach to these disorders is based on a few metabolic screening tests, in particular ammonia, lactate, amino acids, and organic acids. It is important that the biologic fluids are collected simultaneously at the time of the acute attack. Flow charts for the differential diagnosis and diagnostic approach to acute neurological manifestations such as coma, ataxia, and psychiatric aberrations are presented in Figs. B2.7.1–B2.7.3.

course of a nonspecific intercurrent illness, minor surgery, accident, or even immunization may initially be misinterpreted as encephalitis, but represent a conspicuous feature of several metabolic disorders. In glutaric aciduria type I (GA1), a dystonic dyskinetic movement disorder is caused by the acute destruction of the basal ganglia, specifically the striatum. The acute encephalopathic crisis in GA1 typically occurs between the ages 6 and 18 months; affected children may have had mild neurological abnormalities prior to the acute episode and frequently are macrocephalic. Almost half of the patients with Wilson disease present with neurological symptoms, usually after the age of 6 years. Dysarthria, incoordination of voluntary movements, and tremor are the most common signs. There may be involuntary choreiform movements, and gait may be affected.

Acute hemiplegia may be a presenting symptom; it has been reported in patients with organic acidurias, in particular propionic aciduria and methylmalonic aciduria, as well as phosphoglycerate kinase deficiency. Some patients with propionic acidemia present a basal

G. F. Hoffmann
University Children's Hospital, Ruprecht-Karls-University,
Im Neuenheimer Feld 430, D-69120 Heidelberg, Germany
e-mail: georg.hoffmann@med.uni-heidelberg.de

Differential Diagnosis of Metabolic Coma

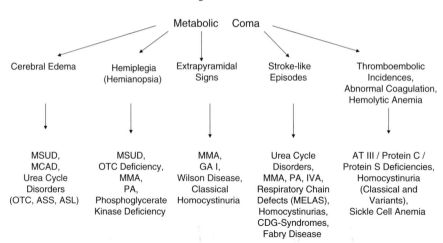

Fig. B2.7.1 Differential diagnosis of metabolic coma. *ASS* argininosuccinate synthetase deficiency, citrullinemia; *ASL* argininosuccinate lyase deficiency, argininosuccinic aciduria; *AT* antithrombin; *CDG* congenital disorders of glycosylation; *GAI* glutaric aciduria type I; *IVA* isovaleric aciduria; *MCAD* medium-chain acyl-CoA dehydrogenase; *MELAS* (mitochondrial encephalopathy, lactic acidosis and stroke-like episodes); *MMA* methylmalonic aciduria; *MSUD* maple syrup urine disease; *OTC* ornithine transcarbamylase deficiency; *PA* propionic aciduria

Differential Diagnosis of Metabolic Causes of Acute Ataxia ? Coma

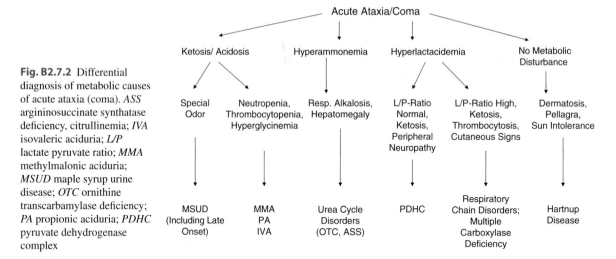

Fig. B2.7.2 Differential diagnosis of metabolic causes of acute ataxia (coma). *ASS* argininosuccinate synthatase deficiency, citrullinemia; *IVA* isovaleric aciduria; *L/P* lactate pyruvate ratio; *MMA* methylmalonic aciduria; *MSUD* maple syrup urine disease; *OTC* ornithine transcarbamylase deficiency; *PA* propionic aciduria; *PDHC* pyruvate dehydrogenase complex

ganglia picture indistinguishable from those of GAI or Lesch–Nyhan disease.

Acute stroke-like episodes and strokes occur in several metabolic disorders (Table B2.7.1). They are the hallmark feature of the mitochondrial encephalopathy, lactic acidosis, and stroke-like episodes, (MELAS) syndrome, a disorder caused by mutations in the tRNA$^{Leu(UUR)}$ gene in the mitochondrial DNA. In total, 80% of patients carry the mutation 3243A > G. Acute

episodes may present initially with vomiting, headache, convulsions, or visual abnormalities and may be followed by hemiplegia or hemianopia. The morphological correlates are true cerebral infarctions, but there is no evidence of vascular obstruction or atherosclerosis and they do not correspond to vascular territories. Stroke-like episodes (metabolic stroke) are also observed in other metabolic disorders such as the congenital disorders of glycosylation, and methylmalonic

Fig. B2.7.3 Differential diagnosis of metabolic causes of acute psychiatric manifestations (coma). *ASS* argininosuccinate synthatase deficiency, citrullinemia; *ASL* argininosuccinate lyase deficiency, argininosuccinic aciduria; *LPI* lysinuric protein intolerance; *MSUD* maple syrup urine disease; *OTC* ornithine transcarbamy-lase deficiency

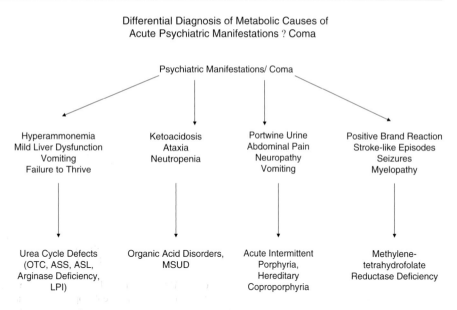

Differential Diagnosis of Metabolic Causes of Acute Psychiatric Manifestations ? Coma

Psychiatric Manifestations/ Coma

Hyperammonemia Mild Liver Dysfunction Vomiting Failure to Thrive	Ketoacidosis Ataxia Neutropenia	Portwine Urine Abdominal Pain Neuropathy Vomiting	Positive Brand Reaction Stroke-like Episodes Seizures Myelopathy
Urea Cycle Defects (OTC, ASS, ASL, Arginase Deficiency, LPI)	Organic Acid Disorders, MSUD	Acute Intermittent Porphyria, Hereditary Coproporphyria	Methylene-tetrahydrofolate Reductase Deficiency

Table B2.7.1 Metabolic causes of stroke and stroke-like episodes

Homocystinuria
Mitochondrial encephalomyopathy
   Pyruvate dehydrogenase deficiency
   Pyruvate carboxylase deficiency
   Respiratory chain disorders
   Leigh disease
Urea cycle disorders
   Carbamoylphosphate synthetase deficiency
   Ornithine carbamoyltransferase deficiency
   Arginosuccinate synthase deficiency
   Arginosuccinate lyase deficiency
   Arginase deficiency
Congenital disorders of glycosylation
Fabry disease
Menkes disease
Sulfite oxidase deficiency
Purine nucleotide phosphorylase deficency
Vanishing white matter disease

and propionic acidurias. Strokes may of course be absent in affected members of families with the MELAS syndrome; some have migraine-like headaches as the only manifestation of the disease, while others manifest only diabetes or are asymptomatic. Classic cerebral strokes as well as cardiovascular accidents may also be caused by various metabolic disorders that cause vascular disease such as classical homocystinuria, the thiamine-responsive megaloblastic anemia syndrome, and Fabry disease. Vascular changes resulting from altered elastic fibers are the cause of ischemic cerebral infarctions in Menke disease. True thromboembolic events may be caused by defects in the anticoagulant systems, such as antithrombin III, protein C, or protein S deficiencies.

Acute ataxia (Fig. B2.7.2) or psychiatric manifestations (Fig. B2.7.3) can be the leading signs of several organic acidurias and late-onset MSUD. In these instances, the metabolic derangement is most often associated with ketoacidosis (see also Chap. B2.2). A rather confusing finding in some patients with organic acidurias is the presence of ketoacidosis in combination with hyperglycemia and glycosuria mimicking diabetic ketoacidotic coma. In late-onset MSUD, a special odor may be noticed. In organic acidurias such as methylmalonic aciduria, propionic aciduria, or isovaleric aciduria, moderate to severe hematological manifestations are common, and have led astute observers to suspect an organic acidemia. These disorders are usually characterized by neutropenia and, especially in infancy, thrombocytopenia. Recurrent infections, particularly mucocutaneous candidiasis, may be a common finding. The specific diagnosis may be obtained through the analysis of amino acids in plasma and organic acids in urine.

Urea cycle disorders, such as OTC deficiency, argininosuccinic aciduria, citrullinemia, arginase deficiency, or lysinuric protein intolerance may present in childhood or adolescence with acute or recurrent episodes of hyperammonemia (Chap. B2.6). Clinical features may include acute ataxia or psychiatric symptoms such as hallucinations, delirium, dizziness, aggressiveness, anxiety, or schizophrenia-like behavior. In addition there may be hepatomegaly, liver dysfunction, and failure to thrive. The correct diagnosis will be missed unless ammonia levels are determined in plasma at the time of acute symptoms. Hyperammonemia may be moderate or mild (150–250 μmol/L) even when the child is in deep coma, and especially the late-onset forms of urea cycle disorder such as OTC deficiency can be easily overlooked and misdiagnosed as schizophrenia, encephalitis, or even intoxication. Diagnostic procedures should include analyses of plasma amino acids, urinary organic acids, and orotic acid.

Mitochondrial diseases manifest in the CNS primarily in high energy consuming structures such as basal ganglia, capillary endothelium, and the cerebellum. Whereas disturbed function of the cerebellum and the basal ganglia leads to characteristic disorders of movement, disturbed capillary function results in fluctuating neurological signs from stroke-like episodes to nonspecific mental deterioration and progressively accumulating damage of both grey and white matter. Acute ataxia in association with peripheral neuropathy is frequently found in patients with pyruvate dehydrogenase deficiency. Moderate or substantial elevation of lactate with a normal lactate/pyruvate-ratio and absence of ketosis supports this diagnosis. Acute ataxia associated with a high lactate/pyruvate-ratio is suggestive of multiple carboxylase deficiency or respiratory chain defects. In the latter, thrombocytosis is often observed in contrast to the thrombocytopenia associated with organic acidurias.

Some inborn errors of metabolism, like Hartnup disease, may present with clinical symptoms of recurrent acute ataxia without causing general metabolic disturbances. Typical additional symptoms like skin rashes, pellagra, and sun intolerance may lead to analysis of the urinary amino acid which provides the specific diagnosis. The characteristic pattern is of an excess of neutral monoamino-monocarboxylic acids in urine with (low) normal concentrations in plasma.

Acute intermittent porphyria and hereditary coproporphyria usually present with recurrent attacks of vomiting, abdominal pain, unspecific neuropathy, and psychiatric symptoms. These disorders have to be excluded in the differential diagnosis of suspected psychogenic complaints and hysteria. Diagnosis can be made by specific analyses of porphyrins. Patients affected with disorders of the cellular methylation pathway such as methylenetetrahydrofolate reductase deficiency may also present with psychiatric symptoms. These often resemble acute schizophrenic episodes, but they may respond to folate therapy. Homocysteine is elevated in plasma, and a positive Brand reaction in the urine may be the first abnormal laboratory finding. Other neurological features include stroke-like episodes, seizures and myelopathy. Diagnosis is made by analysis of amino acids and homocysteine in plasma and CSF. Methyltetrahydrofolate in CSF is greatly reduced.

B2.8 Emergency Treatment of Inherited Metabolic Diseases

Georg F. Hoffmann and William L. Nyhan

Key Facts

> Timely and correct intervention during the initial presentation of metabolic imbalance and during later episodes precipitated by dietary indiscretion or intercurrent illnesses is the most important determinant of outcome in inherited metabolic diseases at risk for acute metabolic decompensation.
> Patients should be supplied with an emergency letter, card, or bracelet containing instructions for emergency measures and phone numbers.
> Logistics of therapeutic measures should be repeatedly evaluated by the specialist team with the family and the primary care physician(s).

The most critical challenge in many inherited metabolic diseases is the timely and correct intervention during acute metabolic decompensation in the neonatal period or in later recurrent episodes. Fortunately, there is only a limited repertoire of pathophysiological sequences in the response of infant to illness, and consequently, a limited number of therapeutic measures are to be taken. Three major groups of disorders at risk for acute metabolic decompensation that require specific therapeutic approaches in emergency situations can be delineated (see Fig. B1.1).

- Disorders of intermediary metabolism that cause *acute intoxication* through the accumulation of toxic molecules.

G. F. Hoffmann (✉)
University Children's Hospital, Ruprecht-Karls-University,
Im Neuenheimer Feld 430, D-69120 Heidelberg, Germany
e-mail: georg.hoffmann@med.uni-heidelberg.de

- Disorders in which there is *reduced fasting tolerance*.
- Disorders in which there is *disturbed energy metabolism*.

A preliminary differentiation of these three groups should be possible with the help of basic investigations, available in every hospital setting, namely the determination of acid–base balance, glucose, lactate, ammonia, and ketones, as discussed in previous chapters. With this information, appropriate therapy can be initiated even before a precise diagnosis is known. In instances, especially during the initial manifestation of a metabolic disease, i.e., when the exact diagnosis is not yet known, measures must be quick, precise and not halfhearted, and every effort must be undertaken to obtain the relevant diagnostic information within 24 h or sooner, i.e., results of acylcarnitines in dried blood spots or plasma, amino acids in plasma, and organic acids in urine.

In all instances, provision of ample quantities of fluid and electrolytes is indispensible. Differences in the therapeutic approach relate primarily to energy requirements and methods of detoxification (Table B2.8.1).

Remember

Emergency treatment must start without delay.

Table B2.8.1 Emergency treatment: energy needs in Infants

Disorders requiring anabolism (acute intoxication):
  60–100 kcal/kg/day
Organic acidurias, maple syrup urine disease, urea cycle disorders⇒ glucose 15–20 g/kg/day + fat 2 g/kg/day
always: + insulin, starting with 0.05 U/kg/h, Adjustments are made dependent on blood glucose (useful combination is 1 U/8g glucose)
early: central venous catheterization
Disorders requiring glucose stabilization (reduced fasting tolerance):
Fatty acid oxidation defects, glycogen storage disease type I, disorders of gluconeogenesis, galactosemia, fructose intolerance, tyrosinemia I ⇒ glucose 7–10 mg/kg/min≈ 10 g/kg/day
Disorders requiring restriction of energy turn-over (disturbed energy metabolism):
PDHC deficiency⇒ reduce glucose supply: 2–3 mg/kg/min≈ 3 g/kg/day
  Add fat: 2–3 g/kg/day
Electron transport chain (oxphos) disorders ⇒ glucose 10–15 g/kg/day

B2.8.1 Acute Intoxication (Fig. B1.1)

In diseases, in which symptoms develop because of *"acute intoxication,"* rapid reduction of toxic molecules is a cornerstone of treatment. In disorders of amino acid catabolism, such as maple syrup urine disease, the classical organic acidurias, or the urea cycle defects, the toxic compounds may be derived from exogenous as well as endogenous sources. In addition, to stopping the intake of natural protein until the crisis is over but no longer than (12 to) 24 (to 48) h, reversal of catabolism and the promotion of anabolism and consequently reversal of the breakdown of endogenous protein is a major goal.

In patients, known to have a disorder of amino acid catabolism, who develop an intercurrent illness and manifestations of metabolic imbalance, such as ketonuria in a patient with an organic aciduria, primary emergency measures at home for 24–48 h consist of frequent feedings with a high carbohydrate content and some salt (Table B2.8.2), and reduction, even to zero, of the intake of natural protein. In diseases such as maple syrup urine disease, the individual amino acid mixture devoid of the amino acids of the defective pathway is continued. Detoxifying medication such as carnitine in the organic acidurias, benzoate, phenylacetate, and arginine or citrulline in the hyperammonemias is employed. During this time period, patients should be reassessed regularly regarding state of consciousness, fever, and food tolerance. If the intercurrent illness continues into the third day, symptomatology worsens, or if vomiting compromises external feedings, admission to hospital is mandatory.

Table B2.8.2 Oral administration of fluid and energy for episodic acute intercurrent illness in patients with metabolic disorders

Age (years)	Glucose polymer/maltodextrin solution		
	(%)	(kcal/100 mL)	Daily amount
0–1	10	40	150–200 mL/kg
1–2	15	60	95 mL/kg
2–6	20	80	1,200–1,500 mL
6–10	20	80	1,500–2,000 mL
>10	25	100	2,000 mL

Adapted from Dixon and Leonard (1992). Oral substitution should only be given during minor intercurrent illnesses and for a limited time of 2–3 days. Intake of some salt should also be provided. The actual amounts given have to be individually adjusted, e.g., according to a reduced body weight in an older patient with failure to thrive

In the hospital, therapy must be continued without interruption. In most instances, an intravenous line is essential, but nasogastric administration, for instance, of amino acid mixtures in maple syrup urine disease is very useful. The management of many of these infants is greatly simplified by the early placement of a gastrostomy. This can usually be discontinued after infancy.

> **Remember**
>
> Calculations for maltodextran/dextrose, fluid and protein intake should be based on the expected and not on the actual weight!

Large amounts of energy are needed to achieve anabolism, e.g., in neonates >100 kcal/kg b.w./day. In a sick baby, this can usually be accomplished only by hyperosmolar infusions of glucose together with fat through a central venous line. Insulin should be started early, especially in the presence of significant ketosis or in maple syrup urine disease, to enhance anabolism. One approach is to use a fixed ratio of insulin to glucose (Table B2.8.1). The administration of lipids intravenously can often be increased to 3 g/kg, if serum levels of triglycerides are monitored.

Acute episodes of massive ketoacidosis, as seen in methylmalonic or propionic aciduria, require especially vigorous supportive therapy. Large amounts of water, electrolytes, bicarbonate, and high doses of intravenous carnitine must be infused together with glucose. Blood concentrations of electrolytes and bicarbonate are determined and an intravenous infusion started before taking time for history and physical examination. Following a bolus of 20 mL/kg of ringer lactate or normal saline, intravenous fluid should contain 75–150 mEq/L of isotonic $NaHCO_3$ (75 with massive ketosis, 150, if coma or HCO_3<10 mEq/L). Carnitine supplementation should be given at 300 mg/kg intravenously. Electrolytes and acid–base balance are checked q6h. Serum sodium should be ≥138 mmol/L. The $NaHCO_3$ content of the infusion is reduced, after the serum HCO_3 has become normal, but the same rate of infusion is continued until ketonuria has subsided. Some children with these disorders benefit from implantation of a venous port to facilitate blood sampling and intravenous infusions.

Forced diuresis with large amounts of fluids and furosemide is especially useful in the methylmalonic acidurias in removing methylmalonate from the body.

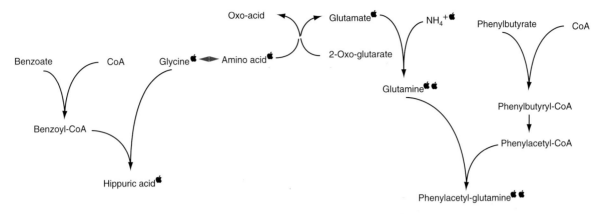

Fig. B2.8.1 Pharmacological detoxification of ammonia. The apple symbols represent nitrogens. Conjugation of glycine with benzoate yields hippurate; conjugation of phenylacetate with glutamine yields phenylacetylglutamine and these are the end products excreted. One nitrogen is excreted with each molecule of hippuric acid and two with phenylacetylglutamine

Detoxification in the organic acidurias depends of the ability to form esters such as propionylcarnitine, which are preferentially excreted in the urine, thus removing toxic intermediates. In these disorders, tissue stores of carnitine are depleted. Carnitine is given to restore tissue supply, but its major utility is to promote detoxification by the formation and excretion of carnitine esters. It is given intravenously in doses of 200–300 mg/kg. Carnitine is less well tolerated enterally. Oral doses of >100 mg/kg are employed, but the dose may have to be reduced in some patients.

In isovaleric aciduria it is useful to add glycine to the regimen to promote the excretion of isovalerylglycine (500 mg/kg).

In maple syrup urine disease, the major element of therapy is to harness the forces of anabolism to lay down accumulated leucine and other branched-chain amino acids into protein. This is done by the provision of mixtures of amino acids lacking leucine, isoleucine and valine. The use of intravenous mixtures is very efficient, and essential in a patient with intractable vomiting, but these are expensive and not generally available. Enteral mixtures are mixed in minimal volume and dripped over 24 h in doses of 2 g/kg of amino acids. Often even a vomiting patient will tolerate a slow drip. Since concentrations of isoleucine are much lower than those of leucine, concentrations of amino acids must be measured at least daily and when the concentrations of isoleucine become low isoleucine is added to the enteral mixture. In many patients valine must also be added before the leucine concentration is lowered adequately.

The pharmacological approach to the detoxification of ammonia in urea cycle defects, and also in those organic acidurias that present with hyperammonemia is the provision of alternative methods of waste nitrogen excretion (Fig. B2.8.1). Benzoate is effectively conjugated with glycine to form hippurate, which is then excreted in the urine. Similarly, phenylacetate is conjugated with glutamine to form phenylacetylglutamine, which is efficiently excreted. Administered orally, phenylbutyrate is converted to phenylacetate. In a metabolic emergency with an as yet unknown diagnosis and a documented hyperammonemia ≥200 μmol/L (350 μg/dL) and in relapses of known patients benzoate and phenylacetate should be given intravenously (Table B2.8.3), along with arginine. Especially during combined intravenous supplementation of benzoate and phenylacetate electrolytes must be checked regularly to avoid hypernatremia. A dose of 400 mg sodium benzoate corresponds to 2.77 mmol and therefore to 2.77 mmol of sodium. In some situations, enteral phenylbutyrate or benzoate along with arginine may be adequate. In urea cycle defects, carnitine administration is also recommended (50–100 mg/kg). Zofran (0.15 mg/kg i.v.) appears to be especially effective against hyperemesis, which can accompany hyperammonemia.

Hyperammonemias may require extracorporal dialysis for detoxification. This should be considered at ammonia levels > 600 μmol/L (1000 μg/dL). Hemodialysis has been repeatedly shown to be more effective than exchange transfusions, peritoneal dialysis, or arteriovenous hemofiltration. This is an argument for the transport of such an infant, if the necessary logistics cannot be promptly organized locally.

In aminoacidopathies, other than maple syrup urine disease, such as phenylketonuria, the homocystinurias

Table B2.8.3 Emergency treatment of hyperammonemic crises

Drug	Loading dose over 1–2 h (mg/kg)	Intravenous daily dose	Preparation
Na-benzoate	250	250(–500) mg/kg	1 g in 50 mL 5–10% of glucose
Na-phenylacetate[a]	250	250(–600) mg/kg	1 g in 50 mL 5–10% of glucose
L-arginine	250	250 mg/kg in OTC, CPS, and in as yet unknown disease – 500 mg/kg in ASS, ASL	1 g in 50 mL 5–10% of glucose
Folic acid		0.1 mg/kg q.day	
Pyridoxine		5 mg q.day	

OTC ornithine transcarbamylase deficiency; *CPS* carbamylphosphate synthetase deficiency; *ASS* argininosuccinate synthetase deficiency; *ASL* argininsuccinate lyase deficiency
[a]In a known patient, not vomiting, it may be possible to employ oral or gastric Na-phenylbutyrate

or the tyrosinemias, the toxic metabolites lead primarily to chronic organ damage rather than a metabolic emergency. Hepatorenal tyrosinemia may lead to a crisis of hepatic insufficiency. The rationale and principles of therapy remain the same as described earlier in the metabolic emergencies, but hypercaloric treatment through central catheters is seldom indicated. Glucose should be administered in accordance with endogenous glucose production rates together with fat. Oral therapy should be resumed as soon as possible including medication and the appropriate amino acid mixture. Patients with tyrosinemia type I should be treated with nitisinone (NTBC) as soon as possible. NTBC is a potent inhibitor of *p*-hydroxyphenylpyruvate dioxygenase; it blocks the genesis of the highly toxic fumarylacetoacetate and its derivatives (see Chap. C2).

In patients with galactosemia or fructose intolerance, toxic metabolites derive predominantly from exogenous sources. Once the diagnosis is suspected or made, therapy consists of the elimination of the intake of galactose and fructose. However, if intravenous alimentation devoid of galactose and fructose is begun without suspicion of the underlying metabolic disorder, gradual reintroduction of oral feeding will lead to protracted disease courses with varying and complicated symptomatology until the diagnosis is made. Patients with galactosemia or fructose intolerance require energy to stabilize and maintain blood glucose.

B2.8.2 Reduced Fasting Tolerance
(Fig. B1.1)

Patients with defects of fatty acid oxidation and gluconeogenesis, such as medium chain acyl-CoA dehydrogenase deficiency and glycogen storage disease type I,

require vigorous administration of glucose in amounts sufficient to restore and maintain euglycemia. Frequent monitoring of blood glucose is essential if symptomatic hypoglycemia is to be avoided. The patient seen first in an emergency room following a convulsion and found to have little or no measurable glucose in the blood is usually treated first with enough hypertonic glucose to restore euglycemia. It is acceptable to follow that with infusion of 5% glucose and water, but glucose levels should be obtained promptly and the concentration changed to 10% or higher, as required to keep the sugar elevated.

Supplementation of carnitine in suspected or proven defects of fatty acid oxidation is currently controversial. At least, restoration of levels of free carnitine appears indicated. A dose of 100 mg/kg is usually adequate. Disorders of carbohydrate metabolism do not need detoxifying treatment.

Long-term management of patients with disorders of fatty acid oxidation is best served by avoidance of fasting. Diagnosed patients should have written instructions that if anorexia or vomiting precludes oral intake, the patient must be brought to hospital for the intravenous administration of glucose. Supplemental cornstarch is a useful adjunct to chronic therapy in disorders of carbohydrate metabolism and of fatty acid oxidation.

B2.8.3 Disturbed Energy Metabolism
(Fig. B1.1)

The "*disorders of disturbed energy metabolism*" include defects of the pyruvate dehydrogenase complex (PDHC), the Krebs cycle, and the respiratory electron transport chain. These disorders are characterized by chronic multisystemic disease rather than acute metabolic emergency. The situation calling for emergency treatment is the occasional occurrence of life threatening acidosis and lactic acidemia. Therapy in this situation calls for vigorous treatment of the acid–base balance as outlined earlier. An issue is the fact that patients with PDHC deficiency are glucose sensitive. Glucose infusions can result in a further increase in lactate. In fact it is advisable to test all patients with lactic acidemia for the lactate response of lactate to glucose. In sensitive patients, intravenous glucose may be employed at rates well below the endogenous glucose production rate (Table B2.8.1). The correction of metabolic acidosis may require high amounts of sodium bicarbonate. In as many as 20% of children with mitochondrial disease the acute decompensation may be complicated by renal tubular acidosis, and this may increase the requirement for sodium bicarbonate. Regardless of the cause, levels of lactate can be lowered by dialysis or the administration of dichloroacetate. Dichloroacetate activates the PDHC in brain, liver, and muscle. Although levels of lactate have been shown to improve, the overall outcome may not be altered.

In patients with mitochondrial disease, replacement of cofactors is commonly undertaken. Evidence in support of the argument is a positive response to biotin in multiple carboxylase deficiency and to riboflavin in some patients with multiple acyl-CoA dehydrogenase deficiency. It is common practice to prescribe a combination of coenzyme Q_{10}, vitamin E, and a balanced B-vitamin supplement called "B50." B50 contains a combination of thiamine, riboflavin, niacin, pyridoxine, biotin, folate, B_{12}, and pantothenic acid. If a measured deficiency in blood carnitine is found, or if urinary excretion of carnitine esters is high, the patient is treated with L-carnitine.

The ultimate goal of therapy is not simply to reverse the metabolic emergency but to prevent irreversible damage to the patient´s brain. The diseases leading to acute intoxication, such as maple syrup urine disease, the classical organic acidurias, and the urea cycle defects, carry the greatest risk of major sequelae. Additional supportive therapeutic measures are used informally in some centers to enhance this goal. These include mannitol for the treatment of cerebral edema, which may also enhance detoxification through increased diuresis. Increased intracranial pressure may be monitored neurosurgically. Overall supportive care is critical in patients in intensive care units, with special vigilance for the detection and prompt treatment of infection.

In summary, the metabolic emergency calls for prompt diagnostic and therapeutic measures, which follow the principles of adequate energy supply, the promotion of anabolism and the use of pharmacological, and if necessary extracorporal detoxification. These are the determinants of success in handling the metabolic emergencies of inborn errors of metabolism.

Key References

Dixon MA, Leonard JV (1992) Intercurrent illness in inborn errors of intermediary metabolism. Arch Dis Child 67:1387–1391

Nyhan WL, Barshop BA, Ozand PT (2005) Atlas of metabolic diseases, 2nd edn. Hodder Arnold, London

Nyhan WL, Rice-Kelts M, Klein J, Barshop BA (1999) Treatment of the acute crisis in maple syrup urine disease. Arch Pediatr Adolesc Med 152:593–598

Prietsch V, Ogier de Baulny H, Saudubray JM (2006) Emergency treatments. In: Fernandes J, Saudubray JM, van den Berghe G, Walter JH (eds) Inborn metabolic diseases – diagnosis and treatment, 4th edn. Springer, Berlin, pp 71–79

Prietsch V, Lindner M, Zschocke J, Nyhan WL, Hoffmann GF (2002) Emergency management of inherited metabolic disease. J Inherit Metab Dis 25:531–546

Patient Care and Treatment

B3

William L. Nyhan and Georg F. Hoffmann

Care and treatment of patients with an inherited metabolic disease require both a detailed knowledge of the natural history of the diseases and a comprehensive understanding of the molecular basis and the pathophysiological consequences of gene defects. Continuous sympathetic company and guidance of patients and their families are essential for optimal outcome. Inherited metabolic diseases are chronic conditions that involve various different organ systems and often show progressive pathology. In addition, several genetic aspects such as passing on a disease to one's children, implications of consanguinity, the possibility of carrier detection, and prenatal or preimplantation diagnosis, can create a severe psychosocial burden for individuals and families as a whole. This implies the need for an equally diverse multidisciplinary approach to care and treatment.

Primary correction of the genetic defect, i.e., gene or molecular therapy, has not yet been established for any inherited metabolic disease. Treatment is usually aimed at circumventing or neutralizing the genetic block, e.g., through the reduction of dietary phenylalanine in phenylketonuria. In addition, symptomatic treatment of the disease, such as medication for seizures or a portable electric wheel chair, is essential for outcome and improved quality of life of the patient and the family. The aim is to help the affected individual to achieve optimal development during childhood and maximal independence, social integration, and self-esteem as an adolescent and adult. This goal can only be achieved by a multidisciplinary approach. Care and treatment of the patient and the family should involve different medical specialties as well as associated professions such as dieticians, nurses, psychologists, physiotherapists, social workers, speech therapists, and teachers. Families may gain valuable emotional support and much practical advice by meeting other affected families. Ideally, a specialist in inherited metabolic diseases coordinates all aspects of care and treatment of the patient in close collaboration with the local family doctor or pediatrician.

The objective of this book is not to provide a detailed coverage of the diverse issues of the long-term care and treatment of inherited metabolic diseases. Treatment is discussed in detail where it is practically relevant for physicians particularly the emergency situation in which there is an acute presentation of a metabolic disorder. There is also a section on anesthesia, a subject seldom considered, but of major importance for patients with a variety of inherited metabolic diseases.

Key Reference

Blau N, Hoffmann GF, Leonard J, Clarke JTR eds (2005) Physician's Guide to the Treatment and Follow-up of Metabolic Diseases. Springer, Berlin Heidelberg New York

W. L. Nyhan
Department of Pediatrics, University of California, UCSD
School of Medicine, 9500 Gilman Drive, La Jolla, CA 92093, USA
e-mail: wnyhan@ucsd.edu

G. F. Hoffmann et al. (eds.), *Inherited Metabolic Diseases*,
DOI: 10.1007/978-3-540-74723-9_B3, © Springer-Verlag Berlin Heidelberg 2010

Anesthesia and Metabolic Disease

B4

William L. Nyhan

Key Facts

> Succinylcholine persistence in patients with butyrylcholinesterase variants; they may fail to breathe long after the surgery is completed. Artificial ventilation must continue.

> Instability of the atlantoaxial joint in patients with mucopolysaccharidoses may lead to disaster during anesthesia. These patients should have surgical procedures in centers with anesthesiologists who have experience in dealing with these patients, and preoperative evaluation of the cervical spine and cord is mandatory.

> (Long) fasting must be avoided in disorders of fatty acid oxidation and in Refsum syndrome. The provision of ample amounts of glucose in these disorders prevents hypoglycemia, rhabdomyolysis, and the crises of Refsum syndrome.

> Catabolism is inherent in surgery; it is magnified by fasting. It can be minimized in patients with organic acidemia or urea cycle defects by the provision of parenteral glucose.

> Urea cycle defects may also be amenable to the provision of intravenous arginine during the procedure. Intravenous benzoate/phenylacetate provides an alternate mode of waste nitrogen excretion.

> Preoperative preparation of patients with homocystinuria, especially those who are B_6 responsive, is designed to minimize levels of homocystine during the procedure.

> Malignant hyperthermia is seen in response to inhalation anesthetics and succinylcholine. It is usually the result of mutations in the RYR1 gene. Rhabdomyolysis in disorders of fatty acid oxidation may mimic malignant hyperthermia. Malignant hyperthermia may follow anesthesia in a variety of myopathies, especially central core disease and King–Denborough syndrome.

B4.1 General Remarks

Special considerations for anesthesia and surgery were dramatized by the recognition, more than 50 years ago, that genetically determined variants in *butyrylcholinesterase*, the cholinesterase found in serum leads to prolongation of the action of *succinylcholine*, the agent used in surgery for relaxation of muscle. Patients with deficient activity of this enzyme remain paralyzed and unable to breathe for long after the surgery is completed. Testing for these variants, of which there are a number, is done spectrophotometrically in the presence of the inhibitor, dibucaine, and the percentage of inhibition is called the dibucaine number. Management of the patient with this problem is simply to continue assisted ventilation until the succinylcholine is broken down. All carboxylic acid esters will ultimately be hydrolyzed despite the absence of specific esterase activity.

Remember

Ideal presurgical procedure is to obtain the butylcholinesterase dibucaine number. Then the anesthesiologist can plan to continue ventilation until the succinylcholine has broken down as a result of the action of other esterases.

W. L. Nyhan
Department of Pediatrics, University of California, UCSD School of Medicine, 9500 Gilman Drive, La Jolla, CA 92093, USA
e-mail: wnyhan@ucsd.edu

G. F. Hoffmann et al. (eds.), *Inherited Metabolic Diseases*, DOI: 10.1007/978-3-540-74723-9_B4, © Springer-Verlag Berlin Heidelberg 2010

B4.2 Mucopolysaccharidoses

The great risk of anesthesia in mucopolysaccharidosis (MPS) is the result of instability of the atlantoaxial joint. This is a particular problem in Morquio disease, but patients with MPS II and VI are also at risk. Deaths have been recorded as complications of anesthesia. Careful positioning is required and hyperextension of the neck must be avoided. General anesthesia should be undertaken in these patients only in centers in which anesthesiologists have had experience with patients with these diseases. In preparation for surgery the patient or parents should be asked about previous problems with anesthesia, obstructive sleep apnea, or transient paralysis that might be an index of cervical instability. The patient should be examined for evidence of cord compression, kyphoscoliosis, and excessive upper respiratory secretions. The blood pressure should be determined, and an EKG and echocardiogram. Recent roentgenograms of the chest and of the cervical spine should be reviewed. Those with kyphoscoliosis should have pulmonary function studies. Sleep studies may be useful. Those with evidence or history of cord compression should have an MRI of the spine. Intubation and induction of anesthesia may be difficult because of limited space; smaller tubes than usual may be required. Visualization may be limited by macroglossia, micrognathia, and immobility of the neck. It may be necessary to immobilize the neck with a halo brace or plaster to avoid damage to the cervical cord. Thick secretions may lead to postoperative pulmonary problems. Recovery from anesthesia may be slow, and postoperative obstruction of the airway has been observed. Wherever possible, local anesthesia is preferable, but in young or uncooperative patients such as those with Hunter or Sanfilippo diseases, this may not be possible. General anesthesia is preferable to sedation, because of the need to control the airway.

> **Remember**
>
> The instability of the atlantoaxial joint is the major anesthetic issue in MPS, but macroglossia and micrognathia, may interfere with intubation. Thick secretions may cause postoperative problems.

B4.3 Avoidance of Hypoglycemia

Patients with many metabolic diseases are at risk for the development of hypoglycemia. For these patients, the usual fasting prior to general anesthesia and surgery could be disastrous. The objective of management is the maintenance of euglycemia: a concentration of glucose in the blood above 4 mmol/L. Relevant disorders include the disorders of fatty acid oxidation (Chap. B2.5), glycogen storage diseases, disorders of gluconeogenesis, such as fructose 1,5-diphosphatase deficiency, hyperinsulinism, and ketotic hypoglycemia (Chap. B2.4). In each instance, the patient's history and tolerance of fasting should be known prior to making plans for surgery. Most patients with disorders of fatty acid oxidation do not become hypoglycemic until they have fasted more than 12 h, while some patients with glycogenosis or hyperinsulinism cannot tolerate a 4-h fast.

Patients undergoing short or minor procedures can be scheduled for noon or later and given glucose. Patients receiving overnight nasogastric glucose should have intravenous glucose started before the nasogastric administration is discontinued. Every patient should be receiving 10% glucose intravenously well prior to the time that hypoglycemia would be expected to begin; and intravenous glucose should be discontinued only after the patient has demonstrated an ability to eat and retain sources of oral sugar. The canula should not be removed until the possibility of vomiting has been excluded. In general, 10% glucose should be employed at rates approximating 2,500 mL/m^2/24 h. This would be equivalent to 150 mL/kg in infants under 1 year, 100 mL/kg, 1–2 years; 1,200–1,500 mL, 2–6 years; and 1,500–2,000 mL, over 6 years of age. Rates must be readjusted on the basis of determined levels of glucose in the blood.

B4.4 Rhabdomyolysis and Myoglobinuria in Disorders of Fatty Acid Oxidation/ Refsum Disease

General anesthesia and the stress of surgery have each been thought responsible for the acute breakdown of muscle that has been observed in patients with abnormalities of fatty acid oxidation. These triggers of the acute attack are particularly notable for the myopathic form of carnitine palmitoyl transferase (CPT) II deficiency. They may do the same in any disorders of fatty acid oxidation, especially long-chain hydroxyacyl-CoA dehydrogenase (LCHAD) deficiency (Chap. C6). Renal failure may be a complication of myoglobinuria. The best answer to preventive anesthesia and surgery in these patients is an ample supply of glucose and water and the avoidance of fasting. This is accomplished by early placement of an intravenous line so that the patient is fasting not more than 6 h. In the presence of myoglobinuria, intravenous glucose should be 10% or higher; adjunctive insulin may be helpful in maintaining euglycemia. Surgery and anesthesia may also induce a metabolic crisis in Refsum disease via mobilization of phytanic acid in fat stores. The same preventive approaches apply.

> **Remember**
>
> The avoidance of fasting and the provision of parenteral glucose are essential for the prevention of myoglobinuria in disorders of fatty acid oxidation. These precepts will also prevent crises in Refsum syndrome.

B4.5 Organic Acidemias: Maple Syrup Urine Disease

The objective in the management of anesthesia and surgery in patients with organic acidemia is the minimization of catabolism. This objective is met best by avoiding anesthesia and surgery, if at all possible, until the patient is in an optimal metabolic state and well over any infections. In preparation for the procedure, metabolic balance should be ascertained by checking the urine for ketones, the blood for ammonia, pH and electrolytes, and in the case of maple syrup urine disease (MSUD), the plasma concentrations of amino acids. Catabolism is minimized by the administration of glucose and water in the regimen employed for hypoglycemia. In MSUD, a dose of the amino acid supplement, either 1/3 of his/her daily dose or at least 0.25 g/kg, is given as late prior to anesthesia as feasible. This would be a place for

intravenous preparations of amino acids designed for the treatment of MSUD. Following the procedure, intravenous glucose should be continued until the oral route is clearly feasible and the electrolytes are stable. A patient with MSUD may be maintained for a while with intravenous amino acids or in their absence with a nasogastric drip of a mixture of amino acids containing no isoleucine, leucine, or valine; blood concentrations of amino acids should be monitored. Mixtures of amino acids containing no sugar, fat, or minerals that can be made in minimal volume and dripped so slowly that they are tolerated by patients usually thought of as requiring nothing by mouth are available.

> **Remember**
>
> Catabolism can be minimized by the provision of parenteral glucose. Patients with MSUD can best avoid catabolic elevation of leucine as a consequence of surgery by the provision of mixture of amino acids, which do not contain the offending branched-chain amino acids. This is quite successfully done with intravenous mixtures, but these are seldom widely available.

B4.6 Urea Cycle Defects

In disorders of the urea cycle, the objective is the avoidance of hyperammonemia by the minimization of catabolism. The approach is as outlined for organic acidemias, except that it is the ammonia that must be carefully monitored.

In addition, patients whose usual medication includes arginine or citrulline should be given intravenous arginine. The patient's usual dose is employed, diluted 2.5 g in 50 mL 10% glucose, and piggybacked via syringe pump to the glucose infusion. In patients receiving sodium benzoate or phenylbutyrate or both, the intravenous mixture of benzoate–phenylacetate is employed, again in a dilution of at least 2.5 g of each per 50 mL and given by piggyback pump. For short procedures, these medications can be begun in the postoperative period. For a longer procedure or one particularly likely to induce catabolism, and certainly in the presence of hyperammonemia, they can be given intraoperatively.

B4.7 Homocystinuria

Patients with cystathionine synthase deficiency are predisposed to the development of thrombosis. This may create an added risk for general anesthesia. Those who are pyridoxine responsive can be prepared for surgery by titrating values for homocysteine and homocystine with added B_6 until an optimal preoperative level is achieved. Nonresponders may be treated with betaine in quantities to achieve minimal concentrations.

B4.8 Malignant Hyperthermia

Malignant hyperthermia is a genetically determined response to inhalation anesthetics or succinylcholine in which rapidly escalating fever and generalized muscle spasm may be fatal. Prognosis has improved with preanesthetic identification and the discovery that dantrolene is specifically therapeutic. Hyperthermia is often a late sign. The earliest manifestation is an increase in end-tidal CO_2. Extreme spasm of the masseter may make insertion of a laryngoscope impossible (jaws of steel). Muscle rigidity is generalized. The skin becomes hot to the touch.

Lactic acid accumulates and there is a mixed metabolic and respiratory acidosis. Hypoxia, hypercarbia, and metabolic acidosis accompany rhabdomyolysis. Ventricular tachycardia, pulmonary edema, or disseminated intravascular coagulation may ensue; as well as cerebral edema and renal failure.

The RYR1 gene on chromosome 19q 13.1 is mutated in heterozygous fashion in a majority of patients. Very many different mutations have been identified over the 106 exons. The RYR1 protein is an integral part of the structure in the sarcolema/reticulum involved in the voltage dependent Ca++ channel. Rows of RYR1 bind to tetrads of the dihydropyridine receptor (DHPR) and mutations in DHPR genes have also been found in patients with malignant hyperthermia.

Malignant hyperthermia has also been encountered following anesthesia in a variety of muscular dystrophies, including Duchenne. It is particularly found in central core disease and King–Denborough syndrome (KDS). Central core disease gene mutations have been linked to RYR1.

Reference

Cole CJ, Lerman J, Todres ID (2009) A practice of anesthesia for infants and children. Elsevier, Philadelphia, pp 847–866

Approach to the Patient with Cardiovascular Disease

C1

Joachim Kreuder and Stephen G. Kahler

Key Facts

> Metabolic disorders are associated with a wide variety of cardiovascular manifestations, including cardiomyopathy, dysrhythmias and conduction disturbances, valvular heart disease, vascular disorders, and pulmonary hypertension.

> Most metabolic cardiomyopathies result from disorders of energy production, mostly involving other organs, particularly skeletal muscle and liver.

> Taken as a group, the disorders of fatty acid oxidation and of oxidative phosphorylation are the most common causes of metabolic cardiomyopathies; another important group is disorders of glycogen metabolism, especially Pompe disease.

> In some metabolic disorders, the cardiac manifestations may be late, subtle, or secondary to metabolic derangements in other organs.

> Valvular dysfunction and infiltrative cardiomyopathy occur as a late complication in many lysosomal storage disorders.

> Myocardial dysfunction is common in hemochromatosis, a metabolic cardiomyopathy most easily prevented.

> Symptomatic coronary heart and cerebrovascular disease during childhood is restricted to severe defects of low-density lipoprotein metabolism.

> Peripheral vascular disease is prominent in homocystinuria. Disorders of lipoproteins metabolism possess a significant long-term, but modifiable burden of premature atherosclerosis to a large number of children.

> Pulmonary arterial hypertension may be a quite rare complication in a few metabolic diseases, especially glycogen storage disease I.

C1.1 General Remarks

A substantial number of metabolic disorders significantly contribute to cardiovascular morbidity because of a direct relationship between the inborn error and outcome or a genetic predisposition resulting from interrelations between gene variants and environmental factors.

Clinical manifestations of metabolic cardiovascular disease are mainly determined by the site of involvement. Cardiomyopathies may present with reduced exercise capacity, edema, tachypnea and dyspnea, or increased frequency of respiratory infections. Palpitations and syncopes are typical clinical features of cardiac rhythm disorders. In some cases, sudden cardiac death due to ventricular tachycardia or fibrillation may be the first manifestation. Metabolic vascular disorders may present as stroke-like episodes, coronary heart disease with angina pectoris or myocardial infarction, peripheral thrombembolism, or tuberous xanthoma. In pulmonary hypertension, reduced exercise capacity, exercise-induced cyanosis, or syncope are the main clinical features.

J. Kreuder (✉)
Department Pediatric Cardiology, University Children's Hospital, Feulgenstrabe 12, 35385 Giessen, Germany
e-mail: joachim.g.kreuder@paediat.med.uni-giessen.de

G. F. Hoffmann et al. (eds.), *Inherited Metabolic Diseases*,
DOI: 10.1007/978-3-540-74723-9_C1, © Springer-Verlag Berlin Heidelberg 2010

As in all metabolic disorders the family history reflects the various patterns of inheritance, including differing penetrance, maternal inheritance of some mitochondrial disorders, and acceleration from one generation to the other. Family examination by echocardiography and electrocardiography is especially important in cardiomyopathies and cardiac channellopathies.

The age at presentation may be another important key to diagnosis in cardiac metabolic disorders. Overt cardiomyopathy within the first year of life has a much higher association with inborn metabolic diseases than in older age groups.

C1.2 Cardiomyopathy and Cardiac Failure

In epidemiological studies, 5–10% of cardiomyopathies in children result from identified or suspected inborn errors of metabolism. However, a comprehensive diagnostic approach including biochemical analysis of cardiac biopsies revealed a metabolic disease in up to 22% of all the affected children. These conditions constitute a less frequent proportion of cardiomyopathy among adults, where ischemic heart disease and diabetic cardiomyopathy have become two of the major causes in the developed countries. During infancy and early childhood, metabolic disorders represent a more frequent cause of cardiomyopathy than in the older children and adolescents.

Approximately, 5% of the inborn metabolic disorders are associated with cardiomyopathy. These disorders can be conveniently divided into those in which the cardiac manifestations are primary or prominent (Table C1.1) and those in which they are less common or less significant (Table C1.2). Rarely, the heart is the only affected organ, as described in cardiac phosphorylase kinase deficiency and certain mitochondrial disorders.

The type of metabolic involvement may determine the age at clinical presentation. Pompe disease [severe lysosomal type II glycogen storage disease (GSD)] usually presents in infancy, whereas cardiomyopathy in other lysosomal storage diseases becomes symptomatic during later childhood. Defects of fatty acid oxidation are likely to present in infancy; mitochondrial disorders may manifest at any age.

C1.2.1 Special Aspects of Cardiac Metabolism

The major fuels for the heart are glucose and fatty acids. The heart, like skeletal muscle, maintains a reserve of high-energy phosphate compounds (e.g., phosphocreatine) as well as glycogen. Before birth the heart uses less fatty acids, more glycolysis, and tolerates anaerobic metabolism more readily than after the neonatal period. This transition period after birth sometimes leads to the appearance of a cardiomyopathy that was clinically silent before then. After a few weeks, the metabolism of the heart relies on both the fatty acids and glucose for fuel; if glucose becomes limiting (during hypoglycemia) the heart can function well, whereas hypoglycemia in the newborn period may lead to significant impairment of cardiac function and dilatation of the heart. During times of increased energy demand and greater cardiac output there is increased utilization of fatty acids and glucose. Long-chain fatty acids, which require carnitine for transport into the mitochondria, are the usual forms present in the blood. Medium-chain fatty acids, which enter the mitochondria directly, can be used to provide fuel to the heart and other organs, if there is a problem with long-chain fatty acid oxidation. Furthermore, during times of metabolic stress the myocardium switches to use more glucose than at other times, and so provision of continuous glucose during times of cardiac dysfunction can be beneficial.

The heart, because it relies more than the other tissues on fatty acid oxidation, may be particularly vulnerable to disturbances of this major energy source. Disturbances of cellular function affecting a small group of cells can have a devastating effect if the region affected is part of the conduction pathways or is able to influence them.

C1.2.2 Patterns and Pathophysiology of Metabolic Cardiac Disease

From a functional point of view, cardiomyopathies during infancy and childhood may be categorized as a hypertrophic, dilated, hypertrophic–hypocontractile (mixed type), restrictive, or noncompaction type.

Table C1.1 Metabolic disorders with cardiomyopathy as a presenting or early symptom

Disorder	Hypertrophic type	Dilated type	Mixed type	Noncompaction type	Tachyarrhythmias	Conduction disorders	Organic Acids	Carnitine Level	Acylcarnitine Profile	Diagnostic Tissues	Specific treatment	Comments
Disorders of fatty acid oxidation and the carnitine cycle												
Carnitine transporter deficiency	+	++	+		+		+	↓↓	+	F, M, W, D	Carnitine	
Carnitine–acylcarnitine translocase deficiency	+	+	++	++			+	↓	++	F, W	Low fat, high carbohydrate diet, MCT. Carnitine, if low	
Carnitine palmitoyl-CoA transferase II deficiency	++	+	++	++			+	↓	++	F, M, L, W, D	Low fat, high carbohydrate diet, MCT. Carnitine, if low	Heterozygote may have symptoms, be vulnerable to malignant hyperthermia
Very-long-chain acyl-CoA dehydrogenase deficiency	++	+	+	+			++	↓	++	F, W, D	Low fat, high carbohydrate diet, MCT. Carnitine, if low	
Long-chain hydroxyacyl-CoA dehydrogenase/ trifunctional enzyme deficiency	++		+	++			++	↓	++	F, W, D	Low fat, high carbohydrate diet, MCT. Carnitine, if low	HELLP syndrome in pregnant heterozygotes
Multiple acyl-CoA dehydrogenase deficiency	++	+					++	↓	++	F and M	Low fat, high carbohydrate diet, Riboflavin, D,L-3-hydroxy-butyrate, carnitine	
Mitochondrial disorders												
Complex I–V deficiencies	++	+	++	+	+	+	+			F, H, L, M, D	High fat, low carbohydrate diet, vitamins, antioxidants, cofactors	Heart block or sudden death may occur. May have lactic acidosis and increased lactate/pyruvate ratio
Kearns-Sayre syndrome	+				+	++				F, M, D		Typical heteroplasmic deletions of mitochondrial DNA
Barth syndrome	+		+	++	+		++			B, D	Pantothenic acid	Specific isolated left ventricular noncompaction. Increased monolysocardio-lipin as a biochemical marker suitable for screening
Disorders of amino and organic acid metabolism												
Propionic aciduria, Methylmalonic aciduria, Cbl C defect		+	+		+		++	↓↓	++	F, L, W	Protein-modified diet carnitine, OH-cobalamin	Cardiomyopathy unrelated to metabolic decom-pensation or nutritional status; may be present-ing symptom. QT prolongation may be the first sign

(continued)

Table C1.1 (continued)

Disorder	Hypertrophic type	Dilated type	Mixed type	Noncompaction type	Tachyarrhythmias	Conduction disorders	Organic Acids	Carnitine Level	Acylcarnitine Profile	Diagnostic Tissues	Specific treatment	Comments
b-Ketothiolase deficiency malonic aciduria	+		+				++	↓	++	F, W	Protein-modified diet, carnitine, bicarbonate. High carbohydrate, low fat diet, carnitine	
Lysosomal storage disorders												
Lysosomal glycogen storage disease (severe form – Pompe)	++		++	+						W, F, M, D	Enzyme replacement	Macroglossia, severe cardiomyopathy, and skeletal myopathy. Characteristic ECG
MPS I (Hurler type)		+	+							W, F, U, D	Enzyme replacement, hematopoietic stem cell transplantation	Early cardiac manifestation due to coronary vascular involvement
Disorders of glycogen metabolism												
GSD type III (debrancher deficiency)	++		+							F, M, L		
GSD type IV (brancher deficiency)	++		+							W, F, M, L		Severe liver disease. Neuropathy, dementia in adult form
Phosphorylase b kinase deficiency	++		+							H		Rapidly fatal. Very rare cardiac glycogenosis
Disorders of glycoprotein metabolism	+	+	+							B, F		Abnormal subcutaneous fat distribution, psychomotor retardation, pericardial effusion
Hemochromatosis	+	+	+		+	+				P, D	Phlebotomy	Restrictive cardiomyopathy occasionally
Nutrient deficiency												
Secondary carnitine deficiency	+	+	+				+	↓↓		P, M, and U	Carnitine	Underlying causes should be clarified
Selenium deficiency		+			+	+				E	Selen	Additional pancreatic insufficiency
Thiamine deficiency/ dependency		+								P, E, and U	Thiamine	Lactic acidosis

Diagnostic tissues commonly used. *D* DNA (leukocytes and other tissues); *E* erythrocytes; *F* fibroblasts; *H* heart; *L* liver; *M* skeletal muscle; *P* plasma; *U* urine; *W* white blood cells (leukocytes)
++ Usually and prominently abnormal; + mildly abnormal

With the exception of mitochondrial disorders, each metabolic disease is preferentially associated with a functional type of cardiomyopathy by echocardiography, which helps to focus the differential diagnosis.

Hypertrophy can be the result of accumulated material stored in the myocardium (e.g., glycogen), the heart's response to poor functioning of the contractile apparatus (abnormalities of structural proteins), or impaired

Table C1.2 Disorders in which cardiovascular involvement is usually mild or late – symptoms are recognized after systemic illness or involvement of other organs

Disorder	Comments and special issues
MAD deficiency (mild, including SCHAD deficiency)	Biochemically similar to severe forms, but onset later and symptoms milder or intermittent. Cardiomyopathy similar to fatty acid oxidation defects (Table C1.1)
Friedreich ataxia	Mitochondrial damage may be due to iron accumulation. Diabetes common
Mucopolysaccharidoses – general pathology	Myocardial thickening, especially septum and LV wall. Aortic and mitral valve thickening and regurgitation, narrowing of aorta, and coronary, pulmonary, renal arteries
MPS I-S, I-H	Infiltration, thickening of septum, LV wall, severe systolic dysfunction (10% of patients)
MPS II	EFE, MS, AS, AR, MR, infarction
MPS VI	MV, AV calcification, stenosis
Gaucher disease	Myocardial thickening due to infiltration; pulmonary arterial hypertension
Fabry disease	Infiltration leading to LVH; MV prolapse, thickening
Fucosidosis	Myocardial thickening due to infiltration
Sialidosis	MR, CHF, pericardial effusion
Mucolipidosis II, III	Aortic regurgitation, myocardial thickening due to infiltration, CHF
Aspartylglycosaminuria	MR, aortic thickening
Homocystinuria	Hypercoagulability, strokes. MV prolapse

AR aortic regurgitation; *AS* aortic stenosis; *CHF* congestive heart failure; *EFE* endocardial fibroelastosis; *LV* left ventricle; *LVH* left ventricular hypertrophy; *MR* mitral regurgitation; *MS* mitral stenosis, *MV* mitral valve

energetics (mitochondrial disorders). Dilatation results when the abnormal or poorly functioning heart is unable to contract adequately due to impaired energy production or toxic intermediates like acids or oxidizing mitochondrial components, and begins to stretch out of shape. This type preferentially occurs in the disorders of carnitine availability and in some of the organic acidurias. The hypertrophic–hypocontractile (mixed) type presents the transition from the hypertrophic to the dilated type and may occur in the late stages

of disorders of fatty acid oxidation, oxidative phosphorylation, and storage disorders.

> **Remember**
>
> In general, the most adaptive response of the heart in metabolic disorders is hypertrophy, with or without dilation and systolic dysfunction.

Pure restrictive cardiomyopathy is extremely rare in children with metabolic cardiomyopathy, but restrictive ventricular performance is observed in endomyocardial fibroelastosis. The noncompaction type mimicking the morphological appearance of the embryonic myocardium represents a nonspecific myocardial response to a variety of stimuli. From a metabolic view, noncompaction appearance is suggestive for Barth syndrome or defects of oxidative phosphorylation.

Beyond direct damage of myocardial cells, coronary vasculopathy due to mucopolysaccharidoses, oligosaccharidoses, or lipoprotein disorders may induce dilated cardiomyopathy.

C1.2.2.1 Endocardial Fibroelastosis

Endocardial fibroelastosis describes a condition peculiar to infants and young children, in which there is significant thickening and stiffening of the endocardium. The basis for this response is not yet known. It can occur in disparate conditions ranging from viral myocarditis to carnitine transporter deficiency, Barth syndrome, severe mucopolysaccharidosis I (Hurler syndrome), and mucopolysaccharidosis VI (Maroteaux–Lamy syndrome). It is a predictor of poor outcome.

C1.2.3 Inborn Errors of Metabolism that Cause Cardiomyopathy

C1.2.3.1 Disorders of Fatty Acid Oxidation and the Carnitine Cycle

Disorders of fatty acid oxidation involving long-chain fatty acids often present as cardiomyopathy. Sometimes the onset is abrupt or overwhelming particularly in the newborn period. Sudden death may occur, presumably reflecting arrhythmia or apnea. Liver involvement (manifest as fasting hypoketotic hypoglycemia, hyperammonemia, or a Reye-like syndrome) and skeletal muscle involvement are common. Very-long-chain acyl-CoA dehydrogenase (VLCAD) and carnitine palmitoyl-CoA transferase II (CPT II) deficiencies are probably the most common; long-chain hydroxyacyl-CoA dehydrogenase (LCHAD)/trifunctional protein and carnitine–acylcarnitine translocase (CACT) deficiencies present similarly. The metabolic pathways and skeletal muscle aspects of these conditions are discussed in Chap. C6. MCAD deficiency, the most common disorder of fatty acid oxidation (and a cause of carnitine depletion), is unusual for a fatty acid oxidation disorder, in that cardiomyopathy is an extremely uncommon feature, but dysrhythmias and sudden death are real concerns.

Disease Info: Defects of Long-Chain Fatty Acid Oxidation

VLCAD Deficiency

Very-long-chain acyl-CoA dehydrogenation is the first step of β-oxidation (Figure in Chap. C6) in the mitochondria, after synthesis of the acyl-CoA (e.g., palmitoyl-CoA) catalyzed by CPT II. It is easy to understand why impairment of this step can lead to severe organ dysfunction, especially in heart, liver, and skeletal muscle. Cardiac symptoms (congestive failure with feeding difficulties and tachypnea), if they occur, are likely to occur in infants and young children, and there may be concurrent liver dysfunction. Cardiac hypertrophy, especially of the left ventricle, is common. ECG may show increased voltages. Urinary organic acids may show increased dicarboxylic acids; plasma or blood spot acylcarnitine analysis shows elevation in C14:1 species. Enzyme assay can be done on fibroblasts and lymphocytes. Treatment involves avoiding fasting, limiting essential long-chain fats to the amount needed for growth, and providing medium-chain lipids and other foods as calorie sources in place of long-chain fatty acids. Although the total plasma carnitine level is often low, chronic carnitine supplementation has not led to documented improvement.

LCHAD/Trifunctional Enzyme Deficiency

Many infants with long-chain 3-hydroxyacyl-CoA dehydrogenase deficiency present with cardiomyopathy, sometimes in the newborn period. This is one of the common disorders of cardiac fatty acid oxidation. Liver dysfunction may be severe, including cirrhosis, and there may be significant skeletal muscle involvement. Urine organic acids reveal increased saturated and unsaturated dicarboxylic and hydroxyl species. Plasma carnitine level may be low; acylcarnitine analysis shows increased hydroxy forms of C16:0, C18:1, and C18:2. Additional findings that are unusual for other disorders of fatty acid oxidation are lactic acidosis, pigmentary retinopathy (in older children and adults), and peripheral neuropathy. Absence of deep tendon reflexes and toe-walking have been reported.

In the late-onset form, dominated by intermittent muscle symptoms, there may be asymptomatic ventricular hypertrophy. Treatment is similar to that in VLCAD deficiency.

Multiple Acyl-CoA Dehydrogenase Deficiency

Infants with the severe form of multiple acyl-CoA dehydrogenase deficiency (MADD), especially the subgroup without malformations, often have cardiomyopathy. Hypotonia, encephalopathy, overwhelming acidosis, and metabolic derangements resulting from impairment of multiple pathways for the degradation of fatty acids and amino acids are common features. The diagnosis is usually established by analysis of urinary organic acids (dicarboxylic aciduria, including ethymalonic, adipic, and glutaric acids) or plasma/blood acylcarnitines (increased median- and long-chain species), and confirmed by enzyme analysis, western blot in fibroblasts, or mutation analysis. Carnitine depletion is common. Severely affected patients are treated with a low-fat, high-carbohydrate diet, avoidance of fasting, provision of abundant carnitine, and riboflavin (50–100 mg/days), but response to therapy is often poor. Administration of D,L-3-hydroxybutyrate (100–800 mg/kg/days) has been shown to induce regression of myocardial systolic dysfunction and hypertrophy.

Disease Info: Defects of the Carnitine Cycle

CACT Deficiency

Most patients with translocase deficiency have had severe disease in early infancy, including acute cardiac events (shock, heart failure, and cardiac arrest). Arrhythmias can be prominent. There may be ventricular hypertrophy. There is significant hepatic and skeletal muscle dysfunction (hyperammonemia and weakness). Total blood carnitine level may be low, especially the free fraction. Acylcarnitine analysis shows mainly long-chain species C16:0, C18:1, and C18:2, reflecting their synthesis by CPT I, and accumulation. Emergency management includes provision of glucose, restriction of long-chain fats, and supplementation with medium-chain lipids and carnitine (see also Chap. B2.8). Despite this, neonatal fatality is common.

CPT II Deficiency

The severe neonatal/infantile form of CPT II deficiency leads to severe cardiac, skeletal muscle, and liver dysfunction, resulting in circulatory shock, heart failure, hypoketotic hypoglycemia, hyperammonemia, and coma. Dysmorphic features and renal dysgenesis may be present, reminiscent of the cystic malformations that occur in glutaric aciduria type II or pyruvate dehydrogenase deficiency (see also Chap. D2).

Plasma and tissue carnitine levels are low, especially free carnitine. Acylcarnitine analysis shows long-chain species, as in translocase deficiency.

Arrhythmias represent a common feature of CPT II deficiency. Long-chain acylcarnitines, long-chain acyl-CoAs, and long-chain free fatty acids all have detergent effects on membranes, so an accumulation might have disruptive effects. On the other hand, the relative deficiency of free carnitine adversely affects the ratio of free CoASH to acyl-CoA, and the plasma and tissue deficiency of carnitine would impair fatty acid oxidation. The true magnitude of the contribution of long-chain acylcarnitines to arrhythmias in CPT II deficiency (and related disorders) is neither not known nor is the true risk of carnitine administration in a desperately ill child with this disorder. Therapy like this for CACT deficiency is somehow

effective in the infantile form, whereas patients with the neonatal type responds poorly to therapy.

Mild CPT II deficiency, among the most common fatty acid oxidation disorders is typified by recurrent rhabdomyolysis and does not present with significant cardiac involvement. Most of these patients harbor at least one copy of a mild CPT II mutation allowing higher residual activity than in the severe infantile form.

Disease Info: Carnitine Transporter Deficiency

A deficiency of the plasma membrane carnitine transporter leads to severe carnitine depletion by a few months to several years of age. In the most extreme cases it can present as neonatal hydrops. There is hypertrophy of the left ventricle, hepatomegaly with hepatic dysfunction (hypoglycemia, hyperammonemia and increased transaminases), hypotonia, and developmental delay. The ECG may show high, peaked T waves and left ventricular hypertrophy. Total plasma carnitine is exceedingly low, often less than $5\,\mu mol/L$, and the acylcarnitine profile shows no abnormal species. In contrast to specific elevations in other disorders of fatty acid oxidation the quantities of all acylcarnitines may be very low, suggesting the diagnosis. Dicarboxylic aciduria is rarely observed. Endomyocardial biopsy (if done – not needed for diagnosis) can show lipid infiltration and, in some cases, endocardial fibroelastosis.

The milder, later onset form may present with cardiac dilatation, abnormal ECG, and hepatomegaly. Skeletal muscle strength may appear to be normal on static testing, but endurance is poor. Muscle biopsy shows lipid storage. Urinary organic acids are usually unremarkable. Diagnosis is confirmed by demonstrating markedly reduced (<10% of controls) carnitine transport in fibroblasts. Heterogeneous mutations have been found in the *SLC22A5* gene encoding the OCTN2 carnitine transporter.

In this autosomal recessive condition, the fractional excretion of carnitine in the urine approaches 100%, as the renal carnitine reabsorptive transport system is the same as that for most other tissues. Accordingly, carnitine must be provided frequently. Intravenous carnitine (during an acute crisis) can be given in a dose of 300 mg/kg/days, as a continuous infusion. Oral carnitine should be given four times daily. The oral dose for children is 100–200 mg/days and for adults 2–4 gm/days, but some patients have required much more to maintain satisfactory plasma levels. The maximal oral dose is usually set by intestinal tolerance, while diarrhea does not occur with parenteral use. If treatment started before irreversible organ damage occurs, the cardiomyopathy improves dramatically, and the heart size returns to normal. Skeletal weakness may also improve, although muscle carnitine levels remain low (2–4% of normal). The long-term prognosis is favorable as long as children remain on carnitine supplements. However, recurrence of cardiomyopathy or sudden death from arrhythmia even without cardiomyopathy have been reported in patients discontinuing carnitine supplementation.

Secondary Carnitine Deficiency

Secondary carnitine deficiency occurs in a large number of settings, discussed in Chap. C6. Even with low plasma levels the cardiac uptake of carnitine is usually sufficient to avoid symptoms. However, there are occasional premature infants receiving long-term total parenteral nutrition (TPN) without carnitine supplementation who become profoundly depleted after a few months. The need for carnitine in infants may exceed their synthetic capability, as an infant needs sufficient carnitine for the increasing mass of muscle and other tissues, whereas adults need only to replace what is lost. A lower renal threshold for carnitine in a sick infant may also become pathophysiologically relevant.

Infants with severe carnitine depletion may have poor cardiac output and dilated cardiomyopathy. The plasma carnitine level may be less than 10 µmol/L. One would expect hypoglycemia from liver carnitine depletion, but this does not occur because of the continuous high-dose glucose of the TPN. Carnitine supplementation (15–30 mg/kg/days IV, given with the TPN infusion) leads to rapid improvement in blood levels and cardiac function.

Severe carnitine depletion can occur in the setting of renal Fanconi syndrome (as in cystinosis and mitochondrial dysfunction) or treatment with the antibiotic pivampicillin. Although very low plasma carnitine levels

are found for a short time during episodes of illness with MCAD deficiency and glutaric aciduria type I, they are not usually associated with cardiomyopathy.

C1.2.3.2 Mitochondrial Disorders

The mitochondrial disorders are discussed in general terms in the Chaps. B2.3 and D1. About 40% of patients with mitochondrial disorders suffer from cardiac involvement in terms of cardiomyopathy or dysrhythmias, leading to earlier presentation and much worse prognosis for survival compared to noncardiac affected patients. Involvement of other organs is common, especially the brain, eye (and eye movements), skeletal muscle, liver, and kidney. However, isolated cardiac deficiency of oxidative phosphorylation represents a substantial part of mitochondrial cardiomyopathies. In about 50% of cardiac manifestations, cardiomyopathy shows the hypertrophic pattern, followed by the mixed hypertrophic-dilated, the dilated, and the noncompaction pattern. Disturbances of cardiac rhythm such as complete heart block or bundle branch block affect about 15–25% of these patients and sudden death may occur, sometimes as the first indication of a mitochondrial disorder. A diagnosis in this situation may be possible if tissues for mitochondrial studies (especially heart, skeletal muscle, and skin) are acquired rapidly after death.

The most common defects of the respiratory chain complexes were complex I, complex IV, and combined deficiencies. An apparent correlation between specific defects of the respiratory chain complexes and cardiac involvement is not possible. Lactic acidosis with an increased ratio of lactate/pyruvate is common, but not obligatory. Mutations of mitochondrial protein-encoding genes, tRNA and rRNA, and deletions/duplications are only found in a minority of pediatric patients with mitochondrial disorders suggesting that mutations of nuclear genes are the leading cause for these diseases (for details of distinct genetic lesions in mitochondrial disorders, see www.mitomap.org).

The Kearns–Sayre syndrome is the prototypical mitochondrial disorder in which there is progressive disturbance of conduction. Most patients represent nonfamilial heteroplasmic deletions of mitochondrial DNA. Cardiac symptoms include hypertrophic or dilated cardiomyopathy, atrial or ventricular arrhythmias, Wolf–Parkinson–White syndrome, and other preexcitation syndromes. Progressive heart block may necessitate pacemaker placement. Major noncardiac symptoms include retinitis pigmentosa, ophthalmoplegia, ataxia, myopathy, and increased CSF protein, with onset before age 20. Many other manifestations may occur, including deafness, seizures, diabetes or other endocrinopathy, renal and gastrointestinal symptoms, and lactic acidosis. Similar manifestations with later onset are typical of chronic progressive external ophthalmoplegia-plus (CPEO-plus).

Other clinical entities of mitochondrial DNA disorders are likely to have cardiac involvement including Leigh syndrome, MERFF, and MELAS. Mutations in nuclear genes which are also associated with the appearance of cardiomyopathy may affect both the structural proteins (part of the respiratory chain complexes, e.g., NDUFS2 and NDUFV2 in complex I) as well as nonstructural proteins responsible for the assembly of respiratory chain complexes (e.g., SCO2 and SURF1), mtDNA stability (e.g., POLG), iron homeostasis (e.g., frataxin), mitochondrial integrity (e.g., tafazzin = G4.5), or mitochondrial metabolism (e.g., PDH E1-α-subunit).

Sengers syndrome, Barth syndrome, and Friedreich ataxia represent other nuclear encoded diseases of the oxidative energy production with neuromuscular involvement. Sengers syndrome (autosomal recessive) is characterized by hypertrophic cardiomyopathy, congenital cataracts, and exercise-induced lactic academia. Deficiency of adenine-nucleotide-translocator ANT1 most probably due to transcriptional or posttranscriptional lesions was found to be associated with Sengers syndrome.

Disorders of oxidative phosphorylation are often attempted before treating with a high-fat, low-carbohydrate diet and supplemental vitamins (especially coenzyme Q, carnitine, and riboflavin in complex 1 deficiency), antioxidants, electron acceptors, cofactors, and metabolic intermediates (e.g., creatine, arginine in acute MELAS manifestation, see Chap. D1). Response to metabolic therapy is highly variable and a matter of continuing debate.

In some cases, metabolic therapy can be directed to the pathobiochemical substrate like inherited primary coenzyme Q deficiency or copper-histidine supplementation in SCO2 deficiency.

Disease Info: Barth Syndrome

Barth syndrome is an X-linked recessive condition that is similar to many mitochondrial oxidative phosphorylation diseases. Neutropenia, cardiomyopathy, and increased urinary excretion of 3-methylglutaconic acid, 3-methylglutarate, and 2-ethylhydracrylate – compounds suggestive of mitochondrial dysfunction – occur. Noncompaction pattern is typical, but not exclusive for the cardiac involvement in Barth syndrome may occur independent of the other features. The onset is typically in infancy, but there may be spontaneous improvement in later childhood. Biopsy of skeletal muscle or heart shows abnormal mitochondria, which may be abnormal in shape and contain inclusion bodies and dense, tightly packed concentric cristae. Lactic acidosis may be prominent. The molecular defect in Barth syndrome is attributed to the G4.5 or tafazzin (TAZ) gene, which encodes a mitochondrial transacylase involved in the remodeling of cardiolipin. Deficiency of the TAZ protein results in reduced levels of cardiolipin and increased monolysocardiolipin content, which can serve as a biochemical marker for this disease.

At least one patient has had a dramatic and sustained response to treatment with pantothenic acid, a precursor of coenzyme A. Pantothenol was ineffective.

Disease Info: Friedreich Ataxia

This disorder presents with slowly progressive spinocerebellar dysfunction in children and young adults. Cardiomyopathy, cardiac dysrhythmias, and diabetes are common. The genetic defect is usually a trinucleotide expansion in the frataxin gene. The mechanism of cellular injury appears to be related to iron accumulation within mitochondria. Beyond deficient energy production, cellular damage leading to apoptosis may be due to peroxidative damage to mitochondrial membranes.

Remember

Serial echocardiography, 24h-ECG, and measurement of BNP/NT-proBNP are valuable tools to supervise metabolic therapy.

In roughly half the patients idebenone, a coenzyme Q analog, is beneficial to reduce myocardial hypertrophy and rhythm disturbances.

C1.2.3.3 Disorders of Amino and Organic Acid Metabolism

Two common organic acid disorders, propionic aciduria and methylmalonic aciduria, in the branched-chain amino acid catabolic pathway, may present with a cardiomyopathy, from birth to a few years of age. The onset may be subtle or sudden. Cardiac failure with dilatation, poor contractility, and rhythm disturbances including ventricular electric instability or bradycardia, may occur.

Remember

Prolongation of normalized QT (QTc) time may be the first sign of cardiac involvement in organic acidurias and should initiate regular cardiac surveillance by echocardiography and measurement of BNP/NT-proBNP blood levels

Cardiomyopathy may also occur in β-ketothiolase deficiency (isoleucine degradation), methylhydroxybutyryl-CoA dehydrogenase deficiency (isoleucine degradation), and malonic aciduria.

The basis for this cardiomyopathy is not known. In some cases it has occurred in children being treated successfully for the metabolic disorder and in a few it has been the presenting symptom. Suggested causes include primary toxicity of metabolites accumulating as a result of the underlying enzymopathy and nutritional deficiency of carnitine or of some other nutrients.

Treatment is directed at correcting the metabolic derangement (e.g., diet and carnitine) and providing appropriate supportive care.

C1.2.3.4 Lysosomal Storage Disorders (Infiltrative Cardiomyopathies)

In this subgroup, the myocardium may become thickened because of accumulated material, particularly within lysosomes. Because of mechanical interference, accumulation initially results in isolated diastolic dysfunction, but may progress to severe systolic failure. In most cases, echocardiography shows global concentric ventricular hypertrophy.

Disease Info: GSD II (Pompe Disease and Lysosomal Acid α-Glucosidase Deficiency)

Pompe disease is among the most common primary metabolic cardiomyopathies and the leading lysosomal disorder in which there are severe cardiac manifestations. In the classical infantile form, symptoms appear in early infancy and the disorder progresses rapidly. Weakness, floppiness, and macroglossia may be apparent within a few months. Cardiac manifestations include shortness of breath and poor feeding. Chest X-ray shows cardiomegaly, echocardiography concentric symmetric hypertrophy with or without outflow tract obstruction, ECG left axis deviation, short PR interval, high QRS voltages, and inverted T waves. Peripheral blood leukocytes may show vacuoles and there is often pathological excretion of oligosaccharides in the urine. Enzyme assay can be performed on mixed leukocytes and purified lymphoytes. Dried blood spot on Guthrie cards is available in some laboratories and may be applied to newborn screening programs. Reduced α-glucosidase activity in a blood sample should be confirmed by enzyme measurement in fibroblasts, muscle biopsy, or by DNA analysis. Muscle biopsy shows a major accumulation of PAS-positive material and membrane-bound (i.e., in lysosomes) accumulation of glycogen in electron microscopy.

Infants with infantile Pompe disease often succumb in a few months due to cardiac failure or arrhythmias, but may survive for 2 or 3 years. Enzyme replacement therapy has recently become available with encouraging results.

Patients with the late-onset form have higher residual activity of α-glucosidase. They present beyond the first year of life with progressive weakness, whereas cardiomyopathy is rare and much less severe (see Chap. C6).

Cardiomyopathy with lysosomal glycogen storage, but normal α-glucosidase activity is observed in X-linked Danon disease, which is caused by mutations of the gene encoding lysosome-associated membrane protein 2.

Other Infiltrative Cardiomyopathies

In men with Fabry disease, there may be thickening of the left ventricle. This can also occur in the heterozygous women of this X-linked disorder, perhaps reflecting skewed lyonization. Coronary artery disease is also common in Fabry disease. The mucopolysaccharidoses and fucosidosis may be complicated by storage in the septum and posterior wall of the left ventricle. Lysosomal storage in the heart may also occur in Gaucher disease.

C1.2.3.5 Disorders of Glycogen Metabolism

Glycogen Debrancher Deficiency (Cori or Forbes Disease, GSD III)

In type IIIa GSD there is involvement of liver, and skeletal or cardiac muscle; in the less common type IIIb there is only hepatic disease, manifest as fasting hypoglycemia, increased transaminases, and rarely mild lactic acidosis. The cardiomyopathy in type IIIa usually does not cause symptoms before adulthood, but outflow tract obstruction and heart failure occur occasionally. During childhood, there may be ventricular hypertrophy on ECG and echocardiography

Glycogen Brancher Deficiency (Anderson Disease, GSD IV)

The usual form of this disorder manifests hepatomegaly and cirrhosis. The deficiency of the branching enzyme activity leads to the accumulation of an amylopectin-like glycogen (also known as polyglucosan bodies), which incites an inflammatory response. Rare, severely affected patients may have heart involvement in childhood with ventricular hypertrophy and secondary dilatation. Liver transplantation is curative for the liver disease. The heart condition may be ameliorated as well, as shown by improved cardiac function and the lessening of storage.

Intramyocardial polyglucosan bodies may also be observed in phosphofructokinase deficiency (GSD7), mutations of the PRKAG2 gene encoding the α-2 subunit of AMP-activated protein kinase, and unclassified polysaccharidoses of the heart and skeletal muscle.

C1.2.3.6 Disorder of Glycoprotein Metabolism

The heart is quiet frequently involved in organ dysfunction in patients with congenital diseases of glycosylation (CDG) leading to early death within the first year of life in a substantial number of patients. Hypertrophic cardiomyopathy is associated with type Ia CDG disorder (phosphomannomutase deficiency), dilated appearance was found in nonclassified forms. Specific therapy is not available.

Disease Info: Hemochromatosis

Hereditary hemochromatosis (HH) characterized by iron deposition and tissue injury in multiple organs is among the most common genetic metabolic diseases in many parts of the world, occurring as often as in 1 in 300 persons. In all types of HH, iron overload results from impairment of the hepcidin–ferroportin regulatory pathway. The most common of the inherited forms (>95%) is autosomal recessive type 1 or *HFE*-related HH. Two mutant alleles of the HFE gene that regulates the expression of the iron-regulatory hormone hepcidin account for essentially all cases. Homozygotes for C282Y are at highest risk; compound heterozygotes C282Y/H63D are at less risk; and homozygotes for H63D are at minimal risk for iron overload. The clinical penetrance of C282Y homozygosity for iron overload-related diseases is up to 30% in men and 2% in women in fourth to sixth decade and very rare before adulthood. In total, 25–35% of C282Y homozygotes may not develop iron overload.

HH is difficult to recognize clinically, because its early symptoms of fatigue and depression do not point to iron overload. Hepatic dysfunction and hepatomegaly are common, manifested by mild elevation of transaminases (see also Chap. C2). Pancreatic dysfunction may lead to diabetes and adrenal dysfunction to Addison disease. Darkening of the skin from iron may be mistaken for the effects of Addison disease. Arthropathy is common.

Cardiomyopathy has an insidious onset and may be attributed to diabetes. Compared to the normal population, cardiomyopathy is 306-fold more frequent in patients with HH. The cardiomyopathy usually results in biventricular dilatation. Ventricular thickening is an early finding; a restrictive form occurs occasionally. Arrhythmias (ventricular ectopic beats, tachycardias, ventricular fibrillation, and heart block) may occur.

Raised transferrin-iron saturation (>45%) and ferritin levels are the usual biochemical markers for iron overload; definitive diagnosis, formerly done by liver biopsy, is now generally achieved by molecular testing, although biopsy may be needed to assess the degree of liver injury.

As hemochromatosis is a recessive disease, parents and all siblings must be tested. Molecular genetic testing to identify C282Y (and H63D) mutants is the first step of cascade testing, followed by iron studies in C282Y homozygotes and C282Y/H63D heterozygotes.

A distinct, but rare disorder is juvenile or type 2 hemochromatosis (JH), in which there are similar findings, but the onset is in childhood. Autosomal recessive JH is caused by mutations in the gene of hepcidin-regulating protein hemojuvelin or the hepcidin gene itself.

Type 3 and 4 HH are caused by mutations in the transferring receptor 2 gene or the ferroportin gene. Symptoms in these subtypes also manifest in the fourth to fifth decade.

HH is treated by phlebotomies whose frequency is targeted by serum ferritin levels (<300 ng/mL in men und 200 ng/mL in women). Tissue damage, such as cardiomyopathy and hepatic fibrosis, may not be reversible, so early diagnosis is essential.

C1.2.3.7 Nutrient-Deficiency Cardiomyopathies

Thiamine

Thiamine (vitamin B_1), as thiamine pyrophosphate, is essential for the function of several decarboxylases of 2-oxoacids, including pyruvate, the branched-chain oxoacids, and 2-oxoglutarate. Severe thiamine deficiency leads to beriberi, a form of cardiac and peripheral vessel dysfunction characterized by loss of peripheral vascular tone, edema, tachycardia, cardiac dilatation, and heart failure. Brain damage (Wernicke's encephalopathy) reminiscent of Leigh disease may occur, and other organs may become damaged. Thiamine deficiency can occur in patients with organic acidurias

receiving limited diets. In this setting, lactic acidosis has been the presenting feature, reflecting impaired activity of pyruvate decarboxylase, the first step in the pyruvate dehydrogenase complex. Deficiency of thiamine resulting from thiamine transport defects (autosomal recessive) typically results in anemia (usually megaloblastic, but may be sideroblastic or aplastic), sensorineural deafness, and diabetes; tachycardia and edema may occur in the most severely affected infants. Diagnosis is made by measuring blood or urine thiamine content.

Selenium

Selenium in the amino acid selenomethionine is a component of several proteins, and cofactor, particularly for glutathione peroxidase. Selenium deficiency, especially when it occurs with vitamin E deficiency, impairs the antioxidant function of various pathways. There may also be increased vulnerability to cardiotropic enteroviruses. Selenium deficiency is a common cause of cardiomyopathy in the Keshan district of China, where there is insufficient selenium in soil and foods. Manifestations include cardiac dilatation, dysrhythmias, and ultrastructural changes. The condition may be fatal unless treated. Pancreatic insufficiency may also develop.

Selenium deficiency may also occur in developed countries. It has been observed following prolonged parenteral nutrition and in patients with small bowel disease. Patients with many forms of heart disease, including ischemic heart disease and HIV cardiomyopathy, have lower selenium levels than controls, raising the possibility that selenium depletion may play a role. Selenium deficiency is diagnosed by the measurement of erythrocyte selenium, along with glutathione (total and reduced), and glutathione peroxidase; it is treated with sodium selenite, 60–100 µg/days.

C1.2.4 Investigations for Metabolic Cardiomyopathies

Laboratory tests to investigate a suspected metabolic cardiomyopathy should focus initially on obtaining information rapidly to determine if there is a specific treatment for the disorder. At the same time, supportive care to ease myocardial workload should be instituted and preparations made for invasive testing is needed.

Cardiomyopathy may be the presenting or dominant clinical feature, but careful searching often reveals other signs of a multisystemic disease as well as abnormal metabolites in blood or urine. Clinical features may include dysmorphic features, neurological and muscular symptoms, and skeletal findings and signs of liver dysfunction. In inborn errors of metabolism that impair energy production or produce toxic metabolites, congestive heart failure often occurs in the setting of an acute metabolic decompensation triggered by intercurrent infections, surgery, fasting, or physical exertion. Since these inciting events may suggest an alternative etiology like e.g., viral myocarditis; it is important to include laboratory testing of blood and urine as part of the initial evaluation.

Initial laboratory tests include complete blood count, glucose, blood gas analysis, plasma lactate, amino acids, carnitine, and acylcarnitine profile, electrolytes, transaminases, creatine kinase, urea, creatinine, and uric acid. Troponin I and BNP or proNT-BNP levels reflect the extent of myocardial damage, ischemia and overlaod, independent from their etiology (Table C1.3).

Lactate is often elevated in patients with cardiac failure simply reflecting poor perfusion. In such a setting the lactate/pyruvate ratio is likely to be elevated and not

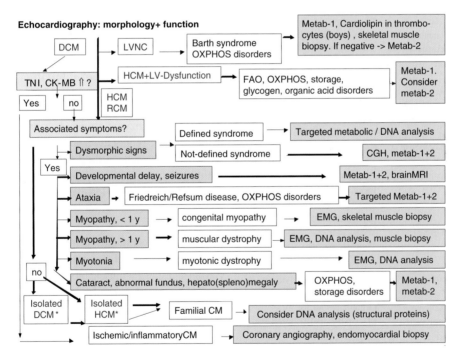

Fig. C1.1 Algorithm for the diagnostic approach to cardiomyo-pathies. *DCM* dilated cardiomyopathy; *HCM* hypertrophic cardiomyopathy; *HDCM* hypertrophic–hypocontractile (mixed type) cardiomyopathy; *LVNC* left ventricular noncompaction; *OXPHOS* mitochondrial; *RCM* restrictive cardiomyopathy; *TNI* troponin I. *Metab-1* first-line investigations (Table C1.3); *Metab-2* second-line investigations (see Table C1.4); *Blue type* echocardiographic types of CM; *Blue background* early routine examinations; *Green background* potentially associated symptoms; *Red frame* suspected etiology; *Yellow background* recommended investigations. *In the case of isolated CM, complete first-line metabolic investigations should be performed in all children younger than 3 years. Otherwise well-defined secondary cardiomyopathies with recognizable etiology (e.g., hypertensive CM and anthracycline-induced CM) were not included in this algorithm

Table C1.3 First-line investigations in suspected metabolic cardiomyopathy

Examination	Criteria/suspected disorder (examples)
Additional clinical symptoms	
Dysmorphic features	Coarse facial appearance, cloudy corneas, slow growth
Muscular symptoms	Weakness, hypotonia, cramps, myotonia
Neurological findings	Encephalopathy, developmental delay, seizures
Liver and spleen involvement	Organ size, ascites, liver skin signs
Skeletal findings	Dysostosis multiplex
Blood	
Complete blood count	Vacuoles, lysosomal storage disease
Blood gas analysis, lactate	Defects in oxidative phosphorylation
Sodium, potassium, calcium, phorphorus	Renal involvement (tubular)
Urea, creatinine, uric acid	Renal involvement (glomerular)
Creatine kinase	Myopathy
Alanine and aspartate aminotransferases	Liver involvement
Carnitine (free and total)	Carnitine transporter deficiency
Acylcarnitine profile	Defects in fatty acid oxidation
Amino acids	Organic aciduria, tyrosinemia
Transferrin isoelectric focusing	CDG syndromes
Acid α-glucosidase	Pompe disease
Cholesterol, triglycerides	Lipoprotein disorders
Troponin I	Myocardial ischemia
BNP/pro-NT-BNP	Ventricular overload/dysfunction
Urine	
Protein, electrolytes	Proteinuria, electrolyte loss (renal involvement)
Organic acids	Organic acidurias
Glycosaminoglycanes	Mucopolysaccharidoses
Oligosaccharides	Oligosaccharidoses
Eye	
Lens	Cataract, defects in oxidative phosphorylation
Retina	Storage disease, defects in oxidative phosphorylation
Other organs	
Abdominal ultrasound	Hepatic or renal involvement

BNP, brain-type natriuretic peptide; *NT*, N-terminal

per se suggestive of disturbed oxidative phosphorylation (see Chap. B2.3). Renal tubular function can be assessed by checking for wasting of amino acids, phosphate, and bicarbonate, resulting in a Fanconi syndrome or isolated renal tubular acidosis. Urinary organic acids with increased Krebs cycle intermediates and lactate may be suggestive of mitochondrial dysfunction, while prominent 3-methylglutaconic acid suggests Barth syndrome (type II) or defective oxidative phosphorylation, especially complex V deficiencies (type IV). Distinct organic acidurias may present with their typical excretion pattern. Hepatic dysfunction may be reflected by increases in transaminases, bilirubin and ammonia, hypoglycemia, an abnormal amino acid profile, and reduced coagulation factors. Consideration should be given to determine thiamine, selenium, vitamin E, and glutathione levels when nutritional deficiencies are suspected..

Abdominal ultrasound and eye examination should be included in the initial diagnostic workup.

Encephalopathy, hypoglycemia, metabolic acidosis, and neuromuscular symptoms have been proposed as key entry points to diagnostic algorithms and second-line tests in suspected metabolic cardiomyopathy [for detailed algorithms see Cox (2007)].

Second-order investigation (Table C1.4) include analysis of additional metabolites, targeted genetic analyses, and enzyme studies in fibroblasts, lymphocytes, or tissue (e.g., fatty acid oxidation and lysosomal enzymes). The echocardiographic type of cardiomyopathy and some ECG findings may allow to near the diagnostic approach. However, the substantial heterogeneity of echocardiographic and ECG findings has to be considered.

Morphological studies including ultrastructural examination as well as biochemical investigations of endomyocardial and skeletal muscle biopsies should be performed in all cases, which unresolved etiology after the noninvasive work up.

Remember

Skeletal biopsy should be performed in all the infants with hypertrophic or hypertrophic–hypocontractile phenotype due to the high probability of defective oxidative phosphorylation, even in the absence of lactic acidemia

Cardiac restricted defects of glycogen metabolism or oxidative phosphorylation will only be detected by direct endomyocardial analysis. (See section Chaps. B2.3 and D1).

C1.2.5 Principles of Treatment in Metabolic Cardiomyopathy

Treatment should be directed to the specific metabolic defect as well as to the functional state of the myocardium. Signs of acute metabolic disturbance like hypoglycemia and metabolic acidosis should be corrected as soon as possible. In metabolic acidosis, carnitine supplementation may help to restore intermediate metabolism by replenishing low free carnitine levels, binding acid compounds, and liberating acyl coenzyme A from CoA-species. For disorders of the intermediary metabolism, there are several guiding principles for treatment. Diet should reduce the intake of nonmetabolizable substrates and offer alternative, metabolizable energy sources and nutrients (e.g., substitution of long-chain by medium-chain fatty acids in VLCAD deficiency, D,L-3-hydroxy-butyrate in MADD). Fasting should be avoided by use of night feeding or continuous tube feedings during infancy, supplemented cornstarch at bedtime may provide sufficient carbohydrate supply through the night in older children. Dietary supplements can reduce secondary toxicity (e.g., carnitine in organic acidurias and antioxidants in defects of oxidative phosphorylation). In some cases, residual enzyme activity can be enhanced by the use of pharmacologic doses of vitamin cofactors (e.g., riboflavin in MADD). Enzyme replacement therapy has emerged as a new therapeutic option, at least in terms of myocardial function and morphology, in several lysosomal storage diseases like Gaucher disease, Pompe disease, Fabry disease, and MPS I, II, and VI. Beneficial effects of hematopoetic stem cell transplantation have been observed in MPS I and VI. In certain cases of severe cardiomyopathy, preceding enzyme replacement is an essential requisite for succeeding hematopoetic stem cell transplantation.

In systolic myocardial failure, conventional therapy with ACE inhibitor, β-adrenergic receptor blockers, spironolactone, and other diuretics should be instituted as soon as possible. Digoxin may be introduced in the presence of atrial flutter or fibrillation, but may also be beneficial in pure dilated forms. Independent from the morphologic pattern, efficient reduction of β-adrenergic sympathetic activity may be crucial for the long-term prognosis especially in cardiomyopathies due to defective energy production. In hypertrophic cardiomyopathy with isolated diastolic dysfunction, β-blocking agents or calcium antagonists should be at least introduced when outflow tract obstruction exists.

In the case of severe myocardial failure, extracorporal membrane oxygenation or ventricular assist devices offer the potential for patient's survival during diagnostic workup and in initiating a specific metabolic therapy. Unloading conditions largely facilitate myocardial recovering and bridge the time until specific and nonspecific treatment works efficiently. If advanced heart failure is accompanied by ventricular dysynchronia, implantation of a biventricular pacemaker may be considered. Heart transplantation may only be an option in cardiac restricted metabolic cardiomyopathies or well-controlled generalized metabolic diseases.

C1.3 Dysrhythmias and Conduction Disturbances

Disturbances of the cardiac rhythm due to metabolic disorders are often combined with overt cardiomyopathy, but may also proceed morphological and functional abnormalities of the myocardium and be the first, in some cases even fatal clinical manifestation. Routine ECG may show preexcitation in respiratory chain disorders, Pompe and Danon disease. Prolongation of QTc interval which increased with age has been observed in about 70% with propionic acidemia. Prolonged repolarization of the myocardium may predispose propionic acidemia patients to ventricular fibrillation or *torsades de pointes* and be the cause of the increased rate of sudden death in these patients.

All FAO disorders that affect cardiac metabolism are another disease group in which rapid ventricular dysrhythmias (e.g., fibrillation, *torsades de pointes*) can occur. LCHAD, VLCAD, and CPTII deficiencies possess the greatest risk for ventricular tachycardia, probably due to the accumulation of potentially arrhythmogenic long-chain acylcarnitines. Even in MCAD deficiency that usually does not affect the myocardium, ventricular tachycardia has been observed in adulthood.

In addition to the specific metabolic therapy, tachyarrhythmias should be treated by β-receptor blockers,

Table C1.4 Second-line investigations in suspected metabolic cardiomyopathy

Abnormalities	Second-line investigation
Clinical symptoms	
Dysmorphic features	
Blood	Acylcarnitines (if not done before), chromosome analysis, CGH array
Urine	Organic acids, mucopolysaccharides, oligosaccharides (if not done before), free sialic acid
Ataxia	
Blood	Phytanic acid
DNA	Frataxin gene mutations
Developmental delay	
Blood	Lactate/pyruvate ratio (L/P) (preferentially after glucose load), NH_3
CSF	Lactate + pyruvate, amino acids
Urine	Free sialic acid
Cranial MRI, MR spectrosopy	
Muscular symptoms	See below
ECG	
AV block	mtDNA analysis
Pre-excitation	mtDNA analysis
Blood	
High lactate + hypoglycemia	
Blood	Lactate/pyruvate ratio (L/P), NH_3
During acute hypoglycemia	
Blood	Insulin, GH, free fatty acids, β-OH-butyrate, amino acids, acylcarnitines
Urine	Ketones, organic acids
With high ketones and uric acid	Amylo-1,6-glucosidase (debrancher enzyme) (GSD III) (liver, muscle, fibroblasts)
Persistent high lactate	
Blood	Lactate/pyruvate ratio (L/P), acetoacetate/β-OH-butyrate ratio
L/P >25:1:	Assays for respiratory chain enzymes (skeletal muscle biopsy, fibroblasts) mtDNA analysis (blood, fibroblasts)
L/P < 15:1	Pyruvate dehydrogenase activity (fibroblasts)
CSF	Lactate + pyruvate, amino acids, protein
Cranial MRI, MR spectrosopy	
Moderate creatine kinase ⇑ (<10× of normal), proximal or generalized muscle weakness	
Blood	Lactate + pyruvate + L/P ratio (preferentially after glucose load)
Urine	Lactate, organic acids, oligosaccharides (if not done before)
Electrophysiology	EMG, NCV, EEG
Skeletal muscle biopsy	(Ultrastructural) morphology, histochemistry, enzyme studies
DNA	According to biopsy studies (mtDNA, nDNA)
High creatine kinase ⇑ (>10× normal), proximal and limb girdle muscle weakness	
Man: DNA if negative: skeletal muscle biopsy	Dystrophin gene mutation analysis (ultrastructural) morphology, immunohistology, histochemistry, enzyme studies
Woman: skeletal muscle biopsy	See above
Moderate creatine kinase ⇑ (<10× normal), scapulo-peroneal muscle weakness + contractures (w/o AV block)	
DNA	Lamin A/C (autosomal dominant), Emerin (X-chromosomal)
If negative: skeletal muscle biopsy	See above
Moderate creatine kinase ⇑ (<10× normal), myotonia	
DNA	Number of CTG repeats in DMPK gene
Liver enzymes ⇑ (w/o hepatomegaly)	
Blood	Lactate/pyruvate ratio (L/P) (preferentially after glucose load), NH_3, ferritin
Liver biopsy	(Ultrastructural) morphology, immunhistology, histochemistry, enzyme studies

CGH comparative genomic hydridization; *mtDNA* mitochondrial DNA; *nDNA* nuclear DNA; *EMG* electromyogram; *NCV* nerve conduction velocity; *EEG* electroencephalogram; w/o with or without propafenone, sotalol, or amiodarone as indicated. In some cases, implantable converters may be indicated due to sustained ventricular tachycardia or symptomatic arrhythmias.

AV and ventricular conduction disturbances and bradycardia are typical sign of the Kearns–Sayre syndrome and other mitochondrial disorders with cardiac manifestation.

Remember

Because of the potentially rapid progression, pacemaker implantation should be considered early in patients with neuromuscular disorders such as Kearns–Sayre syndrome who have second degree AV block or fascicular block, even when they are asymptomatic.

AV block may also occur in MPS II and VI and Fabry disease.

Remember

In contrast to their benefit for ventricular function, long-term enzyme replacement therapy, now available in MPS I, MPS II, and MPS VI, and allogeneic hematopoetic stem cell transplantation seem to have no or low benefit for the preexisting valvular lesions and may only result in abbreviated progression of valvular changes.

The mucolipidoses, especially mucolipidosis I (sialidosis), can be complicated by mitral regurgitation. The lipidoses, especially Gaucher disease and Farber disease, may infrequently show storage in the connective tissues of the valves, causing thickening and subsequent calcification of the aortic and mitral valves, and the development of nodules. The chordae tendineae may develop similar deposits. Functionally, there may be aortic or mitral stenosis or regurgitation. Stiffening and calcification of the aortic and mitral valves occurs in alkaptonuria, a disorder of tyrosine catabolism that causes darkening (ochronosis) and stiffening of cartilaginous tissues.

C1.4 Metabolic Disorders and Valvular Abnormalities

Several metabolic disorders are associated with valvular dysfunction late in the course of the disorder. Thickening of the valves, sometimes with calcification, especially the aortic and mitral, occurs in several lysosomal storage disorders, including Hurler (MPS I-H), Scheie (MPS I-S), Hunter (MPS II), Sanfilippo (MPS III), Morquio (MPS IV), and Maroteaux–Lamy (MPS VI) syndromes. Mitral and aortic regurgitation can be observed in more than 50% of MPS patients, especially in MPS I, II, and VI: aortic and mitral stenosis and mitral valve prolapse are less frequent. As a rule, prevalence of valvular abnormalities largely depends on the age of the patients. In some cases, postcapillary pulmonary hypertension may also develop. Therefore, serial color Doppler echocardiography in regular intervals is required in patients with MPS to assess ventricular function and the progression of cardiac abnormalities with age.

C1.5 Thrombembolic and Vascular Disorders

Morphological and functional abnormalities of blood vessels occur in several metabolic disorders. Tortuosity of vessels is particularly prominent in Menkes syndrome. Angiokeratomata of the umbilicus, buttocks, and genitalia are a feature of X-linked Fabry disease, where they appear in adolescence. In fucosidosis (autosomal recessive) they appear in the first few years.

Hypercoagulability is a prominent aspect of homocystinuria and the CDG syndromes which can lead to major occlusions of cerebral vessels or multiple small cerebral infarcts. Strokes are also a frequent feature in mitochondrial disorders, perhaps as a consequence of endothelial dysfunction and gradual vascular occlusion. Migraine with stroke and stroke-like episodes without residua or with persistent hemiplegia may all occur in mitochondrial disorders, particularly MELAS.

Beyond lipoprotein disorders, coronary atherosclerosis is accelerated in Fabry disease (including some heterozygous females), and in some mucopolysaccharidoses. In MPS I, infiltration of small and precapillary arteries by storage material may result in severe ischemic cardiomyopathy in infants and young children.

C1.5.1 Lipoprotein Disorders

The long-term sequelae of lipoprotein disorders (Table C1.5) lead to atherosclerotic vascular disease in all the arterial beds. Plasma elevation of low-density lipoprotein cholesterol (LDL-C), very low-density lipoproteins, lipoprotein(a), and reduced levels of high-density lipoprotein cholesterol (HDL-C) are well-known risk factors for coronary heart and cerebrovascular disease. LDL-metabolism may be impaired by mutations of the hepatic cell-surface LDL-receptor (familial

hypercholesterolemia) or by mutations in the receptor that recognizes apolipoprotein B100 protein on the surface of LDL particles (familial defective apo B-100), which may present with myocardial infarction and cerebrovascular disease even during the second decade in untreated homozygotes or severe compound heterozygotes. Therefore, screening and treatment of affected children have to take into account the severity of the phenotype, the long-term risk of developing vascular disease and available evidence of clinical benefit in a group of diseases that are mostly asymptomatic within childhood and adolescence.

Fasting LDL-C and HDL-C levels should at least be determined in children with a positive family history for premature cardiovascular events in parents or grandparents below the age of 60 years or with risk-burden diseases like diabetes mellitus, chronic kidney disease, after orthotopic heart transplantation, or after Kawasaki

Table C1.5 Genetic lipoprotein disorders with significantly increased cardiovascular risk

Disorder	Inheritance	Prevalence	LDL-C (mg/dL)	HDL-C (mg/dL)	TG (mg/dL)	Genetic lesion	Risk of atherosclerosis (age at clinical presentation)
Familial hypercholesterolemia							
Heterozygous	AD	1:200–1:500	>135	n-↓	Normal	LDL-receptor	↑–↑↑ (Early to mid adulthood)
Homozygous	AD	1:1,000,000	>425	<35	Normal	LDL-receptor	↑↑↑ (Starting in first decade)
Familial defective apo B-100							
Heterozygous	AD	1:500–1:700	>135	n-↓	Normal	Apo B-100	↑ (Mid to late adulthood)
Homozygous	AD	1:1,000,000	>320	<35	Normal	Apo B-100	↑↑–↑↑↑ (Starting in second decade)
Familial combined hyperlipidemia[a]	AD	1:20–1:50	150–250	n-↓	150–400	Polygenic	↑–↑↑ (Mid to late adulthood)
Familial dysbeta-lipo-proteinemia	AR	1:10,000	>130	n-↓	> 270	apoE-2/-2	↑↑ (Early to mid adulthood)
Apolipoprotein A–I deficiency	AR	<1: 100,000	N	<10	n	Apo A-I	↑–↑↑ (Early to mid adulthood)
Sitosterolemia	AR	1:1,000,000 (homozygous)	Sitosterol↑, campesterol↑	N	Normal	ABCG5, ABCG8	↑↑–↑↑↑ (Starting in first decade)

AD autosomal dominant; *AR* autosomal recessive; *LDL-C* LDL-cholesterol; *TG* triglycerides; *HDL-C* HDL-cholesterol
[a]Prevalence is age dependent

disease. Age-dependent normal levels of LDL-C and HDL-C, stratification by underlying diseases and the assessment of additional risk factors [hypertension, overweight, impaired glucose tolerance, smoking, reduced HDL-C, and elevated lipoprotein(a)] may promote gradual treatment goals.

Remember

Lifestyle modification like diet and exercise and a lipid-lowering medication should aim for levels of LDL-C ≤100 mg/dL in the high-risk group, ≤130 mg/dL in patients with moderate risk, and ≤160 mg/dL in patients with a low, but increased risk of epidemiological evidence.

Statins as HMG-CoA-reductase inhibitors are the first-line drugs to lower increased LDL-C to target levels in children ≥10 years. Ezetimibe inhibiting intestinal cholesterol absorption via the membranous Niemann–Pick C1-like 1 protein and LDL apheresis are additional options in severe hyperlipoproteinemia.

C1.6 Pulmonary Hypertension

Pulmonary arterial hypertension (PAH), a chronic vasculoproliferative disorder of the pulmonary arterial vasculature, has been associated with a few inborn metabolic disorders. PAH is defined as a mean arterial pressure ≥25 mmHg at rest, pressure values between 21 and 24 mmHg were recently classified as borderline PAH. In GSD Ia, PAH may be a late complication observed in about 10% of these patients during adolescence and adulthood. Abnormal production of serotonin and its release from thrombocytes has been suggested to be the most probable cause for pulmonary vasoconstriction and remodeling of the vessel wall in GSD Ia. Several cases of unexplained PAH have been reported in association with Gaucher disease. Liver disease, splenectomy, capillary plugging by Gaucher cells, and enzyme replacement therapy could all play a role in the development of PAH.

PAH may also be a rare manifestion of multisystemic mitochondrial respiratory chain disorders. Preceding liver disease and young age have been consistently found in these patients. Recurrent episodes of cyanosis or oxygen dependency due to pulmonary vasoconstriction result from the marked muscular thickening and intimal proliferation of the medium and small pulmonary arteries.

Table C1.6 Investigation in pulmonary arterial hypertension

Aim/methods	Parameter	Value
Screening of $_pH$		
Echocardiography	Tricuspid valve regurgitation	Normal <2.5 m/s
		Borderline 2.5–2.8 m/s
		Abnormal >2.8 m/s
Verification of suspected pulmonary hypertension		
Right heart catherization	Pulmonary artery pressure pulmonary vasodilator studies including oxygen, nitric oxide, inhaled iloprost	Baseline hemodynamics changes of pulmonary arterial pressure and resistance (especially Rp/Rs ratio)
Main differential diagnosis		
Disorders of the respiratory system	Spirometry, oxygen diffusion capacity Chest HR-CT, sleep studies	
Grading of pulmonary hypertension		
Echocardiography	Right atrium area, TAPSE, Tei-index, left ventricular eccentricity index	
Exercise testing	6-Min walk test, spiroergometry	
Assessment of additional risk factors	Homocysteine	>12 μmol/L
	Lipoprotein (a)	>30 mg/dL
	Genetic thrombophilic factors	FV-Leiden mutation (1691G > A), Prothrombin variation 20210G > A, MTHFR variation 677C > T

Rp/Rs ratio pulmonary arterial resistance/systemic arterial resistance; *HR-CT* high-resolution computer tomography; *TAPSE* tricuspid annular plane systolic excursion

Early detection of increased pulmonary pressure is crucial to initiate medical therapy (e.g., endothelin antagonists, phosphodiesterase inhibitors, systemic, or inhaled prostacyclin analogs).

> **Remember**
>
> Routine echocardiographic assessment of right ventricular performance and pulmonary pressure should be included in the follow-up of patients with metabolic disorders at risk for PAH.

Suspicion for PAH should be verified by right heart catherization and measurement of pulmonary artery pressures including vasodilator studies. Assessment of pulmonary function and additional risk factors as well as exercise testing and echocardiographic grading of pulmonary pressures and right ventricular function complete the diagnostic spectrum (Table C1.6).

Key References

Böhles H, Sewell AC (eds) (2004) Metabolic cardiomyopathy. Medpharm Scientific Publishers, Stuttgart

Cox GF (2007) Diagnostic approaches to pediatric cardiomyopathy of metabolic genetic etiologies and their relation to therapy. Prog Pediatr Cardiol 24(1):15–25

Lipshultz SE, Colan SD, Towbin JA, Wilkinson JD (eds) (2007) Idiopathic and primary cardiomyopathy in children. Progress in pediatric cardiology, vol 23 and 24/1. Elsevier, Amsterdam

Liver Disease

Georg F. Hoffmann and Guido Engelmann

Key Facts

> Liver disease is a common and important sequel of inherited metabolic diseases.

> Defects in the degradation of fatty acids, fructose, galactose, and glycogen as well as of gluconeogenesis, ketogenesis, ammonia detoxification, or oxidative phosphorylation can lead to significant liver disease.

> Specific symptoms of these disorders reflect response to the demand on the pathway affected; it includes pathological alterations of blood ammonia, glucose, lactate, ketone bodies, and pH.

> Specific symptoms are often obscured by consequences of rather nonspecific responses of the liver to injuries that lead to hepatocellular damage, decreased liver function, cholestasis, and hepatomegaly.

> Other inherited diseases interfere primarily with hepatic cell integrity; these are Wilson disease, tyrosinemia type I, cystic fibrosis, α1-antitrypsin deficiency, and deficiencies of biosynthetic pathways, such as in cholesterol biosynthesis, peroxisomal disorders, CDG syndromes, and defects in bile acids synthesis. Very striking physical involvement of the liver with relatively little functional derangement is seen in lysosomal storage disorders.

> The diagnostic laboratory evaluation of liver disease must be broad, especially in neonates, and initiated early. Successful outcome depends very much on early institution of specific therapy. In addition to the increasing therapeutic options for individual disorders, pediatric liver transplantation has developed into a well-established procedure, with the best outcome rates of ≥90% in liver-based metabolic disorders.

C2.1 General Remarks

Despite the complex interrelated functions of the liver in intermediary metabolism, the hepatic clinical response to inherited metabolic disease is limited and often indistinguishable from that resulting from acquired causes, such as infections or intoxications. The diagnostic laboratory evaluation of liver disease must therefore be broad. Careful evaluation of the history and clinical presentation should include a detailed dietary history as well as a list of all medications, the general appearance of the patient, somatic and psychomotor development, signs of organomegaly, neurological signs, and an ophthalmologic examination. In combination with the results of routine clinical chemical investigations (Table C2.1), this should lead to the suspicion of an inborn error of metabolism, the initiation of specific metabolic tests (Table C2.2), and to a provisional grouping into one of the four main clinical presentations (A – jaundice/cholestatic liver disease, B – liver failure/hepatocellular necrosis, C – cirrhosis, or D – hepatomegaly).

The family and personal history of the patient can especially be helpful in acquired as well as inherited liver disease. Routes of infection may become obvious. Linkage of symptoms to oral intake of food or drugs

G. F. Hoffmann (✉)
University Children's Hospital, Ruprecht-Karls-University,
Im Neuenheimer Feld 430, D-69120 Heidelberg, Germany
e-mail: georg.hoffmann@med.uni-heidelberg.de

G. F. Hoffmann et al. (eds.), *Inherited Metabolic Diseases*,
DOI: 10.1007/978-3-540-74723-9_2, © Springer-Verlag Berlin Heidelberg 2009

Table C2.1 First line investigations in disease of the liver

Alanine and aspartate aminotransferases (transaminases)
Lactate dehydrogenase
Cholinesterase
Alkaline phosphatase
γ-Glutamyltranspeptidase

Bilirubin, conjugated and unconjugated
Bile acids

Coagulation studies: PT, PTT, factors V, VII and XI
Albumin, prealbumin

Urea nitrogen, creatinine, uric acid, CK
Glucose
Ammonia

Hepatitis A, B, C
Cytomegalovirus, EBV, herpes simplex, toxoplasmosis, HIV
Viral cultures of stool and urine

Abdominal ultrasound (gall bladder before and after meal, hepatic tumor)
Ultrasound of the heart (vitium cordis, peripheral pulmonary stenosis)

In infancy
Rubella, parvovirus B19, echovirus and a variety of enterovirus subtypes
Bacterial cultures of blood and urine

PT prothrombin time; *PTT* partial thromboplastin time; *EBV* Epstein–Barr virus; *HIV* human immunodeficiency virus

Table C2.2 Second line investigations in suspected metabolic liver disease

Plasma/serum
   Copper, ceruloplasmin
   α-Fetoprotein
   Cholesterol, triglycerides
   Serum iron and ferritin, transferrin, and transferrin saturation
   Lactate, pyruvate, 3-hydroxybutyrate, acetoacetate
   Free fatty acids
   Amino acids
   Free and total carnitine, acylcarnitine profile
   α1-Antitrypsin activity and PI phenotyping
   Lysosomal enzymes

Urine
   Amino acids
   Ketones
   Reducing substances/ sugars (galactosemia, fructose intolerance)
   Organic acids (incl. specific assays for orotic acid and succinylacetone)
   Individual bile acids (bile acid synthesis defects)
   Copper in 24 h urine

Sweat chloride (cystic fibrosis)
In infancy
   Galactose-1-phosphate uridyl transferase (galactosemia)
   Chromosomes (especially when liver disease is accompanied by malformations suggesting trisomy 13 or 18)
   Free T_4 and TSH (hypothyroidism)
   Transferrin isoelectric focusing (CDG syndromes)
   Very long-chain fatty acids (peroxisomal disorders)

may almost be diagnostic in fructose intolerance, paracetamol intoxication, or accidental poisoning.

Another important key to diagnosis is the age at presentation. During the first 3 months of life, the majority of patients with liver disease, including those with inherited metabolic diseases present with conjugated hyperbilirubinemia. Later in infancy, the presentation becomes broader (Fig. C2.1).

Only a few well-defined inherited diseases cause unconjugated hyperbilirubinemia: hemolytic anemias or impaired conjugation of bilirubin resulting from a recessive deficiency of UDP-glucuronyl transferase in Crigler–Najjar syndrome types 1 and 2 or due to a dominantly inherited mild reduction of UDP-glucuronyl transferase in *Gilbert syndrome* (bilirubin, 1–6 mg/dL). The latter is a benign condition manifesting in neonates only, if they are afflicted by a second hemolytic disorder, such as glucose-6-phosphatase deficiency. In later life, mild jaundice aggravated by fasting or intercurrent illness is the only symptom, and the condition is often uncovered accidentally. *Crigler–Najjar syndrome type 1*, usually defined as bilirubin > 20 mg/dL or >360 μmol/L

that does not react on phenobarbitone therapy, leads to severe nonhemolytic jaundice. Severe neurological damage and death due to kernicterus is a common sequel. Patients with *Crigler–Najjar type 2* have bilirubin levels of up to 20 mg/dL. Liver transplant has proven successful in a number of patients, and in future, Crigler–Najjar syndrome type 1 will certainly be an attractive candidate for hepatocyte transplantation and gene therapy (Table C2.3).

Pediatric liver transplantation has developed into a well-established procedure. Patients with cholestatic or liver-based metabolic diseases have the best outcome rates of ≥90% without significant decline after the first year after transplantation. Further progress can be expected from auxiliary partial orthotopic transplantation, when there is no significant fibrosis and the objective of treatment is the replacement of the missing enzyme, e.g., in Crigler–Najjar syndrome type 1 or urea cycle disorders.

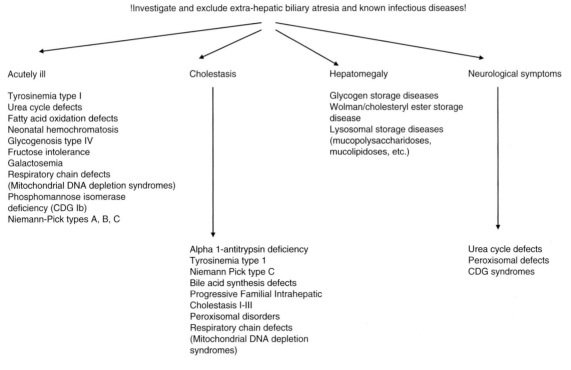

Fig. C2.1 Differential diagnosis of metabolic liver diseases in infants

Table C2.3 Hepatic diseases that may be cured by liver transplantation

Disease	Timing
Acute Wilson disease	If no response to therapy
Neonatal hemochromatosis	Soon if no response to antioxidant cocktail
α-1 Antitrypsin deficiency	In early infancy if cholestasis deteriorates
Urea cycle disorders	Early in the course to prevent further crises
Tyrosinemia Type I	Early in the course if no response to therapy
PFIC I-III	If pruritus and portal hypertension develops
Primary hyperoxaluria	Liver transplantation before development of renal impairment
	Combined LTX/NTX when CCR < 20
Crigler–Najjar Type 1	Before school age, consider liver cell or auxiliary transplantation
Cystic fibrosis	If cholestasis deteriorates and portal hypertension develops
Glucogenosis Type I	In adolescents when risk of malignancy

Questionable: organoacidurias, glucogenosis IV, mitochondriopathies

C2.2 Cholestatic Liver Disease

C2.2.1 Cholestatic Liver Disease in Early Infancy

Cholestatic liver disease may aggravate or prolong physiological neonatal jaundice. It becomes obviously pathological when conjugated hyperbilirubinemia is recognized (conjugated bilirubin > 15% of total). An important early sign is a change in the color of the urine from colorless or only faintly yellow to distinctly yellow or even brown. The significance of this finding is often missed, as this color is similar to adult urine. Of course, by this time the sclerae are yellow – with chronic direct hyperbilirubinemia, the skin becomes yellow and may have a greenish hue. Cholestasis frequently causes pale or acholic stool. A colored stool, however, does not exclude cholestasis.

Remember

A stool specimen should always be looked at in the first visit of jaundiced neonates with conjugated hyperbilirubinemia.

Transient conjugated hyperbilirubinemia can be observed in neonates, especially premature infants, after moderate perinatal asphyxia. It is associated with a high hematocrit and a tendency to hypoglycemia and has an excellent prognosis, if the pathological conditions described later have been excluded.

Remember

Cholestatic liver disease in infancy may be the initial presentation of cystic fibrosis, Niemann–Pick disease type C and tyrosinemia type I.

Biliary obstruction. Infants with cholestatic liver disease often appear well. Early differentiation between biliary atresia, a choledochal cyst, and a "neonatal hepatitis syndrome" is most important. Biliary atresia accounts for 20–30% of neonatal cholestasis syndromes. Structural cholestasis can also be due to intrahepatic bile duct paucity. The syndromal form is *Alagille syndrome*, in which a dominantly inherited dysplasia of the pulmonary artery occurs with distinctive dysmorphic features and paucity of intrahepatic bile ducts resulting in cholestatic liver disease. Intrahepatic bile duct paucity can appear without any other dysmorphies. Routine clinical chemical investigations can seldom differentiate between biliary obstruction and neonatal hepatitis syndrome, although low albumin concentrations and decreased coagulation unresponsive to vitamin K point to a longer disease course such as in prenatal infections or inherited disorders.

Remember

The differentiation between biliary obstruction and neonatal hepatitis syndrome must be vigorously pursued by ultrasonographic, possibly radioisotopic, studies and by liver biopsy, as surgical correction of extrahepatic biliary atresia or a choledochal cyst disorders must be performed as early as possible to minimize intrahepatic biliary disease.

Disease Info: α1-Antitrypsin Deficiency

α1–Antitrypsin is one of the most important inhibitors of proteases (e.g., elastase, trypsin, chymotrypsin, thrombin, and bacterial proteases) in plasma. Different protein variants of α1–antitrypsin are differentiated by isoelectric focusing. The Z variant is characterized by a glutamine to lysine exchange at position 342 in the protein. It alters the charge and tertiary structure of the molecule and is associated with reduced enzyme activity. The frequency of this particular allele is very high in Caucasians; 5% of the population of Sweden is MZ heterozygotes and 2% of the United States. The frequency of the homozygous Pi-ZZ phenotype is 1 in 1,600 in Sweden and 1 in 6,000 in the United States. Normal serum levels of α1-antitrypsin are from 20 to 50 μmol/L, and in the ZZ phenotype, 3–6 μmol/L. Patients with values below 20 μmol/L should have PI phenotyping.

Cholestatic liver disease occurs in 10–20% of infants with the Pi-ZZ α1-antitrypsin phenotype, which in turn accounts for 14–29% of the neonatal hepatitis syndrome, once infectious and toxic causes have been excluded. Bleeding may occur as a result of deficiency of vitamin K with prompt response to intravenous vitamin K. The stool is acholic. Low serum α1-antitrypsin and genetic phenotyping usually leads to the diagnosis. In the acute stages, liver biopsies of infants with α1-antitrypsin deficiency may show giant cell hepatitis with PAS-positive diastase-resistant granules.

Some patients with α1-antitrypsin deficiency, who had no history of neonatal cholestasis, develop cirrhosis eventually and may present with unexplained liver failure. These patients have had the Pi-types ZZ, MZ, and S. In addition, hepatomas and hepatocellular carcinomas have been described in ZZ and MZ phenotypes.

A major proportion of patients with α1-antitrypsin deficiency remain free of liver disease throughout their life. In adulthood, 80–90% of patients with the Pi-ZZ phenotype develop destructive pulmonary emphysema. α1-Antitrypsin is protective of the lung, because it is an effective inhibitor of elastase and other proteolytic enzymes, which are released from neutrophils and macrophages during inflammatory processes. Children with the rare Pi null variant may have severe emphysema early in their life. Intravenous infusions of α1-antitrypsin have been shown to impede the development of emphysema in the affected individuals.

In *dysmorphic infants with cholestasis*, very long-chain fatty acids, as well as chromosomes, should be investigated as peroxisomal diseases, and trisomies 13 and 18 are associated with the neonatal hepatitis syndrome and biliary atresia (trisomie 18). Alagille syndrome has been discussed earlier.

A group of inherited metabolic diseases characterized by *progressive intrahepatic cholestasis* starting in infancy is becoming more recognized. These are the *defects in bile acid biosynthesis*. Unfortunately the necessary laboratory facilities to diagnose these treatable disorders are only available in a few laboratories worldwide. Four different enzyme defects in the modification of the steroid nucleus of bile acids have been elucidated. Malabsorption of fat-soluble vitamins is pronounced and results in spontaneous bleeding and rickets. The level of alkaline phosphatase is often highly elevated, but this feature is not diagnostic. Determination of total bile acids is not helpful. More widespread availability of fast atom bombardment mass spectrometry for rapid analysis of urine samples will hopefully result in a quicker recognition of these disorders in the future. After diagnosis, there is a good clinical and biochemical response to supplementation with bile acids, such as cholic acid in combination with chenodesoxycholic or ursodeoxycholic acids.

Remember

After exclusion of other diseases, infants with cholestatic liver disease should be examined for the treatable defects of bile acid biosynthesis, which requires determination of individual bile acid metabolites.

C2.2.2   Cholestatic Liver Disease in Later Infancy and Childhood

After 3 months of age, the initial clinical and biochemical presentation usually allows a clearer suspicion and differentiation of inherited metabolic liver disease than in neonates. In patients with α1-antitrypsin deficiency, cholestatic liver disease gradually subsides before 6 months of age. In later infancy, three distinct metabolic diseases present with cholestatic liver disease (Table C2.4).

Table C2.4 Differential diagnosis of metabolic cholestatic liver disease (conjugated hyperbilirubinemia)

Age of presentation	Diseases to be considered	Additional findings
<3 Months	α1-Antitrypsin deficiency	⇓ α1-Globulin, ⇓ α1-antitrypsin
	Cystic fibrosis	⇑ Sweat chloride
	Tyrosinemia type I	⇑ AFP
	Niemann–Pick type C	Foam cells in marrow
	Peroxisomal diseases	Encephalopathy
	Bile acid synthesis defects	Prominent malabsorption
>3 Months	Progressive familial intrahepatic cholestasis (e.g., Byler disease)	Progressive cirrhosis
	Rotor syndrome	Normal liver function
	Dubin–Johnson syndrome	Normal liver function

Known infectious diseases should have been ruled out by laboratory tests listed in Table C2.1 and extrahepatic biliary disease by imaging techniques

Disease Info: Progressive Familial Intrahepatic Cholestasis (Byler Disease)

Progressive familial intrahepatic cholestasis (PFIC) is a genetically heterogeneous group of autosomal recessive liver disorders, characterized by cholestasis that progresses to cirrhosis and liver failure before adulthood. Symptoms start later in infancy with jaundice, pruritus, growth failure, and conjugated hyperbilirubinemia. Liver function slowly deteriorates, and terminal liver failure usually occurs before 15 years. Liver transplantation has become the treatment of choice, but may be complicated by postoperative intractable diarrhea and pancreatitis. PFIC may be caused by a deficiency of several hepatobiliary transporters. The term Byler disease is generally used for PFIC type 1 caused by a deficiency of a P-type ATPase that is required for ATP-dependent amino phospholipid transport and encoded by the ATP8B1 gene on chromosome 18q21. Other PFIC types are linked to the ABCB11 gene on chromosome 2q24 (PFIC2) and the ABCB4 gene on chromosome 7q21.1 (PFIC3). PFIC4 is sometimes used as a term for 3β-hydroxy-Δ5-C27-steroid oxidoreductase deficiency, a bile acid synthesis defect (see earlier) caused by mutations in the HSD3B7 gene on chromosome 16p12-p11.2, which has a similar phenotype. Patients with PFIC or the clinically similar bile acid synthesis defects have normal serum levels of γ-glutamyltransferase (GGT).

A different type of PFIC can be distinguished from the defects of bile acid synthesis or secretion by high serum GGT activity and liver histology that shows portal inflammation and ductular proliferation in an early stage. The histologic and biochemical characteristics of this subtype resemble those of the mdr2$^{-/-}$ knockout mice very closely. Lack of MDR3 mRNA negative canalicular staining for MDR3 p-glycoprotein was demonstrated in the liver of patients. One patient was found to be homozygous for a frameshift deletion; another patient was homozygous for a nonsense arg957-to-ter mutation. Interestingly, a heterozygous mother of an affected child experienced recurrent episodes of intrahepatic cholestasis of pregnancy.

The age of presentation (Table C2.6) as well as associated features (Table C2.7) may be helpful in directing the investigations. Jaundice is usually present, but more important and characteristic features are elevated liver transaminases and markers of hepatic insufficiency, such as hypoglycemia, hyperammonemia, hypoalbuminemia, decrease of vitamin K dependent, and other liver-produced coagulation factors. Failure to thrive is mostly present. Deranged liver function may result in spontaneous bleeding or neonatal ascites, indicating end-stage liver disease.

> **Remember**
>
> Encephalopathy associated with severe liver failure is not necessarily obvious, especially, not in neonates and young infants.

Disease Info: Dubin–Johnson and Rotor syndromes

Dubin–Johnson and Rotor syndromes are both autosomal recessively inherited disorders characterized by isolated conjugated hyperbilirubinemia. Patients are usually asymptomatic except for jaundice. Bilirubin levels can range from 2 to 25 mg/dL (34–428 µmol/L). Both the conditions are rare and can be differentiated by differences in urinary porphyrins and appearance of the liver, which is deeply pigmented in Dubin–Johnson syndrome and unremarkable in Rotor syndrome. Excretion of conjugated bilirubin is impaired in both the disorders. The gene involved in Dubin–Johnson syndrome is the canalicular multispecific organic anion transporter on chromosome 10. The gene defect in Rotor syndrome has not yet been identified.

C2.3 Fulminant Liver Failure

C2.3.1 Fulminant Liver Failure in Early Infancy

The differential diagnosis in this age group is wide, ranging from toxic or infectious causes to several inherited metabolic diseases (Table C2.5). Mortality is high.

Acute disease may progress rapidly to hepatic failure. In severely compromised infants, routine clinical chemical measurements do not help to differentiate acutely presenting inherited metabolic diseases from severe viral hepatitis or septicemia, although disproportionate hypoglycemia, lactic acidosis, and/or hyperammonemia all point to a primary metabolic disease. Furthermore, it is not uncommon for septicemia to complicate and aggravate inherited metabolic diseases. Help in the differential diagnosis may come from the judgment of liver size. Decompensated inherited metabolic diseases are often accompanied by significant hepatomegaly due to edema, whereas rapid atrophy can develop in fulminant viral hepatitis or toxic injury.

In babies with acute hepatocellular necrosis, rapid diagnosis of the inherited metabolic diseases listed in Tables C2.5 and C2.7 is essential as specific therapy is available for most and must be initiated as soon as possible. Metabolites accumulating in galactosemia (galactose-1-phosphate) and hereditary fructose intolerance (fructose-1-phosphate) have a similar toxicity particularly for the liver, kidneys, and brain but are usually differentiated by different clinical settings (different age groups) in which first symptoms occur. Determination of amino acids in plasma and urine and analysis of organic acids in urine (particularly succinylacetone, dicarboxylic acids, and orotic acid) should elucidate the presence of hepatorenal tyrosinemia, fatty acid oxidation defects, and urea cycle disorders.

Table C2.5 Differential diagnosis of fulminant liver failure (acute or subacute hepatocellular necrosis)

Age of presentation	Diseases to be considered	Additional findings
<3 Months	Neonatal hemochromatosis	⇑⇑⇑ Ferritin, ⇑⇑⇑ AFP
	Galactosemia	Cataracts, urinary reducing substance
	Tyrosinemia type I	⇑⇑ AFP
	Urea cycle defects	⇑⇑⇑ Ammonia
	Respiratory chain defects	⇑⇑ Lactate
	Long-chain fatty acid oxidation defects	⇑ Lactate, ⇑ urate, ⇑ CK, ⇑ ammonia, (cardio-) myopathy, myoglobinuria
	Niemann–Pick types A, B, C	Foam cells in marrow
	Phosphomannose isomerase deficiency (CDG Ib)	⇓ Transferrin isoforms
3 Months–2 years	Fructose intolerance	⇓ Glucose
	Tyrosinemia type I	⇑⇑ AFP
	Fatty acid oxidation defects	⇓ Glycose, ⇑ uric acid, ⇑ CK, ⇓ ketones, ⇑ lactate, ⇑ ammonia
	Respiratory chain defects	⇑ Lactate
	Urea cycle defects	⇑⇑⇑ Ammonia
>2 Years	Wilson disease	Corneal ring, hemolysis, renal tubular abnormalities, neurologic degeneration
	α1-Antitrypsin deficiency	⇓ α1-Globulin, ⇓ α1-antitrypsin
	Fatty acid oxidation defects	⇓ Glucose, ⇑ uric acid, ⇑ CK, ⇓ ketones, ⇑ lactate, ⇑ ammonia
	Glycogenoses type VI/IX	± ⇓ Glucose, ⇑ transaminases, ⇑ lactate, ⇑ CK
	Urea cycle defects	⇑⇑⇑ Ammonia

Known infectious diseases should have been ruled out by laboratory tests listed in Table C2.1 and extrahepatic biliary disease by imaging techniques

Table C2.6 Age at presentation as a clue to the cause of hepatic failure in infancy

0–7 days	Herpes simplex type 1 and 2
	mtDNA depletion
	Neonatal hemochromatosis
1–4 weeks	Infections
	Galactosemia
	Tyrosinemia
4–8 weeks	Hepatitis B (vertical transmission)
2–6 months	Bile acid synthesis defects
0.5–1 year	Hereditary fructose intolerance
	mtDNA depletion
	Wolcott Rallison syndrome
	Viral hepatitis
	Autoimmune

Disease Info: Galactosemia

Galactosemia is caused by a deficiency of galactose-1-phosphate uridyltransferase (GALT). Clinical symptoms usually start after the onset of milk feeds on the third or fourth day of life and include vomiting, diarrhea, jaundice, disturbances of liver function, or sepsis and may progress untreated to death from hepatic and renal failure. Whenever galactosemia is suspected, adequate blood and urine tests should be initiated (galactose and galactose-1-phosphate in serum, erythrocytes, or dried blood spots; enzyme studies in erythrocytes) and a lactose-free diet should be started immediately. Galactose in urine is not detected by standard stix tests based on the glucose oxidase method (Clinistix® and Tes-tape®) and there is a strong argument for the continued use of the older methods of screening urine for reducing substances (Benedict or Fehling test and Clinitest®), which also detect galactose. Urinary excretion of galactose depends on the dietary intake and will not be detectable 24–48h after discontinuation of milk feedings. On the other hand, babies with severe liver disease from any cause may have impaired galactose metabolism and gross secondary galactosuria. After discontinuing galactose for 2–3 days, a baby with galactosemia begins to recover. Cataracts may have developed in only a few days (Fig. C8.2, Chap. C8) and slowly clear after removal of the toxic sugar.

Table C2.7 Neonatal liver failure

Disorder	Additional clinical features
Mitochondrial hepatopathy, often mtDNA depletion	Muscular hypotonia, multi-system disease, encephalopathy, ↑↑ lactate
Neonatal hemochromatosis	Hepatocellular necrosis, cirrhosis, ↑↑ ferritin, ↑↑ AFP, transaminases may be low
Galactosemia	Onset after milk feeds, jaundice, renal disease, cataracts
Fatty acid oxidation disorders	(Cardio)myopathy, hypoketotic, hypoglycemia, ↑ lactate
Urea cycle disorders	↑↑ Ammonia, encephalopathy
Niemann–Pick type C	Jaundice, hypotonia, hepatosplenomegaly
Glycosylation disorders (CDG, especially type Ib)	Hepatomegaly, hepatocellular dysfunction, protein losing enteropathy, multi-system disease

Rarely: α_1-Antitrypsin deficiency, bile acid synthesis disorders

> **Remember**
>
> In any baby who has received milk and developed liver disease, the investigation should include determination of the enzymatic activity of galactose-1-phosphate uridyl transferase in erythrocytes, regardless of the results of neonatal screening.

> **Remember**
>
> Urinary elevations of succinylacetone may be small in young infants, and repeated analyses with special requests for specific determination by stable isotope dilution may be warranted in patients in whom clinical suspicion is strong.

Genetic defects of fatty acid oxidation and of the respiratory electron transport chain have become recognized as causes of rapidly progressive hepatocellular necrosis in infancy. Defects of fatty acid oxidation are suggested in prolonged intermittent or subacute presentations by myopathy, cardiomyopathy, hypoketotic hypoglycemia, hyperuricemia, elevation of CK, moderate lactic acidosis, and dicarboxylic aciduria (see also Chap. B2.5). Defects of the respiratory chain causing hepatocellular necrosis are characterized by additional variable multiorgan involvement, especially, of the bone marrow, pancreas and brain, moderate to severe lactic acidosis, and ketosis (see also Chaps. B2.3 and D6). During acute hepatocellular necrosis in infancy, these differentiating features may be masked by generalized metabolic derangement. Repeated determinations of metabolites such as lactate, pyruvate, 3-hydroxybutyrate, acetoacetate, free and total carnitine, and analysis of acylcarnitines in addition to determinations of amino acids in blood and organic acids in urine should therefore be performed in any baby with progressive hepatocellular necrosis. If the clinical and biochemical presentation is suggestive of a defect of fatty acid oxidation or of the respiratory chain, appropriate enzymatic confirmation in muscle and liver, or molecular studies of nuclear or mitochondrial DNA, should be sought (see also Chaps. B2.3, D6, and B2.5). If results are negative, they should be followed up by investigating defects of fatty acid oxidation in patients initially thought to have a defect of the respiratory chain, and vice versa. Small infants with primary defects of fatty acid oxidation may present with overwhelming lactic acidosis and infants with severe liver disease due to defects of the respiratory chain with hypoketotic hypoglycemia and dicarboxylic aciduria.

> **Remember**
>
> When cardiomyopathy is present, lactic acidosis may be due to heart failure and poor perfusion.

Disease Info: Neonatal Hemochromatosis

Neonatal hemochromatosis should be considered in the differential diagnosis of rapidly progressive hepatocellular necrosis in infancy. As neonatal hemochromatosis has occurred in several diseases with known origin, such as prenatal infection, tyrosinemia type I, congenital hepatic fibrosis, or Down syndrome, neonatal hemochromatosis can be thought to present a clinicopathological entity rather than an individual disorder. However, in approximately 100 reported infants who presented with liver disease from birth, no known cause could be defined and extrahepatic siderosis and occurrence in siblings suggested a primary genetic disorder of fetoplacental iron handling. Diagnosis is by exclusion of other causes and demonstration of increased concentrations of serum iron, ferritin ($>2,000\,\mu g/L$), and α-fetoprotein as well as decreased concentrations of transferrin. Complete or near complete saturation of iron-binding capacity is suggestive and demonstration of extrahepatic siderosis appears to be especially characteristic. The latter can be assessed by minor salivary gland biopsy or an MRI of the liver. Successful treatment depends on early recognition and successful management of hepatic failure, rapid referral to a transplant center, and if the patient does not recover quickly, early liver transplantation (Table C2.3). Some authors recommend an antioxidant cocktail in patients with neonatal hemochromatosis as well as Desferrioxamine. The outcome with and without this cocktail is extremely variable. Iron storage is not permanently disturbed as survivors with and without transplantation do not develop permanent iron-storage disease.

C2.3.2 Fulminant Hepatic Failure in Later Infancy and Childhood

Fulminant hepatic failure in later infancy or early childhood may present in a similar fashion to that in neonates with elevated transaminases, hypoglycemia, hyperammonemia, decrease of coagulation factors, spontaneous bleeding, hypoalbuminemia, and ascites. Mortality is high with liver transplantation sometimes the only therapeutic option (Table C2.3). On liver biopsy hepatocellular necrosis is obvious. Renal tubular dysfunction or rickets is indicative of an inherited metabolic disease. In combination with early infancy insulin-dependent diabetis mellitus, *Wolcott Rallison syndrome* (OMIM #226980) should be looked for by mutation analysis. The association of acute hepatocellular necrosis with a prominent noninflammatory encephalopathy suggests a diagnosis of Reye syndrome; many patients with this syndrome are now found to have inherited metabolic disease.

The commonest form of acute hepatocellular necrosis in older children is acute or decompensated chronic viral hepatitis. A small or rapidly decreasing liver size is a strong argument against an inherited metabolic disease. Autoimmune disease must also be taken into consideration. Autoantibodies are present in the majority of affected children, and there usually is an increase in IgG, serum protein, and autoantibodies.

Disorders of fatty acid oxidation and urea cycle defects should be high on the list of differential diagnosis of children presenting with acute hepatocellular necrosis. If disproportionate hyperammonemia or hypoketotic hypoglycemia has been observed, vigorous emergency measures should be promptly initiated and diagnostic confirmation sought by specialized metabolic investigations (Chap. B2.8). Both are potentially lethal in the acute episode.

Tyrosinemia type I and fructose intolerance are usually diagnosed in infancy or early childhood; urea cycle and fatty acid oxidation defects can cause acute hepatic dysfunction at any age.

In later childhood, Wilson disease and α1-antitrypsin deficiency are important metabolic causes of severe hepatocellular necrosis. In the Asian race, *citrullinemia type II* (citrin deficiency) is relatively common. Courses may be subacute or chronic, and initial presentation is variable, ranging from isolated hepatomegaly, jaundice or ascites to a chronic active hepatitis-like picture or acute liver failure. Hemolysis, when present, may be an important clue to Wilson disease.

Disease Info: Tyrosinemia Type I

Tyrosinemia type I (fumarylacetoacetase deficiency) usually presents with pronounced acute or subacute hepatocellular damage, and only occasionally with cholestatic liver disease in infancy. Patients who have an acute onset of symptoms very quickly develop hepatic decompensation. They may have jaundice and ascites along with hepatomegaly. There may be gastrointestinal bleeding. Several infants have been noted by their mothers to have a peculiar sweet cabbage-like odor. Generalized renal tubular dysfunction occurs, leading to glucosuria, aminoaciduria, and hyperphosphaturia. Very low levels of phosphate in serum are common findings, as are hypoglycemia and hypokalemia. In some patients the diagnosis of tyrosinemia type I can be difficult, as increases of tyrosine and methionine occur in many forms of liver disease. A highly elevated α-fetoprotein is very suggestive, but again not proof. Very high elevations of α-fetoprotein are also seen in neonatal hemochromatosis, which should be differentiated on the basis of gross elevations of iron and ferritin. Diagnostic proof of tyrosinemia type I comes from the demonstration of succinylacetone in urine and confirmation of the enzyme defect in fibroblasts or biopsied liver.

If tyrosinemia type I does not become symptomatic until later in infancy, patients usually follow a less rapid course. Vomiting, anorexia, abdominal distension and failure to thrive, rickets, and easy bruising may be the presenting features, and there is usually hepatomegaly. Although transaminases may be normal or only slightly elevated, prothrombin time and partial thromboplastin time are usually markedly elevated, as is α-fetoprotein, which may range from 100,000 to 400,000 ng/mL. Individual patients may present with different clinical pictures, such as with acute liver disease and hypoglycemia as a Reye-like syndrome. They may present with isolated bleeding and undergo initial investigation for coagulation disorders before hepatic disease is identified.

Renal tubular disease in tyrosinemia type I is that of a renal Fanconi syndrome with phosphaturia, glucosuria, and aminoaciduria (Chap. C4). There may be proteinuria and excessive carnitine loss. Renal tubular loss of bicarbonate leads to systemic metabolic acidosis. The affected infants have been observed to develop vitamin D resistant rickets at less than 4 months of age.

Beyond infancy, neurologic crises very similar to those of acute intermittent porphyria are a more common cause of admission to the hospital than hepatic decompensation. Succinylacetone inhibits phorphobilinogen synthase (the enzyme affected in acute intermittent porphyria); increased urinary excretion of delta-aminolevulinate and porphobilinogen occurs during neurological crises. About half of the patients experience such crises, starting with pains in the lower extremities, followed by abdominal pains, muscular weakness, or paresis and paresthesias. Head and trunk may be positioned in extreme hyperextension, suggesting opisthotonus or meningismus. Systemic

signs include hypertension, tachycardia, and ileus. Symptoms can continue for up to a week and slowly resolve. These episodes should be much less frequent, now that there is therapy for this disorder. Intellectual function is usually not compromised in tyrosinemia type I.

In the natural disease course, most children with tyrosinemia type I die in their early years, most of them before 1 year of age. Chronic liver disease is that of macronodular cirrhosis. Splenomegaly and esophageal varices develop and are complicated by bleeding. A common complication is hepatocellular carcinoma, which may first be suspected because of a further rise in the level of α-fetoprotein. Liver or combined liver–kidney transplantation was the only promising option of treatment until the advent of 2(2-nitro-4-trifluoro-methylbenzoyl)-1,3-cyclohexanedione (NTBC). Nowadays, liver transplantation in tyrosinemia type 1 is only necessary in nonresponders to NTBC therapy. The drug is a potent inhibitor of p-hydroxyphenylpyruvate dioxygenase, thus preventing the formation of the highly toxic fumarylacetoacetate, and its products succinylacetoacetate and succinylacetone. Vigorous compliance is most important as hepatic malignancy may develop rapidly after a short interruption of or inconsistent treatment. If the treatment is instituted early, hepatic and renal function slowly improve to normal, and neurological crises are prevented. Concentrations of succinylacetone, α-fetoprotein, and delta-aminolevulinate gradually decrease to near normal values.

The differential diagnosis of the patient with elevated levels of tyrosine in the blood include tyrosinemias type II and III and transient neonatal tyrosinemia. *Tyrosinemia type II* (tyrosine aminotransferase deficiency), known as the Richner–Hanhart syndrome, results in oculocutaneous lesions, including corneal erosion, opacity, and plaques. Pruritic or hyperkeratotic lesions may develop on the palms and soles. About half of the patients described have had low-normal to subnormal levels of intelligence, but this may reflect bias of ascertainment.

The phenotype of *tyrosinemia type III* (p-hydroxyphenylpyruvate dioxygenase deficiency) is similar. It may include neurological manifestations such as psychomotor retardation and ataxia but also remain asymptomatic. As treatment with NTBC in patients with tyrosinemia type I shifts the metabolic block from fumarylacetoacetate hydrolase to *p*-hydroxyphenylpyruvate dioxygenase or from tyrosinemia type I to tyrosinemia type III, treatment with NTBC must be supplemented by dietary treatment with a phenylalanine- and tyrosine-reduced diet, which is the rational approach to treatment in tyrosinemias type II and III.

Metabolic investigations or neonatal screening, particularly in premature infants sometimes detects tyrosinemia and hyperphenylalaninemia not due to a defined inherited metabolic disease. The protein intake is often excessive, especially, when an evaporated milk formula is being used. This form of tyrosinemia is thought to result from physiological immaturity of *p*-hydroxyphenylpyruvate dioxygenase and is a warning that protein intake should be moderate during the first weeks of life. Relative maternal vitamin C deficiency may play a role. This condition is sometimes associated with prolonged jaundice and feeding problems and can cause diagnostic confusion.

Disease Info: Hereditary Fructose Intolerance

Symptoms develop in hereditary fructose intolerance when fructose or sucrose is introduced into the diet. The recessively inherited deficiency of fructose-1-phosphate aldolase results in an inability to split fructose-1-phosphate into glyceraldehyde and dihydroxyacetone phosphate. Fructose-1-phosphate accumulates in liver, kidney, and intestine. Pathophysiological consequences are hepatocellular necrosis and renal tubular dysfunction, similar to what occurs in galactosemia. There is an acute depletion of ATP caused by the sequestration of phosphate and direct toxic effects of fructose-1-phosphate.

Depending on the amount of fructose or sucrose ingested, infants may present with isolated asymptomatic jaundice or with rapidly progressive liver failure, jaundice, bleeding tendency, and ascites, suggesting septicemia or fulminant viral hepatitis; hepatosplenomegaly, if present, argues against the latter diagnosis. Postprandial hypoglycemia develops in 30–50% of the patients affected with fructose intolerance and may progress to coma and sudden death. Most patients present subacutely with vomiting, poor feeding, diarrhea, or sometimes failure to thrive. Pyloric stenosis and gastroesophageal reflux are common initial diagnoses. The clinical picture may be more blurred in later life and laboratory findings may be unrevealing.

Hereditary fructose intolerance deserves consideration as a cause of renal calculi, polyuria, and periodic or progressive weakness or even paralysis. A major clue to diagnosis may be an accurate dietary history that will reveal an aversion to fruits and sweets.

Characteristic clinical chemical laboratory features include elevated transaminases, hyperbilirubinemia, hypoalbuminemia, hypocholesterolemia, and a decrease of vitamin K dependent, liver-produced coagulation factors. There is an occasional pattern of consumption coagulopathy. In addition, patients may have hypoglycemia, hypophosphatemia, hypomagnesemia, hyperuricemia, and metabolic acidosis in a renal Fanconi syndrome with proteinuria, glucosuria, aminoaciduria and loss of bicarbonate, and high urine pH despite acidosis. In these circumstances detecting fructose in the urine is virtually diagnostic of the disease, but it may be absent. Elevated plasma levels of tyrosine and methionine in combination with markedly elevated excretion of tyrosine and its metabolites in urine may misleadingly suggest a diagnosis of tyrosinemia type I.

The prognosis in hereditary fructose intolerance depends entirely upon the elimination of fructose from the diet. After withdrawal of fructose and sucrose, clinical symptoms and laboratory findings quickly reverse. Vomiting stops immediately, and the bleeding tendency stops within 24 h. Most clinical and laboratory findings become normal within 2–3 weeks, but hepatomegaly will take longer time to resolve.

The excellent response to treatment supports a presumptive diagnosis of fructose intolerance. Confirmation of diagnosis should first be attempted by molecular analysis. Several frequent mutations are known, such as A149P in Caucasians. An intravenous fructose tolerance test can usually not be performed any longer in diagnostically difficult cases as there are no i.v. preparations of fructose available. Demonstration of the enzyme defect in liver tissue may be necessary in exceptional constellations.

Mitochondrial DNA depletion syndromes are increasingly identified as causes of rapidly progressive liver disease. Forms known so far are caused by defects in the deoxyguanosine kinase, polymerase-γ (POLG), MPV17, recessive Twinkle helicase (PEO1) genes, as well as in the EIF2AK3 gene.

Disease Info: Alpers Disease

In patients with Alpers disease, liver failure mostly occurs later in the course of disease, often triggered by the use of valproic acid. Mutation in the POLG gene results in defects in respiratory chain complexes I and IV. Despite fulminant liver failure, aminotransferases typically are only mildly elevated. Most patients with Alpers disease present at preschool or school age with neurological symptoms like seizures or even epileptic state and epilepsia partialis continua. Patients' history usually reveals mild and then progressive psychomotor development. However, liver failure may develop before significant neurological disease. If in an unclear situation a therapeutic liver transplantation is being considered, mutation analysis of the POLG gene should be pursued as soon as possible. Alpers syndrome due to mutations in the POLG gene can be considered a contraindication for transplantation as the children will continue to develop a progressive fatal encephalopathy.

Disease Info: Wilson Disease

Wilson disease, or hepatolenticular degeneration, is characterized by the accumulation of copper in various organs and low serum levels of ceruloplasmin. Clinical manifestations are highly variable, but hepatic disease occurs in ≈80% of the affected individuals. This is usually manifest at school age, rarely before 4 years of age. About half of the patients with hepatic disease, if untreated, will develop neurological symptoms in adolescence or adulthood. In other patients with Wilson disease, neurological manifestations are the presenting symptoms.

One extreme of the clinical spectrum of Wilson disease is a rapid fulminant course in children over 4 years of age progressing within weeks to hepatic insufficiency manifested by icterus, ascites, clotting abnormalities, and disseminated intravascular coagulation. This is followed by renal insufficiency, coma, and death, sometimes without diagnosis.

Wilson disease can also present with a picture of acute hepatitis. Nausea, vomiting, anorexia, and jaundice are common presenting complaints, and the episode may subside spontaneously. In the presence of splenomegaly, the diagnosis may appear to be infectious mononucleosis. Recurrent bouts of hepatitis and a picture of chronic active hepatitis in children above the age of 4 years are suggestive of Wilson disease. These patients experience anorexia and fatigue. Hepatosplenomegaly is prominent. In some patients isolated hepatosplenomegaly may be discovered accidentally. Any hepatic presentation of Wilson disease leads to cirrhosis; the disease may present as cirrhosis. The histological picture is indistinguishable from chronic active hepatitis. Terminally there may be hepatic coma or a hepatorenal syndrome.

Hemolytic anemia may be a prominent feature of Wilson disease in children, and its presence is very suggestive of the diagnosis. Renal tubular disease is subtle; a generalized aminoaciduria often displays an unusually high excretion of cystine, other sulfur-containing amino acids and of tyrosine. Later there may be a full-blown Fanconi syndrome, and patients may develop renal stones or diffuse nephrocalcinosis.

In adults, the onset of Wilson disease is classically neurological, predominantly with extrapyramidal signs. Choreoathetoid movements and dystonia reflect lenticular degeneration and are frequently associated with hepatic disease. This picture has been associated with poor prognosis. Progression tends to be much slower in patients presenting with parkinsonian and pseudosclerotic symptoms, such as drooling, rigidity of the face, and tremor. Speech or behavior disorders, and sometimes frank psychiatric presentations, can occur in children. The lack of overt liver disease can make diagnosis difficult. Dementia develops ultimately in untreated patients.

The availability of effective treatment for Wilson disease by copper-chelating agents makes early diagnosis crucial. A key finding is the demonstration of Kayser–Fleischer rings around the outer margin of the cornea as gray–green to red–gold pigmented rings (Fig. C2.2). Slit lamp examination may be required. The rings are difficult to be seen in green–brown eyes. They are pathognomonic in neurological disease, but they take time to develop and are absent in most children who present with hepatic disease.

Biochemical diagnosis of Wilson disease may sometimes be difficult. The diagnosis is usually made on the basis of an abnormally low serum ceruloplasmin, liver copper content, and urine copper content plus mutation analysis. In 95% of patients, ceruloplasmin is below 20 mg/dL (200 mg/L) (control children 25–45 mg/dL). However, intermediate and even normal values have been reported in patients. Levels of copper in the serum are usually elevated, but measurement of urine copper is more reliable. Urinary excretion of copper is increased to >100 µg/day (1.6 µmol/day in about 65% of patients) (control children < 30 µg/day (0.5 µmol/day)). Further increase in urinary copper excretion can be provoked by loading with 450 mg of D-penicillamine 12 h apart while collecting urine for 24 h. Controls excrete less than 600 µg (9.4 µmol)/day, whereas in Wilson disease excretion ranges from 1,600 µg (25 µmol) to 3,000 µg (47 µmol)/day. The most sensitive test is the measurement of the concentration of copper in the liver, and this test may be required for diagnosis. Disposable steel needles or Menghini needles should be used. Patients with Wilson disease usually have highly elevated concentrations of copper in the liver (>250 µg (4 µmol) of copper per gram of dry weight; heterozygotes 100–200 µg/g, controls < 50 µg (0.8 µmol)). Elevated concentrations of copper in the liver may also be found in children with extrahepatic biliary obstruction or cholestatic liver disease.

Liver histology is not specific. Rodamin or other staining techniques for copper are not sensitive in childhood Wilson and therefore do not contribute to the diagnosis. As 80% of patients with Wilson's disease show at least one of the 200 known mutations in the ATP7B gene, molecular diagnosis of Wilson disease is a helpful tool in confirming the diagnoses.

Once the diagnosis of Wilson disease is established, family members (particularly sibs) should be thoroughly examined. Examination of liver tissue will be necessary in the case where an asymptomatic sibling has a low ceruloplasmin level, elevated liver enzymes and high copper urine, which can be consistent with heterozygosity as well as homozygosity. Early diagnosis must be vigorously pursued, as the best prognosis has been demonstrated following early treatment of asymptomatic patients.

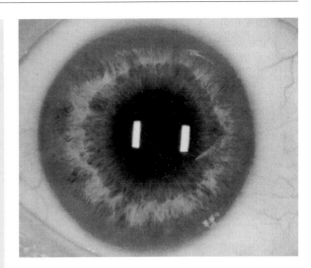

Fig. C2.2 Kayser–Fleischer ring in Wilson disease. Courtesy of Prof. Dr. Wolfgang Stremmel, Heidelberg, Germany

Remember

The association of liver disease with intravascular hemolysis and renal failure is highly suggestive of Wilson disease as are bouts of recurrent hepatitis and a picture of chronic active hepatitis in children above the age of 4 years.

C2.4   Cirrhosis

Cirrhosis is the end stage of hepatocellular disease. The list of diseases that can result in cirrhosis and failure of the liver is extensive and includes infectious, inflammatory and vascular diseases, biliary malformations, as well as toxic and finally metabolic disorders. Cirrhosis can result from most of the diseases discussed in this chapter. Exceptions are primary defects of bilirubin conjugation and some of the storage disorders that lead to hepatomegaly.

Glycogenosis type IV, branching enzyme deficiency, can cause primarily cirrhotic destruction of the liver. In Wilson disease, and even more frequently in α1-antitrypsin deficiency, a cirrhotic process may be quiescent for a long period with no evidence of signs or symptoms of liver disease. Patients may be recognized following family investigations, during investigations of an unrelated disease, or the disease may remain unrecognized until decompensation leads to full-blown liver failure. Specific metabolic diseases leading to cirrhosis are listed in Tables C2.8 and C2.9.

Table C2.8 Differential diagnosis of cirrhosis

Age of presentation	Diseases to be considered	Additional findings
<1 Year	Glycogenosis type IV	Myopathy
	Galactosemia	Cataracts, urinary reducing substance
	Neonatal hemochromatosis	⇑⇑⇑⇑ iron, ⇑⇑⇑ ferritin, ⇑⇑⇑ AFP, ⇓ transferrin
	Tyrosinemia type I	⇑⇑⇑ AFP
>1 Year	α1-Antitrypsin deficiency	⇓ α1-Globulin, ⇓ α1-antitrypsin
	Wilson disease	Corneal ring, hemolysis, renal tubular abnormalities, neurologic degeneration
	Tyrosinemia type I	⇑ AFP

Known infectious and autoimmune diseases should have been ruled out by laboratory tests listed in Table C2.1 and extrahepatic biliary disease by imaging techniques

Table C2.9 Chronic hepatitis or cirrhosis in older children

Disorder	Clinical features
Wilson disease	Neurological and renal disease, corneal ring
Hemochromatosis	Hepatomegaly, cardiomyopathy, diabetes mellitus, diabetes insipidus, hypogonadism
α_1-Antitrypsin deficiency	Failure to thrive, ↓ α_1-antitrypsin
Tyrosinemia type I	Coagulopathy, renal disease, failure to thrive, ↑ AFP
Hereditary fructose intolerance	Symptoms after fructose intake: hypoglycemia, renal disease, failure to thrive, ↑ urate
Transaldolase deficiency	Hepatosplenomegaly, cirrhosis (single patient)
Cystic fibrosis	Failure to thrive, recurrent airway infections
Coeliac disease	Failure to thrive, diarrhea, small stature

Remember

α1-Antitrypsin should be quantified in any child, adolescent, or adult in the differential work-up of cirrhosis.

As cirrhosis progresses, signs and symptoms of decompensation eventually emerge. Regardless of the primary disease patients develop weight loss, failure to thrive, muscle weakness, fatigue, pruritus, steatorrhea, ascites, or anasarca, as well as chronic jaundice, digital clubbing, spider angiomatoma and epistaxis, or other bleeding (Table C2.10). Complications of cirrhosis include portal hypertension, bleeding varices, splenomegaly, and encephalopathy. Terminally there may be hepatic coma. Liver transplantation provides the only realistic therapy. In some cases bridging to transplantation with an albumin dialysis or liver cell transplantation may be indicated.

Table C2.10 Signs and symptoms of liver cirrhosis

General	Malnutrition, failure to thrive, muscle wasting, hypogonadism, elevated temperature, frequent infections
CNS	Lethargy progressing to coma, behavioral changes, depression, intellectual deterioration, pyramidal tract signs, asterixis
Gastrointestinal tract	Nausea and vomiting, splenomegaly, caput medusa, hemorrhoids, epistaxis hematemesis, abdominal distension, steatorrhea, ascites
Kidney	Fluid and electrolyte imbalance, progressive renal insufficiency
Skin	Jaundice, flushing, pruritus, palmar erythema, spider angiomatoma, digital clubbing

Disease Info: Glycogenosis Type IV

Infants with this rare form of glycogen storage disease often present around the first birthday with findings of hepatic cirrhosis, an enlarged nodular liver and splenomegaly. Hypotonia and muscular atrophy are usually present and may be severe. Treatment is symptomatic and palliative. Transplantation of the liver is curative in predominant liver disease; untransplanted patients usually succumb to complications of cirrhosis before the age of 3 years. Cardiomyopathy and myopathy are often present.

The disorder is due to a deficiency of the branching enzyme α-1,4-glucan: α-1,4-glucan-6-glucosyl transferase that leads to a decrease in the number of branch points making for a straight chain of insoluble glycogen like starch or amylopectin. The content of glycogen in liver is not elevated, but the abnormal structure appears to act like a foreign body causing cirrhosis. The diagnosis can be established by enzyme assay of leucocytes, cultured fibroblasts, or liver.

α1-Antitrypsin deficiency (see textbox chapter C2 page 4) is an important cause of neonatal cholestasis as well as of chronic active hepatitis (v. r.). In patients with α1-antitrypsin deficiency manifesting cholestatic liver disease in infancy, cholestasis gradually subsides before 6 months of age and patients become clinically unremarkable. However, 20–40% of these children develop hepatic cirrhosis in childhood.

Remember

About 50% of apparently healthy children with the homozygous Pi-ZZ phenotype have subclinical liver disease, as indicated by elevated levels of aminotransferases and γ-glutamyltranspeptidase.

In the presence or absence of a history of neonatal cholestasis or hepatits, α1-antitrypsin should be quantified in any child, adolescent, or adult with unexplained liver disease.

C2.5 Hepatomegaly

Hepatomegaly is often the first clinical sign of liver disease. Two clinical aspects are helpful to the diagnostic evaluation of the patient: first, the presence or absence of splenomegaly and second, the consistency and structure of the enlarged liver.

Remember

Splenomegaly, especially hepatosplenomegaly, is the hallmark of storage diseases.

Functional impairment of the liver, such as decreases of coagulation factors and serum albumin or impaired glucose homeostasis, is usually absent in lysosomal storage diseases, and aspects of liver cell integrity are unremarkable. Exceptions are Niemann–Pick diseases, both the types A/B and C (Table C2.11). In lysosomal storage diseases, the liver and spleen are firm but not hard on palpation. The surfaces are smooth and the edges easily palpated. The liver is not tender. There may be a protuberant abdomen and umbilical hernias. Hepatosplenomegaly may lead to late hematological complications of hypersplenism. A presumptive diagnosis of lysosomal storage disease is strengthened by involvement of the nervous system and/or mesenchymal structures resulting in coarsening of facial appearance and skeletal abnormalities. Macroglossia makes a

Table C2.11 Differential diagnosis of hepatomegaly

Age of presentation	Diseases to be considered	Additional findings
<3 Months	Lysosomal storage diseases, specifically	Splenomegaly
	Wolman disease	Adrenal calcifications
	CDG syndrome type I	Lipodystrophy, inverted nipples
	Defects of gluconeogenesis	$\Downarrow$ Glucose, $\Uparrow$ lactate
	Mevalonic aciduria	Severe failure to thrive, splenomegaly, anemia
3 Months–2 years	Glycogen storage diseases	$\pm \Downarrow$ Glucose, $\Uparrow$ lactate, $\Uparrow$ lipids, myopathy
	Defects of gluconeogenesis	$\Downarrow$ Glucose, $\Uparrow$ lactate
	Lysosomal storage diseases	Splenomegaly
	α1-Antitrypsin deficiency	$\Downarrow \alpha$1-Globulin, $\Downarrow \alpha$1-antitrypsin
>2 Years	Hemochromatosis	Diabetes mellitus, hypogonadism
	Cystic fibrosis	Pulmonary involvement, malnutrition, $\Uparrow$ sweat chloride
	Lysosomal storage diseases, specifically	Splenomegaly
	Niemann–Pick, type B	Pulmonary infiltrates
	Cholesterol ester storage disease	Hypercholesterolemia
	Glycogenosis type VI/IX	$\pm \Downarrow$ Glucose, $\Uparrow$ lactate, $\Uparrow$ CK
	Fanconi–Bickel syndrome	Fanconi syndrome

storage disorder virtually certain. In addition, slow gradual progression is evident.

The diagnostic work-up for lysosomal storage disorders in a patient with hepatosplenomegaly may start with the investigation of mucopolysaccharides and oligosaccharides in urine. Positive results are followed up with confirmatory enzymatic studies. If mucopolysaccharides and oligosaccharides are negative, lymphocytes are investigated for vacuoles (D5 – Pathology). If negative, bone marrow is investigated for storage cells. If storage cells are found, corneal clouding is sought with a slit lamp. If both are present, N-acetylglucosaminylphosphotransferase is determined to make a diagnosis of mucolipidoses II or III. If corneal clouding is not present, potential enzymes to be determined are sphingomyelinase (Niemann–Pick type I, A and B), acid lipase (Wolman), and cholesterol uptake and storage (Niemann–Pick type II or C). If there are neither pathological urinary screening results nor storage cells but peripheral neuropathy, the activity of ceramidase is determined seeking a diagnosis of Farber disease. Histological, histochemical, electron microscopical, and chemical examinations may be required of biopsied liver (D5 – Pathology).

Any acutely developing liver disease due to infectious, inflammatory, toxic, or metabolic origin may cause hepatomegaly as a result of edema and/or inflammation. In these disorders, other manifestations of the disease have usually led to consultation, and hepatomegaly is discovered during physical examination. On palpation, the liver may feel firm but not hard and the surface is smooth. The liver may be tender. Clinical or routine clinical chemical studies (Table C2.1) are likely to reveal abnormalities which direct further diagnostic evaluation. Inherited metabolic diseases considered in this category have been discussed under acute or subacute hepatocellular necrosis (Table C2.5).

If the enlarged liver feels hard, is not tender, and has sharp or even irregular edges, a detailed evaluation of causes of cirrhosis should be performed even in the presence of unremarkable liver function tests. A hard irregular or nodular surface is virtually pathognomonic of cirrhosis. Metabolic causes of silent liver disease associated with hepatomegaly, which may lead to quiescent cirrhosis are Wilson disease and α1-antitrypsin deficiency. Another important metabolic disorder is hemochromatosis, in which hepatomegaly may be the only manifestation in adolescence and young adulthood. Although this disease usually does not progress to hepatic failure, as does Wilson disease, early recognition and initiation of treatment allows the prevention of irreversible sequels.

In patients with persistent isolated hepatomegaly, additional findings are helpful in the differential diagnosis and should be specifically sought (Table C2.12). Defects of gluconeogenesis result in severe recurrent fasting hypoglycemia and lactic acidosis (Table C2.13). Of the three enzymatic *defects of gluconeogenesis*,

Table C2.12 Differential diagnosis of metabolic causes of hepatomegaly

Additional findings	Suggestive disorder
Cardiomyopathy	Glycogenosis III, hemochromatosis, phosphoenolpyruvate carboxykinase deficiency, disorders of fatty acid oxidation and of oxidative phosphorylation
Muscular weakness	Glycogenoses III, IV, VI, and IX, fructose intolerance, disorders of fatty acid oxidation and of oxidative phosphorylation
Enlarged kidneys	Glycogenosis I, Fanconi–Bickel syndrome
Renal Fanconi syndrome	Glycogenoses I and III, Wilson disease, fructose intolerance, tyrosinemia type I, Fanconi–Bickel syndrome, mitochondrial disorders
Hemolytic anemia	Wilson disease, fructose intolerance
Fasting intolerance, hypoglycemia	Glycogenoses I and III, fructose-1,6-diphosphatase deficiency, disorders of fatty acid oxidation and of oxidative phosphorylation
Diabetes mellitus, hypogonadism	Hemochromatosis
Neurologic deterioration (Kayser–Fleischer ring)	Wilson disease
Early onset emphysema	α1-Antitrypsin deficiency
Susceptibility to infections	Glycogenoses Ib/c
Malnutrition	Cystic fibrosis
Lipodystrophy, inverted nipples	CDG syndrome type I
Isolated	Glycogenosis Typ IX

Table C2.13 Hepatomegaly plus hypoglycemia

Disorder	Clinical features
Glycogen storage disease I	Hepatocellular dysfunction, large kidneys, ↑↑↑ triglycerides, ↑ urate, ↑ lactate
Glycogen storage disease III	Short stature, skeletal myopathy
Fanconi–Bickel disease	Tubulopathy, glucose/galactose intolerance
Disorders of gluconeogenesis	↑ Lactate
Glycosylation disorders (CDG, e.g., type Ib)	Hepatomegaly, hepatocellular dysfunction, protein losing enteropathy, multisystem disease

hepatomegaly is a consistent finding in fructose-1, 6-diphosphatase deficiency, while patients with deficiency of pyruvate carboxylase or phosphoenolpyruvate carboxykinase tend to present with lactic acidemia and multisystem disease without hepatomegaly.

Confronted with an infant or young child with a moderately enlarged smooth, soft liver and otherwise completely unremarkable history and physical examination, investigations may be postponed until confirmation of persistence of hepatomegaly on repeat clinical examinations a few weeks later. If unexplained hepatomegaly persists or additional indications of liver disease develop, a liver biopsy should be obtained for histological and electron microscopic investigation. Additional tissue should be frozen at −80°C for biochemical analyses. Patients with hepatomegalic glycogenoses may present with a moderately enlarged smooth, soft liver and otherwise completely unremarkable history and physical examination in infancy and early childhood. Similarly, patients with hemochromatosis may present with hepatomegaly without additional symptoms in late childhood and adolescence.

Disease Info: Hemochromatosis

Recessively inherited hemochromatosis is one of the most common genetic disorders in Caucasians; prevalence rates are between 2 and 5/1,000. Hepatomegaly is the most frequent early manifestation. Usually it develops in adolescence or young adults. Additional symptoms that may be present include diabetes milltus, hypogonadism, skin pigmentation, recurrent epigastric pain, cardiac arrhythmias, and congestive heart failure.

Hemochromatosis is usually considered as an adult disorder; however, early manifestations are being increasingly recognized in adolescents and children.

The value of early diagnosis cannot be overemphasized, because optimal outcome can be achieved through treatment of pre- or oligo-symptomatic patients, before the onset of irreversible damage. Laboratory investigations of symptomatic patients reveal increased concentrations of iron and ferritin in serum, as well as increased saturation of transferrin of 77–100%. The diagnosis of hemochromatosis is made by determination of the iron content of the liver. Molecular methods are now available, as there are only two major mutations that account for nearly all the mutant alleles.

C2.5.1 The Glycogenoses

Isolated hepatomegaly is found in several glycogen storage diseases. The combined frequency varies considerably according to the ethnic background and approximates 1:20,000–1:25,000 in Europe. The original description was by von Gierke in 1929, and glycogenoses were the first inborn errors of metabolism defined enzymatically by Cori and Cori in 1952. The current classification of the glycogenoses has been extended to nine entities. Glycogenosis type 0, also referred to as aglycogenosis, is the deficiency of glycogen synthetase. As the glycogen content in the liver is actually reduced, it is not a storage disorder but a disorder of gluconeogenesis (see also Chap. B2.4). The symptoms of glycogenoses types II, V, VII, and sometimes IV are primarily those of muscle disease.

Advances in techniques of enzymatic and molecular diagnosis may provide definitive diagnosis without requiring liver biopsy. However, quantitative determination of the glycogen content of the liver is still necessary in the work-up of many patients with suspected glycogen storage disease. Glucagon challenges may be helpful in glycogenoses I and III (see (D8) Function Tests-Monitored Prolonged Fast and Glucagon Stimulation).

Disease Info: Glycogen Storage Disease Type I

Glycogen storage disease type I results from a deficiency of any of the proteins of the microsomal membrane-bound glucose-6-phosphatase complex. In classic Ia glycogen storage disease (von Gierke disease), glucose-6-phosphatase is deficient. Type Ib is due to defective microsomal transport of glucose-6-phosphate, Ic to defective transport of phosphate, and Id due to defective transport of glucose. Molecular studies contradict types Ib and Ic as separate entities. They are both caused by mutations in the glucose-6-phosphate translocase and should be taken together as glycogen storage disease type I b/c or type non-a. A variant type Ia results from a deficiency of the regulatory protein; this has so far only been reported in a single patient.

The hallmark of von Gierke disease is severe fasting hypoglycemia with concomitant lactic acidosis, elevation of free fatty acids, hyperlipidemia, elevated transaminases, hyperuricemia, and metabolic acidosis. Lactic acidosis may be further aggravated by ingestion of fructose and galactose, as the converted glucose is again trapped by the metabolic block in the liver. Affected patients may be symptomatic in the neonatal period, when there may be hepatomegaly, hypoglycemic convulsions, and ketonuria. However, the condition often remains undiagnosed until hypoglycemic symptoms reappear in the course of intercurrent illnesses or, when the infant begins to sleep longer at night, at 3–6 months of age. Infants are chubby in appearance, but linear growth usually lags. The liver progresses slowly in size. An immense liver down to the iliac crest is generally found by the end of the first year when the serum triglycerides reach very high levels. Because of the accumulation of lipid the liver is usually soft and the edges may be difficult to palpate. With increasing activity of the child at around the first birthday, the frequency of hypoglycemic symptoms tends to increase. As in any of the diseases that cause severe hypoglycemia, convulsions and permanent brain injury or even death may occur. However, many children are quite adapted to low glucose levels, and in the untreated state, the brain may be fuelled by ketone bodies and lactate. Unusual patients may remain clinically asymptomatic of hypoglycemia until up to 2 years of age. Increased bleeding tendency may result in severe epistaxis and multiple hematomas, and abnormal hemostasis and persistent oozing may complicate traumatic injuries or surgery.

Patients with glycogen storage disease type I non-a (type Ib/c) develop progressive neutropenia and impaired neutrophile functions during the first year of life. As a result, recurrent bacterial infections result including deep skin infections and abscesses, ulcerations of oral and intestinal mucosa, and diarrhea. In the second or third decade inflammatory bowel disease may develop.

In the presence of a suspicion of glycogen storage disease type I, diagnosis is ascertained by liver biopsy. Hepatocytes are usually swollen because of extensive storage of glycogen and lipids. The structure of the glycogen stored is normal. Care must be taken to obtain enough liver to allow the assay of glucose-6-phosphatase and, if need be, associated transport proteins. Primary molecular diagnosis of glycogen storage disease type Ia and Ib/c is becoming increasingly available. This is helpful in obviating liver biopsy.

Several late complications have been observed in patients with type I glycogen storage diseases despite treatment. Most patients have osteoporosis and some have spontaneous fractures. Hyperuricemia may result in symptomatic gout after adolescence. Xanthomas may develop. Pancreatitis is another consequence of hypertriglyceridemia. Multiple hepatic adenomas develop, sometimes to sizable tumors. They are usually benign; however, malignant transformation has occurred. Renal complications include a Fanconi syndrome, hypercalciuria, nephrocalcinosis, and calculi. Microalbuminuria may be followed over time by proteinuria, focal segmental glomerulosclerosis, intestitial fibrosis, and renal failure. Pulmonary hypertension is a rare, although very serious, complication in adult patients.

Disease Info: Glycogen Storage Disease Type III

Glycogen storage disease type III results from a deficiency of the debranching enzyme, amylo-1,6-glucosidase. The physical and metabolic manifestations of liver disease are usually less severe than in type I glycogenosis, and fasting intolerance gradually diminishes over the years. The predominant long-term morbidity of this disease is myopathy. In infancy it may be impossible to distinguish type I and III on clinical grounds. Hypoglycemia and convulsions with fasting, cushingoid appearance, short stature, and nosebleeds characterize either disease. However, in contrast to type I glycogenosis, concentrations of uric acid and lactate are usually normal. The transaminases are elevated. Creatine phosphokinase level is elevated as well. This may be the earliest evidence of myopathy.

In glycogen storage disease type III, glycogen accumulates in muscle as well as in the liver. In approximately 85% of patients, both the liver and muscle are affected, and this is referred to as glycogenosis type IIIa. When the deficiency is only found in the liver, it is referred to as IIIb.

With time in many patients the major problem is a slowly progressive distal myopathy. It is characterized by hypotonia, weakness, and muscle atrophy. It is often notable in the interossei and over the thumb. Some patients have muscle fasciculations, suggestive of motor neuron disease, and storage has been documented in peripheral nerves. Weakness tends to be slowly progressive. Ultimately the patient may be wheel-chair bound. Rarely, the myocardium may be involved as well with left ventricular hypertrophy or even clinical cardiomyopathy.

Several functional tests have been designed to differentiate glycogen storage disease type I from type III. Following a glucose load the initially elevated blood lactate will decrease in glycogenosis type I. In type III, lactate levels are usually normal but rise postprandially. In type I gluconeogenesis is blocked and alanine concentration is increased. In type III, gluconeogenesis is overactive, resulting in significantly lowered concentrations of alanine. One of the most useful tests is a glucagon challenge 2–3 h after a meal, which will yield a good response in GSD type III (but no increase in glucose in GSD type I). After a 14-h fast, glucagon will not usually provoke a rise in blood glucose in GSD type III, as all the terminal glycogen branches have been catabolized (see E7 – Function Tests, Monitored Prolonged Fast and Glucagon Stimulation). Finally, the diagnosis of glycogenosis type III is proven by demonstrating the deficiency of the debranching enzyme amylo-1,6-glucosidase in leukocytes, fibroblasts, liver, or muscle. Prenatal diagnosis is possible through enzyme analysis in amniocytes or chorionic villi.

Defects of the phosphorylase system are sometimes listed as two or even three separate groups of glycogen storage diseases. When done this way, the category type VI is then restricted to rare primary defects of hepatic phosphorylase, type VIII to impaired control of phosphorylase activation, and type IX to deficient activity of the phosphorylase kinase complex. The phosphorylase kinase complex consists of four different tissue-specific subunits. By far the most common of these defects is an X-linked recessive defect of the α-subunit of phosphorylase kinase, which affects ≈75% of all patients with defects of the phosphorylase system (type IXa).

Disease Info: Glycogen Storage Diseases Type VI, VIII, and IX

The clinical symptoms of defects of the phosphorylase system, types VI, VIII, and IX glycogenoses, are similar to, but milder than in, types III or I. Hepatomegaly is a prominent finding, and may be the only indication of a glycogen storage disease. Muscle hypotonia, tendency to fasting hypoglycemia, lactic acidosis, elevation of transaminases, and hypercholesterolemia are mild and may be normal after childhood.

Following a glucose or a galactose load in glycogenoses type VI, VIII, and IX blood lactate will show pathological increase from normal or only moderately elevated levels. Overactive gluconeogenesis results in lowered concentrations of plasma alanine. The response to the administration of glucagon even after a 12–14h fast is usually normal. Diagnosis of glycogenoses type VI, VIII, and IX can be proven by demonstration of the enzyme deficiency in the affected tissue, liver, or muscle. Primary molecular diagnosis has greatly facilitated the diagnostic process.

The rare hepatic glygogenosis with renal Fanconi syndrome (Fanconi–Bickel syndrome, glycogen storage disease type XI) was shown to be due to a primary defect of the liver-type facilitated glucose transport. Hepatomegaly with glycogen storage, intolerance to galactose, failure to thrive and consequences of full-blown Fanconi syndrome are usually obvious in early childhood.

Remember

Type I glycogenosis is the most serious of all hepatic glycogenoses because it leads to a complete blockage of glucose release from liver, impairing both glucose production from glycogen and gluconeogenesis.

Key References

Green A (ed) (1994) The liver and inherited diseases. J Inher Metab Dis 14(Suppl 1)

Kelly DA (ed) (2004) Diseases of the liver and biliary system. Blackwell, UK

Suchy FJ (ed) (2007) Liver disease in children, 3rd edn. Cambridge University Press, Cambridge, MA

Gastrointestinal and General Abdominal Symptoms

Stephen G. Kahler

Key Facts

> Vomiting is typical of the organic acidurias and hyperammonemic syndromes.
> Pain and constipation occur in the porphyrias and familial fevers.
> Pancreatitis occurs with many organic acidurias, lipid and fatty acid disorders, and defects of oxidative phosphorylation.
> Malabsorption and diarrhea can be due to disorders of digestive enzymes, especially disaccharidases, defects of carrier proteins, and mitochondrial dysfunction.
> Ascites occurs in many lysosomal disorders.

C3.1 General Remarks

Gastrointestinal manifestations of metabolic disorders include vomiting, diffuse abdominal pain, pancreatitis, slowed transit time and constipation, maldigestion and malabsorption (which may result in diarrhea), and ascites. These symptoms may occur as part of a systemic disorder of intermediary metabolism in which other symptoms predominate, or as the major or exclusive symptoms.

C3.2 Vomiting

Vomiting is a characteristic feature of many disorders of intermediary metabolism, including those characterized by acidosis (the organic acidurias), hyperammonemia due to disorders of the urea cycle, and fatty acid oxidation defects (Table C3.1). Initial laboratory investigations for vomiting, including acid–base balance, lactate, ammonia, and urinary organic acids, can point the way to a diagnosis.

Chronic or recurrent vomiting in infancy, leading to formula changes before the underlying acidosis is discovered, is a common event in the organic acidurias due to defects in the metabolism of branched-chain amino acids – propionic, methylmalonic, isovaleric acidurias, etc. (see also Chap. B2.2).

The hyperammonemia of disorders of the urea cycle often provokes vomiting. In severe cases, this will be rapidly followed by deterioration of the level of consciousness, but in milder cases the vomiting can be intermittent. Hyperammonemia can also be prominent in the fatty acid oxidation disorders, especially MCAD deficiency. Symptoms in these disorders occur intermittently and are triggered by fasting or intercurrent infections. The appropriate investigations are discussed in more detail in Chap. B2.5.

Vomiting will lead to alkalosis, so the discovery of acidosis when investigating a vomiting infant or child should immediately raise the possibility of an underlying organic aciduria, or loss of base (e.g., renal tubular acidosis).

Remember

Hyperammonemia can provoke hyperventilation, leading to respiratory alkalosis, so the discovery of alkalosis when acidosis is expected (i.e., during a

S. G. Kahler
Department of Pediatrics, Division of Clinical Genetics, University of Arkansas for Medical Sciences, 4301 W. Markham Street, Little Rock, AR 72205, USA
e-mail: KahlerStepheng@uams.edu

G. F. Hoffmann et al. (eds.), *Inherited Metabolic Diseases*,
DOI: 10.1007/978-3-540-74723-9_C3, © Springer-Verlag Berlin Heidelberg 2010

work-up for suspected sepsis, especially in an infant) should immediately lead to measurement of the blood ammonia level.

C3.2.1 Cyclic Vomiting of Childhood (Ketosis and Vomiting Syndrome)

Vomiting is a prominent feature of a relatively common and poorly understood condition characterized by ketosis and abdominal pain, and triggered by fasting, often in the setting of infection – otitis, etc. In some children, episodes can also be provoked by strenuous exercise. Typically episodes begin in the second year and usually end the latest with puberty. The abdominal pain may be intense, similar to that which occurs in diabetic ketoacidosis. Urinary organic acid analysis shows prominent ketosis, but no pathological metabolites, and acylcarnitine analysis shows prominent acetylcarnitine. Treatment with intravenous glucose usually results in rapid resolution of symptoms. Phenothiazine antiemetics are of limited use, but ondansetron can be quite beneficial. Reassurance that this condition is difficult but not dangerous is helpful. Very few patients with this pattern of symptoms have been shown to have deficiencies of β-ketothiolase or succinyl-CoA:3-oxoacid CoA transferase. Abdominal migraine appears to be the

explanation in others. However, there remain a substantial number of children with this syndrome for whom a coherent explanation has not yet been found. Impaired uptake of ketones into peripheral tissues has been suspected. This disorder is sometimes confused with ketotic hypoglycemia, but the blood glucose level is not abnormally low, the patients do not have the slight body build of many children with ketotic hypoglycemia, and the treatments for ketotic hypoglycemia (avoiding fasting, cornstarch at bedtime, etc.) do not seem to be particularly beneficial in cyclic vomiting.

C3.3 Abdominal Pain

Crampy abdominal pain occurs with intestinal dysfunction – malabsorption, infectious diarrhea, etc., or mechanical problems, while diffuse pain is often due to an inflammatory response. Metabolic disorders are usually not considered until several episodes of abdominal pain have occurred without an obvious explanation. This section will address diffuse abdominal pain; pancreatitis is discussed separately. Abdominal pain due to the disorders discussed below is often intense, and may lead to surgical exploration for suspected appendicitis. Recent advances in imaging may help in lessening unnecessary surgery. On the other hand, when the patient has a metabolic disorder associated with recurrent abdominal pain, the physician must be careful during each episode that appendicitis or another surgical problem is not being attributed to the metabolic disorder.

C3.3.1 The Porphyrias

The porphyrias are disorders of the synthesis of heme, a component of cytochromes as well as hemoglobin. Diffuse or colicky abdominal pain and constipation occur in three of the hepatic porphyrias – acute intermittent, variegate, and hereditary coproporphyria. All three show autosomal dominant inheritance, and enzyme activity is typically ~50% of normal. The dominant porphyrias are among the few dominantly inherited enzymopathies.

Symptoms are uncommon in childhood. Episodes of illness in all three of the dominant porphyrias with abdominal symptoms appear to be related to increased

Table C3.1 Important causes of vomiting in metabolic disorders

Neonatal/early infancy or later, with or without encephalopathy
　　Organic acidurias
　　Urea cycle defects/hyperammonemia syndromes
　　Fatty acid oxidation disorders
With severe abdominal pain
　　Porphyrias (acute intermittent porphyria, coproporphyria, variegate porphyria)
　　As a symptom of associated pancreatitis
With acidosis/ketoacidosis
　　Organic acidurias
With liver dysfunction
　　Organic acidurias (chronic or recurrent)
　　Urea cycle defects/hyperammonemic syndromes
　　Galactosemia
　　Fructose intolerance
　　Tyrosinemia type I
　　Fanconi–Bickel syndrome
　　Fatty acid oxidation disorders (acute)

activity of the first step of porphyrin synthesis, δ-aminolevulinic acid synthase. Although many of the porphyrias intermittently have the characteristic red (or dark) urine, this feature is not always evident, especially in coproporphyria. Many of the porphyrias have prominent photodermatitis, with reddening and easy blistering after sun exposure; hypertrichosis can also occur. In unusual cases, an individual (doubly heterozygous) may have more than one form of porphyria and present with severe symptoms, even in childhood.

Acute intermittent porphyria (which does not have skin lesions) is the commonest form in most populations. It is due to deficient activity of porphobilinogen (PBG) deaminase (also called hydroxymethylbilane synthase and previously known as uroporphyrinogen synthase). The incidence of carriers (heterozygote frequency) is generally thought to be 5–10/100,000, but it may be as high as 1 in 1000 (Northern Sweden). A large proportion (50–90%) has no symptoms. Episodes of mental depression, abdominal pain, peripheral neuropathy, or demyelination may be triggered by ethanol, barbiturates, oral contraceptives or other drugs, or hormonal changes, but often no precipitating factor can be identified.

Hereditary coproporphyria, due to defects in coproporphyrinogen III oxidase (coproporphyrin decarboxylase), is generally milder than acute intermittent porphyria, and is less likely to have neurological symptoms. Onset is unusual in childhood. The rare homozygote may have the onset of symptoms in infancy, with persistent jaundice and hemolytic anemia.

Variegate porphyria is due to protoporphyrinogen oxidase deficiency. The highest incidence is among Afrikaners in South Africa, where the heterozygote frequency is 3 per 1000; about half will have symptoms, typically triggered by medications, and made worse by iron overload (e.g., consider concurrent hemochromatosis). Heterozygotes rarely develop manifestations in childhood, but symptoms can begin as early as in infancy in the rare homozygote or compound

heterozygote. Photosensitivity is more common in variegate porphyria than in hereditary coproporphyria.

The diagnosis of any of the porphyrias can be difficult. Sometimes a positive family history of porphyria or illness suggestive of porphyria (depression, recurrent abdominal pain, etc.) will be present. Dark or red urine can be a major clue. A positive urine screening test (the Watson-Schwartz test or similar reaction) may be present only during acute illness and cannot be relied upon at other times. Urine PBG is quite reliable during times of clinical illness. Comprehensive evaluation of blood, urine, and stool for porphyrins is the most reliable diagnostic approach (see Table C3.2). In the conditions with abdominal pain erythrocyte porphyrins are normal. Determination of enzyme activities or molecular analyses should not be the primary diagnostic measure.

Diffuse abdominal pain also occurs in the familial fevers. *Familial Mediterranean fever* (FMF) is an autosomal recessive condition characterized by episodes of noninfective peritonitis, pericarditis, meningitis (Mollaret meningitis), orchitis, arthritis, and erysipelas-like erythroderma. Onset in childhood is common in the severe forms. Amyloidosis leading to renal failure can develop. FMF is so common in some ethnic groups, including Sephardic and Armenian Jews, and some Arab communities, that pseudodominant pedigrees are regularly encountered. Defects in pyrin (marenostrin), a protein in the myelomonocytic-specific proinflammatory pathway, is the underlying cause. Pyrin downregulates several aspects of the inflammatory response. Diagnosis is based on molecular testing of the FMF gene called MEVF. Most patients respond well to colchicine; interferon-alpha, thalidomide, etanercept, infliximab, and anikara have been helpful.

Autosomal dominant familial periodic fever is a similar disorder, much less common than FMF. It was originally reported in an Irish/Scottish family and called familial Hibernian fever. It is also called

Table C3.2 Characteristic laboratory findings in porphyrias with abdominal symptoms

Disease	OMIM	Enzyme	Urine	Stool
Acute intermittent porphyria	176000	Hydroxymethylbilane synthase	ALA, PBG, ±coproporphyrin	±Protoporphyrin
Hereditary coproporphyria	121300	Coproporphyrinogen oxidase	ALA, PBG, coproporphyrin	Coproporphyrin
Variegate porphyria	176200	Protoporphyrinogen oxidase	ALA, PBG, ±Coproporphyrin	Protoporphyrin, ±Coproporphyrin

ALA delta-aminolevulinic acid; *PBG* porphobilinogen

TNF-receptor-associated periodic fever syndrome (TRAPS) and is caused by mutations in the tumor necrosis factor receptor-1 gene TNFRSF1A.

Abdominal pain and fever also occur in mevalonic aciduria, in the form known as hyper IgD with periodic fever and in hemochromatosis.

C3.4 Pancreatitis

Pancreatitis remains one of the most mysterious of acute life-threatening conditions. Except for mechanical obstruction of pancreatic secretion due to gallstones, the mechanisms of pancreatitis are not understood, even when a precipitating or proximate cause is known, such as chronic ethanol use. Gallstones in children are usually associated with hemolytic disorders; in adults, there is often no obvious cause.

The organic acidurias primarily associated with pancreatitis are in the catabolic pathways for branched-chain amino acids. They include maple syrup urine disease, isovaleric aciduria, 2-methylcrotonyl-CoA carboxylase deficiency, propionic aciduria, methylmalonic aciduria, and β-ketothiolase deficiency. Acidosis, ketosis, vomiting, and abdominal pain are common during episodes of metabolic decompensation in these disorders, so pancreatitis may not be suspected. Conversely, pancreatitis may be the presenting illness in mild forms of these conditions, especially isovaleric acidemia. A search for an underlying organic aciduria (urine organic acids, plasma or blood acylcarnitines, and plasma amino acids) should therefore be part of the initial investigation of pancreatitis (Table C3.3).

Pancreatitis also occurs in disorders of oxidative phosphorylation, especially cytochrome oxidase deficiency, and MELAS syndrome due to mutations in the tRNA leucine gene, and carnitine-palmitoyl-CoA

transferase (CPT) I. Lipid disorders, especially hyperlipidemia due to lipoprotein lipase deficiency, and hypo/abetalipoproteinemia, are also often associated with pancreatitis. Homocystinuria due to cystathionine β-synthase deficiency is the aminoacidopathy most commonly associated with pancreatitis. Depletion of antioxidants (glutathione, vitamin E, selenium, etc.) may play a role in the pathogenesis of pancreatitis. The contribution of mutations in genes which can contribute to pancreatitis in other situations (e.g., CFTR, SPINK1, and PRSS1) is not yet known.

C3.5 Constipation/Slowed Transit/Pseudoobstruction

Constipation and pseudoobstruction occasionally are manifestations of systemic metabolic disease, although in most cases they are due to diet, habit, or intestinal motility abnormalities associated with neuronal dysfunction. The porphyrias are noted for constipation, especially during times of crisis. The syndrome of hyper IgD with fever may have constipation (c.f. FMF, in which diarrhea is more likely). Constipation may also be prominent in the Fanconi–Bickel syndrome of glycogen storage and renal tubular dysfunction and malonyl-CoA decarboxylase deficiency.

In the organic acidurias and hyperammonemias constipation can be troublesome. Altered bowel function may lead to decompensation of the primary metabolic disorder, because of the accumulation of intermediate compounds (e.g., propionate and ammonia) produced by gut flora. Treatment of the constipation can lead to significant improvement in metabolic control. Metronidazole is often used to alter bowel flora, to diminish the production of propionate or methylmalonate in patients with disorders of propionate metabolism

Table C3.3 First-line investigations for pancreatitis

Urinary organic acid analysis
Plasma amino acids
Plasma total homocysteine
Blood spot or plasma acylcarnitine analysis
Blood lipid profile (lipoprotein electrophoresis)
Selenium
Total glutathione
Zinc
Vitamins A, C, E
Calcium

C3.6 Ascites

Ascites is rarely the sole presenting symptom of metabolic disease, but it accompanies several of them. Ascites or hydrops occurs in many lysosomal diseases, including sialidosis (mucolipidosis I), galactosialidosis, sialic acid storage disease, Farber lipogranulomatosis, Gaucher disease, Niemann-Pick disease, mannosidosis, and mucopolysaccharidoses IV-A, VI. In severe or early-onset disorders, the ascites may occur before birth as nonimmune hydrops fetalis. Hydrops is especially common in MPS VII (Sly disease–β-glucuronidase deficiency).

C3.7 Diarrhea

Mitochondrial neurogastrointestinal encephalopathy syndrome (MNGIE) (myo-, neuro-, gastro-intestinal encephalopathy) is a generalized disorder of mitochondrial dysfunction. Onset of intestinal symptoms is in childhood or early mid adult life, and includes chronic diarrhea, stasis, nausea, and vomiting, resulting in impaired growth. Wasting and cachexia may occur. Skeletal growth may be retarded. There is eventual loss of longitudinal muscle, diverticuli (which may rupture), intestinal scleroderma, and pseudoobstruction. Electrophysiologic studies have shown visceral neuropathy with conduction failure. Prokinetic drugs have been generally ineffective. Lactic acidosis is often present. The extraintestinal symptoms are variable but typical of a mitochondrial disorder (see Table C3.4).

In vitro analysis of mitochondrial function reveals a variety of impairments, especially deficiency of complex I or complex IV, or combined deficits. Mitochondrial DNA analysis (liver and muscle) shows depletion and multiple DNA deletions. Recurrences in sibs, high frequency of parental consanguinity, and lack of vertical transmission are consistent with an autosomal recessive inheritance. Mapping of MNGIE to distal 22q has been followed by identification of pathologic mutations in the gene ECGF1 (platelet-derived endothelial growth factor). The gene product is also known as thymidine phosphorylase and gliostatin. Impaired function of this gene leads to impaired mitochondrial DNA synthesis. Mutations in POLG (DNA polymerase gamma) are another cause of MNGIE, but without leukodystrophy.

A similar autosomal recessive condition, whose cause is not known, has been called *oculogastrointestinal myopathy* or familial visceral myopathy with external ophthalmoplegia. There is destruction of the gastrointestinal smooth muscle, whereas the myenteric plexus appears normal. Abdominal pain, diarrhea, diverticuli, and dilatation of the bowel occur. Patients also suffer from a demyelinating and axonal neuropathy, focal spongiform degeneration of the posterior columns, ptosis, and external ophthalmoplegia. The onset is in childhood or adolescence, with death by age 30 in many patients. Most reports of this condition are from the 1980s, and there may be a considerable overlap with MNGIE, which was generally not excluded enzymatically or molecularly.

Chronic diarrhea also occurs in *Menkes disease*, perhaps because of autonomic dysfunction.

C3.8 Maldigestion

Generalized impairment of digestion due to pancreatic problems (e.g., cystic fibrosis) or liver disease is well known. Several disorders of digestion involve primary enzymes of carbohydrate metabolism (Table C3.5). A deficiency typically results in severe watery (osmotic) diarrhea when the affected substrate or its precursors are ingested. There may also be excessive gas production

Table C3.4 Extraintestinal manifestations in mitochondrial neurogastrointestinal encephalopathy syndrome

Organ	Findings
Growth	Slow; cachexia and wasting
Brain	Leukodystrophy
	Increased CSF protein
	Ataxia
Eye	Ophthalmoplegia, ptosis
Ear	Sensorineural deafness
Cranial nerves	Dysarthria, dysphonia, facial palsy
Heart	Heart block
Skeletal muscle	Ragged-red fibers, weakness
Peripheral nerves	Demyelinating neuropathy, axonal degeneration

Table C3.5 Disorders of carbohydrate digestion

Disorder	OMIM	Enzyme	Major substrate
Disaccharide intolerance I	222900	Sucrase/isomaltase	Sucrose
Disaccharide intolerance II – congenital alactasia	223000	β-Glycosidase complex – lactase, glycosylceramidase	Lactose
Disaccharide intolerance III – adult lactase deficiency	223100	β-Glycosidase complex – lactase, glycosylceramidase	Lactose
Trehalase deficiency	275360	Trehalase	Trehalose (mushrooms)
Not recognized	154360	Glucoamylase (maltase) I and II	

and bloating. All are autosomal recessive. The Pearson marrow-pancreas syndrome, usually caused by deletion of mitochondrial DNA, has exocrine pancreatic failure. The same deletion (and pancreas failure) can be found in Kearns–Sayre syndrome. Failure of the exocrine and/or endocrine pancreas and other endocrine organs may occur in a variety of other mitochondrial disorders (see Chap. D1).

C3.8.1 Disaccharide Intolerance I – Sucrase/Isomaltase Deficiency

This deficiency is a rare cause of infantile diarrhea, which becomes evident with the introduction of sucrose in the diet. There are several different mechanisms for enzyme deficiency, including impaired secretion, abnormal folding, deficient catalytic activity, and enhanced destruction.

C3.8.2 Disaccharide Intolerance II – Infantile Lactase Deficiency and Congenital Lactose Intolerance

Congenital lactase deficiency is extremely rare. In nearly all cases, lactase deficiency in infants and young children is *acquired* through infection and loss of the mature brush border.

Congenital lactose intolerance appears to be distinct from congenital lactase deficiency. In the former, there is excessive gastric absorption of lactose (leading to lactosemia and lactosuria), vomiting, failure to thrive, liver dysfunction, and renal Fanconi syndrome. This condition may be fatal if not recognized and treated by elimination of lactose from the diet. Interestingly, lactose becomes well tolerated after 6 months. The basis for this condition is not known.

C3.8.3 Disaccharide Intolerance III – Adult Lactase Deficiency

Adult lactase "deficiency" is a common polymorphism. In fact, declining expression of intestinal lactase during childhood is the usual state, mirroring the declining importance of milk in mammalian nutrition after infancy. In a few regions, including Northern Europe, unfermented milk remains an important dietary component after infancy. The ability to digest milk is clearly an advantage, so among individuals from those regions there are a minority with lactose intolerance. (It may be that the custom of drinking unfermented milk arose because of a chance mutation that interrupted the usual decline in lactase activity with age.) Intestinal lactase activity depends on the summed expression from both the alleles. Differences in lactase expression do not reside in the coding sequence itself but in a *cis*-acting regulatory element.

C3.9 Malabsorption

Malabsorption in metabolic disorders can be due to abnormalities in ion channels, transport molecules, carrier proteins for lipids, or cotransport molecules. Symptoms are attributable to the deficiency of the substance not being properly absorbed (i.e., essential fatty acids and fat-soluble vitamins), and the effects due to abnormally high amounts of the substance within the gut. Ion-channel defects distort the balance of water and electrolytes, leading to diarrhea; abnormalities of transport molecules lead to diarrhea; and deficiency of a cotransport molecule (e.g., intrinsic factor) can have major consequences because of the resulting deficiency of an essential nutrient. First-line investigations for metabolic causes of malabsorption should include stool pH and analysis of reducing substances in stool. Characterization of stool sugars will confirm what has been suggested by the history. A breath hydrogen test after dietary challenge can confirm malabsorption.

C3.9.1 Glucose–Galactose Malabsorption

Glucose–galactose malabsorption is clinically similar to sucrase/isomaltase deficiency –severe life-threatening watery diarrhea from early infancy. Elimination of glucose and galactose from the diet is necessary. Fortunately, fructose is well tolerated so a fructose-based formula is effective. This condition is most often recognized in middle Eastern Arab populations. The defect in the sodium–glucose cotransporter SGLT1 is due to mutations in the solute-carrier (SLC) gene SLC5A1.

C3.9.2 Electrolytes

C3.9.2.1 Chloride Diarrhea

In this recessively inherited form of diarrhea, there is voluminous watery diarrhea with high chloride content (greater than the sum of sodium and potassium), from an early age. Polyhydramnios is common, perhaps universal. The defect is in the brush-border chloride/bicarbonate exchange mechanism. Treatment with sodium and potassium chloride is effective. Mutations have been discovered in the gene SLC26A3.

Defects of the Na^+/H^+ exchange mechanism result in *sodium diarrhea* and metabolic acidosis. The presentation is similar to congenital chloride diarrhea, but the stool electrolyte composition shows high sodium and an alkaline pH. Treatment with oral Na–K–citrate will normalize the electrolyte status of the patient. Mutations have been found in the serine protease inhibitor gene SPINT2.

Microvillus inclusion disease is another recessive cause of intractable diarrhea in infancy, and perhaps the most common noninfectious cause. Jejunal biopsy shows intracytoplasmic inclusions, consisting of brush-border microvilli, suggesting that this is a disorder of intracellular transport, impairing assembly. Mutations have been found in the myosin type 5 gene (MYO5B).

C3.9.3 Protein-Losing Enteropathy

Protein-losing enteropathy, often due to infection or impaired function of intestinal lymphatics, is also a cardinal feature of the congenital disorder of glycosylation *CDG 1B* due to phosphomannose isomerase deficiency. There may be liver disease and a bleeding diathesis. Unlike the other CDG syndromes, mental retardation and severe neurological problems do not occur. Diagnosis is based on isoelectric focusing of transferrin and enzyme assay. Treatment with oral mannose is effective. The CDG syndromes are discussed in greater detail in Chap. C10.

C3.9.4 Amino Acids

The two main disorders of intestinal amino acid transport are those involving tryptophan and methionine.

Tryptophan malabsorption (*Hartnup disease*) occurs as an autosomal recessive disorder that may be clinically silent. The transport of several neutral amino acids in the intestine and kidney are involved, but tryptophan is the one most likely to be limiting. In the absence of adequate niacin in the diet there will be a deficiency of nicotinic acids and nicotinamide, resulting in a pellagra-like rash, light sensitivity, emotional instability, and ataxia. In severe cases, this can progress to an encephalopathy with delirium and seizures. There may be an increase in stool indoles and urinary indican, reflecting the action of intestinal bacteria on the unabsorbed tryptophan. The diagnosis is suggested by finding high urinary levels of the neutral amino acids alanine, serine, threonine, asparagine, glutamine, valine, leucine, isoleucine, phenylalanine, tyrosine, tryptophan, histidine, and citrulline. Plasma levels of these amino acids are normal or slightly low. Mutations have been found in the gene SLC6A19.

A few infants were reported to have *methionine malabsorption*. Clinical manifestations have included white hair, tachypnea, mental retardation, seizures, diarrhea, and a peculiar odor like that of hops drying in an oast house. The urine may show increased alpha-hydroxybutyric acid after a methionine load. The condition appears to be autosomal recessive. No new cases have been reported in several decades.

C3.9.5 Vitamins and Other Small Molecules

Vitamin B_{12}

The intricate story of vitamin B_{12} illustrates the interface between diet, digestion, absorption, and intermediary metabolism. Vitamin B_{12}, synthesized by microbes, is the precursor of substances known as cobalamins. Two forms are essential for human metabolism: Methylcobalamin is a cofactor for the remethylation of homocysteine to methionine, and adenosylcobalamin is used by methylmalonyl-CoA mutase. Defects of the cobalamin pathway can therefore cause problems with either or both of these reactions.

Vitamin B_{12} in food (primarily meat and dairy products) is first released by digestion in the stomach. It binds to specific glycoproteins (r-proteins), especially transcobalamin I (TC I). In the duodenum, the pancreatic proteases act to release B_{12} again, and it now binds to intrinsic factor produced by gastric parietal cells. The intrinsic factor-B_{12} complex (B_{12}–IF) binds to a specific receptor (cubilin) on ileal enterocytes. The receptors internalize the B_{12}–IF, which then dissociates. The absorbed B_{12} is then transported to the bloodstream, coupled to transcobalamin II (TC II). The B_{12}–TC II complex is the main way of distributing newly absorbed B_{12} to the tissues. However, most of the B_{12} in the bloodstream is bound to TC I, as methylcobalamin.

Autosomal recessive genetic defects in intrinsic factor or the ileal receptor system typically lead to megaloblastic anemia with neurologic changes (developmental delay, hypotonia, hyporeflexia, and coma). Onset is usually after the first year. Infants in the first year apparently do not depend on the ileal receptor system for B_{12} uptake, which explains the lack of symptoms in young infants with problems in this system. The receptor defect is the Imerslund–Grasbeck syndrome (megaloblastic anemia I), which may have proteinuria as well as anemia. Defects in TC II, on the other hand, become apparent in the first few months with megaloblastic anemia, failure to thrive, and neurological delay. Congenital B_{12} deficiency can occur in the offspring of vegan/vegetarian mothers who have not had adequate intake of B_{12}. Deficiency of B_{12} will lead to mild methylmalonic aciduria and hyperhomocysteinemia. Infants with congenital B_{12} deficiency may be first recognized by increased propionylcarnitine on newborn screening. Late-onset B_{12} deficiency is usually due to lack of intrinsic factor due to atrophic gastritis, other stomach problem, or an unexplained mechanism. The defects of B_{12} metabolism after uptake from the bloodstream lead to variant forms of homocystinuria, methylmalonic acidemia, or both.

Investigation of suspected B_{12} disorders includes determining erythrocyte indices, plasma homocysteine, acylcarnitine analysis for propionylcarnitine, and urine methylmalonic acid. Serum cobalamin levels are low in defects involving intrinsic factor and gut uptake, but are normal or close to it in TC II deficiency (see also Chap. D8).

Many transporters and their genes are now known – there are at least 360 members of the solute-carrier SLC system, organized into more than 40 groups. Clinical

Table C3.6 Disorders of transport molecules

Disorder	OMIM	Gene/transporter	Nutrient
Glucose/galactose malabsorption	606824	SCL5A1	Glucose, galactose
Thiamine-responsive megaloblastic anemia	249270	SCL19A2/ THTR1	Thiamine
Imerslund–Grasbeck syndrome; Norwegian type megaloblastic anemia	261100	CBN/ Cubulin or AMN	B_{12}–intrinsic factor complex
Systemic primary carnitine deficiency; carnitine uptake defect	212140	SLC22A5/ OCTN2	Carnitine
Acrodermatitis enteropathica	201100	SLC39A4/ ZIP4	Zinc
Hereditary folate malabsorption	229050	SCL46A1/ PCFT/ HCP1	Folate
Unknown		hRFT1	Riboflavin
Unknown		SCL5A6/ SMVT	Biotin, alpha lipoate, pantothenic acid

deficiencies of only a few are known at present. They include SCL19A2 for thiamine, SCL22A5/OCTN2 for carnitine, and SLC39A4 for zinc (Table C3.6).

Key References

Gross U, Hoffmann GF, Doss MO (2000) Erythropoietic and hepatic porphyrias. J Inherit Metab Dis 23:641–661

Hediger MA, Romero MF, Peng JB et al (2004) The ABCs of solute carriers: physiological, pathological and therapeutic implications of human membrane transport proteins. Introduction. Pflugers Arch 447:465–468

Kahler SG, Sherwood WG, Woolf D et al (1994) Pancreatitis in patients with organic acidemias. J Pediatr 124:239–243

Pfau BT, Li BU, Murray RD et al (1996) Differentiating cyclic from chronic vomiting patterns in children: quantitative criteria and diagnostic implications. Pediatrics 97:364–368

Kidney Disease and Electrolyte Disturbances

C4

William L. Nyhan

Key Facts

> Hypochloremic metabolic acidosis with increased anion gap points to classic metabolic disorders, e.g. methylmalonic acidemia.

> Renal tubular acidosis is hyperchloremic and there is no increase in anion gap; differential diagnosis is diarrheal disease.

> Urinary tract stone disease in pediatric populations should suggest an inborn error of metabolism.

> Renal Fanconi syndrome is the common result of several inherited metabolic disorders that cause renal tubular dysfunction.

> Renal tubular alkalosis is characteristic of the Bartter and Gitelman syndromes. Calcium excretion is decreased in Gitelman syndrome; it is normal or increased in the presence of defective genes, which cause Bartter syndrome.

C4.1 General Remarks

Kidney disease and disturbed fluid and electrolyte homeostasis are important sequelae of inherited metabolic disease. They may occur as presenting manifestations. Therapy must be addressed promptly and must be continued.

The most important renal manifestations of inherited metabolic disease are (recurrent) dehydration, renal tubular dysfunction, and/or urinary tract calculi and crystalluria (v.i).

Renal pathology may also lead to failure to thrive, myoglobinuria (Chap. C6), unusual odor (see B1 Table B1.1), and abnormal color (see B1 Table B1.2). Renal cystic disease is seen in Zellweger syndrome, carnitine palmitoyltransferase II deficiency, and multiple acyl-CoA dehydrogenase deficiency (glutaric aciduria type II) due to the deficiency of electron transfer flavoprotein (ETF) and ETF dehydrogenase. Multiple microcysts lead to congenital nephrotic syndrome in CDG-Ia (Table C4.1).

In methylmalonic aciduria, a major subset of patients develops a variety of renal manifestations leading to chronic renal failure. Isolated renal tubular dysfunction may lead to acidosis and hyperchloremia along with proximal renal tubular bicarbonate wasting. It may also be complicated by interstitial nephritis and renal glomerular failure. A hemolytic uremic syndrome has been observed in infants with cobalamin C disease, the combined methylmalonic aciduria and homocystinuria.

Renal disease is also a late complication of glycogenosis type I (von Gierke disease). These patients may develop proteinuria, increased blood pressure, urinary tract calculi, or nephrocalcinosis. Many of these manifestations have been attributed to hyperuricemia. However, there is also glomerulosclerosis and interstitial fibrosis leading to glomerular dysfunction that may end in renal failure.

Remember

Different types of renal pathology, but especially proximal tubular dysfunction (Fanconi syndrome) and focal segmental glomerulosclerosis, can be the result of a primary mitochondrial disorder.

W. L. Nyhan
Department of Pediatrics, University of California, UCSD School of Medicine, 9500 Gilman Drive, La Jolla, CA 92093, USA
e-mail: wnyhan@ucsd.edu

G. F. Hoffmann et al. (eds.), *Inherited Metabolic Diseases*,
DOI: 10.1007/978-3-540-74723-9_C4, © Springer-Verlag Berlin Heidelberg 2010

Table C4.1 Primary Renal Tubular Disorders

Cystinuria: amino acid transport defect
Diabetes insipidus: usually vasopressin receptor defect
Bartter syndrome: electrolyte transport defects in the loop of Henle
Gitelman syndrome: Na/Cl cotransport defect in the distal tubule
Hypophosphatemic rickets: pathological activation of fibroblast growth factor 23
Renal tubular acidosis (RTA) type I: deficient distal tubular H$^+$ secretion
RTA type II: deficient proximal tubular HCO$_3^-$ secretion
RTA type IV: reduced aldosterone effect, usually drug induced

Table C4.2 Recurrent Or Episodic Dehydration

Hyperchloremic acidosis	
Failure to thrive, rickets, polyuria	Renal tubular acidosis
	Cystinosis
Diarrhea	Lactase deficiency
	Sucrase, isomaltase deficiency, Glucose galactose malabsorption
	Acrodermatitis enteropathica
Hypochloremic alkalosis	
Polyuria	Bartter and Gitelman syndromes
Diarrhea	Congenital chloride diarrhea
Diarrhea, hypoproteine-mia, anemia	Cystic fibrosis
Vomiting	Pyloric stenosis, bulimia
Hypernatremia	Nephrogenic diabetes insipidus
	Diabetes insipidus
Hyponatremia, hyperkalemia	Congenital adrenal hyperplasias, adrenal aplasia, hypoplasia, pseudohypoaldosteronism
Hypochloremic acidosis	Propionic acidemia
Increased anion gap, ketoacidosis	Methylmalonic aciduria
	Diabetic ketoacidosis
	Isovaleric acidemia
	3-Oxothiolase deficiency

C4.2 Dehydration

Renal and electrolyte abnormalities present frequently with acidosis and dehydration, and this may be indicative of a metabolic disease (Table C4.2). More commonly, this picture of abnormal clinical chemistry is caused by infectious diarrhea.

Rarely, chronic diarrhea is caused by an inherited disorder of intestinal absorption (C3). Patients with clinical manifestations of dehydration, decreased skin turgor, depressed fontanel, sunken eyes, decreased urine output, or documented acute loss of weight are fortunately regularly assessed by measuring the electrolyte concentrations, acid–base balance, urea nitrogen, and creatinine in the blood. Among the clinical signs of dehydration is poor skin turgor. Not so widely known is the fact that turgor is measured by the relative rate that a pinched up piece of skin becomes restored to its resting state. In fact, in rats, measured weight loss in experimentally induced dehydration had a straight-line correlation with the stop-watched time of the skin to flatten.

Electrolyte analysis in the dehydrated patient with renal disease often reveals hyperchloremic acidosis. The anion gap is not increased. Most commonly, this picture results from acute diarrhea, although chronic diarrhea can lead to chronic acidosis and chronic dehydration. Hyperchloremic acidosis also results from renal tubular acidosis (RTA) (v-i).

Remember

Metabolic acidosis resulting from the classic inborn errors of intermediary metabolism is hypochloremic, and the anion gap is increased (Chap. B2-2).

Acute infectious diarrhea can precipitate an attack of metabolic imbalance in many inborn errors of metabolism, but in these situations the metabolic abnormality predominates and there is an anion gap. Dehydration resulting from inherited disease is also characterized by recurrent or episodic attacks of dehydration.

Remember

Metabolic acidosis with increased anion gap indicates either ketosis (→check ketostix, measure ketones in blood), the presence of pathological organic acids (→examine urinary organic acids, blood lactate), or both.

A combination of the electrolyte pattern and the clinical manifestations permits a ready dissection of the heritable causes of recurrent dehydration. Actually, many of the chronic diarrheas, such as the disaccharidase deficiencies, do not often lead to dehydration. Patients are so accustomed to their problem that they compensate with ample fluid intake. The water intake of infants and children with nephrogenic diabetes insipidus is enormous. These patients often get into trouble when exogenous forces such as intercurrent illness interfere with their ability to compensate. Admission to hospital and a requirement for parenteral fluids, even with fairly trivial surgery, can lead to major morbidity and mortality if physicians do not recognize and supply large quantities of water necessary to maintain these patients.

Hypochloremic alkalosis results from depletion of intracellular potassium resulting from intestinal losses. In small infants, it is the hallmark of pyloric stenosis. Infants with congenital chloride diarrhea and those with cystic fibrosis (CF) both have diarrhea, but those with CF are edematous from hypoproteinemia and pale from anemia. Those with Bartter syndrome and Gitelman syndrome do not have diarrhea. A teenager or adult with bulimia can mimic Bartter syndrome; so can one with chronic laxative abuse.

The adrenal hormone deficiency diseases are readily recognized in those females with ambiguous genitalia. They are often missed in those without, such as male infants with adrenal hyperplasia or infants with absent or hypoplastic adrenals or with pseudohypoaldosteronism. The hyponatremia and renal salt wasting and the hyperkalemia should be giveaways for the diagnosis.

C4.3 Urinary Tract Calculi

Kidney stones or calculi occurring anywhere in the urinary tract represent a common affliction among adults; they are rare in children. In adults, the composition of the stone is usually a salt or a mixture of salts of calcium, calcium oxalate, and calcium phosphate.

> **Remember**
>
> In total, 60–70% of calculi found in pediatric populations result from inborn errors of metabolism (Table C4.3) (Fig. C4.1).

Table C4.3 Urinary Tract Calculi

Stone	Disorder	Enzyme
Cystine	Cystinuria	
Uric Acid	Lesch–Nyhan	HPRT
	PRPP synthetase superactivity	PRPP synthetase
	Glycogenosis I	Glucose-6- phosphatase
	Renal hypouricemia	URAT1 (*SLC22A12* gene)
2,8-Dihydroxyadenine	APRT deficiency	APRT
Xanthine	Xanthinuria	Xanthine oxidase
Oxalate	Oxaluria, glycolic aciduria	Alanine:glyoxylate amino-transferase
	Oxaluria, glyceric aciduria	D-Glycerate dehydrogenase
Calcium salts	Hypercalciuria + uricosuria	Multifactorial
	Wilson disease	P-type ATPase transporter

HPRT hypoxanthine guanine phosphoribosyl transferase; *PRPP* phos-phoribosylpyrophosphate; *APRT* adenine-phosphoribosyltransferase; *ATPase* adenine triphosphatase

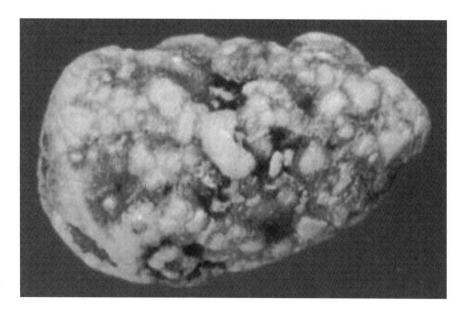

Fig. C4.1 Urinary calculus passed by a hyperuricemic 2-year-old boy with Lesch–Nyhan disease. Reprinted with permission from Nyhan et al. (2005)

Lithiasis in the urinary tract may present with pain, which is referred to as renal colic. This sudden onset pain is of such extreme intensity that it may lead to nausea and vomiting. The pain reflects the movement of a stone along the ureter, and may be well localized by the patient to this curvilinear distribution. Pain may disappear on entry of the calculus into the bladder, only to reappear on entry into the urethra. There may be associated frequency or dysuria. Some patients may have these symptoms as a result of crystalluria as well as with discrete stones. Hematuria can also result from crystalluria or calculi.

Remember

Clinical symptoms in small children with urinary tract calculi are often nonspecific (abdominal pain, nausea, vomiting, and recurrent urinary tract infections). Urinary tract ultrasound is indicated in all children with microhematuria.

Urinary tract infection is a common complication of urinary tract calculi. It may present with pyuria, dysuria, and fever. Infection will usually not disappear until the stone is removed, by passage, lithotripsy, or surgery. Repeated episodes of pyelonephritis and obstruction may lead to renal failure.

Patients with symptoms should not only be examined for the possibility of stones, but also those with diseases in which calculi are common should be monitored. Stones containing calcium are radiopaque, but urate stones (Fig. C4.1) are not; cystine stones are radiopaque but may be difficult to visualize roentgenographically. Ultrasonography is useful in detecting hydronephrosis or hydroureter, but may miss small stones. Intravenous urography is useful in delineating calculi and defining the presence or absence and degree of obstruction. Retrograde pyelography permits visualization without intravenous injection of the dye, but it requires cystoscopy. CT scan may permit detection of radiolucent stones not evident with other methods.

Cystinuria results from mutations in the gene, which is responsible for the cystine transporter of the kidney and intestine. It leads to increased urinary excretion of lysine, ornithine and arginine, as well as cystine. Only cystinuria causes symptoms, all the consequence of its lack of solubility and consequent formation of calculi. Treatment is by ensuring ample fluid throughout the day and also at night to keep cystine soluble. Cystine crystallizes at concentrations above 1,250 μmol/l at pH 7.5. Treatment with penicilliamine is effective by the formation of mixed disulfides with cysteine, which are soluble.

Uric acid stone disease is seen commonly in Lesch–Nyhan disease as well as the other variant hypoxanthine-guanine phosphoribosyltransferase deficiencies. Patients with phosphoribosyl-pyrophosphate (PRPP) synthetase superactivity and with glycogenosis type I also overproduce purine and excrete it as uric acid in large quantities. Deafness is common in patients with PRPP synthetase mutations. Other patients with uric acid calculi have uricosuria as a result of increased urate clearance by the kidney. Some well-defined kindreds have been reported. Most of them have normal blood concentrations of uric acid; some are hypouricemic and some, like the Dalmatian dog, are hyperuricemic. Mutations in the *SLC22A12* gene lead to abnormalities in URAT1, the predominant transporter of uric acid at the apical membrane of the renal tubule.

In interpreting values of uric acid in plasma or serum, it must be remembered that children have an especially high clearance capacity for uric acid and consequently can keep serum levels within normal ranges despite a pathologically increased endogenous production (Table C4.4). Urinary concentrations of uric acid give more reliable results. For diagnostic purposes, a random urine sample should be promptly analyzed for uric acid and creatinine. Age-related control ranges are summarized in Table C4.5.

Table C4.4 Investigations In Children With Renal Stones

Ultrasound scan of renal tract (stones? dilatation?)
Determine urinary oxalate, calcium, citrate, cystine (→ amino acids), uric acid (→ purines)
Urine microscopy
Consider intravenous urography, CT

Table C4.5 Uric Acid Excretion In Control Subjects

Age (years)	<2	2–4	4–8	8–10	10–12	>12
upper limit Ua/Crea	<2[a]	<1.5	<1.3	<1.1	<1.0	<0.8
lower limit Ua/Crea	<0.5[a]	<0.5	<0.4	<0.3	<0.3	<0.3

[a]In very young infants, especially, during the first week of life the standard deviation is extremely high (99th percentile between approximately 0.2 and 2.8)

Fig. C4.2 Massive calcium oxalate material obtained from a 6-month-old patient with hyperoxaluria type II

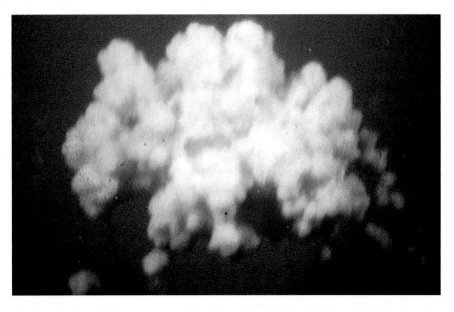

Table C4.5 provides estimates of uric acid/creatinine ratios in morning urine samples (Kaufman et al. 1968), which can be taken as a possible hint to either elevate or reduce excretion of uric acid. A few facts have to be borne in mind when interpreting uric acid excretion in spot urine samples in general and using this table in particular.

The figures are estimated from a continuously falling curve with varying standard deviations at different ages (Kaufman et al. 1968). By that they represent "forced mean values" for the given age group and give an approximation of the normal range of uric acid excretion. Patients with Lesch–Nyhan-Syndrome (HPRT deficiency) seem to be always clearly above those upper limits.

In patients with either "borderline findings" with this proposed uric acid/creatinine ratio or high clinical suspicion of primary or secondary disturbances of uric acid metabolism, a determination of the 24 h excretion corrected for body surface is probably more accurate. 520 ± 147/1.73 m^2/24 h (mean ± 1 SD) is given by Wilcox (1996) based on several previous publications. As an alternative, correction of uric acid excretion for creatinine clearance gives a constant value between 3 and 40 years of age: 0.34 ± 0.11 mg/dL of glomerular filtrate (mean ± 1 SD) according to Wilcox (1996). Glomerular filtrate was estimated from simultaneous measurement of serum creatinine (S_{cr}), urinary creatinine (U_{cr}), and urinary uric acid (U_{ua}) in overnight fasted patients. All the values are in mg/dL, using the following equation:

$(U_{cr}) \times (S_{cr})/(U_{cr})$ = uric acid excreted in mg/dL of glomerular filtrate.

Adenine phosphoribosyltransferase deficiency, common in Japanese, leads to increased excretion of the very insoluble dioxygenated derivative of adenine. Xanthine oxidase deficiency is associated with stones composed of the very insoluble xanthine and with hypouricemia. Xanthine stones are also observed in patients with hyperuricemia treated with allopurinol, but in many it is possible to find a dosage regimen that minimizes or avoids the propensity for stone formation, because hypoxanthine is very soluble.

The two forms of oxaluria, known as type I and type II, are characterized by very early onset renal stone disease (Fig. C4.2) and early renal failure. In type I, there is glycolic aciduria as well as hyperoxaluria, in type 2 there is glyceric aciduria. Successful treatment has combined transplantation of both liver and kidney. Hyperoxaluria and calcium oxalate calculus formation has also been reported in cystic fibrosis.

C4.4 Renal Tubular Dysfunction Fanconi Syndrome

The Fanconi syndrome represents a generalized disruption of renal tubular function in which the proximal tubular reabsorption of amino acids, glucose, phosphate, bicarbonate, and urate is impaired, leading to a generalized aminoaciduria, glycosuria, phosphaturia, uricosuria, and increased urinary pH. As a consequence, there is vitamin D-resistant rickets and osteomalacia.

Remember

Fanconi syndrome is characterized by polyuria and increased urinary excretion of amino acids, glucose, and phosphate (frequently also calcium, urea, and protein). Metabolic acidosis with increased urinary pH is common.

Obligatory polyuria in this syndrome can lead to clinically important dehydration, especially when fluid intake is restricted. Chronic hyperchloremic acidosis may worsen in acute situations. Losses of ions and metabolites in the urine may lead to symptomatic depletion. Thus, hypokalemia may lead to muscle weakness or even paralysis, constipation, and ileus, as well as disturbances of cardiac rhythm and function. Excretion of carnitine may deplete body stores and lead to disturbed fatty acid oxidation and hypoketotic hypoglycemia (Chap. B2-5), muscle weakness, or congestive cardiac failure. Losses of calcium may lead to tetany or convulsions. Hypomagnesemia may similarly develop. Shortness of stature or failure to thrive is seen regularly.

A number of genetically determined diseases lead to the Fanconi syndrome (Table C4.6). The most common of these is cystinosis (v.i.).

Among these disorders, associated syndromic features lead to the diagnosis and the appropriate confirmatory test. Hepatic dysfunction is seen in hepatorenal tyrosinemia, usually as the major clinical feature, and the diagnosis is made by urinary organic acid analysis for succinylacetone. Hepatic dysfunction is also seen along with cataracts in galactosemia and with hypoglycemia in hereditary fructose intolerance. Confirmation of each is by enzyme assay; in the latter liver is required; as an alternative mutational analysis may reveal the common Caucasian mutations. Fanconi syndrome has been reported in glycogenosis I, III, and XI. Type I can be diagnosed clinically by glucagon testing (Chap. D8 – Glucagon Stimulation), by enzyme assay of liver or by mutaion analysis. Currently, we reserve liver biopsy for those in whom mutational analysis does not provide the diagnosis. The clinical chemistry is in characterized by hypoglycemia, lactic acidemia, hyperalaninemia, hyperlipidemia, and hypercholesterolemia. Other renal complications are common in glycogenosis I, including distal renal tubular disease, amyloidosis, nephrocalcinosis, and calculi (v.s.). Renal failure may be a late complication with proteinuria, focal glomerulosclerosis, and interstitial fibrosis. In Lowe syndrome and Wilson disease, the full Fanconi picture is often absent from the urine, but a generalized aminoaciduria is the rule. In Wilson disease, the pattern also includes increased cystine and methionine, indices of the liver dysfunction. In electron transport defects, a variety of patterns of RTA is seen, including the complete Fanconi syndrome. Raised levels of lactate should

Table C4.6 Heritable Causes Of The Fanconi Syndrome

Disorder	Molecular defect or basis	Distinguishing characteristics
Cystinosis	Lysosomal cystine transporter	Corneal deposits, shortness of stature
Hepatorenal tyrosinemia	Fumarylacetoacetate hydrolase	Hepatic dysfunction
Galactosemia	Galactose-1-phosphate uridyltransferase	Hepatic dysfunction, cataracts, mental retardation
Hereditary fructose intolerance	Fructose-1-phosphate aldolase	Hepatic dysfunction, hypoglycemia
Glycogenoses	Glucose-6-phosphatase, amylo-1,6-glucosidase, phosphorylase-b-kinase	Hepatomegaly, hypoglycemia, hyperlipidemia, hypercholesterolemia, lactic acidemia
Fanconi–Bickel syndrome	GLUT2 mutations	Hepatomegaly
Lowe syndrome	OCRL-1 gene on Xq25–26, phosphatidylinositol 4, 5-biphosphate-5-phosphatase	Cataracts, glaucoma, hypotonia, developmental retardation
Wilson disease	P-type ATPase transporter	Hepatic dysfunction, Kayser–Fleischer ring, neurologic dysfunction
Electron transport defects	mtDNA deletions (Pearson, Kearns–Sayre), mtDNA depletion (RRM2B), cytochrome c oxidase, complex III or IV	Lactic acidemia, encephalomyopathy
Drugs	Outdated tetracycline, gentamycin, valproic acid, 6-mercaptopurine, azathioprine	
Heavy metal poison	Cadmium, lead, manganese	
Idopathic	—	

give the major clue. An early lethal mitochondrial DNA depletion syndrome caused by defects in the RRM2B gene characteristically results in the Fanconi syndrome.

In some clearly genetic kindreds with idiopatwhic Fanconi syndrome, a molecular defect has not been found, and these are classified as idiopathic. In addition, an acquired Fanconi syndrome has been observed with a variety of renal insults, including the ingestion of outdated tetracycline, 6-mercaptopurine, and heavy metal poisoning. Deficiency of vitamin D leads to a moderate generalized aminoaciduria, but not usually to the rest of the Fanconi syndrome.

C4.4.1 Cystinosis

Cystinosis is one of the most important causes of the Fanconi syndrome and as such manifests all the features of the syndrome (v.s.). In addition, there are some clinical manifestations that are unique to this disease. Patients generally have fair skin, hair, and irises. Ophthalmic abnormalities include photophobia that is caused by deposits of cystine in the cornea. These refractile crystalline bodies may be seen early by slit lamp. They may lead ultimately to thickened, hazy corneas and may be complicated by corneal ulcers. Crystalline cystine may also be identified in conjunctiva. In addition, there is a characteristic peripheral retinopathy visible as pigmentation and depigmentation. Some adults with the disease have been legally blind.

Hypothyroidism results late from deposition of cystine in the gland. Myopathy may follow cystine deposition in muscle or carnitine depletion because of losses in urine. Some patients have developed diabetes mellitus. Late neuologic abnormalities include tremor, seizures, or mental retardation. Hydrocephalus and cerebral atrophy have been documented. The diagnosis is usually made by the assay of cystine content in leukocytes or cultured fibroblasts. The molecular defect is in the transporter for cystine from lysosomes (Fig. C4.3).

> **Remember**
>
> Cystinosis is a lysosomal transporter defect that causes increased intracellular deposition of cystine crystals. Typical clinical features include failure to thrive, short stature, and renal tubular disease.

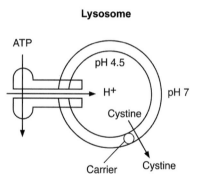

Fig. C4.3 The ATP-dependent lysosomal carrier-mediated efflux of cystine which is defective in patients with cystinosis. Reprinted with permission from Nyhan et al. (2005)

C4.4.2 Renal Tubular Acidosis

Renal tubular acidosis (RTA) includes the Fanconi syndrome and cystinosis (v.s.) (Table C4.7). A small population of patients have RTA without any of the features of the Fanconi syndrome. These patients fail to thrive as infants and display shortness of stature later. Vomiting is frequently encountered in infants, and many infants are anorexic. Infants are often described as irritable or apathetic. Metabolic bone disease manifests itself as rickets and osteomalacia, particularly, in proximal RTA. The diagnosis is often first suggested by roentgenographic examination of the bones of a patient with failure to thrive. Urolithiasis is sometimes seen in older patients with distal RTA.

A lowered serum bicarbonate, with hyperchloremia and a normal anion gap is characteristic. Patients seldom have an HCO_3^- over 19 mEq/L, but values are usually over 10 mEq/L. The serum bicarbonate is the most reliable indicator, as the pH and pCO_2 may change in a crying infant. Relative alkalinity of the urine is often the key to the diagnosis. In distal RTA, the urine pH remains high, and net excretion of acid is low even when the serum bicarbonate is low. In some patients, it may not be readily evident that in an acidotic patient a urinary pH of six may be relative alkalinity. Also, modern clinical chemistry laboratories have largely dispensed pH meters to determine urinary pH, and dipstix may be less than precise.

Defective acidification of the urine leads to renal losses of sodium and potassium and polyuria. Bone resorption leads to hypercalciuria. The serum calcium is normal. Phosphaturia may lead to hypophosphatemia. Alkaline phosphatase may be increased. The excretion of citrate may be low; with hypercalciuria

Table C4.7 Renal Tubular Acidosis

Type I (distal)	Isolated
	With deafness
	Hypergammaglobulinemia (Sjögren)
	Nephrocalcinosis (e.g., hyperparathyroidism, vitamin D poisoning)
	Drugs: amphotericin B, lithium tubulointerstitial disease, renal transplantation, obstruction
Type II (proximal)	Isolated
	Pyruvate carboxylase deficiency
	Methylmalonic acidemia
	Carbonic anhydrase II deficiency (with osteopetrosis)
	Drugs (acetazolamide)
Combined Type IV (distal hyperkalemic)	Isolated
	Carnitine palmitoyl transferase I deficiency
	Mineralocorticoid deficiency
	Pseudohypoaldosteronism
	Hyporeninemic, hypoaldosteronism (diabetes, NSAIDs)
	Drugs (spironolactone, amiloride, ACE inhibitors)

leading to nephrocalcinosis and nephrolithiasis. Renal ultrasonography is useful for early detection.

The distinction of the two major types of RTA, proximal RTA (sometimes called type II) and distal RTA (sometimes called type I), is best made by the assessment of urinary loss of bicarbonate and serum concentration during intravenous or oral loading with $NaHCO_3$ that causes a progressive increase in the serum level. This requires the collection of urine under oil and so maintained until analyzed. The fractional excretion of bicarbonate ($FEHCO_3\%$) is calculated as $UHCO_3/UCreatinine(Cr) \times SCr/SHCO_3 \times 100$, where U and S indicate urine and serum, respectively. The percentage in patients with distal RTA is less than 10, whereas in proximal RTA values of 10–15% are seen when the serum level is 20 mEq/L, and there may be a massive bicarbonaturia, over 15%. Patients with distal RTA and hyperkalemia may have values from 5 to 10%, whereas those with classic hypokalemia usually have values less than 5%. The hyperkalemic patients may represent a generalized tubular dysfunction and are sometimes referred to as type IV. These patients may have hypoaldosteronism, pseudohypoaldosteronism, or hyporeninemic hypoaldosteronism.

Some discrete syndromes are associated with RTA. Pyruvate carboxylase deficiency and methylmalonic aciduria are associated with proximal RTA. A mixed proximal and distal RTA is seen in patients with carbonic anhydrase deficiency in which there is a genetically determined syndrome of RTA, osteopetrosis, and cerebral calcifications. A mixed RTA is also seen in carnitine palmitoyltransferase I (CPTI) deficiency.

C4.4.3 Bartter Syndrome

Bartter syndrome is an uncommon cause of salt-wasting hypokalemic alkalosis in which calcium excretion is normal or increased. It is in this way distinguished from Gitelman syndrome, in which hypokalemic alkalosis is accompanied by hypocalciuria and hypomagnesemia.

Bartter syndrome (type 1) is caused by loss of function mutation in the Na–K–Cl co-transporter gene *SLC 12A*, previously called *NKCC2*, on chromosome 15q15–21, which codes for a protein that mediates electrolyte transport in the loop of Henle, at the site of action of the diuretics, furosemide, and butmetanide. Mutations in this gene have also been found in antenatal Bartter syndrome, in which ultrasonography has revealed fetal nephrocalcinosis in utero. Bartter syndrome is heterogeneous; patients with the typical syndrome have been found in whom the mutation was in the inwardly rectifying potassium channel, ROMK (*KCNJ1*), which recycles reabsorbed K^+ back into the tubule (type 2). The classic syndrome as described by Bartter (type 3) is caused by mutations in the renal chloride channel B gene *CLCNKB*. Infantile Bartter syndrome with sensorineural deafness (type 4) may be caused by mutation in the *BSND* gene or by simultaneous mutations in both the *CLCNKA* and *CLCNKB* genes. Bartter syndrome has also been reported in patients who turned out to have mutations in the calcium-sensing receptor (*CASR*) gene, in which loss of function mutations usually lead to hypocalciuria and secondary hyperparathyroidism, whereas gain of function mutations lead to hypercalciuria and hypocalcemia. In Bartter syndrome, presentation is usually prior to 5 years of age. The initial presentation may be with dehydration and hypovolemia. Some patients present with cramps or weakness in the muscles resulting from the hypokalemia. Some have had convulsions or tetany. Chvostek and Trousseau signs may be positive. There may be polyuria, nocturia, or enuresis.

A craving for salt is common. Some patients display vomiting, and constipation is common.

Shortness of stature or failure to thrive is the rule. Mental retardation has been observed in about two-thirds of the children. Some have had abnormal electroencephalography. Ileus has been observed, and attacks of hypoventilation, both also concomitants of hypokalemic alkalosis. Rickets has been reported rarely. Nephrocalcinosis has been observed in many, especially in those with the so-called antenatal or infantile forms of Bartter syndrome.

Hypokalemia, alkalosis, hyperaldosteronism, and hyperreninemia are regular laboratory findings, as is normal blood pressure. Bartter and colleagues noted unresponsiveness of the blood pressure to intravenous angiotensin II, and hypothesized that increased production of renin was a compensatory response to maintain blood pressure, and that aldosterone production was also stimulated. Volume expansion can reduce levels of renin and aldosterone. Histologically there is hyperplasia of the renal juxtaglomerular apparatus. There is increased renal prostaglandin production. Large urinary losses of sodium and potassium lead to contraction of volume. Hypokalemia is usually profound. The concentration is less than 2.5 mEq/L. Patients are unable to form a concentrated urine, and this isosthenuria does not respond to administration of antidiuretic hormone.

Less common laboratory findings include hypomagnesemia, hypocalcemia, and glucose intolerance without fasting hyperglycemia. Some patients have hyperuricemia, and clinical gout has been observed.

The differential diagnosis of Bartter syndrome includes Gitelman syndrome (see below). It also includes primary hyperaldosteronism, a renin producing tumor and renal artery stenosis, all three of which are differentiated by the presence of hypertension. Chronic diarrhea, especially laxative abuse, and bulimia may mimic Bartter syndrome, as of course may chronic or surreptitious diuretic use.

Remember

Both Bartter syndrome and Gitelman syndrome are characterized by renal loss of salt with hypokalemic alkalosis and hyponatremia. Bartter syndrome is clinically more severe with hypercalciuria and often nephrocalcinosis, failure to thrive, growth retardation, and muscle weakness. Clinical manifestation of the more frequent Gitelman syndrome is mild and often nonspecific; electrolyte changes resemble thiazide therapy.

C4.4.4 Gitelman Syndrome

Gitelman syndrome is a disorder in which depletion of magnesium and potassium lead to hypokalemic alkalosis. It was once thought to be a variant of Bartter syndrome, but it is caused by mutations in the thiazide-sensitive Na–Cl cotransporter gene on chromosome 16q13, referred to as *SLC12A3*, which codes for a transporter that mediates sodium and cloride reabsorption in the distal convoluted tubule. This transporter is the target of the thiazide diuretics used to treat hypertension. At least 17 different nonconservative mutations have been found.

Patients with this disorder present later than those with Bartter syndrome, often in adulthood, and without hypovolemia, but there are patients with findings that overlap both the syndromes.

Episodic muscle weakness has been one presentation. Tetany has been another, often precipitated by intercurrent infectious illness. There may be paresthesias or carpopedal spasm. Patients have been described with a chronic dermatosis, in which the skin was thickened and had a purple–red hue. Erythema of the skin has been observed in experimental magnesium depletion in rats. Prolongation of the QT electraradiographic interval is common; ventricular fibrillation is a rare complication.

In Gitelman syndrome, hypokalemic metabolic alkalosis is accompanied by hypomagnesemia and hypocalciuria. Renal wasting of potassium and magnesium is characteristic. There is increased excretion of sodium, chloride, and magnesium in response to intravenous furosemide, as well as abolition of the hypocalciuria, consistent with a defect in transport in the distal tubule as opposed to the loop of Henle.

C4.5   Investigation for Renal Tubular Dysfunction

Initial clinical chemistry is undertaken to determine serum values for Na, K, Cl, HCO_3, and pH. This will establish the presence or absence of acidosis and whether or not it is hyperchloremic. Other useful blood chemistry data include Ca, PO_4, Mg, alkaline phosphatase, urea, and creatinine.

The urine is studied to assess the presence of a Fanconi syndrome by analysis of glucose, amino acids,

Ca, PO$_4$, and creatinine. Proteinuria or increased amount of retinol-binding protein or *N*-acetylglucosaminidase indicate tubular damage and proximal tubular leak. Decreased urinary concentrating ability may also indicate generalized tubular dysfunction.

In the presence of acidosis, the pH of urine is measured. For this purpose it is important to analyze promptly after passage. NaHCO$_3$ supplements should have been discontinued. In a patient suspected of having RTA in whom acidosis is not present an ammonium chloride load may be useful (Table C4.8).

Table C4.8 Investigations For The Analysis Of Renal Tubular Dysfunction

Initial clinical chemistry
Plasma: Na, K, Cl, HCO$_3$, urea, creatinine, urate, Ca, Mg, PO$_4$, ionized Ca, alkaline phosphatase, parathyroid hormone
Urine: reducing substances,
amino acids, tubular reabsorption of phosphate, Ca/creatinine ratio, albumin/creatinine ratio, retinol binding protein/creatinine ratio,
N-acetyl glucosaminidase/creatinine ratio
Further investigation aimed at a specific cause
Blood lactate and pyruvate
Pyruvate carboxylase-leukocytes or fibroblasts
Leukocyte cysteine
Renal (liver) ultrasound
In the presence of hepatic dysfunction
Plasma: 1.25 – hydroxylvitamin D
Erythrocyte: galactose 1-phosphate uridyltransferase
Urine: organic acids for succinylacetone
DNA: common mutations for hereditary fructose intolerance and glycogenoses Ia, Ib
Plasma: ceruloplasmin, urine, plasma: copper
Roentgenograms: joints (rickets, osteomalacia)
Plasma: renin, aldosterone
Blood or muscle mtDNA
Blood acylcarnitine profile
Urine: toxicology
Muscle biopsy: electron transport chain activity
Liver biopsy: aldolase, GSD I, Fanconi–Bickel
Skin biopsy: phosphatidylinositol-4, 5-bisphosphate 5-phosphatase (Lowe syndrome)

Key References

Nyhan WL, Barshop BA, Ozand PT (2005) Atlas of metabolic diseases, 2nd edn. Hodder-Arnold, London

Kaufman JM, Greene ML, Seegmiller JE (1968) Urine uric acid to creatinine ratio – a screening test for inherited disorders of purine metabolism. J Pediatr 73:583–592

Wilcox WD (1968) Abnormal plasma uric acid levels in children. J Pediatr 128:731–741

Bartter FC, Pronove P, Gill JR Jr et al (1962) Hyperplasia of the juxtaglomerular complex with hyperaldosteronism and hypokalemic alkalosis: a new syndrome. Am J Med 33: 811–828

Birkenhäger R, Otto E, Schürmann MJ et al (2001) Mutation of BSND causes Bartter syndrome with sensorineural deafness and kidney failure. Nat Genet 29:310–314

Schlingmann KP, Konrad M, Jeck N et al (2004) Salt wasting and deafness resulting from mutations in two chloride channels. New Engl J Med 350:1314–1319

Gitelman HJ, Graham JB, Welt LG (1966) A new familial disorder characterized by hypokalemia and hypomagnesaemia. Trans Assoc Am Physicians 79:221–235

Simon DB, Nelson-Williams C, Bia MJ et al (1996) Gitelman's variant of Barter's syndrome, inherited hypokalaemic alkalosis, is caused by mutations in the thiazide-sensitive Na–Cl cotransporter. Nat Genet 12:24–30

Scheinman SJ, Guay-Woodford LM, Thakker RV, Warnock DG (1999) Genetic disorders of renal electrolyte transport. N Engl J Med 340:1177–1187

Simon DB, Bindra RS, Mansfield TA (1997) Mutations in the chloride channel gene, CLCNKB, cause Bartter's syndrome type III. Nat Genet 17:171–178

Neurological Disease

C5

Angels García-Cazorla, Nicole I. Wolf, and Georg F. Hoffmann

Key Facts

> The correct diagnosis of inherited metabolic diseases that affect the nervous system primarily is a major challenge because the same neurological symptoms and often even disease course may be caused by non-metabolic disorders.

> Neurometabolic diseases often start with common and non-specific signs, such as isolated developmental delay/mental retardation, seizures, dystonia, or ataxia. They are especially to be suspected when the course of the disease is progressive or when additional neurological systems or other organs become involved. An important clue is the co-existence of different neurological features that cannot be explained by a "simple" neuroanatomic approach.

> Acute or recurrent attacks of neurological manifestations such as coma, ataxia or abnormal behaviour are major presenting features especially in the late-onset inborn errors of metabolism (see also B2.7).

> The initial diagnostic approach to these disorders is based on a few metabolic screening tests. It is important that the biologic fluids are collected at the time of the acute attack. And always consider treatable disorders first when choosing your plan of investigations.

Remember

Signs and symptoms suggestive of a neurometabolic disorder
Positive family history, consanguinity
Unusual age and/of sequence of neurological symptoms
Slowing/plateau of development, regression
Progressive loss of hearing and/or vision
Simultaneous affection of different neurological systems
Suggestive neuroimaging findings
Involvement of other organs than the CNS

> Metabolic investigations are usually not indicated in children with moderate static developmental delay, isolated delay of speech development in early childhood, occasional seizures, e.g. during fever, or well-defined epileptic syndromes. Other genetic aetiologies outside the metabolic field have also been considered, especially as causes of mental retardation, ataxia, dystonia, and spastic paraplegia.

C5.1 General Remarks

Neurological disease can be considered as the most common and important consequence of inherited metabolic diseases for three reasons. In building and maintaining the structure and function of the brain many more genes are involved when compared to the other organs. Also, the brain seems to possess restricted capabilities for repair. As a consequence even slowly but continuously or repeatedly ongoing insults will

A. García-Cazorla (✉)
Servicio de Neurologia, Hospital Sant Joan de Deu, Passeig Sant Joan de Deu 2, 08950 Esplugues, Barcelona, Spain
e-mail: agarcia@hsjdbcn.org

G. F. Hoffmann et al. (eds.), *Inherited Metabolic Diseases*,
DOI: 10.1007/978-3-540-74723-9_C5, © Springer-Verlag Berlin Heidelberg 2010

result in lasting and often progressive neurological disease. Finally, in the development of modern human societies many physical disabilities from reduced vision or hearing to loss of a limb or even an organ will still allow relatively independent and unimpaired activities and life. On the contrary, mental abilities and capacities are being required at an ever increasing level and even marginal or specific partial inabilities can have profound negative effects on the status and well-being of an individual.

C5.2 History and Neurological Examination

Family history, including possible consanguinity, and age at onset of symptoms are crucial to arrive at a suspicion of a neurometabolic disorder. Five aspects should be specifically kept in mind:

1. *Multi-system involvement*: In patients with neurological diseases of undefined origin, searching for multi-system involvement can be very helpful. This includes special neurological functions, such as vision and hearing, as well as overall growth and physical development. Eye, liver, spleen, heart, kidney, skin and the skeletal system are the most prominently affected organs in inborn errors of metabolism besides the nervous system.
2. *Stability/progression of the disease*: Although neurometabolic disorders classically lead to progressive neurodegenerative disease courses due to organelle dysfunction, e.g. lysosomal and peroxisomal disorders and mitochondriopathies, many of them can present as static or non-progressive neurological dysfunctions. Metabolic disorders affecting small molecules often show a stable neurological course. Examples include creatine deficiency syndromes, 4-hydroxybutyric aciduria, and some defects of purine metabolism. Some CDG disorders have also been proven to be static encephalopathies.
3. *Multi-neurological involvement*: When isolated neurological symptoms persist over time, the diagnosis of an inborn error of metabolism is less likely. Neurometabolic disorders tend to involve more than one system. However, some exceptions have to be kept in mind, including progressive dystonia without additional symptoms in Segawa disease, isolated cerebellar ataxia in some forms of coenzyme Q_{10} deficiency, and isolated mental retardation in creatine transporter (CRTR) defect, some more benign forms of adenylosuccinate lyase deficiency, as well as in some patients with Sanfilippo disease, in particular, type A.

4. *Asymmetry of the symptoms*: Contrary to perceived wisdom, asymmetrical involvement does not argue against neurometabolic diseases. Although the evolution of these disorders tends to result in generalised clinical manifestations, it is common to detect unilateral signs. Examples include unilateral dystonia in Segawa disease, Leigh disease, some cases of GLUT1 deficiency, and unilateral tremor in atypical forms of glutaric aciduria type I.
5. *Fluctuation of symptoms*: In inborn errors of intermediate metabolism symptoms often fluctuate. In neurotransmitter disorders with dopaminergic dysfuncion, dystonia and oculogyric crises may worsen with fatigue and improve with rest; in GLUT1 deficiency, symptoms like epilepsy, ataxia, dysarthria and dyskinesia may worsen with fasting and improve after eating or while resting; in urea cycle disorders, consciousness, hyperkinesia and other symptoms may develop with intercurrent illnesses or fluctuate depending on protein intake.

C5.3 Neurological Regression/ Deterioration

Progressive neurologic and mental deterioration is a very important clinical hallmark of inborn errors of metabolism. In this context, it is helpful to take into consideration the age of onset, presence or absence of epilepsy, other neurologic signs as ataxia or other movement disorders, and the co-existence of non-neurologic symptoms, especially hepatosplenomegaly, bone or retinal involvement. Altered metabolism of complex molecules, defects of energy metabolism and organic acidurias are the main pathophysiological groups involved in neurological deterioration (Zschocke et al. 2004).

It is important to analyse the speed of progression in these disorders. In storage diseases, development usually slows down before reaching a plateau and frank regression starts. Loss of acquired skills follows at variable speed. In slow progressive disorders, it is often difficult to decide whether there is true regression or simply a residual syndrome. Old family photographs or home videos may be helpful. Cerebral imaging may also change only slowly or even be normal, especially at the onset of symptoms. Organic acidurias can manifest with acute and dramatic deterioration, with a plateau (or even partial recovery) later on. This is especially true for glutaric aciduria type I or mitochondrial disorders. The latter may display acute deteriorations with regression, followed by partial recoveries. Over time, the course of these disorders is relentlessly downhill.

There are several non-metabolic disorders giving rise to a degenerative disease course. This is especially true for disorders from the autistic spectrum and Rett syndrome in girls where early development is usually normal, and deterioration may be rapid. Continuous spike-waves during sleep (CSWS) is another differential diagnosis that is amenable to treatment. Sleep electroencephalography (EEG) studies must therefore be performed in all children with regression in addition to metabolic investigations, regardless of whether seizures are present or not. Also in other epileptic encephalopathies, the untreated epilepsy itself, if severe enough, can lead to regression mimicking a neurodegenerative disorder, e.g. Dravet or Lennox–Gastaut syndrome. Differential diagnosis is completely different from a true neurodegenerative disorder. Additional important causes of neurologic and mental deterioration are as follows: side effects of antiepileptic drugs, especially valproate, intoxication by heavy metal contamination (lead and mercury); and the Münchausen-by-proxy syndrome (Table C5.1).

Table C5.1 Important differential diagnoses in regression

Additional Leading Symptom	Disease
Epilepsy	Late-infantile neuronal ceroid lipofuscinosis, Alpers disease, MELAS, MERRF and other progressive myoclonus epilepsies
Ataxia	Late-infantile neuronal ceroid lipofuscinosis, GM_2-gangliosidosis, mitochondrial disorders, cerebrotendinous xanthomatosis, Refsum disease, vitamin E-responsive ataxias
Neuropathy	Metachromatic leukodystrophy, Friedreich ataxia, Refsum disease, vitamin E-responsive ataxias
Retinopathy	Infantile and late-infantile neuronal ceroid lipofuscinoses, juvenile neuronal ceroid lipofuscinosis, PKAN, Refsum disease, mucolipidosis type IV
Cataract	Cerebrotendinous xanthomatosis, α-mannosidosis, Fabry disease
Hepatosplenomegaly	Sandhoff disease, Gaucher disease, Niemann–Pick disease, infantile form of Salla disease
Spasticity	Metachromatic leukodystrophy, adrenoleukodystrophy, Krabbe disease and many others
Dystonia	Glutaric aciduria type I, Wilson disease, biotin-responsive basal ganglia disease
Dysostosis multiplex	Mucopolysaccharidoses, oligosaccharidoses, GM_1-gangliosidosis

Remember

In the differential diagnosis of neurodegenerative disorders, age of onset, additional (leading) symptoms and the dynamics of regression are important clues for differential diagnosis.

Disease Info: Metachromatic Leukodystrophy (MLD)

The classical late-infantile form of this autosomal recessive disorder usually starts between 10 and 25 months with floppiness or gait disturbance. Severe spasticity develops, tendon reflexes are decreased or absent reflecting polyneuropathy. Cerebrospinal fluid (CSF) protein is elevated. Cognition remains relatively intact until late in the course of the disease, seizures are uncommon. Arylsulphatase A activity is severely impaired; excretion of sulphatides is increased. The latter can differentiate between true arylsulphatase A deficiency and pseudodeficiency that occurs in 7–15% of the general population. The juvenile form may present with psychiatric symptoms. If done before neurologic symptoms develop, bone marrow transplantation is a successful treatment, at least for some patients. Magnetic resonance imaging (MRI) shows involvement of the posterior central white matter with sparing of the subcortical areas; the posterior part of the corpus callosum is also usually involved.

Disease Info: X-linked Adrenoleukodystrophy (X-ALD)

This X-chromosomal disorder starts in childhood with progressive gait disturbance and insidious onset of cognitive decline. The course is relentlessly downhill; spasticity and dementia develop. Adrenocortical involvement is not a regular finding in this form that occurs in about half of the affected individuals. About 25% of the patients show another clinical picture with adrenal insufficiency and neuropathy (adrenomyeloneuropathy), 10% have isolated Addison's disease. VLCFA are elevated with an increased ratio of C26:C22. Bone marrow transplantation in presymptomatic boys at risk for developing X-ALD is curative but cannot stop the progress if done after onset of neurological symptoms. Whether Lorenzo's oil may lower the risk of developing the severe childhood form is still under debate (Moser 1997).

Disease Info: GM2-Gangliosidosis

The most common form is due to the absence of hexoaminidase A activity and starts in infancy, also called Tay–Sachs disease, with regression, acoustic startle reaction and hypotonia. Spasticity, blindness, macrocephaly and seizures develop later. A cherry-red spot in the macular region is almost invariably present. Sandhoff disease shows the same neurological symptoms, but can also lead to liver involvement; hexoaminidase A and B activities are absent. The juvenile form of GM2-gangliosidosis can present with ataxia, action myoclonus, dystonia and dementia. Cerebellar atrophy is a frequent neuroradiological finding in this form.

Disease Info: Niemann–Pick Disease Type C (NPC)

In total, 95% of cases in this autosomal recessive disorder are caused by mutations in *NPC1*, which is important for intracellular cholesterol trafficking. The remaining 5% are caused by mutations in *NPC2*. Half of the patients have a cholestatic neonatal icterus, which disappears spontaneously within the first 3 months of life. Some infants go on to develop severe cholestatic liver disease with impaired liver function; they do not display neurologic symptoms. Mental retardation and regression or initial normal development followed by regression in childhood are common. Vertical supranuclear (upward) gaze palsy is a typical symptom, but is usually absent in small children. Cataplexy and epilepsy are common. Hepatosplenomegaly is not always present. If disease starts later in childhood or in adulthood, ataxia and slowly progressing dementia are the leading symptoms. There is great clinical heterogeneity. In cultured fibroblasts, cholesterol esterification is defective, but this test may be normal. Chitotriosidase activity is moderately increased and a useful biochemical marker. Sea-blue histiocytes are found in bone marrow aspirates.

Disease Info: Neuronal Ceroid Lipofuscinoses (NCL)

These disorders, all with autosomal recessive inheritance, show storage of autofluorescent material. There are several forms with onset from neonatal age until adulthood; the retina is involved in almost all. Infantile NCL (Santavuori–Haltia disease) is frequent in Finland, but can also be found in other ethnic groups. Affected infants show an initially normal development, regression becomes apparent at the end of the first year of life with ataxia, loss of vision and myoclonus. EEG shows progressive slowing and in the later stages of the disease isoelectric tracing. The disease is due to absent activity of palmitoylprotein thioesterase 1 (*CLN1*). Mutations in the same gene can give rise to the juvenile form of the disease. Late-infantile NCL (Jansky–Bielschowsky disease) is caused by mutations in the gene coding for tripeptidylpeptidase 1 (TPP1) (*CLN2*). It starts between 2 and 5 years of age with epilepsy, ataxia and regression followed by loss of vision and spasticity. Juvenile NCL (Batten disease) starts with loss of vision due to retinitis pigmentosa around the age of 6. Regression starts thereafter; parkinsonism and epilepsy are additional symptoms. There is a common 1.02 kb deletion in the CLN3 gene coding for a membrane protein with palmitoyl-protein Δ-9 desaturase activity. A useful and simple screening test is looking for lymphocyte vacuolisations in a peripheral blood smear. This should be done in every child with retinitis pigmentosa. CLN8 shows similar symptoms as the late-infantile form is due to *CLN2* mutations; it is caused by mutations in *CLN8* that also lead to progressive epilepsy with mental retardation (EPMR, Northern epilepsy). There is also an adult-onset form of NCL, Kufs disease. The genetic defect(s) is not yet known.

Krabbe Disease

Deficiency of β-galactocerebrosidase gives rise to this disorder. Its infantile form starts around the age of 6 months with irritability, progressive stiffness and opisthotonus. Later, infants become hypotonic because of neuropathy. CSF protein is elevated. Seizures are relatively common. The juvenile form has a less stereotyped clinical picture. Ataxia, dementia, dystonia and loss of vision are frequent symptoms.

Sanfilippo Disease

This autosomal recessive disorder (mucopolysaccharidosis type III) is caused by mutations in four different genes coding for heparan *N*-sulphatase (type A), α-*N*-acetylglucosaminidase (type B), acetyl CoA:-α-glucosaminide acetyltransferase (type C) and *N*-acetylglucosamine 6-sulphatase (type D). Mental retardation and insidious regression become apparent between 2 and 6 years of age. Coarse features may be absent or not very prominent. Urine screening for mucopolysaccharides by glycosaminoglycane electrophoresis should therefore be done in all children with mental retardation and/or regression.

Infantile Neuroaxonal Dystrophy (INAD)

This is a very rare neurodegenerative disorder, which starts at the end of the first or in the second year of life after normal development. First symptoms are stagnation of development, muscle hypotonia and truncal ataxia. Nystagmus and further deterioration follow. Children develop spasticity, optic atrophy and additional evidence of chronic denervation.

Skin biopsy shows spheroid inclusions in nerve endings. Cerebral MRI is remarkable for T2 hyperintense cerebellar cortex; signal of globus pallidum may be hypointense (Fig. C5.1). EEG displays fast rhythms (Fig. C5.2). A large proportion of cases have mutations in *PLA2G6*, a gene coding for a phospholipase A2 (Morgan et al. 2006). The exact pathogenesis of this disorder is not yet understood.

C5.4   Delayed Speech Development

Isolated delay in speech development is frequent. Per se it does not indicate a metabolic disorder and metabolic investigations are not warranted. If speech delay is part of the global developmental delay, investigations should be performed for mental retardation (see later). There are several disorders in which expressive speech is more profoundly affected than overall development. This is the case for creatine deficiency syndromes, 4-hydroxybutyric aciduria and adenylosuccinate lyase deficiency, but it may also be found in mitochondrial disorders, especially when associated with hearing impairment. It is important to evaluate cognitive abilities independently. Equally important is a thorough approach of therapists in order to enable assisted communication or teach simple sign languages. Abnormal speech development may be seen in galactosemia despite treatment.

C5.5   Deafness

Deafness can be caused by a great variety of different genetic and environmental causes. Genetic factors account for at least half of all the cases of congenital deafness. In fact, about 300 independent genes have shown to cause hearing loss. Amongst them, from 77 to 88% are transmitted as autosomal recessive traits, 10–20% as dominant and 1–2% as X-linked. In 20–30% of the cases, other associated clinical manifestations permit the diagnosis of a specific form of syndromic deafness (Nance 2003). Metabolic disorders that exhibit deafness in variable forms (from profound deafness to variable degrees of hypoacusia) belong to this syndromic group (Table C5.2). The hearing loss in metabolic disorders is mostly sensorineural, symmetrical, and

Fig. C5.1 MRI of a child with INAD. (**a**), (**c**) and (**d**) are axial T2w images. In (**a**), cerebellar atrophy is evident, (**c**) demonstrates low pallidal signal, (**d**) some cortical atrophy. In (**b**), the axial FLAIR image displays hyperintensity of the cerebellar cortex

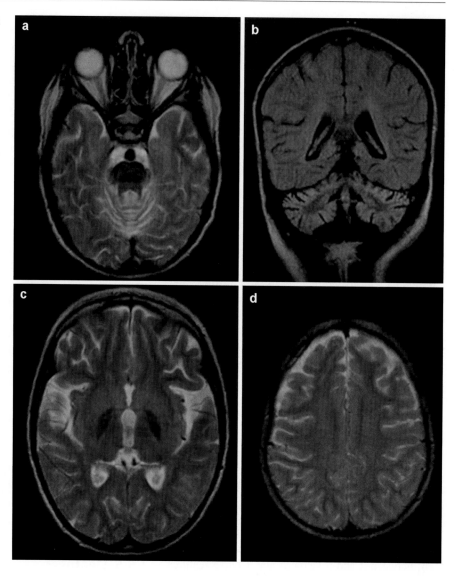

manifests a predominant involvement of high frequencies, although in advanced stages, all frequencies can be affected. Moreover, it is usually progressive, and in general, there is no specific medical treatment except possibly for early therapy in biotinidase deficiency. Cochlear implants have been reported to be effective in mitochondrial encephalopathy, lactic acidosis and stroke-like episodes (MELAS), maternally inherited diabetes and deafness (MIDD), Kearns–Sayre (KSS) and chronic progressive external ophthalmoplegia (CPEO) syndromes. Mitochondrial dysfunction is the most important cause of deafness of metabolic origin (Kokotas et al. 2007). Outer hair cells have a high ATP demand,

do not divide, and receive poor, indirect metabolic support from Deiter cells, especially those at the basal coil, which are the most metabolically active. It is postulated that a drop in the level of ATP results in progressive ionic imbalances in both the outer hair cells and stria vascularis, leading to cell injury and cell death.

Mitochondrial dysfunction is the most important cause of deafness from metabolic disorders. However, the great majority of the mitochondrial causes of deafness are not included in our conventional classification of metabolic disorders. That refers to more than 50 nuclear genes involved in non-syndromic hearing loss. In addition, several rare mutations in the mitochondrial

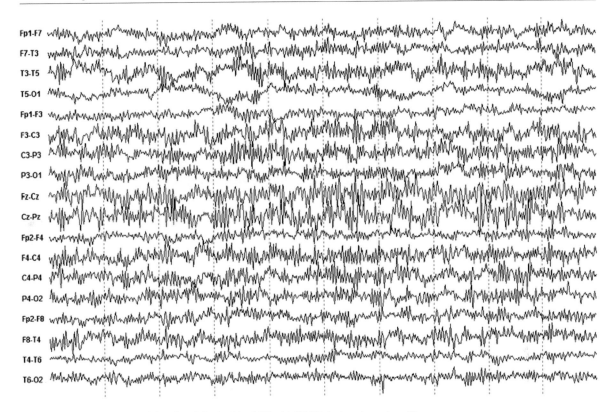

Fig. C5.2 Prominent general fast β-activity in this child with INAD during sleep stage II

MTTS1 and *MTRNR1* genes have been found to be responsible for non-syndromic hearing loss. In contrast, well-known mutations in the mitochondrial DNA such as those associated with NARP, Pearson, MELAS, MERFF or Kearns–Sayre syndromes have multi-system involvement (varying degrees of myopathy, cardiomyopathy and encephalopathy), in addition to, although not always, hearing loss. In MIDD, neurosensory hearing loss is a very prominent component of the clinical picture. MIDD syndrome is caused by mitochondrial DNA rearrangements. Diabetes is non-insulin dependent at onset but progresses to insulin dependency with age. Retinopathy, cardiomyopathy, myopathy, encephalopathy and kidney disease are present in many patients resulting in a phenotypic overlap with MELAS syndrome. On the other hand, mutations in the *OPA1* gene that encodes a dynamin-related GTPase involved in mitochondrial fusion, cristae organisation and control of apoptosis, have been linked to non-syndromic optic neuropathy transmitted as an autosomal dominant trait. However, it can also be responsible for a syndromic association of sensorineural deafness, ataxia, axonal sensory-motor polyneuropathy, chronic progressive external ophthalmoplegia and mitochondrial myopathy characterised by cytochrome c oxidase negative and ragged red fibres. Finally, deafness/dystonia peptide (DDP) is the product of a gene on Xq22 that gives rise to deafness, blindness, retardation and dystonia found in the Mohr–Tranebjaerg syndrome.

Fabry Disease

Both progressive hearing impairment and sudden deafness have been reported in this disorder. Hearing loss on high-tone frequencies has also been found on audiograms in Fabry patients with clinically "normal" audition. Furthermore, the incidence of hearing loss appeared significantly increased in Fabry patients with kidney failure or cerebrovascular lesions. The origin and mechanisms of deafness probably involve the inner ear. Neuropathologic studies have disclosed evidence of glycosphingolipid accumulation in the ear in vascular endothelial cells and in various ganglion cells. More specifically, sudden deafness could also be potentially caused by vascular mechanisms due to the accumulation of glycosphingolipids within lysosomes of endothelial and smooth muscle cells leading to progressive narrowing, ischemia, and frank occlusion in the vessels feeding the cochlea. Middle ear findings of seropurulent effusions and hyperplastic mucosa have been demonstrated in temporal bones of patients. Strial and spiral ligament atrophy in all turns and hair cell loss mainly in the basal turns were also common findings. Nevertheless, the exact pathophysiologic mechanisms of the cochlear involvement deserves further studies (Germain et al. 2002).

The diagnosis is made by enzyme studies (α-galactosidase) in plasma, serum, leukocytes or fibroblasts. Enzyme replacement therapy is available.

C5.5.1 Other Lysosomal Disorders

Many lysosomal disorders can exhibit hypoacusia or deafness due to abnormal lysosomal storage in the inner ear or bone hearing malformations. Here, we outline some of the most involved disorders.

C5.5.2 Mucopolysaccharidoses

Hypoacusia and profound deafness are frequent in mucopolysaccharidoses, in particular, mucopolysaccharidosis type I (MPS I) and Morquio's syndrome (MPS IV). Clinical findings of otitis media with mixed hearing loss are common. Although audition could be

Table C5.2 Differential diagnosis of syndromic deafness

Metabolic disorders and syndromic deafness	Other genetic syndromic deafness

Mitochondrial disorders
  Mutations in *MTTS1* and *MTRNR1*: non-syndromic deafness
	Pendred syndrome
	  Sensorineural deafness, malformations of the inner ear and goiter. Is the most common form of syndromic deafness. Autosomal recessive. Mutations SLC26A4 gene

Mitochondrial DNA mutations (syndromic deafness): NARP, Pearson, Wolfram, MELAS, MERFF, Kearns–Sayre, MIDD, OPA1, DDP	
	Branchio-oto-renal syndrome Sensorineural or mixed. Branchial cleft fistulas, pre-helical pits, deformities of the inner ear, dysplastic or polycystic kidneys Autosomal dominant. Mutations EYE 1 gene
Biotinidase deficiency	Waardenburg syndrome

Lysosomal disorders
  Fabry disease
  Mucopolysaccharidoses
  Sphingolipidoses
  Oligossaccharidoses
Peroxisome biogenesis disorders
	Sensorineural hearing loss, patches of cutaneous dyspigmentation, blue eyes, heterochromia, synophorys, lateral displacement of the inner canthi of the eyes. Genetically heterogeneous, at least eight loci involved

	Usher syndromes Sensorineural deafness with retinitis pigmentosa. Phenotypically and genetically heterogeneous. Autosomal dominant and recessive forms
Purine disorders PRPS (phosphoribosylpyrophosphate deficiency)	
	Jervell, Lange–Nielsen syndromes Sensorineural deafness and prolongation of the QT interval. Autosomal recessive Mutations KVLQT1 potassium channel gene
	Alport syndrome Sensorineural deafness, progressive nephritis, ocular abnormalities. Mutations involving tissue specific polypeptide subunits of collagen encoded by the COL4A genes. Autosomal recessive or X-linked

preserved at initial stages of the disease, hearing loss tends to progress over time from mild and moderate to total deafness. In a mouse model of MPS I, cells with lysosomal storage vacuoles were observed in spiral ligament, spiral prominence, spiral limbus, basilar membrane, epithelial and mesothelial cells of Reissner's membrane, endothelial cells of vessels and some ganglion cells. The number of vacuoles increased with aging. Total loss of the organ of Corti appeared also over time. These age-related changes suggest the necessity of early therapeutic intervention.

Sphingolipidoses such as Krabbe disease and *oligosacccharidoses* such as mannosidoses have also a high incidence of profound neurosensorial deafness.

C5.5.3 Peroxisomal and Purine Disorders

Perceptive deafness, either congenital or as progressive hearing loss, has been reported as a common sequel of peroxisome biogenesis disorders such as Zellweger syndrome and variants, as well as Refsum disease. Phosphoribosylpyrophosphate (PRPS) deficiency is a purine disorder characterised in childhood by a variety of neurological deficits, including inability to walk or talk, abnormal facies and sometimes inherited nerve deafness. In early adulthood it gives rise to gout or stones. PRPS deficiency may also manifest in the carrier female and should be suspected in any seemingly X-linked defect where the mother presents with gout or hyperuricemia and may be deaf. Both the complete and "partial" defects can present as acute renal failure in infancy.

C5.6 Global Developmental Delay/Mental Retardation

Mental retardation is a frequently occurring condition, affecting up to 3% of the population, with a major impact on the life of the affected individual, the family and society. Establishing an etiologic diagnosis is a major challenge as the spectrum of possible causes is enormous and the range of diagnostic investigations extensive and costly. Although the hope that a specific diagnosis will lead to a rational therapy is mostly futile, a specific diagnosis by itself is beneficial by ending the diagnostic odyssey, and providing knowledge of the short- and long-term prognosis, the recurrence risk, treatment options as well as contact with other families. Often it is a great step towards acceptance of the disability (AACAP, 1999).

There are as yet no guidelines available for investigating mental retardation, which have been established in an evidence-based approach. Studies report the yield of different diagnostic approaches between 10 and 81%. With regards to inborn errors of metabolism as a cause of mental retardation studies are not comparable, e.g. with regards of the parameters investigated. Especially those disorders which could lead to unspecific mental retardation (see Table C5.3) were mostly not investigated even in any of the few recent studies. What can be concluded is that inborn errors of metabolism are not a major cause of isolated mental retardation. In these disorders, mostly additional neurological and/or somatic systems are involved guiding the diagnostic process. They are elucidated in other sections of this chapter, e.g. neurodegeneration, movement disorders, etc. Nevertheless, inborn errors of metabolism remain responsible for 1–5% of unspecific mental retardation even in countries offering extended neonatal screening. Metabolic disorders have a high recurrence rate and available prenatal diagnosis,

Remember

- Deafness in metabolic disorders is commonly neurosensorial, symmetrical, progressive and syndromic (associated with other clinical signs)
- Transmission or mixed hypoacusia correspond normally to muco- or oligo-saccharidoses
- Mitochondrial disorders are the most frequent cause of deafness in metabolic diseases
- Always consider the possibility of biotinidase deficiency because of its therapeutic possibilities

Table C5.3 Inborn errors of metabolism presenting with primary mental retardation

Mitochondriopathies
Mucopolysaccharidoses
Creatine deficiency syndromes
Defects of purine and pyrimidine metabolism
(Maternal) phenylketonuria
4-Hydroxybutyric aciduria
Fumaric aciduria
Homocystinuria

furthermore some of them are treatable. Therefore, guidelines considering which metabolic tests to be employed in mental retardation, are badly needed.

The assessment of a person with mental retardation is typically multidisciplinary. Taking a good clinical history and performing a detailed clinical examination (including formal testing, neurological and dysmorphological assessment) by a trained specialist remain the bases and must come before any laboratory testing (Van Karnebeek et al. 2005). Auditory and visual capabilities must also be ascertained (Shevell et al. 2005).

With the present techniques, routine high-resolution chromosome testing is indicated in any child with mental retardation, even in the absence of dysmorphic features. FISH analysis for subtelomeric arrangements, molecular testing for *MECP2*, catch 22, fragile X, Angelman and/or Prader–Willi syndromes should be initiated using selection criteria, such as clinical checklists. Microarray analysis is on the edge of becoming widely available replacing FISH analysis.

Neuroradiological studies have a high yield for relatively unspecific brain abnormalities in patients with mental retardation, such as delayed myelination, but a low relevance in helping to establish a specific diagnosis. It is debatable whether they should be routinely performed as they often involve invasive sedation. They have to be initiated in the presence of specific symptoms such as abnormal brain size, focal neurological findings, epilepsy, skin lesions or neurodegeneration.

Metabolic studies should also not be initiated in the first "diagnostic round", but in the absence of clues for other causes the yield is still sufficiently high (at least 1% in an average population) to recommend testing (see Table C5.4). Neonatal screening programs have decreased the number of mentally retarded persons due to well treatable metabolic diseases. A special issue in testing for metabolic disorders is whether the disorder thought of is potentially treatable. Doing focused or sequential metabolic testing (i.e. based on results of basic tests) can increase the diagnostic yield up to 14%.

Individual relatively homogeneous populations can have a much higher yield of specific metabolic disorders, e.g. the Finnish or the Ashkenazi Jewish population. Parental consanguinity, loss of developmental milestones and/or a previously affected sibling point to a monogenic disorder. In these circumstances, comprehensive metabolic evaluation should be initiated early together with neuroimaging studies, and genetic and ophthalmologic evaluation.

Table C5.4 Checklist of laboratory tests in mental retardation focusing on monogenic disorders

Laboratory tests in unspecific mental retardation without dysmorphic features

Genetic analyses, e.g. chromosomes, consider fragile X syndrome

Basic laboratory tests (blood glucose, lactate, ammonia, acid–base status, blood counts, liver function tests, creatine kinase levels, uric acid)

Thyroid function

Creatine metabolites (urine → creatine transporter (CRTR) deficiency)

Glycosaminoglycanes in urine (by electrophoresis → Sanfilippo disease)

Consider maternal phenylalanine

Consider purines and pyrimidines (urine)

Additional laboratory tests in mental retardation with neurological abnormalities

Consider additional genetic analyses, e.g. Rett syndrome, Angelman syndrome, FISH or microarray analysis

Urine: Simple tests, organic acids, glycosaminoglycans, oligosaccharides, sialic acid

Plasma/serum: quantitative amino acids

Biotinidase activity, if not included in neonatal screening (dried blood spots)

Consider purines and pyrimidines (urine), glycosylation disorders (CDG)

Consider thiamine deficiency

Additional laboratory tests in mental retardation with dysmorphic features

Additional genetic analyses, e.g. microarray analysis

Sterols, peroxisomal studies (very long-chain fatty acids, phytanic acids, plasmalogens)

Transferrin isoelectric focusing for glycosylation studies (CDG)

Consider maternal phenylalanine

Psychomotor retardation and...

Progressive loss of skills or organomegaly: consider lysosomal disorders

Multi-system disorder: consider mitochondrial disorders peroxisomal disorders, glycosylation disorders (CDG)

Progressive myopia, dislocated eye lenses: measure total homocysteine

Abnormal hair: consider Menkes disease

Macrocephaly: check urinary organic acids (glutaric aciduria type I, Canavan disease), lysosomal disorders. MRI is recommended as hydrocephalus must be ruled out. One of the recently identified leukodystrophies, megalencephalic leukodystrophy with Subcortical cysts can only be diagnosed by MRI

(adapted from: Zschocke and Hoffmann (2004))

Remember

- Inborn errors of metabolism are rare causes of isolated non-specific mental retardation.

> - In metabolic disorders presenting with mental retardation, additional neurological and/or somatic systems are involved guiding the diagnostic process.
> - Doing a focused or sequential metabolic testing can increase the diagnostic yield up to 14%.

C5.7 Epilepsy

Epilepsy is an important sign of many metabolic disorders, although metabolic disorders are rarely the underlying cause of epilepsy (Wolf et al. 2005). Convulsions are considered to reflect grey matter involvement in neurodegenerative disorders, but may also be prominent in acute metabolic decompensation, which may be reversible. Seizure semiology or EEG patterns mostly do not depend on the underlying disorder, but are rather determined by age at presentation, although there are exceptions. Seizures in metabolic disorders are more often focal than generalised. In most disorders, their treatment is guided by seizure semiology and age of onset and requires conventional antiepileptic drugs, as in epilepsy due to other causes. Specific therapy – mostly cofactors as in biotinidase deficiency but also dietary treatment as in phenylketonuria – only exists for few metabolic disorders. In these, it must be started early in order to avoid persisting neurologic damage. Therefore, it is of utmost importance to think about metabolic causes of epilepsy early in the course of presentation, especially in neonates and infants, in order to provide adequate treatment.

In otherwise healthy children with febrile seizures or clear-cut epileptic syndromes responding promptly to adequate antiepileptic treatment, metabolic investigations are not warranted. In children with cryptogenic difficult-to-treat epilepsy, metabolic investigations should be initiated. However, it is important to correctly classify the epileptic syndrome and to consider other underlying disorders such as focal cortical dysplasia, which might be difficult to find even with advanced MRI technology or other genetic disorders such as channelopathies or mutations in genes like *ARX* or *CDKL5* instead of repeating or expanding metabolic testing.

One of the most important aspects in the differential diagnosis of epilepsy caused by metabolic disorders is the age of onset of seizures. Diagnoses to consider in a neonate are completely different from possible diagnoses in a school-aged child. Exceptions are mitochondrial disorders in which epilepsy can start at any age. It is also important to look for other symptoms, such as ataxia or dementia. EEG features are sometime of help, but usually non-specific.

C5.7.1 Neonatal Period

The great majority of vitamin-responsive epilepsies start in the neonatal period or early infancy (Surtees et al. 2007). Although rare, they are treatable disorders. Seizures consist of a mixture of partial, massive myoclonus, erratic myoclonus of face and extremities, or sometimes tonic seizures. If myoclonic seizures dominate the clinical pattern, the epilepsy syndrome is called "early myoclonic encephalopathy" (EME). EEG often shows a burst-suppression pattern. Myoclonic jerks may be without EEG equivalent. Among the non-treatable disorders, non-ketotic hyperglycinemia (NKH) is the most frequent. In many cases, the aetiology remains unclear despite adequate investigations. In Table C5.5, treatable and non-treatable epileptic encephalopathies starting in the neonatal period are summarised.

> **Pyridoxine-Dependent Seizures (PDS)**
>
> First described in 1954, the genetic basis of pyridoxine (B_6)-dependent seizures was discovered in 2006. Mutations in *ALDH7A1* encoding antiquitin, which has α-aminoadipic semialdehyde dehydrogenase activity, lead to accumulation of α-aminoadipic semialdehyde and Δ1-piperideine-6-carboxylate. The latter metabolite inactivates pyridoxal-5′-phosphate, which is involved as an essential cofactor in many enzymatic reactions including neurotransmitter metabolism. The classical form of PDS starts within the neonatal period with therapy-resistant seizures, especially myoclonic, but also tonic seizures. Administration of pyridoxine usually has an immediate positive effect; children may become apnoeic. Atypical forms of PDS start later in infancy or show partial effect of conventional antiepileptic drugs. In some children, the response to pyridoxine may initially not occur, and some respond to folinic acid instead. There is no universal protocol for a pyridoxine trial (see below). The disorder can now be unequivocally diagnosed by measuring α-aminoadipic

semialdehyde and pipecolic acid, which are diagnostically elevated in urine and plasma even under treatment. Psychomotor development is better the earlier the pyridoxine treatment is started, but even with adequate and immediate treatment outcome is mostly not entirely normal.

Pyridoxal Phosphate-Dependent Seizures

Mutations in the *PNPO* gene encoding pyridox(am)ine 5-phosphate oxidase lead to decreased levels of pyridoxalphosphate (PLP), the active form of

vitamin B_6, in the CNS. Activity of different enzymes dependent of PLP is reduced, leading to a disturbed metabolism of neurotransmitters and amino acids. Measurement of these metabolites often, but not invariably, gives abnormal results, typically elevations of 3-methoxytyrosine, glycine, threonine as well as lactate, and decreases of homovanillic acid and 5-hydroxyindolacetic acid in CSF. The latter constellation mimics aromatic L-amino acid decaboxylase deficiency. Affected neonates are often born prematurely with signs of foetal or neonatal distress. Seizures start early within the first day of life and are resistant to therapy. They respond

Table C5.5 Epileptic encephalopathies presenting in the neonatal period

Treatable disorders	Treatment	Diagnostic test
Pyridoxine dependency	Pyridoxine (or pyridoxal-5-phosphate) 30 mg/kg (usually 100 mg) as starting dose, then 30 mg/kg/day	Response to pyridoxine; elevated pipecolic acid (CSF, plasma, urine) and α-aminoadipic semialdehyde (urine)
Folinic acid dependency	Folinic acid 2–3 mg/kg/day in 3 doses	Response to folinic acid; elevated pipecolic acid (CSF, plasma, urine) and α-aminoadipic semialdehyde (urine); unknown peak in CSF HPLC
PNPO deficiency	pyridoxal-5-phosphate 30–40 mg/kg/day in 3–4 single doses	Response to pyridoxal 5-phosphate; elevated glycine, threonine, 3-orthomethyldopa, lactate
Phosphoserine aminotransferase deficiency	Serine supplementation	Low CSF and plasma serine and glycine
Urea cycle defects	Appropriate treatment	Hyperammonaemia, plasma amino acids, urine orotic acid
Organic acidurias	Appropriate treatment	Urinary organic acids, acylcarnitines
Holocarboxylase synthetase deficiency	High-dose biotin	Organic acids
Maple syrup urine disease	Appropriate treatment	Plasma amino acids: elevation of leucine,
Not treatable disorders		
Non-ketotic hyperglycinaemia		Elevated CSF:plasma glycine ratio
Zellweger syndrome		Elevated VLCFA
Neonatal adrenoleukodystrophy		Elevated VLCFA
Molybdenum cofactor disease		Sulphite test in fresh urine, fibroblast studies, uric acid
Sulphite oxidase deficiency		Sulphite test in fresh urine, fibroblast studies
GABA transaminase deficiency		GABA in CSF
Adenylosuccinate lyase deficiency		Modified Bratton–Marshall test, purines in urine
Respiratory chain disorders and PDHc deficiency		Lactate elevation in CSF, plasma and urine, activity of respiratory chain enzymes and PDHc in muscle and fibroblasts
Glutamate transporter deficiency		Glutamate oxidation in fibroblasts, genetic studies (sequencing of *SLC25A22*)
Congenital glutamine deficiency		Extremely low levels of plasma, urine and CSF glutamine
Neonatal form of neuronal ceroid lipofuscinosis		Cathepsin D activity

promptly to administration of PLP (30–60 mg pyridoxal 5′-phosphate/kg b.w./day), which needs to be given at least three times per day in order to prevent recurrence of seizures before the next dose. If treatment is not initiated, the disorder leads to severe neurologic deficits and is lethal. If treatment is started in the neonatal period, children may survive without neurologic symptoms.

Non-ketotic Hyperglycinemia (NKH)

NKH is caused by impaired function of the glycine cleavage system, a multienzyme complex, with the P protein subunit being the most frequently affected. Most patients suffer from the classical form starting in the first day of life with seizures including singultus, lethargy progressing to coma and apnoea necessitating artificial ventilation. Glycine concentration in CSF is highly elevated especially in relation to its concentration in plasma (quotient > 0.04). EEG shows a burst-suppression pattern. If children are ventilated, they may survive, but prognosis regarding the neurologic outcome is extremely poor. Development is virtually absent, and refractory epilepsy persists even with dietary restriction of glycine and treatment with sodium benzoate, which lowers also glycine levels in CSF.

C5.7.2 Treatment Protocol in Neonates

Pyridoxal phosphate can be used as first-line treatment as it stops both pyridoxine- and pyridoxal-phosphate-dependent seizures. The recommended dose is 30–60 mg/kg/day in at least three doses. To evaluate efficacy, therapy should be maintained for 5 days. CSF (and urine) studies should be performed before treatment in order to have a biochemical marker, but should not delay treatment. If therapy is successful, the appropriate genetic studies should be performed as well.

If pyridoxal phosphate is not available, pyridoxine (B_6) should be used first: 100 mg in a neonate (or 30 mg/kg) either intravenously or orally in a single dose, preferably with EEG monitoring. High doses may be necessary to control seizures, at least initially. In classical cases, we suggest a starting dose of 100 mg

intravenously. If there is no response within 24 h, the same dose should be repeated (and possibly increased up to 500 mg total) before excluding pyridoxine responsiveness. If there is uncertainty about a partial response, pyridoxine should be continued at 30 mg/kg/day for 7 days before final conclusions are drawn. Also with this medication, CSF, plasma and urine samples should be acquired before treatment; again, this must not delay treatment initiation. The use of vitamins does not preclude the introduction of other vitamins/drugs during this period of time if seizures do not stop. The possibility of late-onset pyridoxine-dependent seizures in children up to 3–4 years of age should be considered (pyridoxal phosphate or pyridoxine may be tried). Folinic acid is effective for the extremely rare folinic acid-dependent seizures in a dose of 2–3 mg/kg/day, which appear also to be due to mutations in *ALDH7A1* encoding antiquitin. It is recommended to maintain the treatment for at least 1 month to test efficacy. If biotinidase cannot be ruled out quickly, e.g. with neonatal screening, biotin: 10–100 mg/day can be administered as well. Urinary organic acids should be analysed before starting treatment. Plasma biotinidase activity will remain diagnostic despite therapy.

Remember

In neonatal-onset epileptic encephalopathy, results of pending metabolic investigations must not be waited for in order to start treatment which must not be delayed. Every neonate with seizures should have a trial with pyridoxine, pyridoxal phosphate (or only pyridoxal phosphate) and folinic acid.

C5.7.3 Infancy

In infancy, several disorders present with epileptic encephalopathy, among them untreated PKU has virtually disappeared in many countries with neonatal screening, biotinidase deficiency, GLUT1 deficiency, infantile neuronal ceroid lipofuscinosis (CLN1), GAMT deficiency (also CRTR deficiency) and Menkes disease. Late-onset forms of pyridoxine dependency may start during infancy and early childhood. In these disorders, seizures are (partially) resistant to treatment with conventional antiepileptic drugs.

GLUT1 Deficiency

Glucose enters the brain by crossing the blood-brain barrier. Its uptake into the brain is mediated by the glucose transporter type 1 (GLUT1). GLUT1 deficiency is characterised by persistent hypoglycorrhachia (glucose CSF/serum quotient < 0.45) in the absence of hypoglycemia and with normal or low lactate in the CSF. Although the neurologic phenotype may vary from case to case, epilepsy starting in infancy is the predominant feature. Clinical manifestations vary from mild to severe and include acquired microcephaly, developmental delay, pyramidal signs, a complex movement disorder with dystonia, ataxia and spasticity, and different forms of seizures, including myoclonic seizures resistant to anticonvulsant drugs. GLUT1 deficiency can be treated effectively with the ketogenic diet. Mutation analysis of *SLC2A1* encoding GLUT1 and measurement of erythrocyte uptake of 3-O-methyl-D-glucose confirm the diagnosis. Mutations are usually de novo, but familial cases have been described.

GAMT Deficiency and Other Creatine Deficiency Syndromes

Creatine is crucial for energy metabolism and is synthesised in a two-step process: the first is mediated by AGAT (arginine–glycine amidinotransferase) and the second by GAMT (guanidinoacetate methyltransferase). Furthermore, a CRTR encoded by a X-chromosomal gene is required for creatine uptake into brain and muscle. Disorders of creatine synthesis or transport produce psychomotor delay and epilepsy, which is frequently refractory to conventional antiepileptic drugs. In all the disorders, low creatine concentration in the brain is demonstrated by a severe decrease or absence of the normal creatine peak in brain MRS (spectroscopy). All disorders of creatine metabolism can be reliably diagnosed by analysis of guanidino compounds in urine or plasma. In GAMT deficiency, guanidinoacetate and other guanidino compounds are elevated. Epilepsy is especially prominent in this defect and includes manifestation as West syndrome. It is resistant to conventional anticonvulsant therapy. GAMT deficiency can be treated by creatine supplementation and a diet enriched in ornithine and low in arginine, the latter in order to lower the guanidino compounds appear to be toxic for the CNS. Diet is efficient for seizure control even if started late in the course of the disease. In AGAT deficiency, creatine must be supplemented. There is no treatment for CRTR deficiency.

Biotinidase Deficiency

Epilepsy often starts at 3 or 4 months of life. West syndrome is the most frequent epileptic syndrome, and conventional antiepileptic drugs are ineffective. Alopecia and (perioral) dermatitis are useful clinical clues. Psychomotor development is severely delayed, and, if untreated, optic atrophy and deafness develop. Lactate is mostly elevated as are 3-methylcrotonylglycine, 3-hydroxyisovaleric, 3-hydroxypropionic and 2-methylcitric acid in urine and other body fluids. Low doses of biotin (5–10 mg/day) stop the seizures. Diagnosis is easily made by measuring biotinidase activity, which is possible in dried blood spots.

Menkes Disease

This is an X-linked condition which starts in early infancy. Neonatal period is usually normal. First symptom is often epilepsy with refractory focal seizures and even focal status epilepticus or West syndrome. Development is severely delayed, muscle hypotonia profound. Spasticity develops later. Hairs are abnormally brittle and steely; the microscopical aspect is that of pili torti. Copper and ceruloplasmin are low. The genetic defect involves a copper-transporting ATPase (*ATP7A*). Copper deficiency also involves other structures, especially bones and connective tissue. Bone fractures and subdural haematomas sometimes evoke the diagnosis of non-accidental injuries. In the cranial MRI, cerebral vessels show increased tortuosity (Fig. C5.3). Treatment consists of subcutaneous copper-histidine, but its effects are only marginal if started after manifestation of the disease.

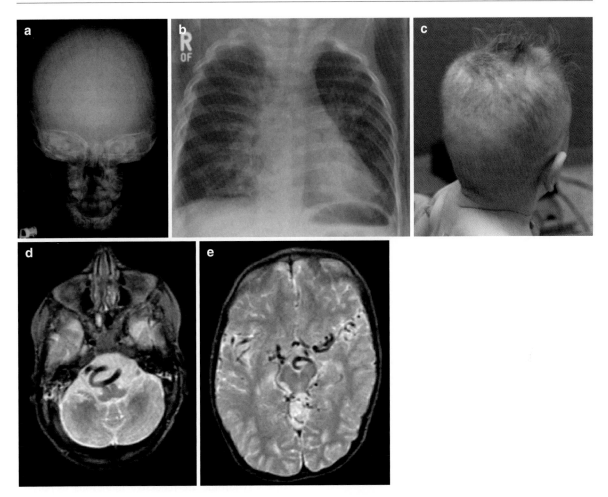

Fig. C5.3 Menkes disease. In this infant with Menkes disease, wormian bones in the lambda and sagittal sutures are seen (**a**), (**b**) depicts a serial rib fracture of ribs 4–8 on the right, another frequent finding. Hairs are steely and fragile and were never cut (**c**). The MRI at the age of 4 shows tortuous and enlarged vessels in these axial T2w images (**d**) and (**e**)

C5.7.4 Childhood and Adolescence

In this age group, late infantile (CLN2) and juvenile (CLN3) forms of neuronal ceroid lipofuscinoses (NCL) and mitochondrial disorders are the most common neurometabolic conditions with prominent seizures. If MRI shows stroke-like lesions in the occipital or temporal regions, a mitochondrial disease is the most probable diagnosis. Alpers disease and also MELAS may manifest with refractory status epilepticus in a previously normal child, a difficult clinical situation. Regarding antiepileptic therapy, drugs should be chosen depending on the epileptic syndrome with the exception of valproic acid, which must not be used in mitochondrial disease, especially Alpers disease, as the risk of fatal liver failure is high.

Late Infantile Neuronal Ceroidlipofuscinosis (CLN2, Jansky–Bielschowsky)

This autosomal recessive disorder is caused by mutations in the gene coding for TPP1, a lysosomal enzyme important for protein degradation. The disease starts between age 2 and 5 years, usually with progressive ataxia and epilepsy. Generalised tonic–clonic seizures are frequent in the beginning; later on myoclonic and focal clonic seizures are seen. Epilepsy is difficult to treat, especially myoclonus. Dementia proceeds quickly. The retina is also involved, and due to pigmentary retinopathy vision deteriorates. EEG shows background changes and spikes with slow photic stimulation, which can trigger seizures (Fig. C5.4). MRI displays cerebellar and less supratentorial atrophy and mild white matter changes.

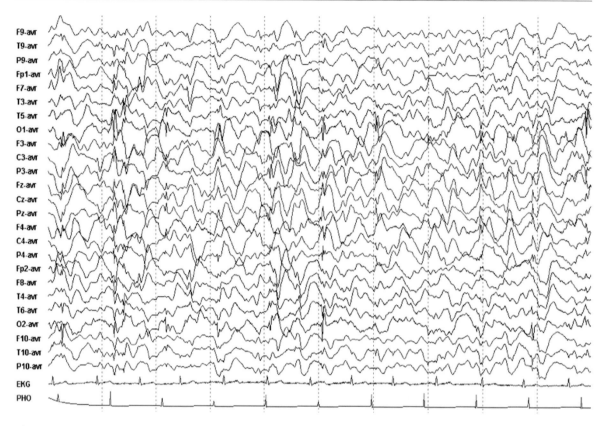

Fig. C5.4 Slow photic stimulation triggers posterior spikes in this child with late-infantile neuronal ceroid lipofuscinosis

Alpers Disease

This autosomal recessive disorder starts at any age from infancy to young adulthood, most frequently in childhood. First symptom is often refractory status epilepticus in a previously healthy child with normal or almost normal development. EEG in this phase shows rhythmic high-amplitude delta with superimposed (poly) spikes (RHADS) involving either left or right posterior region (see Fig. C5.5). Liver function at that stage is usually normal. If status epilepticus is survived, most children develop a relentlessly downhill course with refractory seizures, especially epilepsia partialis continua, optic atrophy and dementia. Some children have a more stable course with almost complete recovery after status. Administration of valproic acid almost invariably triggers liver failure. If liver transplantation is done, neurologic outcome is extremely poor and survival short. Liver failure can also develop without valproic acid. The most frequent cause of

Alpers syndrome are recessive mutations in polymerase γ 1 (*POLG1*), an enzyme that is involved in mtDNA maintenance. mtDNA is depleted in liver. In some patients, lactate and protein are elevated in CSF; in others, all investigations including activity of respiratory chain enzymes in muscle remain repeatedly negative.

The progressive myoclonic epilepsies are a group of genetic disorders where epilepsy with myoclonic and generalised seizures appears in combination with cognitive deterioration and usually also ataxia. Myoclonus is often exaggerated by external stimuli, such as light, sound, or touch, and they are very difficult to treat. This group of disorders comprises Unverricht–Lundborg disease, which has a more benign long-term course (mutations in Cystatin B, *CSTB*, formerly known as EPM1), Lafora disease (80% of patients carry mutations in *EPM2A*, Laforin; another gene involved is *EPM2B* or *NHLRC1*), myoclonic epilepsy with ragged red fibres (MERRF; mutations in *MTTK* which is located in the

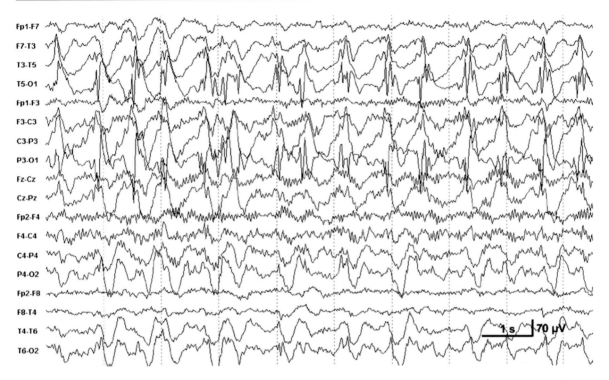

Fig. C5.5 RHADS over the left posterior region at manifestation of Alpers disease; the child was compound heterozygous for two mutations in *POLG1*

mtDNA), some forms of the NCL, and the most frequent being late infantile NCL, sialidosis (neuraminidase deficiency; a cherry red-spot is common) and dentatorubral-pallidoluysian atrophy (DRPLA).

> **Remember**
>
> Only a few metabolic epilepsies beyond the neonatal period are amenable to causal treatment of a metabolic cause. In the majority of patients, conventional antiepileptic drugs must be used according to the seizure type. Valproic acid must be avoided in children with Alpers disease and other mitochondrial disorders as it can trigger fatal liver failure (Table C5.6).

C5.8 Movement Disorders

Our understanding of pediatric movement disorders is rapidly evolving, stimulated by progress in the discovery of monogenic neurogenetic disorders and the development of structured diagnostic and therapeutic approaches in the light of age-dependant physiological development and pathophysiological responses of gross and fine motor functions. Again a logical series of investigations should be followed with the primary aim of early diagnosis of treatable conditions.

C5.9 Ataxia

Ataxia is defined as an inability to maintain normal posture and smoothness of movement while force and sensation are intact. There are many variations in the clinical phenotype, ranging from findings of pure cerebellar dysfunction to mixed patterns of CNS (extrapyramidal pathways, brainstem and/or cerebral cortical participation) or peripheral nervous system involvement. A wide range of molecular defects has been identified, among them classical metabolic disorders (Parker et al. 2003), as well as also other neurogenetic defects. It is important to first consider the (partially) treatable disorders that give rise to ataxia, including vitamin E

Table C5.6 Checklist of laboratory tests in epilepsy focusing on monogenic disorders

---

Laboratory tests in epilepsy with neonatal onset

Basic laboratory tests (blood glucose, lactate, ammonia, acid–base status, calcium, magnesium)

Pipecolic acid and 5-aminoadipic semialdehyde (pyridoxin-dependent seizures)

CNS and plasma amino acids (non-ketotic hyperglycinemia, serine biosynthesis defects, congenital glutamine deficiency)

Neurotransmitters (PNPO deficiency)

CSF GABA (GABA transaminase deficiency)

Sulphite test (molybdenum cofactor deficiency and sulphite oxidase deficiency)

VLCFA (peroxisomal disorders)

Laboratory tests in epilepsy with infantile onset (<1 year)

Basic laboratory tests (blood glucose, lactate, ammonia, acid–base status, calcium, magnesium)

CSF and plasma glucose (GLUT1 deficiency)

Amino acids (PKU)

CSF lactate (mitochondrial disorders)

Organic acids (biotinidase deficiency, MHBD deficiency, organic acidurias)

Biotinidase activity

Creatine, creatinine and guanidinoacetate in urine (creatine synthesis defects and CRTR defect)

Copper and ceruloplasmin (Menkes disease)

VLCFA (peroxisomal disorders)

Purines and pyrimidines in urine

Consider lysosomal studies (e.g. CLN1, Tay–Sachs disease)

Pipecolic acid and 5-AASA (pyridoxine-dependent seizures)

Laboratory tests in epilepsy with onset in late infancy and childhood (and usually additional signs and symptoms as ataxia or regression)

Basic laboratory tests (lactate, ammonia, acid–base status)

CSF lactate (mitochondrial disorders)

CSF and plasma glucose (GLUT1 deficiency)

Creatine, creatinine and guanidinoacetate in urine (creatine synthesis defects and CRTR defect)

Lysosomal studies (e.g. CLN2)

Pipecolic acid and 5-AASA (pyridoxine-dependent seizures) for atypical late-onset cases, also consider therapeutic trial

Purines and pyrimidines in urine

---

deficiency, biotinidase deficiency, abetalipoproteinemia, thiamine-responsive pyruvate dehydrogenase deficiency, cerebrotendinous xanthomatosis and primary coenzyme Q_{10} deficiency. A pragmatic approach classifies ataxias according to their clinical evolution: intermittent or episodic, stable or progressive.

C5.9.1 Intermittent/Episodic Ataxias

These are mainly defects of intermediary metabolism. Ataxia is a frequent sign during acute or subacute decompensation of amino acid (especially MSUD), organic acid and urea cycle disorders. Defects of energy metabolism presenting with intermittent ataxia may involve exclusively the nervous system and are often more difficult to diagnose. Lactate may be elevated only intermittently with clinical abnormalities. Intermittent ataxia can be seen in Hartnup disease; additional symptoms are pellagra-like skin changes, photic dermatitis and psychiatric symptoms. Carbohydrate-sensitive ataxia is a feature of mild pyruvate dehydrogenase deficiency and occurs only in boys. GLUT1 deficiency may present with intermittent ataxia as the only finding, mimicking other episodic ataxias. Ataxia is usually worse before meals. Some children improve greatly with frequent carbohydrate-rich snacks and do not need ketogenic diet. Mild forms of biotinidase activity may also give rise to intermittent ataxia. The so-called "episodic ataxias" may be mistaken for metabolic disorders, although they belong to the channelopathies. Correct diagnosis is important, as effective treatment exists also for these disorders. As a rule, metabolic parameters may be normal between bouts of ataxia; testing is therefore mandatory when patients are symptomatic and usually involves CSF investigations also. An important non-metabolic differential diagnosis for intermittent ataxia is that of intoxication, especially with benzodiazepines and other centrally acting drugs.

C5.9.2 Non-Progressive Ataxia

Non-progressive ataxias are mostly secondary to cerebellar malformations, e.g. in Joubert syndrome. True metabolic causes of non-progressive ataxias include CDG type Ia and other types of congenital glycosylation defects, Marinescu–Sjögren syndrome, 4-hydroxybutyric aciduria deficiency and L-2-hydroxyglutaric aciduria. In CDG Ia, MRI displays cerebellar atrophy (Poretti et al. 2008) or hypoplasia is usually accompanied by brainstem hypoplasia. Mitochondrial disorders rarely show non-progressive ataxia.

C5.9.3 Progressive Ataxia

Many neurometabolic and neurodegenerative disorders involve the cerebellum and are accompanied by a more or less prominent ataxia, which is most often progressive. In some disorders, ataxia is the most prominent sign and these are usually called the heredoataxias. Friedreich's ataxia is part of this group, albeit not a classical metabolic disorder, also the vitamin E-responsive ataxias. Ataxia is a prominent symptom in Refsum disease, cerebrotendinous xanthomoatosis and mevalonic aciduria. The relatively recent group of ataxias with coenzyme Q_{10} deficiency consists of several disorders without clear molecular defect. Infantile neuroaxonal dystrophy (INAD) is a rare neurodegenerative disorder starting in the second year of life with ataxia, hypotonia and nystagmus.

Remember

The rare treatable causes for progressive ataxia should be checked in all the patients by determining – vitamin E levels, phytanic acid, possibly Q_{10} levels in mononuclear cells or muscle, and if clinical manifestations are suggestive, also sterols.

Non-metabolic disorders are another frequent cause of hereditary progressive ataxia. An important group of the DNA repair disorder – ataxia telangiectasia (AT) is the most frequent example. Ataxia with oculomotor apraxia (AOA) 1 and 2 also belong to this group; α-fetoprotein is elevated in AT and AOA2, making for a simple and cheap screening test in progressive ataxias; it belongs to the initial evaluation of an ataxic child.

Friedreich Ataxia

Friedreich ataxia (FRDA) is the most common spinocerebellar degeneration. Onset is before the age of 25, usually before the age of 16. It is an autosomal recessive disorder, and virtually all the affected individuals carry expanded GAA repeats in the gene coding for frataxin, which appears to be involved in mitochondrial iron homoeostasis and iron sulphur centre regulation; oxidative stress is probably increased. The main clinical signs associated with ataxia are pes cavus, spinocerebellar degeneration (polyneuropathy and pyramidal tract lesion) and cardiomyopathy. MRI is usually normal, but may show spinal atrophy later in the disease. Metabolic investigations are normal. The effect of antioxidant therapy with idebenone, a coenzyme Q_{10} homologue, is still under debate; cardiac hypertrophy may improve, but neurologic symptoms appear to remain constant, although there might be an effect with higher doses.

C5.9.4 Vitamin E-Responsive Ataxias (AVED, Ataxias with Isolated Vitamin E Deficiency)

Vitamin E deficiency results from recessive mutations in the gene for α-tocopherol transfer protein (*TTP1*). Laboratory findings include low-to-absent serum vitamin E and high serum cholesterol, triglycerides, and β-lipoprotein. High doses of vitamin E (400–1200 IU/day) improve neurologic function. This disorder can start from childhood to adulthood. MRI is usually normal. Retinitis pigmentosa, peripheral neuropathy and pyramidal signs may be present; cardiomyopathy is rare. *Abetalipoproteinemia* (Bassen–Kornzweig disease) is a rare disorder resulting from a dysfunction in the microsomal triglyceride transfer protein (*MTP*) gene. Acanthocytosis in peripheral blood smears is a constant finding. Decreased serum LDL and VLDL and increased HDL cholesterol levels together with low triglyceride levels are also present.

Refsum Disease

Accumulation of phytanic acid is the laboratory hallmark of this disorder, which is due to mutations in the genes coding for phytanoyl-CoA-hydroxylase (*PAHX* or *PHYH*) or peroxin 7 (*PEX7*). Affected patients have peripheral neuropathy and retinits pigmentosa, sometimes cardiac involvement and impaired hearing. Ichthyosis and multiple epiphyseal dysplasia are possible associated symptoms. The disease starts usually in adolescence or late childhood. Plasmapheresis may be required to effectively lower phytanic acid levels, and a diet without phytanic acid or chlorophyll should be followed.

Cerebrotendinous Xanthomatosis (CTX)

This autosomal recessive disorder is caused by mutations in *CYP27A*, which is coding for sterol 27-hydroxylase. Progressive ataxia and involvement of pyramidal tracts start in childhood or adolescence, sometimes later. Characteristic features are bilateral cataracts. Neonatal liver disease and chronic diarrhoea are other early symptoms. Xanthomata may appear only late. Cholestanol is elevated in this disorder. Therapy is with chenodeoxycholic acid and HMG-CoA-reductase inhibitors in order to lower cholestanol levels.

Coenzyme Q$_{10}$-Responsive Ataxias and Defects of Coenzyme Q$_{10}$ Biosynthesis

Coenzyme Q$_{10}$ deficiency may produce ataxia as the only neurologic manifestation. Q$_{10}$ levels should be measured in muscle or mononuclear cells. High-dose coenzyme Q$_{10}$ supplementation is effective in some. The genetic background of ataxias with Q$_{10}$ deficiency remains obscure in many cases. It may be secondary to other genetic defects as aprataxin deficiency in AOA1. Recently, mutations in *CABC1* (also called *ADCK3*) could be identified in patients with autosomal recessive ataxia and epilepsy. The protein encoded by this gene is involved in biosynthesis of Q$_{10}$. The other known defects in Q$_{10}$ biosynthesis – affected genes are PDSS1, PDSS2 and COQ2 – do not give rise to isolated or predominant ataxia, but to multi-system involvement including renal disease.

Remember

Treatable causes of ataxia (vitamin E deficiency, abetalipoproteinemia, coenzyme Q$_{10}$ deficiency and possibly also cerebrotendinous xanthomatosis) should be routinely checked in patients with (progressive) ataxia. Intermittent ataxias are often due to metabolic disorders. Important differential diagnoses for the latter are channelopathies and intoxications (Table C5.7).

Table C5.7 Checklist of Laboratory Investigations in Ataxia

Basal laboratory investigations (including blood gases, lactate, ammonia and albumin)
Plasma amino acids
Urinary amino acids
Urinary organic acids
CSF and plasma glucose
CSF lactate (and pyruvate)
Vitamine E
Cholesterol
Coenzyme Q$_{10}$
Sterols
Phytanic acid
Transferrin electrophoresis or MS/MS
α-Fetoprotein
Consider lysosomal studies if regression
Consider genetic testing for inherited ataxias

C5.10 Dystonia, Parkinsonism, Chorea

Movement disorders in inborn errors of metabolism include dystonia, secondary parkinsonism, chorea, tremor, myoclonus and tics (Fernández-Alvarez et al. 2001). Different movement disorders may co-exist in the same patient with a metabolic disease. However, dystonia is the predominating type of movement disorder in patients with inborn errors of metabolism. In general, diseases causing parkinsonism in adults may produce dystonia in children.

When the movement disorder is associated with intercurrent illnesses, onset is usually abrupt and generalised (i.e. in glutaric aciduria type I). In other cases, movement disorders develop late in the course of the disease, with focal onset and progressive generalisation, causing major disability and wheelchair dependency (i.e. homocystinuria, Niemann–Pick C disease and GAMT deficiency). Although other signs of neurological dysfunction usually co-exist, some inborn errors of metabolism can initially present as isolated dystonia (Segawa syndrome, panthothenate-kinase-associated neurodegeneration (PKAN), Leigh syndrome, pyruvate dehydrogenase deficiency, and juvenile form of metachromatic leukodystrophy (MLD).

C5.10.1 Dystonia

Clinically, the term dystonia is used for both a symptom (sustained, abnormal muscular contraction causing

Table C5.8 Dystonias

Primary dystonia	Lesch–Nyhan disease
	MELAS
Pure	3-Methylglutaconic aciduria
Idiopathic generalised torsion dystonia (DYT1)	Methylmalonic acidemia
Transient idiopathic infantile dystonia	Mucopolysaccharidoses
Paroxysmal kinesiogenic choreoathetosis	Niemann–Pick disease
Paroxysmal non-kinesiogenic dystonia	2-Oxyglutaric aciduria
Paroxysmal exercise-induced dystonia	
	Pterin defects
Dystonia "Plus"	GTP cyclohydrolase I deficiency
Infantile parkinsonism-dystonia	6-pyruvoyltetrahydropterin synthase deficiency
Myoclonic dystonia (DYT11)	Sepiapterin reductase deficiency
Dopa-responsive dystonia (DYT5)	Dihydropteridine reductase deficiency
Tyrosine hydroxylase deficiency	Propionic acidemia
Aromatic L-amino acid decarboxylase deficiency	Pyruvate dehydrogenase deficiency
Hereditary myoclonic dystonia (DYT11)	Sulphite-oxidase deficiency
Rapid-onset dystonia-parkinsonism	Tyrosinemia type I
Juvenile parkinsonism	Triose phosphate isomerase deficiency
	Vitamin E deficiency
Dystonia secondary to metabolic disease	Wilson disease
Biotinidase deficiency	
Cerebral folate deficiency syndrome	*Other genetic causes of dystonia*
Creatine deficiency syndromes (guanidinoacetate	Ataxia-oculomotor apraxia
methyltransferase deficiency)	Ataxia-telangiectasia
Ethylmalonic aciduria	Benign familial chorea
4-Hydroxybutyric aciduria	Infantile and juvenile Batten disease
D-2-Hydroxyglutaric aciduria	Dentato-pallidoluysian atrophy
L-2-Hydroxyglutaric aciduria	Dystonia and sensorineural deafness
Niemann–Pick C	Familial dystonic-amyotrophic paraplegia
Fucosidosis	PKAN (Hallervorden–Spatz) disease
Galactosemia	Hereditary non-progressive athetoid hemiplegia
Glutaric aciduria type I	Huntington disease
GLUT1 deficiency	Intranuclear neuronal inclusion disease
Hartnup disease	Machado–Joseph disease (striatonigral autosomal
Homocystinuria	dominant degeneration)
Infantile Gaucher disease	Myocionic hereditary dystonia with nasal malformations
Juvenile GM2 and GMI gangliosidosis	Neuroaxonal dystrophy
Juvenile metachromatic leukodystrophy	Olivocerebellar atrophy
Keratan sulphaturia	Pelizaeus–Merzbacher disease
Krabbe leukodystrophy	Progressive calcification of the basal ganglia
Leber hereditary optic neuropathy plus dystonia	Progressive pallidal degeneration
Leigh syndrome	Rett syndrome

fluctuating tone and abnormal posturing) and a group of disorders, which hereafter will be distinguished from the symptom by the term primary dystonia. Whereas the group of primary dystonias consists only of five entities with an additional seven dystonias "plus", a wide range of neurogenetic and neurometabolic disorders can cause secondary dystonias (Tables C5.8 and C5.9).

In many different metabolic diseases dystonia is a major feature (Assmann et al. 2003). In fact, almost all neurometabolic disorders can cause dystonia at some stage, but glutaric aciduria type I, Leigh syndrome and other mitochondrial cytopathies are among the most frequent.

If dystonia is focal, has progressed slowly, or remained isolated over time, it is unlikely to be due to an inborn errors of metabolism. In contrast, if dystonia appears abruptly, settles rapidly, is generalised and postural from the very first stages of the disease, then a metabolic cause should be strongly considered. GLUT1 deficiency can cause paroxysmal exercise-induced

Table C5.9 Checklist of laboratory tests in dystonia

1) Treatable causes of dystonia:
   Biogenic amines, pterines, glucose and folate in the CSF
   Plasma amino acids and total homocysteine in blood
   Creatine and guanidinoacetate compounds in urine
   Copper (plasma and urine), ceruloplasmin (plasma)
   Plasma biotinidase activity

2) Pure dystonia:
   Biogenic amine metabolites in the CSF
   DYT-1 gene

3) Dystonia associated with other neurologic signs:
   Parkinsonism: Biogenic amines and pterines in the CSF,
   copper and ceruloplasmin, lactate, pyruvate, plasma
   amino acids (consider respiratory chain activity and
   mitochondrial DNA study), consider *PANK2* gene
   depending on MRI and other clinical findings,
   juvenile parkinsonism genes
   Myoclonus: urine organic acids, DYT5 gene, consider
   mitochondrial and lysosomal investigations
   Developmental delay and spasticity: uric acid plasma and
   urine, purines in urine, lactate, pyruvate, plasma
   amino acids, organic acids, depending on other data
   consider mitochondrial and lysosomal investigations
   Cerebellar ataxia: organic acids in urine, plasma and
   urine amino acids, plasma vitamin E with cholesterol
   and triglyceride studies, consider mitochondrial
   investigations, aprataxin gene (if oculomotor apraxia)
   and immunological studies (ataxia-telangiectasia),
   depending on other data consider Niemann–Pick C
   studies and spinocerebellar inherited diseases

4) Abrupt generalised dystonia (especially in a catabolic
   state):
   Organic acids (including glutaric and 3-hydroxyglutaric
   acids), lactate, pyruvate, plasma amino acids
   (consider other mitochondrial and PDH studies)

5) Dystonia associated with other signs:
   Visceral signs: lysosomal investigations, urine organic
   acids
   Ocular signs: if optic atrophy gen LHON, if oculomotor
   apraxia gen aprataxin, if ocular telangiectasia,
   immunologic studies and gen ataxia-telangiectasia, if
   retinitis pigmentosa, plasma vitamin E, mitochondrial, lysosomal investigations
   Deafness: plasma biotinidase activity, glycosaminoglycans and oligosaccharides in urine, consider
   mitochondrial investigations and dystonia/deafness
   gene

dyskinesia and also complex movement disorders with elements of dystonia, ataxia and spasticity, even without epilepsy (García-Cazorla et al. 2008).

Obviously, in all the cases it is important to consider first those inborn errors of metabolism for which some effective therapeutic intervention is possible, such as dopa-responsive dystonia syndromes (Segawa disease and other neurotransmitter deficiencies), creatine deficiency syndromes, cerebral folate deficiency syndrome, Wilson disease, homocystinuria, biotinidase, vitamin E and GLUT1 deficiencies.

Inherited Disorders of Biogenic Amines

The disorders of dopamine and serotonin synthesis are aromatic L-amino acid decarboxylase deficiency, tyrosine hydroxylase deficiency and disorders of tetrahydrobiopterin (BH_4) synthesis. In contrast to classical forms of BH_4 deficiency Segawa disease (GTP cyclohydrolase I deficiency) and sepiapterin reductase deficiency present without hyperphenylalaninemia and are not detected by neonatal screening for phenylketonuria. Childhood-onset dystonia or parkinsonism-dystonia is the hallmark of functional dopamine deficiency and the most suggestive clinical symptom of pediatric neurotransmitter diseases. In very young infants, the symptoms are less specific, patients often presenting with truncal hypotonia, restlessness, feeding difficulties or motor delay. Hypokinesia, increased limb tone, oculogyric crises, ptosis and faulty temperature regulation are also some of the common signs. Segawa disease, also called dopa-responsive dystonia, is an autosomal dominant disease characterised by progressive dystonia that normally appears during the first decade of life, is not associated with cognitive impairment and has a dramatic and lifelong responsiveness to levodopa. Tyrosine hydroxylase, amino acid decarboxylase and sepiapterin deficiencies may also respond in different degrees to levodopa. The most important biochemical investigations for the diagnosis of these neurological diseases are cerebrospinal fluid investigations for neurotransmitter metabolites and pterins (see later). Timely diagnosis is especially important for those conditions with specific treatments.

Glutaric Aciduria Type I

Glutaric aciduria type I is an autosomal recessive disease caused by the deficiency of glutaryl-CoA dehydrogenase. Classically, patients have an abrupt presentation, usually between 6 and 18 months of age, with encephalitis-like symptoms following an acute illness. Later psychomotor regression and abnormal movement disorders appear; dystonic or choreo-athetotic movements, focal, segmental or generalised, present as twisting and torsion postures of hands and feet in a child otherwise alert, with profound hypotonia of the neck and trunk and stiff arms and legs. Typically T2-weighted MRI shows frontotemporal atrophy and high signal in the striatum. Macrocephaly is present in about 70% of the cases. In a minority of cases, the onset is insidious with slowly developing psychomotor delay, hypotonia and dystonic posturing. Urine organic acid analysis reveals elevations of glutaric and 3-hydroxyglutaric acids. Isolated slight increases of 3-hydroxyglutaric acid only or normal values of both the acids have been described. Increased ratios of acylcarnitines to free carnitine in plasma and urine as well as elevations of glutaryl-carnitine in body fluids can also be detected. Treatment consists of a diet combined with oral supplementation of L-carnitine and an intensified emergency treatment during acute episodes of intercurrent illness. This strategy has significantly reduced the frequency of acute encephalopathic crises in early diagnosed patients. Anticholinergic drugs and botulinum toxin type A have proved beneficial as symptomatic treatment for severe movement disorders.

Lesch–Nyhan Disease

Lesch–Nyhan disease is caused by the X-linked recessive deficiency of the purine salvage enzyme hypoxanthine-guanine phosphoribosyltransferase (HPRT). Affected patients exhibit over-production of uric acid, a characteristic neurobehavioural syndrome that includes mental retardation, recurrent self-injurious behaviour and a complex spectrum of motor disturbances. Pathogenesis of the neurologic and behavioural features remains incompletely understood but has been related to dopaminergic function in the basal ganglia. All patients exhibit profound motor disabilities. Extrapyramidal and pyramidal signs typically begin to develop between 6 and 18 months of age. The most prominent feature of the motor syndrome in all patients is dystonia affecting all parts of the body. Less than half of the patients also had chorea less severe than dystonia, and it typically emerged only with stress or excitement (Jinnah et al. 2006). Other movement disorders as tremor, opisthotonus and extensor spasms of the trunk may

also be apparent. A small number of patients with alternating variants of HPRT did not display abnormal behaviour; so enzyme assay is indicated in any patient with the neurologic features of this disease. Allopurinol is indicated for renal manifestations but does not improve neurological symptoms. Levodopa, dopaminergic agonists, dopamine-depleting agents have been used to treat movement disorders without convincing results. Pimozide, haloperidol, fluphenazine and risperidone have been used to control self-injurious behaviour; baclofen and benzodiazepines may be useful to control spasticity.

Wilson Disease

This is an autosomal recessive disorder due to a defect in the copper adenosine triphosphatase transporter (ATP7B) resulting in abnormal deposition of copper in liver, brain and other tissues. Hepatic abnormalities are the first manifestations of the disease in 50% and can co-exist with neurological forms. Neurological manifestations usually appear after the age of 10 years, although onset of neurological symptoms in patients as young as 4 years has been reported. In children, neurological symptoms may begin insidiously. Dysarthria, incoordination of voluntary movements and tremor are common symptoms, as are dystonia or a rigid-akinetic syndrome. There may be involuntary choreiform movements, and the gait may be affected. Psychiatric manifestations and behaviour disorders are also common. Ocular abnormalities are usually silent but have a great diagnostic value. The Kayser–Fleischer ring (see Fig. C2.2 Chap. C2) is practically pathognomonic for the disease and precedes the appearance of neurological abnormalities. MRI usually shows hypointensity on T1-weighted and hyperintensity on T2-weighted sequences in the lenticular nuclei, thalami, brainstem, claustrum and white matter (Fig. C5.6). The contrast between the normal low intensity of the red nuclei and substantia nigra and the abnormal high-intensity signal in the midbrain tegmentum results in the "face of the giant panda sign". Plasma ceruloplasmin and copper levels are decreased, whereas cupruria is augmented. Because of frequent side effects and initial neurologic deterioration with penicillamine therapy, the

Fig. C5.6 Wilson disease Axial T2w images of an adolescent demonstrating (**a**) symmetric hyperintense signal changes and atrophy of caudate nucleus and putamen and (**b**) hyperintense signal changes in the midbrain. The "sign of the giant panda" is marginally visible in this patient

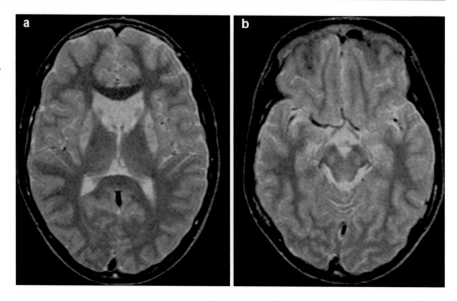

less toxic substances trientine or zinc have gradually replaced penicillamine over the past few years as the first-line treatment for Wilson disease. Initial zinc therapy for asymptomatic/presymptomatic patients and maintaining zinc therapy in patients after long-term chelation seem to be safe and effective.

Panthothenate-Kinase-Associated Neurodegeneration

The disease is caused by mutation in the gene for pantothenate kinase 2 (*PANK2*) located on chromosome 20. It is characterised by a progressive movement disorder, mainly consisting of dystonia or parkinsonism, usually associated with dementia and pyramidal tract signs. The most specific pathological findings include dysmyelination and deposition of iron-staining pigments in the pallidum and the pars reticulata of the substantia nigra, axonal swelling in the cerebral cortex and basal ganglia, increased lipofuscin deposition and, in a few cases, Lewy bodies. In the early onset form, there is an initial silent period, then unstable gait appears and regression begins between 5 and 10 years. Dystonia (often in the upper limbs, trunk and oromandibular muscles) may be an early manifestation but may not be apparent until 1 year after onset of regression. Retinopathy and acanthocytosis are common. Progressive deterioration leads to death between 11 and 15 years of life. Dystonia in the lower limbs and oromandibular

muscles is the main sign in juvenile onset cases followed by intellectual deterioration, seizures and ataxia. Parkinsonism is the predominant clinical manifestation in late-onset (adult) cases. MRI shows bilateral T2 high signal in the medial part of the pallidum surrounded by a larger zone of markedly low signal, the so-called eye-of-the-tiger image (Fig. C5.7). In some cases, only a markedly decreased signal of the pallidum without central hyperintensity is found. If MRI is done early in the course of the disease, the typical hypointense signal may not be present on MRI. The pallidum may be hyperintense instead, mimicking a mitochondrial disorder. Only symptomatic treatment is available.

Remember

- Dystonia is a major symptom in many neuro-metabolic diseases and is usually associated with other neurological signs.
- If dystonia is associated with intercurrent illnesses, appears abruptly and is suddenly generalised or if it is focal but has a progressive generalisation, it is very probably caused by a metabolic disorder.
- CSF studies are necessary if first-line examinations have not detected the aetiology. Also, L-dopa should be tried, especially when CSF analysis reveals low values of dopamine metabolites.

C5.10.2 Parkinsonism or Rigid Akinetic Syndrome

Metabolic disorders causing the rigid-akinetic syndrome as the main clinical symptom include: (1) neurotransmitter deficiencies (especially early onset forms) such as tyrosine hydroxylase, aromatic L-amino acid decarboxylase and pterin defects; (2) early onset disorders of energy metabolism such as pyruvate carboxylase deficiency or some mitochondrial DNA defects and (3) panthothenate-associated neurodegeneration (PKAN). In Wilson disease onset of neurological symptoms in childhood is exceptional. However, as Wilson disease is a treatable disorder, copper studies are still strongly recommended from early school age.

C5.10.3 Chorea

The term chorea is a derived from the Greek word "choreia" for dancing and refers to involuntary rapid spasmodic movements of the face, neck and proximal limb muscles. It may extend to the oropharyngeal muscles generating swallowing difficulties.

Choreic movements appear in glutaric aciduria type I (in the context of severe acute dyskinetic syndrome), Lesch–Nyhan disease, PKAN and homocystinuria and Niemann–Pick C among others (Table C5.10).

Table C5.10 Differential diagnosis of chorea

Benign familial chorea
Canavan disease
Dentatorubropallidoluyisian atrophy
Familial inverted choreoathetosis
Friedreich ataxia
Galactosemia
Glutaric aciduria I
Guanidinoacetate methyltransferase deficiency
Homocystinuria
Huntington chorea
Infantile NCL
Lesch–Nyhan syndrome
Neuroacanthocytosis
Niemann–Pick C
Mutations in *NKX2.1*
PKAN
Pontocerebellar hypoplasia type 2
Propionic acidemia
Pterin defects
Wilson disease

C5.10.4 Spasticity

Spasticity is a very common clinical situation in pediatric and adult neurology. It refers to dysfunction of the motor system in which certain muscles are continuously contracted. This contraction gives rise to muscle stiffness interfering with voluntary movements. Control of voluntary movements is achieved through the upper motor neurons in the brain motor cortex, which send their axons via the corticospinal tract to connect to lower motor neurons in the spinal cord. Spasticity is the result of damage to upper motor neurons or to the corticospinal tract. Symptoms may vary from mild stiffness to severe muscle spasms and include hypertonia, brisk deep tendon reflexes, pathological reflexes, clonus and weakness. Depending on the affected anatomical region, spasticity may be more evident or restricted to the lower extremities (spastic diplegia or paraplegia) to one side of the body (spastic hemiplegia) or affecting all four limbs (spastic quadriplegia or tetraparesis).

In children, most events related to motor damage occur during late pregnancy and delivery such as prematurity, neonatal asphyxia, birth trauma or infections. The consequent clinical manifestations are usually grouped under the general term cerebral palsy. In contrast, traumatic injury to and infections of the CNS that take place later on as well as genetic conditions (including inborn errors of metabolism), may also result in spasticity. Since some of these metabolic disorders are treatable and offer family genetic counselling it is important to include them in the diagnostic approach of spasticity.

Spasticity in metabolic disorders is in general associated with involvement of additional neurological functions or organs. It may appear acutely and related to signs of metabolic intoxication such as loss of consciousness or vomiting. However, some disorders can start with isolated spastic paraparesis such as X-linked adrenoleukodystrophy(X-ALD), homocysteine remethylation defects, HHH syndrome (hyperammonemia, hyperornithinemia and homocitrullinuria), arginase deficiency and Segawa disease.

The main components of the motor system (motor neurons and myelin) are extremely vulnerable to inborn errors of metabolism. This is the reason why disorders of both intermediary metabolism and complex molecules may exhibit spasticity. Disorders that interfere with myelin metabolism, defects in energy production or small toxic molecules often cause pyramidal tract lesions. In fact, almost all progressive neurometabolic diseases end up manifesting different degrees of spasticity. This section will deal with those inborn errors of metabolism in which spasticity is the dominant or one of the most prominent signs in the clinical picture (Sedel et al. 2007).

Remember

- The possibility of an inborn error of metabolism should be considered in every child with the diagnosis of cerebral palsy but without a history of perinatal or postnatal brain injury (prematurity, hypoxia, infections and traumatic brain injury).
- In inborn errors of metabolism, spasticity tends to be syndromic or complicated (other neurological signs and/or other organs are involved). However, in some cases spasticity may remain isolated for a long time.
- Spasticity is probably the most common neurologic sign in neurometabolic disorders. It is therefore important to search carefully for other associated clinical signs.

C5.10.5 Treatable Inborn Errors of Metabolism with Prominent Di/Tetraparesis:

Urea cycle disorders such as arginase deficiency, result in progressive spasticity, seizures and mental retardation with relatively mild hyperammonemia. HHH syndrome (hyperammonemia, hyperornithinemia and homocitrullinuria) is a disorder of ornithine transport between cytoplasm and mitochondria that causes progressive spastic diplegia in addition to other signs of neurologic dysfunction. Routine investigation should include plasma ammonia and amino acids (both in plasma and urine) (Scaglia et al. 2006). Therapeutic strategies include diet and ammonia-lowering agents.

Biotinidase deficiency may also manifest with progressive spastic paraparesis. It may improve with biotin (5–20 mg/day). Measurement of plasma biotinidase activity reveals the diagnosis.

Homocysteine remethylation defects can lead to demyelination of the pyramidal tracts and produce a subacute combined degeneration of the spinal cord. It is important to measure plasma amino acids, total homocysteine and

folate concentration in every patient with isolated spasticity, as it may be the only clinical sign over a long period. The combination of betaine (up to 10 g/day in 3 doses), folic acid (5–10 mg/day) and hydroxycobalamin (0.5–1 mg/day orally or 1 mg i.m. monthly) is not as effective as it is in resolving other neurological or psychiatric symptoms related to this same defect.

Cerebral folate deficiency is characterised by low CSF 5-methyltetrahydrofolate concentration and early psychomotor delay, microcephaly, movement disorders, ataxia and spastic paraplegia; clinical improvement follows high doses of folinic acid (3–5 mg/kg/day). It is not clear if this syndrome is an inborn error of metabolism, because these patients were shown to have autoantibodies against folate receptors suggesting an acquired autoimmune mechanism. Furthermore, there are secondary causes of cerebral folate deficiency such as Aicardi–Goutières, Rett syndrome and mitochondrial disorders.

Cerebrotendinous xanthomatosis is a sterol disorder that may present with progressive spasticity from the second decade of life. Early diagnosis and appropriate treatment may obviate this complication. Other clinical signs such as neonatal liver disease, cataracts or peripheral neuropathy are often present. Elevated levels of plasma cholestanol and bile acid precursors (in plasma or urine) are diagnostic. Treatment with chenodeoxycholic acid (750 mg/day) and statins improve and even reversal the neurological disability.

Dopamine synthesis defects especially GTPCH I deficiency may exhibit pyramidal signs, and, in some cases, lower limb dystonia can mimic spastic paraparesis. Therefore, CSF study and a trial of levodopa should be advisable in all patients with unexplained spastic paraparesis or dystonic cerebral palsy.

Vitamin E deficiency (see also Ataxia). Spasticity may appear together with peripheral neuropathy and retinitis pigmentosa. Laboratory findings include low-to-absent serum vitamin E and high serum cholesterol, triglycerides, and β-lipoprotein. High doses of vitamin E (400–1200 IU/day) improve neurologic function.

Remember

- Measure ammonia, amino acids, biotinidase activity, total homocysteine, folate, cholestanol and vitamin E, in all patients with spasticity of unknown origin
- Consider a trial of L-dopa and CSF studies to measure neurotransmitters and folate

C5.10.6 Progressive Spasticity Associated with Multiple Neurologic Signs, Irritability and Global Deterioration

This is a group of heterogeneous disorders that usually manifest a complex neurological picture in which progressive spasticity is one of the main features. Peripheral neuropathy, visual, auditory and visceral involvement are frequently present. Brain MRI may disclose specific white matter patterns that can be very helpful in the diagnostic approach.

In *lysosomal disorders,* some of the most representative diseases giving rise to spasticity are Krabbe disease, MLD, MPS III, fucosidosis and mannosidoses. *X-linked adrenomyeloneuropathy* can present with spasticity as an isolated sign for a long time, whereas in *adrenoleukodystrophy* of childhood, cognitive and behavioural problems may appear before the motor disturbances. Brain MRI is usually very helpful in diagnosis approach.

In *mitochondrial disorders*, pyramidal tract involvement is also frequent, however, other signs and symptoms often guide the diagnostic approach.

Neuroaxonal dystrophy and related *high brain iron disorders* are due to mutated PLA2G6, encoding a phospholipase A2. They manifest progressive neurological regression and distended axons (spheroid bodies) in the nervous system as well as high basal ganglia iron. Progressive spastic paraparesis, extrapyramidal signs and usually dementia, retinitis pigmentosa and optic atrophy are present.

Some cerebral organic acidurias such as *Canavan disease* (high urine and brain MRS N-acetylaspartate) or *L-2-hydroxyglutaric aciduria* are examples of childhood leukodystrophies exhibiting different degrees of progressive spasticity and well-defined brain MRI patterns.

Remember

- Check nerve conduction, visual, auditory function, skeleton examination (X-ray), urine glycosaminoglycans/ oligosaccharides, in patients with multiple neurological signs and progressive spasticity.
- Some brain MRI specific patterns can give the diagnostic clue.
- Consider the possibility of a brain iron disorder in a patient with progressive spasticity, especially if episodes of regression are triggered by infectious events, and even in the absence of specific brain MRI findings (basal ganglia involvement).

C5.10.7 Spastic Tetraparesis Associated with Ichthyosis

This association is typical of *Sjögren–Larsson syndrome* (fatty alcohol NAD oxidoreductase deficiency). The skin alteration consists of yellowish-brown hyperkeratosis (ichthyosis). Glistening dots are present in the macular fundus. Mental retardation is also present. Cutaneous signs may remain isolated for a long time and spastic tetraparesis can appear in adulthood. High leukotriene B_4 in urine, enzymatic activity in fibroblasts or leukocytes and mutation analysis are the diagnostic tools. Zileuton improves the cutaneous symptoms and may ameliorate the neurological disease (Gordon 2007).

Multiple sulphatase deficiency combines features of mucopolysaccharidosis, MLD and ichthyosis, starts in infancy and is usually fatal in early childhood. Glycosaminoglycans are increased in urine, and enzyme studies show deficiencies of many sulphatases (Tables C5.11 and C5.12).

C5.11 Neuroradiology

Imaging of the brain is one of the most important diagnostic tools in this field. Morphological evaluation can be done best with MRI where brain structures can be adequately viewed. Cranial computer tomography (CCT) is still important when looking for calcifications or in the emergency situation when MRI takes too long in an instable patient. Proton MR spectroscopy (^{1}H-MRS) is a powerful tool to assess the main cerebral metabolites and is diagnostic for some disorders.

Interpretation of cerebral imaging studies is not easy, and care should be taken that in patients with the diagnosis or suspicion of an inborn error of metabolism, images should be reviewed personally together with a neuroradiologist experienced in this field.

Table C5.11 Differential diagnosis of spasticity

Clinical signs associated to spasticity	Disorders
Additional neurological signs	
Peripheral neuropathy	CTX, mitochondrial disorders (axonal neuropathy), biotinidase deficiency, β-mannosidosis, sialidosis type I, Krabbe disease, MLD, homocysteine remethylation defects, vitamin E deficiency
Leukoencephalopathy	Krabbe disease, MLD, Cannavan disease, L-2-hydroxyglutaric aciduria, X-ALD, homocysteine remethylation defects, some mitochondrial disorders, multiple sulphatase deficiency, Schindler disease
Ataxia	CTX, cerebral folate deficiency, biotinidase deficiency, HHH syndrome, some mitochondrial disorders, L-2-hydroxyglutaric aciduria
Movement disorders	Dopamine synthesis defects, cerebral folate deficiency, mitochondrial disorders, brain iron disorders
Epilepsy	Homocysteine remethylation defects, cerebral folate deficiencies, mitochondrial disorders, sialidosis, Schindler disease, multiple sulphatase deficiency, Canavan disease, L-2-hydroxyglutaric aciduria
Microcephaly	Cerebral folate deficiency, homocysteine remethylation defects, arginase deficiency, mitochondrial disorders
Macrocephaly	Cerebral organic acidurias, MPS
Developmental delay/mental retardation	In all of them except GTPCH I (dominant) and sialidosis type I
Additional non-neurological signs	
Visceral	Urea cycle disorders (liver involvement, cyclic vomiting), CTX (diarrhoea), X-linked adrenoleukodystrophy (adrenal insufficiency), most lysosomal disorders (organomegaly)
Cutaneous signs	CTX (xanthomas), multiple sulphatase deficiency and Sjoegren–Larsson (ichthyosis), biotinidase deficiency (alopecia, dermatitis), X-linked ALD (melanoderma), sialidosis II (angiokeratoma)
Ocular signs	Homocysteine remethylation defects, (retinitis pigmentosa, optic nerve atrophy), CTX (cataracts), biotinidase deficiency, (optic neuropathy), Sjoegren–Larsson (retinopathy), cerebral folate deficiency (optic atrophy), different lysosomal disorders (cherry red spot), brain iron disease, mitochondrial disorders, vitamin E deficiency (retinitis pigmentosa)

CTX Cerebrotendinous xantomatosis; *MLD* metachromatic leukodystrophy; *X-ADL* X-linked adrenoleukodystrophy

"Normal" MRIs should be re-evaluated as some abnormalities escape detection by neuroradiologists unfamiliar with metabolic disorders. In infancy, normal brain maturation – the process of myelination which is more or less completed at the age of 24 months at least in the MRI – has to be taken into account; there may be subtle abnormalities. The signal of mature, myelinated white matter is dark in T2w images and bright in T1w images. In infants (and patients with hypomyelination), myelination is assessed best using T1w sequences; it is complete in T1 images at the age of 9 months. After that age, T2w images are most informative regarding progress of myelination and also involvement of white matter in metabolic and non-metabolic disorders.

Remember

Neuroimaging should be repeated if new neurologic symptoms appear, if there is clincal regression and also if the first study has been during the first 2 years of life to assess whether myelination has been completed.

A pattern recognition approach greatly facilitates differential diagnosis. In this approach, affected structures are analysed and compared with known disorders. It is a powerful method not only for established disorders, but also for the differentiation of new disorders, especially leukoencephalopathies (Lyon et al. 2006,

Table C5.12 Checklist of Laboratory Tests in Spasticity

Treatable causes of spasticity
  Plasma ammonia, plasma and urine amino acids.
  Biotinidase activity (plasma)
  Folate and total homocysteine (blood)
  Cholestanol (plasma), bile acid precursors (urine and
    plasma)
  Vitamin E, triglycerides, cholesterol and fractions,
    erythrocyte morphology (plasma)
  Folate and biogenic amine metabolites in the CSF
Progressive spasticity with signs of neurologic deterioration
  First consider treatable disorders
  Glycosaminoglycans, oligosaccharides, sialic acid (urine)
  Lysosomal enzymes (blood)
  Very long-chain fatty acids (plasma)
  Lactate, pyruvate (plasma)
  Organic acids (urine)
  Consider PLA2G6 mutation depending on clinical and
    MRI findings
Spasticity with icthyosis
  Glycosaminoglycans in urine
  Enzymatic activity of fatty alcohol NAD oxidoreductase
    in fibroblasts
Other non-metabolic causes of spasticity
  Hereditary diseases: spinocerebellar atrophy, familiar
    spastic paraparesis
  Infections: AIDS, HTLV-1
  Immunologic disorders: multiple sclerosis
  Malformations: Arnold–Chiari, cervical/lumbar
    spondylosis
  Cerebral palsy (prematurity, hypoxia, infections)
  Neoplasm

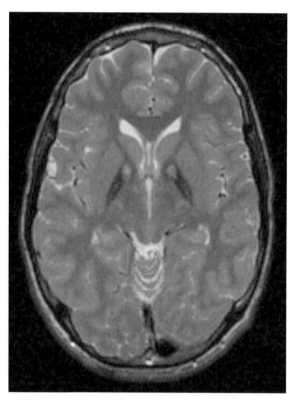

Fig. C5.7 PKAN. This axial T2w image displays the pathognomonic eye-of-the-tiger sign, a hypointense pallidum with central hyperintense gliosis

Schiffmann R et al. 2004). Typical and diagnostic patterns include the classical form of X-ALD, Canavan disease, INAD (Fig. C5.1), PKAN (Fig. C5.7) or L-2-hydroxyglutaric aciduria. Table C5.13 gives an overview of cerebral structures affected in important inborn errors of metabolism. The most obvious differentiation is between affected grey or white matter. If grey matter is involved, it must be discriminated between cortex, deep grey matter structures (basal ganglia and thalamus) and cerebellar grey matter, also between prolonged (hyperintense signal) or decreased (hypointense signal) T2 abnormalities. If primarily white matter is involved, differentiation must be made between the location of affected white matter (subcortical/arcuate fibres, central, periventricular, corpus callosum and brainstem), the gradient (symmetry, anterior vs. posterior white matter, central vs. peripheral white matter and rostral vs. caudal white matter) and other general characteristics of white matter involvement (contrast enhancement, vacuolisation or cysts, calcifications, swelling and small vs. large and isolated vs. confluent lesions).

In cerebral ^{1}H-MRS, four main physiological metabolites can be assessed easily: choline, creatine and phosphocreatine, N-acetylaspartate (NAA) and myo-inositol. Lactate is not normally visible in CNS spectra. Concentration of these metabolites has traditionally been expressed as relation to creatine, but it should be properly quantified. Metabolite levels are age related; adequate control groups are therefore important. ^{1}H-MRS is diagnostic for creatine deficiency syndromes, Canavan disease, ribose-5-phosphate isomerase deficiency (accumulation of polyols in the CNS) and probably complex II deficiency where CNS succinate is elevated (Table C5.14). All these disorders are rare and can also be diagnosed by biochemical analysis of body fluids. Complete absence of

Table C5.13 MRI findings in inherited metabolic disorders

Grey matter	
Cerebellar atrophy	Unspecific; present in many metabolic and degenerative conditions
High T2w signal of cerebellar cortex	INAD, Marinescu–Sjögren syndrome, CoQ$_{10}$ deficiency, mitochondrial disorders
Basal ganglia and thalamic involvement (symmetrical)	
long T2	Mitochondrial disorders, Wilson's disease, organic acidurias, Alpers disease (may be unilateral)
short T2 (pallidum)	PKAN, INAD
short T2 (thalamus)	INCL, Tay–Sachs disease, Krabbe disease
Dentate involvement	L-2-hydroxyglutaric aciduria, cerebrotendinous xanthomatosis
Cerebral atrophy	Unspecific, present in many neurodegenerative disorders
Stroke-like lesions	MELAS, Alpers disease, urea cycle disorders
Polymicrogyria	Zellweger disease
Cobblestone lissencephaly	Walker–Warburg syndrome and other O-glycosylation defects
White matter	
Delayed myelination	Unspecific, present in many inherited and acquired conditions
Hypomyelination	Tay–Sachs disease, INCL, Salla disease, non-metabolic disorders (e.g. Pelizaeus–Merzbacher disease)
Early involvement of subcortical white matter	Galactosemia, L-2-hydroxyglutaric aciduria
Central white matter/centrum semiovale	Krabbe disease, metachromatic leukodystrophy, X-ALD, phenylketonuria, Lowe syndrome, disorders of cytosolic methyl group transfer, various other disorders
Miscellaneous	
Subdural effusions	Glutaric aciduria type I, Menkes disease
Elongated and tortuous arteries	Menkes disease
Reduced opercularisation	Glutaric aciduria type I
Agenesis of the corpus callosum	PDHc deficiency, mitochondrial disorders
Caudothalamic cysts	Zellweger syndrome, glutaric aciduria type I
Calcifications	Mitochondrial disorders (especially Kearns–Sayre syndrome), folate deficiency, other disorders (e.g. Aicardi-Goutières syndrome)

Table C5.14 Typical ^{1}H-MRS abnormalities in inherited metabolic disorders

^{1}H-MRS finding	Disease
Absent creatine peak	Creatine synthesis (GAMT, AGAT) and transport (CRTR) deficiencies
Elevated lactate	Mitochondrial disorders, pyruvate dehydrogenase deficiency, other IEMs, non-metabolic conditions (ischemia, infection, neoplasia)
Elevated polyols	Ribose-5-phosphate isomerase deficiency
Strongly increased NAA	Canavan disease
Absent NAA	Putative NAA synthesis defect
Increased choline	Demyelination (e.g. metachromatic leukodystrophy, X-ALD)
Increased succinate	Complex II deficiency
Increased lipids	Sjögren–Larsson syndrome

cerebral NAA which is a neuronal and axonal marker has been described in one single child; the metabolic defect has not yet been elucidated. This disease is not amenable to biochemical diagnosis. One of the questions ^{1}H-MRS can answer is whether lactate is elevated in the CNS, which is possible even with normal CSF lactate levels. This may be the only metabolic indicator of a mitochondrial disorder, hence the importance of ^{1}H-MRS for neurometabolic disorders.

As a minimal protocol, MRI should include axial T1w, T2w and FLAIR images and sagittal Tw1 images. If there are cerebellar abnormalities, coronar T2w or FLAIR images should be acquired. Diffusion-weighted imaging is part of many routine studies nowadays and should always be done if stroke-like episodes or "metabolic stroke" is suspected (Roach et al. 2008). Fibre-tracking is a novel method to depict connections within the CNS. If possible, ^{1}H-MRS should be done together with conventional MR imaging, at least one single voxel. Optimally, voxels of interest in ^{1}H-MRS should be located in the basal ganglia, in the centrum semiovale, in the cortex (usually in the occipital cortex) and also in the cerebellum (Barkovich et al. 2005; van der Knaap et al. 1999).

C5.12 Neurophysiology

Neurophysiologic studies are important for diagnosis and follow-up in neurometabolic disorders, especially if epilepsy or neuropathy are part of the clinical picture. There are few pathognomonic or typical findings. Of major interest for neurometabolic disorders are EEG, electroretinography (ERG), measurement of nerve conduction velocities and evoked potentials. Electromyography (EMG) is done if myopathy or motor neuropathy are suspected. It can reveal myotonia-like discharges as typical finding in juvenile type II glycogenosis.

EEG may be of value in the diagnosis of several neurometabolic disorders. In INAD, it shows a pronounced, diffuse fast β–activity in the absence of medication, especially in stage I and II sleep which helps in the diagnosis of this rare disorder (Fig. C5.2). In late-infantile neuronal ceroid lipofuscinosis, slow photic stimulation leads to occipital spikes (Fig. C5.4) and may even trigger focal occipital seizures. In the infantile form, EEG shows early a slowing of the background, later in the course an isoelectric tracing. In the neonatal manifestation of maple syrup urine disease, EEG displays comb-like rhythms. A burst-suppression pattern is not specific and may be found in different epileptic encephalopathies with neonatal onset the most frequent being non-ketotic hyperglycinemia. In patients with homocystinuria, centrotemporal spikes are often present resembling the epileptiform potentials in benign epilepsy with centrotemporal spikes. If cortical abnormalities are present, EEG reflects their localisation and quality – in cobblestone lissencephaly, it shows generalised β-activity, usually of high amplitude. In Alpers disease, EEG is very valuable in the early stage of the disease and diplays, albeit not in all patients, RHADS, usually over the posterior regions (Fig. C5.5).

Somatosensory evoked potentials (SSEP) are helpful in delineating posterior column involvement, e.g. in FRDA or cobalamin deficiency. Giant SSEP are found in some of the progressive myoclonic epilepsies including late infantile neuronal ceroid lipofuscinosis. Visual evoked potentials help to detect early involvement of the optic nerve, e.g. in mitochondrial disorders, INAD or Alpers disease. ERG is important in detecting retinal involvement,which is of use in the differential diagnosis of neurodegenerative disorders. Retinal involvement is part of the NCL, but also of panthotenate-associated neurodegeneration (PKAN), mitochondrial disorders and many others (see also Chap. C8).

C5.13. Diagnostic Lumbar Puncture

In an increasing number of encephalopathies of unknown origin metabolic investigations of CSF can be instrumental in identifying the underlying neurometabolic disorder. As there is still widespread uncertainty about when to perform specialised CSF investigations and what to investigate in many patients remain undiagnosed, although they often have recognisable phenotypes. As a consequence futile diagnostic searches continue, and the often available rational therapy cannot be instituted. On the other hand, a lumbar puncture should only be performed in the diagnostic work-up of a suspected neurometabolic disorder after basic analyses have been carried out in blood and urine (see Table C5.15) and after the results of neuroimaging studies have been carefully evaluated. There is no place for a selective screening in CSF. Reliable results of specialised CSF investigations can only be obtained if the appropriate protocol is strictly adhered to. This should be discussed beforehand with the neurometabolic laboratory (see (D2) Biochemical Studies).

White cell hexosaminidase, sphingomyelinase, palmitoylprotein thioesterase activity, aryl sulphatase,

Table C5.15 Investigations for neurometabolic diseases in blood and urine

Blood/plasma/serum: Full blood count and reticulocytes, usual chemistry profile including Ca, P, alkaline phosphate, creatinine, uric acid, copper, ceruloplasmin, T3, T4, TSH, thyroid binding globulin, prolactin
Amino acids, total homocysteine, lactate and pyruvate, ammonia, biotinidase, very long-chain fatty acids, pristanic acid, pipecolic acid, transferrin isoelectric focussing
Urine: Organic acids, lactic acid, uric acid (urate/creatinine ratio, guanidino compounds, sulphite, purines and pyrimidines, bile acid intermediates, mucopolysaccaccharides, oligosaccharides, sialic acid), creatinine (preferably 24-h urine)
Blood or urine: Acyl-carnitine esters

glucocerebrosidase, galactocerebrosidase, fucosidase and tripeptidyl peptidase activity

The diagnosis of monogenic defects of neurotransmission is almost exclusively based on the quantitative determination of the neurotransmitters and/or their metabolites in CSF, i.e. the amino acids glutamate, glycine and γ-aminobutyric acid (GABA), the acidic metabolites of the biogenic monoamines, dopamine, serotonin, epinephrine and norepinephrine, and individual pterin species. In other neurometabolic disorders, results of CSF investigations are important, although not exclusive part of the diagnostic work-up, e.g. GLUT1 deficiency, mitochondriopathies and serine synthesis disorders.

Remember

Whenever CSF investigations are performed, the analysis should include quantitative determination of lactate, pyruvate and amino acids, the latter by methods especially suited for CSF, in addition to cells, glucose, protein, immunoglobulin classes, specific immunoglobulins and an evaluation of the blood-brain barrier (Table C5.16).

Preprandial plasma amino acids, serum glucose and blood lactate should always be determined at the time of the lumbar puncture, as ratios are highly informative for a large number of disorders and almost indispensable for the diagnosis of some disorders, e.g. non-ketotic hyperglycinemia (CSF glycine almost always > 30 μM and glycine CSF/plasma ratio > 0.04), glucose transport protein deficiency (glucose CSF/plasma ratio < 0.45) and defects of serine synthesis (CSF serine < 14 μM and serine CSF/plasma ratio < 0.2). Unreported blood contamination of CSF is the most common cause for an erroneous diagnosis of non-ketotic hyperglycinemia. Because amino acids and glucose change dramatically after a meal, timing of the lumbar puncture and blood taking should not be post- but pre-prandial, i.e. at least 4–6h after a meal.

Table C5.16 Investigations for neurometabolic diseases in CSF

Cells, protein, immunoglobulin classes and glucose (plus plasma glucose and evaluation of blood-brain barrier)
Lactate (plus preprandial blood lactate)
Amino acids (plus preprandial plasma amino acids)
Biogenic amine metabolites
Individual pterin species
5-Methyltetrahydrofolate

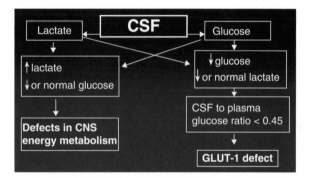

Fig. C5.8 Evaluation of CSF/blood results of glucose and lactate

Blood should be taken first as glucose may rise stress related during the lumbar puncture.

Figure C5.8 depicts an algorithm for the interpretation of pathological CSF/plasma results of glucose and lactate. Glucose and lactate must be looked together. Pathologically altered ratios may indicate a disease intrinsic to the CNS. Elevations of CSF lactate together with a reduction in glucose results from inadequate aerobic energy production, e.g. in mitochondriopathies but more commonly in the course of CNS infections. In contrast, reduced levels of CSF glucose in GLUT1 deficiency is accompanied by low normal or even reduced levels of lactate. Post-prandial or stress-related elevated blood glucose is the most common cause of a reduced CSF/blood ratio for an erroneous suspicion of GLUT1 deficiency.

Take Home Messages

> Neurological disease can be considered as the most common consequence of inborn errors of metabolism.
> A structured diagnostic approach should be based on:
  -Age-dependant physiological developments
  -Predominant neurological manifestation (mental retardation, epilepsy, motor disturbances)
  -Therapeutic possibilities.
> A high level of suspicion and close interaction between paediatric neurologist and specialist for inborn errors of metabolism are indispensable to effectively and timely identify patients in whom neurological disorders are the presenting and/or main symptoms of an inborn error.

Key References

American Academy of Child and Adolescent Psychiatry Working Group on Quality Issues (1999) Practice parameters for the assessment and treatment of children, adolescents, and adults with mental retardation and comorbid mental disorders. J Am Acad Child Adolesc Psychiatry 38(12 Suppl):5S–31S

Assmann B, Surtees R, Hoffmann GF (2003) Approach to the diagnosis of neurotransmitter diseases exemplified by the differential diagnosis of childhood-onset dystonia. Ann Neurol 54(Suppl 6):S18–24

Barkovich AJ (2005) Magnetic resonance techniques in the assessment of myelin and myelination. J Inherit Metab Dis 28:311–343

Fernández-Álvarez E, Aicardi J (2001) Movement disorders in children. Mac Keith Press, London

García-Cazorla A (2008) Neurometabolic diseases: guidance for neuropaediatricians. Rev Neurol 47(Suppl 1):S55–63

Germain DP, Avan P, Chassaing A, Bonfils P (2002) Patients affected with Fabry disease have an increased incidence of progressive hearing loss and sudden deafness: an investigation of twenty-two hemizygous male patients. BMC Med Genet 11(3):10

Gordon N (2007) Sjögren-Larsson syndrome. Dev Med Child Neurol 49:152–154

Jinnah HA, Visser JE, Harris JC et al (2006) Lesch-Nyhan Disease International Study Group. Delineation of the motor disorder of Lesch-Nyhan disease. Brain 129:1201–1217

Kokotas H, Petersen MB, Willems PJ (2007) Mitochondrial deafness. Clin Genet 71:379–391

Lyon G, Fattal-Valevski A, Kolodny EH (2006) Leukodystrophies: clinical and genetic aspects. Top Magn Reson Imaging 17:219–242

Morgan NV, Westaway SK, Morton JEV et al (2006) PLA2G6, encoding a phospholipase A2, is mutated in neurodegenerative disorders with high brain iron. Nat Genet 38:752–754

Moser H (1997) Adrenoleukodystrophy: phenotype, genetics, pathogenesis and therapy. Brain 120:1485–1508

Nance WE (2003) The genetics of deafness. Ment Retard Dev Disabil Res Rev 9:109–119

Parker CC, Evans OB (2003) Metabolic disorders causing childhood ataxia. Semin Pediatr Neurol 10:193–199

Poretti A, Wolf NI, Boltshauser E (2008) Differential diagnosis of cerebellar atrophy in childhood. Eur J Pediatr Neurol 123:155–167

Roach ES, Golomb MR, Adams R et al (2008) Management of stroke in infants and children. Stroke 39:1–48

Scaglia F, Lee B (2006) Clinical, biochemical, and molecular spectrum of hyperargininemia due to arginase I deficiency. Am J Med Genet C Semin Med Genet 142:113–120

Schiffmann R, van der Knaap MS (2004) The latest on leukodystrophies. Curr Opin Neurol 17:187–192

Sedel F, Fontaine B, Saudubray JM (2007) Hereditary spastic paraparesis in adults associated with inborn errors of metabolism: a diagnostic approach. J Inherit Metab Dis 30: 855–864

Shevell M, Ashwal S, Donley D et al (2003) Practice parameter: evaluation of the child with global developmental delay. Neurology 60:367–380

Surtees R, Wolf N (2007) Treatable neonatal epilepsy. Arch Dis Child 92:659–661

van der Knaap MS, Breiter SN, Naidu S et al (1999) Defining and categorizing leukoencephalopathies of unknown origin: MR imaging approach. Radiology 213:121–133

Van Karnebeek CDM, Jansweijer MCE, Leenders AGE et al (2005) Diagnostic investigations in individuals with mental retardation. Eur J Hum Genet 13:6–25

Wolf NI, Bast T, Surtees R (2005) Epilepsy in inborn errors of metabolism. Epileptic Disord 7:67–81

Zschocke J, Hoffmann GF (2004) Vademecum Metabolicum. Manual of metabolic paediatrics, 2nd edn. Schattauer, Stuttgart

Metabolic Myopathies

C6

Stephen G. Kahler

Key Facts

> The metabolic disorders which affect muscle can cause chronic weakness and hypotonia, or episodic exercise intolerance cumulating in rhabdomyolysis, or both. Rhabdomyolysis disorders can be conveniently separated according to tolerance of short, intense exercise compared to longer, milder efforts.

> Most metabolic disorders which affect skeletal muscle do so by altering energy metabolism. Muscle at rest uses fatty acids as the main energy source.

> During intense exercise, there will be anaerobic glycolysis and utilization of muscle glycogen. During sustained exercise, fatty acids become the source of fuel. Exercise, fasting, cold, infections, and medications may elicit symptoms.

> Important causes of metabolic myopathy include adenosine monophosphate (myoadenylate) deaminase deficiency, and disorders of glycolysis, glycogenolysis, fatty acid oxidation, and oxidative phosphorylation. In many cases other organs are involved.

> Diagnosis requires careful attention to dietary and exercise history, and appropriate laboratory investigations. Exercise testing, electromyogram, and muscle biopsy can provide essential information.

> Treatment depends on avoiding precipitating factors and optimizing muscle energetics.

C6.1 General Remarks

Many metabolic disorders cause muscle dysfunction or damage (Table C6.1). The pathophysiological basis in most is impairment of energy production when stressed, particularly by exercise, cold, fasting, or infection (especially of viral origin). In some situations, the problem is confined to skeletal muscle, but in many there is cardiac involvement as well. Liver, brain, retina, and kidney, all of which have significant energy requirements, may also be involved. Even more extensive or patchy involvement, e.g., pancreas and bone marrow, is a characteristic of the mitochondrial disorders where heteroplasmy may occur (see also Chaps. B2.3 and D6).

C6.1.1 Special Aspects of Skeletal Muscle Metabolism

Skeletal muscle relies on different fuel sources at different times and circumstances. Fatty acids are the primary fuel at rest. Glucose from the blood and derived from muscle glycogen is used during short-term intensive

S. G. Kahler
Department of Pediatrics, Division of Clinical Genetics, University of Arkansas for Medical Sciences, 4301 W. Markham Street, Little Rock, AR 72205, USA
e-mail: KahlerStepheng@uams.edu

G. F. Hoffmann et al. (eds.), *Inherited Metabolic Diseases*,
DOI: 10.1007/978-3-540-74723-9_C6, © Springer-Verlag Berlin Heidelberg 2010

Table C6.1 Major presentations of metabolic myopathies?

	Enzyme (position- in pathway – Fig. C1)	Rhabdomy-olysis	Hypotonia, weakness	Cramps	Worsened by fasting?	Worsened by exercise?	Worsened by cold?	Worsened by infection?	Incr. Baseline CK
RHABDOMYOLYSIS AND MYOGLOBINURIA PRESENTATION									
Intense exercise not tolerated; second wind phenomenon		++	+	++		++			+
GSD type V	Muscle phosphorylase (II)	++	+	++		++			+
GSD type IX	Muscle phosphorylase kinase (II)	+	+	+		+			+
GSD VII	Muscle phosphofructokinase (8)	+	+	+		+	++		++
PGK deficiency	Muscle phosphoglycerate kinase (III)	++		++		++			++
PGAM deficiency	Phosphoglycerate mutase (III)	++		++		++			++
β-Enolase deficiency	β-Enolase (III)	++		++		++			+
LDH deficiency	Lactic dehydrogenase M subunit (12)	++				++			
Myoadenylate deaminase deficiency	Muscle AMP deaminase	+	+	+		+			-
Short, intense exercise tolerated; prolonged exercise not tolerated		+	+	++	++	++	++	++	+
Translocase deficiency	Carnitine-acylcarnitine translocase (22)								
CPT II deficiency	Carnitine palmitoyltransferase II (23)	++			++	++	++	++	
VLCAD deficiency	Very-long chain acyl-CoA dehydrogenase (24)	++	+		++	+		+	+
LCAD deficiency	Long-chain acyl-coA dehydrogenase (24)								
LCHAD/trifunctional enzyme deficiency	Long-chain 3-hydroxyacyl-CoA dehydrogenase (26)	++							
MCAD deficiency	Medium-chain acyl-CoA dehydrogenase (24)	-	(+)		++	+	-	++	
SCAD deficiency	Short-chain acyl-CoA dehydrogenase (24)		++						
Hydroxyacyl-CoA dehydrogenase (short-chain hydroxyacyl-CoA dehydrogenase) deficiency		++						+	
HYPOTONIA AND WEAKNESS		+	++		+	+			+
Carnitine transporter deficiency	Plasma membrane carnitine transporter (20)		++		++				+
Secondary carnitine depletion			++			+	+		
Mild multiple acyl-CoA dehydrogenase deficiency (MADD) deficiency	Electron-transfer flavoprotein (ETF) or ETF dehydrogenase ETF-QO		+						
Lysosomal glycogen storage disease (Pompe)	Lysosomal α-glucosidase		++						++
GSD type III	Glycogen debrancher (II)	+	++	+					++
GSD type IV	Glycogen brancher enzyme (I)		+						
Neutral lipid storage disease I	Comparative gene identification-58		+						+
Neutral lipid storage disease II	ATGL		+						+
MITOCHONDRIAL MYOPATHIES	Many disorders and mechanisms. (See Chap. B2.3 and Fig. B2.3.2	+	++	+		+	+	+	+
Coenzyme Q deficiency	Several known gene defects and mechanisms	+	++						

See text for details about specific disorders

D DNA (predominant or common mutation); *E* erythrocytes; *F* fibroblasts; *H* heart; *K* kidney; *L* liver; *M* muscle; *W* leukocytes. This list is only a guide. Which tissue is required and which test is to be done depends on the laboratory performing the test, and in some cases on which organs are affected

++ Often present or abnormal; + occasionally present or abnormal

[a]Hepatic dysfunction with encephalopathy is a "Reye-like syndrome"W

Abnormal EMG	Muscle biopsy	Organic acids	Carnitine level	Acylcarnitine profile	Cardiomy-opathy	Hepatic dysfunc-tion[a]	Encephal-opathy[a]	Diagnostic tissues	Comments
+	+								Disorders of glycogenolysis and glycolysis; AMP deficiency
	+							M	Occ. severe infantile form. Proximal > distal
	+			One form				M	Four syndromes, two involving skeletal muscle
+	++				+			M and E	Hemolytic anemia, rare, hyperuricemia. Muscle cannot utilize glucose – worse after glucose, high-CHO meal. Severe infantile form with cardiomyopathy
	++	-					++	M	Hemolytic anemia. Neurologic abnormalities. X-linked
-	++	-						M	Very rare
-	++	-						M	Very rare
	-	-						M	Very rare. Lactate does not rise after ischemic exercise when pyruvate is elevated. Uterine stiffness
+	++							L	Impaired ammonia production with ischemic exercise
+	++	++	+	++	++	++	++		Disorders of fatty acid oxidation and carnitine-assisted transport into mitochondria
	+	+	++	++	++	++	+	F	
	++	+	?	++	++	++	+	F, M, L, and W	Heterozygote may have symptoms, be vulnerable to malignant hyperthermia. Lactic acidosis. Sensori-motor neuropathy.
++		++	++	++	++	++	++	F, W, and L	
								F, W, and L	Uncommon; see text
	++	++	++	++	++	++	++	F, M, L, and D	HELLP syndrome in pregnant heterozygote
	+	++	++	+	++	++	++	F, L, W, and D	Myopathy is minimal; this is the commonest disorder of fatty acid oxidation. Most early cases called systemic carnitine deficiency
+		++				++	++	F, M, and L	Rare. Extremely variable
					++	++		F, M, and L	Very rare
+	+		+		+	+			Carnitine deficiency or depletion; Pompe disease; glycogen brancher and debrancher deficiencies
+	++	+	??		++	++	+	F, M, L, and K	
+	+	+	??		+	++	+		Occurs in many settings
+	+	++	+	++	++	++	++	F, M, and L	Mild forms exist – may respond to riboflavin
++	++				++			W, M, and F	Variable. Macroglossia, severe cardiomyopathy in infantile Pompe form
	++				Most, but sx rare	++		E, F, H, L, M, and W	Liver ± muscle. Distal > proximal.
	++				+	++		L, M, W, E, F, and D	Severe liver disease. Neuropathy, dementia in adult form
+	++							M	Ichtyosiform nonbullous erythroderma
+	++				+			M	Hepatomegaly
+	++	+	+	+	++	+	++	M, W, L, H, and F	Several syndromes. See Table D6.3. Lactate /pyruvate ratio usually increased
	+				+	+	+	M	Renal tubular dysfunction, ataxia. Myopathic forms allelic with MADD

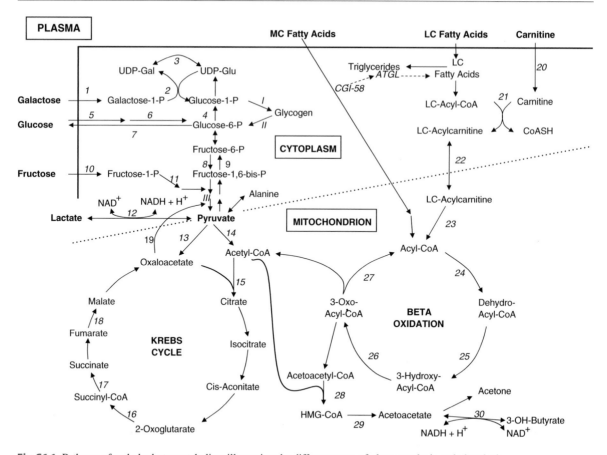

Fig.C6.1 Pathway of carbohydrate metabolism illustrating the different steps of glycogenolysis and glycolysis

exercise. Fatty acids predominate again during prolonged exercise and during fasting. Impairment of muscle energy metabolism will lead to clinical symptoms. The history of events that elicit the symptoms is a guide to the likely area of the biochemical defect.

Triglycerides are stored in the cytoplasm as droplets close to the mitochondria. The mobilization of free fatty acids from the lipid droplets depends on hormone sensitive lipases and involves the hydrolase ATGL and its activator protein comparative gene identification-58 (CGI-58), two recently identified causes of lipid storage myopathies (Fig. C6.1).

Resting muscle in the fed state uses fatty acids as the primary fuel; glucose is stored as muscle glycogen (in the cytoplasm). Preformed high-energy phosphate compounds and muscle glycogen, in addition to glucose and fatty acids in the blood stream, are a source of energy for short-term intense activity. Lactate is the end product of anaerobic glycolysis. Impaired ability to utilize muscle glycogen (e.g., glycogen storage diseases (GSD) III – debrancher deficiency, V – muscle phosphorylase

deficiency, and muscle phosphorylase kinase deficiency) results in significant limitation when the patient attempts short, intense exercise. There will be diminished production of pyruvate and hence lactate. The situation is magnified, if the muscle being tested is deprived of oxygen and continuous fuel by a tourniquet. This is the principle of the ischemic exercise test (see Chap. D8).

Defects of glycolysis in muscle, e.g., deficiencies of muscle phosphofructokinase (PFK), phosphoglycerate kinase (PGK), phosphoglycerate mutase (PGAM), β-enolase, and lactate dehydrogenase (LDH), can cause symptoms similar to muscle phosphorylase deficiency. The pathways of glycogenolysis and glycolysis are shown in Fig.C6.1.

When sustained muscle activity is initiated there is an initial reliance on glucose and glycogen as a fuel source. Metabolic disorders affecting these pathways typically cause symptoms at this time. After a few minutes glycogen stores will be depleted, and fatty acids become more important as a fuel. The carnitine cycle and the β-oxidation spiral of fatty acid oxidation are essential at this point, so defects in these pathways can result in easy fatigability and impaired tolerance of sustained exercise.

C6.1.2 Basic Patterns of Metabolic Myopathies

The two major distinct syndromes of muscle metabolic disorders are exercise intolerance and rhabdomyolysis (with or without myoglobinuria), and weakness (with or without hypotonia). Rhabdomyolysis can be further divided into syndromes where it occurs during strenuous exercise and those where it occurs afterwards.

> **Remember**
>
> Major symptoms of myopathies are weakness, hypotonia, exercise intolerance, and rhabdomyolysis.

Rhabdomyolysis, the destruction of skeletal muscle cells, often results from failure of energy production, leading to an inability to maintain muscle membranes. The hallmark of rhabdomyolysis is elevation of muscle enzymes in the blood, particularly creatine kinase (CK or CPK). This elevation can persist for several days after an acute event. Chronic elevation of CK indicates continuous damage.

Rhabdomyolysis during short-term intensive exercise is a primary feature of the disorders of carbohydrate metabolism, especially muscle phosphorylase (McArdle disease). After a period of intense pain with or without cramping, however, there may be considerable relief and ability to continue exercise, called the "second wind" phenomenon, as the muscle switches to increased use of fatty acids for fuel. Patients with McArdle disease will also benefit from glucose administration before exercise, because they are able to utilize glucose. In contrast, patients with a metabolic block in glycolysis, e.g., in PGK, cannot utilize neither glucose nor glycogen. Glucose administration even diminishes the concentrations of the alternative fuels triglycerides and ketone bodies ("out of wind" phenomenon).

Postexercise cramps and rhabdomyolysis are the more common pattern in fatty acid disorders, especially deficiencies of carnitine palmitoyltransferase (CPT) II, very long-chain acyl-CoA dehydrogenase (VLCAD), long-chain hydroxyacyl-CoA dehydrogenase (LCHAD), and short-chain hydroxyacyl-CoA dehydrogenase

(SCHAD) (see also Chap. B2.5), and mitochondrial oxidative phosphorylation disorders. Rhabdomyolysis may also be a chronic feature of the various muscular dystrophies, which are usually disorders of the structural proteins of muscle (dystrophin, actin, tropomyosin, the dystroglycan complex, etc).

> **Remember**
>
> Short, intense exercise stresses glycolysis and glycogen utilization.
>
> Prolonged exercise requires adequate utilization of fatty acids.
>
> Fasting, cold, infection, and medications can worsen many myopathies.

Myoglobinuria is an extreme result of rhabdomyolysis. When muscle cells lyse myoglobin is released. Visible myoglobin in the urine indicates extensive damage. Typically, there is no myoglobin in the urine if the CK is <10,000 IU, so the absence of myoglobinuria provides no reassurance regarding absence of rhabdomyolysis.

Myoglobinuria is an emergency situation, as the pigment may precipitate in the renal tubules, leading to renal failure, which may become irreversible. Severe rhabdomyolysis can raise the serum potassium level dangerously high, leading to cardiac rhythm disturbances. Accordingly, dark urine in a patient suffering from muscle symptoms (pain, weakness, cramping, etc) must be tested for myoglobin using a specific test (to distinguish the pigment from hemoglobin). Hemoglobinuria most often accompanies hematuria, readily detectable by finding erythrocytes on microscopic analysis of the urine. Intravascular hemolysis will occasionally result in hemoglobinuria, without hematuria.

Myoglobinuria is treated with diuresis, and careful monitoring of electrolyte, fluid status, and urine output, until the myoglobinuria resolves. Investigation of the underlying cause of myoglobinuria begins at the same time as its treatment.

Chronic weakness and hypotonia are typical features of disorders of endogenous triglyceride catabolism, glycogen breakdown, carnitine availability, fatty acid oxidation, and oxidative phosphorylation. Important causes include lysosomal GSD (acid maltase deficiency – Pompe disease), glycogen debrancher deficiency, carnitine transporter defect and secondary carnitine deficiencies,

VLCAD, LCHAD, SCHAD deficiencies, and mitochondrial myopathies. Chronic weakness may certainly result from rhabdomyolysis and consequent muscle destruction from any cause, especially if recurrent.

C6.2 Approach to Metabolic Myopathies

The most urgent issues in the assessment of myopathy are to determine if there is weakness so severe to impair respiration, if there is sufficient damage to lead to myoglobinuria, and if there is cardiac involvement. Hepatic involvement, often manifest as hypoglycemia and fasting intolerance, occurs in many metabolic disorders, particularly those involving glycogen or fatty acid metabolism. A toxic encephalopathy, including cerebral edema, may also develop.

The history of muscle dysfunction may be easy to elicit from an adult or a child (or the parents), but may be difficult with infants. Hypotonia and weakness may first become evident as developmental delay. Careful assessment may then reveal that social, fine motor, and language skills are appropriate for age, and the only area of delay is in gross motor skills.

As a young child grows older, problems with exercise intolerance and easy fatigability become easier to detect, particularly if there is an unaffected older sibling to serve as a reference point for the parents. Occasionally, a child with a muscle disorder is thought to be "seeking attention" or malingering, but careful history and observation can usually eliminate this possibility quickly. Laboratory tests that convincingly demonstrate ongoing muscle injury (e.g., elevated CK) are most persuasive.

Disorders made worse by fasting may not be evident in infancy, as most infants are fed frequently. An inability to tolerate intense or prolonged exercise will not be evident in infancy, and perhaps not until adulthood. Rhabdomyolysis in response to cold also may not become evident until adolescence or adulthood. Rhabdomyolysis triggered by infection (usually viral), or fasting, may present in infancy as sudden weakness, accompanied by dark urine. Rhabdomyolysis is often quite painful, but may be painless.

Some conditions that are not yet completely characterized can cause severe and potentially fatal rhabdomyolysis in children, particularly in the setting of viral infection. Children with such conditions, like children with named disorders of fatty acid oxidation or mitochondrial dysfunction, need to be monitored carefully during infections.

The history of exercise can provide preliminary guidance in determining the most likely causes of a myopathy. An inability to perform sudden intense exercise suggests a problem with glycogenolysis or glycolysis, while inability to perform at a sustained level suggests a problem with fatty acid oxidation.

Many mitochondrial disorders of oxidative phosphorylation first become apparent because of skeletal muscle weakness. Even isolated myopathies can occur. Rhabdomyolysis is uncommon. Mitochondrial disorders may have prominent muscle involvement. Mitochondrial disorders can involve any organ at any age. Other organs commonly affected include the brain, retina, extraocular muscles, heart, liver, kidney, pancreas, gut, and bone marrow. Systemic growth may be impaired. Mild hypertrichosis often accompanies systemic lactic acidosis. Despite the diversity of mitochondrial dysfunction there are several common syndromes in which many patients can conveniently be grouped. They include MERRF, MELAS, and infantile myopathy (Chap. D6).

Two very rare neutral lipid storage diseases could be recently identified. Neutral lipid storage disease type I or Chanarin–Dorfman syndrome manifests as a slowly progressive proximal myopathy sparing the axial muscles. The hallmark of the disorder is an ichthyosiform nonbullous erythroderma. Neutral lipid storage disease type II is due to mutations in the activator gene ATGL, again leading to a lipid myopathy associated with cardiac dysfunction and hepatomegaly.

C6.2.1 Genetics

Most metabolic myopathies, like most other metabolic disorders, are inherited in an autosomal recessive manner. All disorders of fatty acid oxidation and most disorders of glycogen and glucose metabolism are inherited this way. However, other mechanisms including one form of phosphorylase b kinase deficiency, and PGK deficiency, autosomal dominant (heterozygous CPT II deficiency), mitochondrial maternal transmission, and sporadic mitochondrial disorders occur. Specifics of inheritance are mentioned when appropriate in the discussion of the various disorders.

Because of the highly variable nature of most metabolic disorders of muscle, all siblings of patients should be checked for the condition which is in the family. If the disorder may be dominant, X-linked, or mitochondrially inherited other appropriate relatives should also be examined carefully.

C6.2.2 Physical Examination

The general physical examination of a patient suspected of myopathy includes assessment of growth and development, and particular attention to other organs. The muscles should be examined for bulk and regional (proximal and distal) or local evidence of wasting, texture and consistency, and tenderness. Deep tendon reflexes, which are generally preserved in myopathies, but lost in peripheral neuropathies, should be tested carefully. Attention should be especially directed to extraocular movements and the retina, the tongue, the heart, and the size and character of the liver.

C6.2.3 Laboratory Investigations

Laboratory investigation of suspected myopathies should be undertaken during the acute episode if possible, and later repeated as indicated. Routine serum electrolytes, measurement of glucose, urea and creatinine, and "muscle enzymes" including CK, LDH including isoforms, aldolase, SGOT (ALT), SGPT (AST), total and free carnitine, plasma or blood spot acylcarnitines profile, plasma lactate and pyruvate, phosphate, calcium, thyroid hormone, plasma and urine amino acids, and urine organic acids, may all provide useful information.

Following the assessment of the first-order laboratory tests, further tests may be warranted. Functional testing using ischemic exercise (for suspected glycogen storage and glycolytic disorders, and adenosine monophosphate deaminase deficiency) can be most helpful (see Chap. D8). Graded exercise or bicycle ergometry may help pinpoint the metabolic error, or define the general area of impairment, if history and blood tests have not done so. A "diagnostic fast" to evoke abnormal metabolites or provoke symptoms should only be done if information cannot be obtained by another method – challenges are better put to fibroblasts or tissue samples. However, a fast under controlled circumstances can provide valuable information regarding how long it is safe for a particular child to fast when healthy (see Chap. D8).

Third-order tests include electromyogram (often coupled with nerve conduction studies), chest X-ray, electrocardiogram, echocardiogram, and muscle biopsy (perhaps together with nerve biopsy). Light and electron microscopic examination, and special stains for glycogen, lipid, and various enzymes may all be essential. "Classic" lipid storage is found in four conditions: primary carnitine deficiency due to a deficiency of the carnitine transporter, mild multiple acyl-CoA dehydrogenase deficiency (MADD) with secondary coenzyme Q_{10} deficiency, and the neutral lipid storage diseases types I and II.

Many enzymes can be studied in fibroblasts or lymphocytes, and DNA can be obtained from blood or a buccal brush instead of a tissue biopsy. Mitochondria can be prepared for functional and molecular studies from muscle (the preferred source) but also liver, leukocytes, and other samples. Coenzyme Q is best measured in muscle. Details of these tests are given in (Chap. D5). If an open muscle biopsy is done, a skin biopsy for fibroblast culture and DNA analysis can be taken from the edge of the incision. Some pathologists and mitochondrial laboratories are now able to analyze muscle tissue obtained by needle biopsy. Table C6.1 provides a guide to the principal features of the major metabolic myopathies and the usefulness of the various diagnostic materials.

C6.3 Specific Disorders of Muscle Metabolism

C6.3.1 Exercise Intolerance/ Rhabdomyolysis and Myoglobinuria Presentation

C6.3.1.1 Intense Exercise not Tolerated. Mild, Prolonged Exercise Tolerated. Fasting Tolerated. Dietary Modifications Helpful

Muscle Glycogen Phosphorylase (Myophosphorylase) Deficiency – McArdle Disease (GSD Type V)

This dramatic disorder of muscle glycogen metabolism is a relatively common cause of rhabdomyolysis and myoglobinuria. Although it is inherited in an autosomal recessive manner, most symptomatic patients are men. Symptoms usually begin between late childhood and late middle age. Strenuous exercise leads rapidly to cramping and fatigue, but, after a period of rest (adaptation), exercise is tolerated. Some patients with McArdle disease have chronic progressive weakness and wasting, without pain or cramping.

Exceptional cases include a rapidly fatal form in infants or young children with hypotonia and generalized weakness, a late onset form with chronic weakness, and a late onset form with severe symptoms (pain, cramping, weakness, and muscle swelling), after decades of normal activity. Diagnosis after inadvertent discovery of elevated CK in a child without symptoms has been reported.

Diagnosis is suspected from the symptoms, and response to ischemic exercise. The enzyme is expressed mainly in muscle. Muscle biopsy may show myopathic changes and increased glycogen content.

Specific treatment is generally not needed, as avoiding strenuous exercise prevents symptoms in most patients. A high-protein, low carbohydrate diet has been suggested to improve endurance. Others have found increased carbohydrate intake (glucose and fructose) immediately before exercise to be helpful.

Muscle Glycogen Phosphorylase Kinase Deficiency (Formerly Phosphorylase b Kinase Deficiency, GSD IX)

There have been a few men with deficiency of muscle phosphorylase kinase. Weakness without cramps and cramps without weakness have both been reported. Increased muscle glycogen content, elevation of CK, and rhabdomyolysis have been reported. Enzyme deficiency was demonstrated in muscle. The gene encoding the alpha subunit of phosphorylase (PHKA1) in muscle is on the X chromosome. It is distinct from the liver isoform (also on X). There are also three autosomal components of the glycogen phosphorylase kinase system. Autosomal recessive defects have been found in the beta and gamma peptides. No defects in the three delta subunit isoforms (which are calmodulins) have been reported.

Muscle Glycolytic Disorders

Deficiencies of five glycolytic enzymes in muscle are rare causes of myopathy similar to muscle phosphorylase deficiency. They are PFK, PGK, PGAM, β-enolase, and triosephosphate isomerase (Fig.C6.1). Hemolytic anemia can occur in all. PGK deficiency is X-linked

recessive. Patients may have neurologic problems (mental retardation, behavioral abnormalities, seizures, and strokes). The other disorders are autosomal recessive.

Lactate Dehydrogenase (LDH) Deficiency

Lactate dehydrogenase catalyzes the conversion of pyruvate and NADH to lactate and NAD^+. The enzyme is a tetramer of H and M peptides, produced from LDHB and LDHA genes. Homozygous deficiency of the M protein results in impaired muscle LDH activity. The result is impaired regeneration of NAD^+ for anaerobic glycolysis, and impaired production of lactate (and resulting high levels of pyruvate) with exercise, detectable by the ischemic exercise test (see Chap. D8). Cramps, weakness, and myoglobinuria can occur with strenuous exercise. Deficiency of LDH can result in a "false negative" result if LDH is being measured to assess tissue damage in other situations. No syndrome is attributable to LDHB deficiency.

Adenosine Monophosphate (Myoadenylate) Deaminase Deficiency

This autosomal recessive disorder of purine metabolism is probably the commonest metabolic myopathy, with impaired exercise tolerance, postexercise cramps, and myalgias. Myoglobinuria is uncommon, but CK is often elevated after exercise. Onset of symptoms (usually pain after exercise) ranges from childhood to later adult life. In the US population perhaps 2% are homozygous for deficiency, but most have no symptoms. Because AMP deaminase deficiency is so common, it has sometimes been found coincidentally with a less common muscle disorder that by itself would account for the symptoms, e.g., muscle phosphorylase or PFK deficiency. As the enzyme deficiency will only be discovered by ischemic exercise testing, or specific assay or molecular test, there is a selection bias toward muscle problems.

Many patients discovered to have AMP deaminase deficiency have other symptoms as well, especially neuromuscular disease. Diminished synthesis of AMP deaminase occurs in a variety of situations. This is termed acquired deficiency and does not seem to have a direct genetic basis, and the common mutation is not present at a frequency above the background rate.

AMP deaminase catalyzes the deamination of AMP to IMP (inosine monophosphate) in the purine nucleotide cycle (see Fig. C6.2). During exercise there will be increased production of IMP and ammonia, and maintenance of the adenylate energy charge by preventing AMP accumulation. A decrease in ATP and increase in ammonia will also stimulate glycolysis by increasing the activity of PFK. The increase in IMP may also enhance glycogen phosphorylase. Finally, during intense exercise AMP deaminase moves from the cytosol and becomes bound to myosin, which suggests that it is important in muscle metabolism during such times.

The diagnosis of AMP deaminase deficiency is approached by ischemic exercise ordinarily provoking a rise in blood ammonia level (see Chap. D8). If AMP is deficient, there will be diminished ammonia production. Muscle biopsy may be normal or show some myopathic changes. Specific staining for AMP deaminase is a generally reliable diagnostic test. Enzyme activity in deficient muscle ranges up to 15% of normal; some authorities regard activity >2% as adequate to prevent symptoms. A common mutation accounts for most cases of inherited AMP deaminase deficiency. This common mutation is actually a pair of mutations in linkage disequilibrium, GLN12TER (p.Q12X) and PRO48LEU. The nonsense mutation in exon 2, GLN12TER can result in a severely truncated protein. However, an alternative splicing mechanism allows for phenotypic rescue by production of a shortened but functional protein, with PRO48LEU in exon 3 retained. This may account for the great variability in symptoms

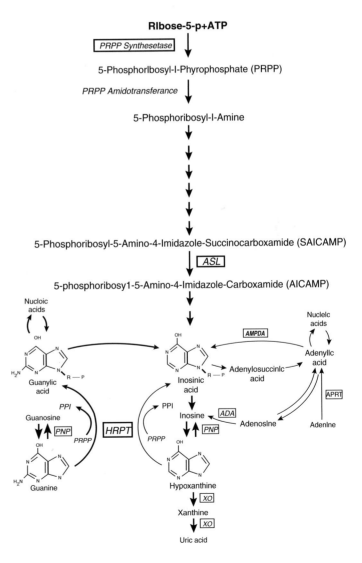

Fig. C6.2 Pathways of synthesis, salvage, and degradation of purines. The enzymatic steps in boxes indicate the sites of the commonly encountered disorders of purine metabolism *AMPDA* muscle adenosine monophosphate deaminase deficiency; *APRT* adenine phosphoribosyltransferase deficiency; *ASL* adenylosuccinate lyase (adenylosuccinase) deficiency; *HPRT* hypoxanthine–guanine phosphoribosyltransferase deficiency; *PNP* purine nucleoside phosphorylase deficiency; *SO* sulfite oxidase deficiency; *XO* xanthine oxidase (xanthine dehydrogenase) deficiency

in homozygotes for this mutation. The allele frequency was 0.13 (Caucasians) and 0.19 (African-Americans) in one study, which accounts for the observed homozygote frequency of about 0.02. Polymorphisms of angiotensin I-converting enzyme may contribute to the variability of symptoms seen with AMP deaminase deficiency.

AMP deaminase deficiency has been found in patients with aldolase deficiency, lactate dehydrogenase M (LDHA) deficiency, and β-enolase deficiency.

C6.3.1.2 Short, Intense Exercise Tolerated, Prolonged Exercise not Tolerated, Fasting Detrimental, Diet Effects Less Pronounced. Symptoms may be Triggered by Infection. Restriction of Long-Chain Fats, with Supplementation of Medium-Chain Lipids, may be Helpful, Especially for Cardiomyopathy

Carnitine-Acylcarnitine Translocase Deficiency

An inability to import long-chain acylcarnitines into the mitochondrial matrix would be expected to cause serious difficulties, especially in cardiac and skeletal muscle, and in the liver. The severe infantile form of translocase deficiency typically does this, starting a day or two after birth. Cardiac (cardiomyopathy, usually hypertrophic) and hepatic dysfunction (hypoglycemia, vomiting, and hyperammonemia) are more prominent than hypotonia and weakness. Urinary organic acids show dicarboxylic aciduria, and the plasma/blood spot acylcarnitine profile is dominated by long-chain species (C16:1, C18:1, and C18:2), which can be formed but not used, and dicarboxylic acylcarnitines.

CPT II Deficiency

CPT II deficiency is the commonest disorder of fatty acid oxidation to cause episodic rhabdomyolysis. CPT II is needed to synthesize long-chain acylcarnitines once they have been translocated into the mitochondria, so the clinical features are similar to translocase deficiency. Prolonged exercise, cold, infection, and emotional stress (which will increase catecholamines

and fatty acid metabolism) may precipitate episodes, which usually do not occur in children. Cardiac involvement is uncommon in this form of CPT II deficiency.

Plasma or blood spot acylcarnitine analysis shows prominent long-chain species, especially saturated and unsaturated C16 and C18 forms, and there may be dicarboxylic aciduria, similar to translocase deficiency.

A severe form of infantile CPT II deficiency also exists. Hepatic encephalopathy with hypoketotic hypoglycemia, severe cardiac involvement, renal malformations, and low plasma and tissue carnitine levels may be present. This form is usually fatal, from cardiac complications. It is discussed in more detail in section (Chap. D1, Cardiac).

Treatment includes avoiding of fasting and providing adequate fuel for the muscles. Medium-chain fatty acids do not need the carnitine system in order to enter the mitochondria, so they can be used in place of long-chain fats as a source of energy.

Although this is an autosomal recessive disorder, heterozygosity for a mutation may be associated with subtle myopathy and risk of malignant hyperthermia (MH) in response to anesthetics or muscle relaxants.

There is a form of CPT I that is solely expressed in muscle. No clinical deficiency has been recognized so far.

VLCAD Deficiency

VLCAD is the first enzyme of the β-oxidation spiral. It is bound to the inner mitochondrial membrane. Deficiency of VLCAD is a common cause of metabolic myopathy and cardiomyopathy. For several years, the enzyme now known as VLCAD was called LCAD (long-chain acyl-CoA dehydrogenase); reports from before about 1993 regarding LCAD deficiency almost always involve what is now called VLCAD. VLCAD utilizes fatty acids of 14–20 carbons. A major source of confusion is that fatty acids called very long chain fatty acids, of chain length >20, are metabolized by a different system altogether, in the peroxisomes.

Impairment of VLCAD will lead to variable skeletal, cardiac, liver, and brain symptoms, including recurrent Reye syndrome with coma, and hypoketotic hypoglycemia. Muscle soreness and episodic rhabdomyolysis may be provoked by infection, cold, fasting, or emotional stress (perhaps mediated by catecholamines). There is usually dicarboxylic aciduria, although during severe metabolic derangement it may be overlooked because of excessive lactic aciduria indistinguishable from a primary defect of the respiratory chain. Carnitine depletion, with low plasma and tissue levels, can occur and acylcarnitine analysis shows prominence of C14:1 (tetradecenoyl) species, derived from oleic acid (C18:1). Hepatic dysfunction may result in hyperammonemia and lipid accumulation. Muscle biopsy may show lipid storage, and the EMG is often myopathic.

VLCAD deficiency, like other disorders of fatty acid oxidation, must be promptly treated during the acute episode with glucose sufficient to maintain the blood glucose level at 6–8 mM or even higher (see also Chap. B2. 8). The use of carnitine supplementation has been controversial on theoretical and experimental grounds, particularly because of fear that long-chain acylcarnitines would accumulate and provoke arrhythmias. However, there are few convincing reports of this actually happening. Long-term management emphasizes adequate calories from carbohydrate, restricting long-chain dietary fats, avoiding fasting and other stressors, and supplementation with medium-chain triglycerides, which will provide a source of fuel that can be metabolized without requiring VLCAD. Triheptanoin, a novel treatment to provide a constant source of ketone bodies for patients with defects of long-chain fatty acid oxidation is showing great promise in preliminary studies.

The enzyme now known as the LCAD is in the mitochondrial matrix. Its major substrates are unsaturated long-chain fatty acids, 12–18 carbons in length. Deficiency is very uncommon; manifestations are similar to other disorders of fatty acid oxidation.

LCHAD (Including Trifunctional Protein) Deficiency

LCHAD deficiency often results in chronic myopathy, with rhabdomyolysis, which may be extensive, particularly during viral infections. Like other disorders of long-chain fatty acids there is often cardiomyopathy and significant liver dysfunction, both of which may be fulminant. The extent of chronic liver dysfunction can be greater than in other disorders, and fibrosis often occurs. There may be Reye-like episodes of hepatic encephalopathy. In addition there may be peripheral neuropathy and retinopathy. The basis for these complications is not yet known.

The enzyme activity called LCHAD is found in an octameric protein ($\alpha 4\beta 4$) called the trifunctional protein, for its ability to catalyze the 2-enoyl-CoA hydration, 3-hydroxyacyl-CoA dehydrogenation, and 3-oxoacyl-CoA thiolysis of long-chain acyl-CoAs. The first two activities reside in the α subunit, and thiolase activity in the β subunit. The two subunits depend on each other for stability. The trifunctional protein is in the mitochondrial inner membrane.

There is some relationship between mutation and symptoms. The commonest mutation (87% in one study), c.1528 G > C (p.E510Q) in the α subunit, usually causes liver dysfunction with hypoketotic hypoglycemia in infancy.

LCHAD deficiency is an autosomal recessive disorder, and carriers are generally symptom free. A particular complication of heterozygous (carrier) status for LCHAD deficiency, especially the p.E510Q mutation, is serious liver disease during pregnancy when carrying an affected infant. The mother may suffer from acute fatty liver of pregnancy (AFLP, with nausea and anorexia, vomiting, and jaundice) or the HELLP syndrome of hypertension or hemolysis, elevated liver enzymes, and low platelets. It may be that the production of abnormal fatty acid metabolites by the fetus overloads the mother's ability to deal with them, on top of the increased fatty acid mobilization that occurs during pregnancy. Prospective studies of women with AFLP or HELLP syndrome, however, have not found an increased number of carriers of LCHAD deficiency, indicating there are other causes for these conditions. Women heterozygous for hepatic CPT I deficiency, which may cause a Reye-like syndrome in homozygotes, may also suffer from AFLP when carrying an affected fetus.

In untreated patients, the urine organic acids reveal increased saturated and unsaturated dicarboxylic and hydroxy species. The plasma acylcarnitine profile typically shows elevation of hydroxy-C18:1 species, which, in combination with an elevation of two of the three long-chain species C14, C14:1, and hydroxy-C16, identifies over 85% of patients with high specificity (<0.1% false positive rate). Blood spot acylcarnitine analysis is not quite as sensitive, because of higher levels of long-chain species in blood samples. Dietary treatment (restriction of long-chain fats and supplementation with medium-chain triglycerides) will lower the long-chain acylcarnitine species, often to normal. Plasma carnitine levels are usually low, especially during acute illness. Carnitine is sometimes given at such times. Its usefulness as a medication for this myopathy (and whether it might provoke arrhythmias in certain situations – see Chap. C1) is a subject of current investigation.

Short-Chain Acyl-CoA Dehydrogenase Deficiency

This enzyme deficiency is extremely variable, having been reported in infants and adults. Muscle symptoms, when present, have ranged from a mild lipid myopathy with low muscle carnitine, to a more severe condition with weakness, poor exercise tolerance, and myopathic EMG. Systemic symptoms of hepatic encephalopathy have occurred. The impaired metabolism of short-chain acyl-CoAs leads to short-chain dicarboxylic aciduria [ethylmalonic and adipic, similar to electron-transfer flavoprotein (ETF) deficiency] and excess butyrate. Acylcarnitine analysis may show increased C4 species.

Hydroxyacyl-CoA Dehydrogenase (HADH) Deficiency

HADH deficiency is a very rare condition, with recurrent rhabdomyolysis, hypertrophic cardiomyopathy, and hypoketotic/hyperinsulinemic hypoglycemia. Mild dicarboxylic and hydroxydicarboxylic aciduria was reported. The enzyme can be assayed in muscle or in mitochondria from skin fibroblasts. This enzyme was previously called SCHAD.

C6.3.2 Weakness and Hypotonia Presentation

C6.3.2.1 Carnitine Transporter Deficiency

The carnitine transport defect is the result of deficient activity of the high-affinity carnitine transporter (OCTN2, encoded by the gene SLC22A5), active in kidney, muscle, heart, fibroblasts, and lymphocytes. Renal fractional excretion of carnitine, calculated in relation to creatinine clearance, approaches 100% (normal <5%). The severe carnitine depletion that

results (plasma levels can be <5 μmol/L, normal ≈ 45 μmol/L) will lead to tissue carnitine depletion as well. Hepatic carnitine depletion results in hypoketotic hypoglycemia. Onset of myopathy and cardiomyopathy can be in the first few months, or not for several years. Urine organic acids are typically normal. Muscle biopsy reveals lipid accumulation, and the muscle carnitine level is extremely low. Response to carnitine supplementation is dramatic, but because of the ongoing renal leak of carnitine, it is extremely difficult to maintain normal plasma carnitine levels or tissue levels, and exercise tolerance may be limited. Oral carnitine supplementation to an amount just short of provoking a fish odor (trimethylamine) by exceeding the oxidizing capacity is the usual approach. Inheritance is autosomal recessive.

C6.3.2.2 Secondary Carnitine Depletion

Adults are able to synthesize all the carnitine they need. The major dietary source of carnitine is meat. The carnitine content of human breast milk is similar to that of plasma. Carnitine deficiency has occurred in several infants on prolonged parenteral nutrition (without added carnitine), with resulting myopathy and cardiomyopathy, impaired ketogenesis, and hepatic steatosis. Carnitine supplementation (intravenous or oral) was rapidly beneficial. This experience suggests that carnitine may be an essential nutrient in the very young, and that routine carnitine supplementation of TPN solutions for infants should be considered.

Severe carnitine depletion can result from a generalized Fanconi syndrome, characteristic of cystinosis, Lowe syndrome, mitochondrial disorders (especially, cytochrome C oxidase deficiency), etc (see also Chap. C4). Recognition of the carnitine depletion usually occurs after the discovery of Fanconi syndrome. Plasma carnitine measurement and determination of the fractional excretion should be part of the investigation of all patients with Fanconi syndrome. Restoration of tissue carnitine levels may take a very long time even after correction of the renal leak, as after transplantation for cystinosis.

Some medications, such as valproic acid and pivampicillin are essentially organic acids and there may be excretion of metabolites as carnitine esters causing significant urinary losses of carnitine as valproylcarnitine or pivaloylcarnitine, and consequently secondary systemic carnitine deficiency. Use of pivampicillin has been linked to life-threatening crisis, especially in patients with an underlying metabolic disorder [e.g., medium-chain acyl-CoA dehydrogenase (MCAD) deficiency].

MCAD deficiency is unusual among fatty acid oxidation disorders for having only minimal skeletal muscle symptoms. Hepatic and cerebral symptoms (Reye-like syndrome, hypoketotic hypoglycemia, and sudden unexplained death) are the usual features. However, carnitine depletion can occur. MCAD deficiency accounts for nearly all the patients described with "systemic carnitine deficiency," before the enzyme deficiency was discovered. This may be the mechanism for chronic weakness and impaired exercise tolerance in some older patients with MCAD deficiency. Long-term carnitine supplementation, whose use in MCAD deficiency is not universally accepted, might be expected to ameliorate this situation. Longitudinal studies have not yet been reported.

C6.3.2.3 2,4-Dienoyl-CoA Reductase Deficiency

This extremely rare disorder has been described in one infant with hypotonia, normal deep tendon reflexes, poor feeding, and failure to thrive. There was plasma carnitine deficiency, and a unique unsaturated acylcarnitine (C10:2) in plasma, shown to be derived from long-chain unsaturated fatty acids.

C6.3.2.4 MADD–ETF OR ETF-Dehydrogenase Deficiency (Synonymously Glutaric Aciduria Type II)

The severe form of this disorder causes overwhelming acidosis shortly after birth. Impairment of the ETF system blocks many different dehydrogenation systems for fatty acids and amino acids degradation. Milder deficiency of the same system can cause a lipid storage myopathy that may not become apparent for years or decades. Gradual onset of weakness and easy fatigability may be overlooked initially, and the history may first suggest an inflammatory myopathy. There may be liver dysfunction. Urine organic acids can show dicarboxylic aciduria, including ethylmalonic, adipic, and glutaric acids. Plasma acylcarnitine analysis shows elevation of short- and medium-chain species. A secondary deficiency of coenzyme Q_{10} (CoQ) may occur. Mitochondrial studies may show deficient activity complex I and II. Response to supplemental riboflavin

(50–100 mg/day), the precursor of the cofactor flavin adenine dinucleotide, is often dramatic in the milder forms. A postulated disorder of riboflavin transport may be the cause of a similar disorder.

C6.3.2.5 Lysosomal GSD Type II (Pompe Disease)

Pompe disease is the severe infantile form of lysosomal α-glucosidase (acid maltase) deficiency. It is one of the most common storage diseases presenting in infancy, and the first one to be identified. The infant typically presents in the first few months with weakness and profound hypotonia. Feeding and respiratory difficulties are common. There is macroglossia, but minimal hepatomegaly. At least 80% have significant cardiac involvement. Progressive weakness and cardiomyopathy usually lead to death within a year. Despite the hypotonia the muscles feel firm or even woody.

There is a spectrum of deficiency of α-glucosidase, with onset of symptoms reported as late as the eighth decade. Various terms, including juvenile and adult onset, are used to describe late-onset patients. The age of onset bears no relation to the rapidity of the course. The older the patient the more likely that symptomatic muscle involvement will be patchy clinically and morphologically. However, enzyme activity will be deficient, regardless of the appearance of the cells. The function of lysosomal glycogen is not known. α-Glucosidase activity can be measured in leukocytes, as well as in muscle or in liver biopsy, or in cultured skin fibroblasts. Muscle biopsy, which is not necessary for diagnosis if enzyme assay can be performed, shows enlarged lysosomes engorged with glycogen, altering the ultrastructure of the cell.

There was no satisfactory treatment of Pompe disease until the development of enzyme replacement therapy. Recombinant α-glucosidase can arrest and even reverse the disease if begun early enough, so early diagnosis is now an urgent matter.

C6.3.2.6 Glycogen Debrancher Deficiency – GSD Type III (Cori or Forbes Disease)

This relatively common disorder of glycogen metabolism results from varying deficiencies of amylo-1,6-glucosidase, 4-α-glucoanotransferase, the debrancher enzyme, a remarkable peptide which has two separate catalytic activities (transferase and glucosidase). There is always liver involvement, but muscle involvement is variable, and does not occur at all in about 15% (GSD IIIb). In infancy and childhood the liver symptoms dominate, with hepatomegaly, hyperlipidemia, and fasting hypoglycemia similar to GSD I. Muscle weakness may not be apparent. After puberty the liver symptoms subside, but the myopathy may persist as weakness, and may worsen with time. CK may be elevated, but may be normal even if there is muscle involvement. There can be distal wasting, myopathic EMG, and peripheral neuropathy. There is usually cardiac involvement (mild) as well.

Diagnosis is suspected from the history. Enzyme assay and gene analysis can be done using fibroblasts, lymphocytes, muscle, or liver. Liver and muscle biopsies are often done to obtain direct information about these organs. Analysis of glycogen structure in muscle or liver can demonstrate abnormalities due to the lack of normal glycogen breakdown. The differences in tissue expression are traceable to alternate splicing of exon 1 of the gene. Differences in phenotype correlate with different mutations. Two mutations in exon 3 account for 90% of patients with GSD IIIb (i.e., no muscle involvement). If these mutations are not present, muscle biopsy must be done to ascertain if there is muscle involvement. Support of the glucose availability is achieved with corn starch, similar to GSD I. Treatment of the myopathy using high-protein meals and high-protein enteral feeds overnight has been attempted, but it does not seem to improve the long-term outlook.

C6.3.2.7 Glycogen Brancher Deficiency – GSD Type IV (Anderson Disease)

Type IV GSD, glycogen brancher deficiency, can cause hypotonia and weakness, but the clinical picture is dominated by hepatic fibrosis and dysfunction. Cardiomyopathy may be significant in the severe infantile form.

C6.3.2.8 Glycogen Synthase Deficiency – GSD type 0

This disorder results in insufficient glycogen reserves in the liver, so that fasting hypoglycemia occurs relatively soon after a meal, and excessive lactate is produced from dietary glucose. One family has been reported with a muscle form of the disease, which caused muscle weakness, reduced exercise capacity, and hypertrophic cardiomyopathy in the first decade.

C6.3.2.9 Mitochondrial Myopathies and Coenzyme Q Deficiency

The mitochondrial myopathies are an extremely heterogeneous group of disorders. Symptoms may be confined to muscle, or may involve other organs, particularly the brain, heart, liver, and kidneys. Symptoms may already be present at birth or not appear for decades. Myopathy is particularly evident in the syndromes of chronic progressive external ophthalmoplegia (CPEO) including the Kearns–Sayre syndrome (KSS) or ophthalmoplegia-plus; mitochondrial encephalomyopathy, lactic acidosis, and stroke-like episodes (MELAS); mitochondrial encephalomyopathy with ragged-red fibers (MERFF); fatal infantile mitochondrial myopathy; depletion of the mitochondrial DNA; and autosomal dominant and recessive mitochondrial myopathies. Molecular defects can be in the mitochondrially encoded tRNAs, mitochondrial- and nuclear-encoded subunits of the oxidative phosphorylation complexes, and many other proteins. Some of the most relevant disorders and etiologies are shown in Table 3, Chap. D6.

Muscle symptoms are generally those of chronic weakness and impaired exercise tolerance. Cramps are unusual. Rhabdomyolysis can occur, particularly, in the setting of sustained exercise or febrile illness. Malignant hyperthermia may occur with anesthesia or muscle relaxants.

Systemic lactic acidosis may be present at rest or elicited with exercise. Some infants will have acidosis from the work of breathing, but be chemically normal with ventilator support. CK may be elevated. Plasma amino acids may show increased alanine. Urinary organic acids may show increased of lactate, citric acid cycle intermediates, and dicarboxylic fatty acids. The plasma carnitine level may be normal or low. Plasma acylcarnitine analysis may show a generalized increase in short- and medium-chain species, especially acetylcarnitine, or be unrevealing.

EMG may be normal or suggest myopathy; nerve conduction studies may reveal a peripheral neuropathy, usually axonal.

Muscle tissue can be analyzed for carnitine content and acylcarnitine species and coenzyme Q level. Muscle biopsy may show dense clusters of abnormal mitochondria, especially near the surface of the cell membrane ("ragged red fibers"), as well as increased lipid, but may be normal (see also Chap. D5). Cells may stain strongly for succinate dehydrogenase (complex II) yet not stain for cytochrome oxidase (COX), particularly in CPEO, KSS, and MERFF. Maternally inherited Leigh syndrome patients may have deficient COX staining, but no ragged-red fibers. Electron microscopy may show abnormal mitochondrial morphology, including paracrystalline inclusions.

Studies of oxidative phosphorylation are best carried out in fresh muscle biopsy tissue. Some laboratories will work with frozen muscle tissue or freshly isolated platelets. Mitochondrial DNA studies are optimally performed from muscle biopsy as well. If there is a heteroplasmic disorder in the mtDNA, other tissues (leukocytes and fibroblasts) can sometimes give a misleading normal result. Mitochondrial myopathies are a subset of the overall group of mitochondrial cytopathies, which are discussed in Chap. D6.

Mitochondrial disorders of oxidative phosphorylation are generally treated with a high-fat, low carbohydrate diet, and supplemental vitamins and antioxidants, especially coenzyme Q (ubiquinone) and riboflavin (which may be quite helpful for complex I deficiency myopathy). Vitamin C, thiamin, vitamin E, vitamin K3 (as an artificial electron acceptor-donor), dichloroacetate, carnitine, and succinate have been used in various situations. Responses are generally subtle, but occasionally a patient responds dramatically to CoQ or other therapies.

The synthesis of coenzyme Q involves nine steps; recessive defects have been discovered in SPSS1, SPSS2, CABC1, COQ2, and APTX. Besides myopathy there may be ataxia, deafness, encephalopathy, liver disease, renal tubular dysfunction, and cardiac valvulopathy, depending on the defect. In many patients suffering from the myopathic form of CoQ deficiency MADD deficiency is the primary defect.

C6.3.3 Myopathies with Major Cardiac Involvement

The cardiac manifestations of several disorders discussed in this chapter, including GSD types II and IV, fatty acid oxidation disorders including carnitine transport defect, deficiencies of carnitine-acylcarnitine translocase, CPT II, VLCAD, and LCHAD/tri-functional enzyme, and mitochondrial disorders are discussed in Chap. C1.

C6.3.4 Malignant Hyperthermia

Malignant hyperthermia (MH) in response to anesthetics occurs in many different situations and myopathies. MH is most commonly due to the failure of regulation of calcium concentration in the sarcoplasmic reticulum. Excess calcium permits continuous muscle contraction, leading to heat generation, and a rise in body temperature. Severe myoglobinuria, irreversible kidney damage, and death from hyperthermia or arrhythmia due to hyperkalemia may occur. For these reasons, all patients with a myopathy must be especially carefully monitored during surgery or any other procedure where anesthesia is used, and the most risky anesthetics (e.g., halothane) and muscle relaxants (e.g., suxamethonium) should be avoided. Premedication with dantrolene can lessen the risk of untoward reactions. Several genes are now known for MH syndromes. MHS1 is due to mutations in the ryanodine receptor RYR1 (with or without central core disease). MHS2 is due to mutations in the alpha subunit of the gated sodium channel IV, SCN4A, also altered in hypokalemic periodic paralysis, paramyotonia congenita, and related disorders. MHS3 is due to mutations in the calcium channel CACNL2A. MHS5 is due to changes in another calcium channel, CACNA1S. All of these conditions can be dominantly transmitted. Patients with muscular dystrophies or the recessive Native American myopathy with cleft palate and congenital contractures are also vulnerable. Even for these high-risk conditions MH does not occur with each exposure to a triggering agent. Of the disorders of intermediary metabolism, which are the primary topic of this book, the greatest risk is to patients with CPT II deficiency (perhaps even in the heterozygous state), and with mitochondrial disorders, but all patients with metabolic myopathy should be regarded as at potential risk for MH.

Key References

Bonnefont J-P, Taroni F, Cavadini P, et al (1996) Molecular analysis of carnitine palmitoyltransferase II deficiency with hepatocardiomuscular expression. Am J Hum Genet 58: 971–978

Bruno C, DiMauro S (2008) Lipid storage myopathies. Curr Opin Neurol 21:601–606

DiMauro S (2007) Muscle glycogenoses: an overview. Acta Myol 26:35–41

DiMauro S, Gurgel-Giannetti J (2005) The expanding phenotype of mitochondrial myopathy. Curr Opin Neurol 18:538–542

Leonard JV, Schapira AH (2000) Mitochondrial respiratory chain disorders I: mitochondrial DNA defects. Lancet 355:299–304

Leonard JV, Schapira AH (2000) Mitochondrial respiratory chain disorders II: neurodegenerative disorders and nuclear gene defects. Lancet 355:389–394

Pestronk A. Washington University Neuromuscular Disease Center website. http://neuromuscular.wustl.edu

Vladutiu GD, Bennett MJ, Smail D et al (2000) A variable myopathy associated with heterozygosity for the R503C mutation in the carnitine palmitoyltransferase II gene. Mol Genet Metab 70:134–141

Psychiatric Disease

C7

Ertan Mayatepek

Key Facts

> Psychiatric manifestations may be the only symptom of inherited metabolic diseases before additional neurological or other clinical signs are recognized.

> Inherited metabolic diseases can manifest acutely as attacks of delirium (visual), hallucinations, mental confusion, hysteria, schizophrenia or psychosis, e.g., in urea cycle disorders, organic acidurias, maple syrup urine disease, porphyrias, methylene tetrahydrofolate reductase deficiency, cobalamin metabolism defects, Morbus Fabry, and metachromatic leukodystrophy.

> In infancy, autistic features may be a leading clinical feature of metabolic diseases, e.g., in urea cycle disorders, inborn errors of biopterin, or purine metabolism.

> Psychiatric manifestations are mostly combined with regression of cognitive functions, e.g., in X-linked adrenoleukodystrophy or mucopolysaccharidosis type III (Sanfilippo).

> Patients with late-onset lysosomal storage disorders may initially present with psychiatric diagnoses such as dementia, psychosis, or emotional illness.

> Psychiatric manifestations can become most important in the long-term management of many patients with metabolic disorders.

E. Mayatepek
Department of General Pediatrics, University Children's Hospital, Moorenstrasse 5, 40225 Düsseldorf, Germany
e-mai: mayatepek@uni-duesseldorf.de

C7.1 General Remarks

Inherited metabolic diseases can manifest as acute attacks of delirium or psychosis as well as intellectual disintegration, mental regression, or chronic psychosis. Being aware of these manifestations allows to initiate appropriate diagnostic investigations and, if available, to institute rationale effective therapy (Table C7.1 and C7.2).

In the course of many neurometabolic diseases, psychiatric manifestations often become of critical importance, and it is most relevant to inform families and to evaluate and treat them appropriately. Typical constellations in early childhood range from severe disturbances of mood and vegetative symptoms in patients with neurotransmitter defects, and Smith–Lemli–Opitz syndrome to hyperactivity in patients with Sanfillipo disease and pterin defects to (auto-) aggressive behavior in Lesh–Nyhan disease. These aspects are beyond the scope of this book, except to stress the necessity of close collaboration with colleagues from child psychiatry in these instances.

C7.2 Acute Psychiatric Manifestations

Acute psychiatric attacks may be the first clinical correlate of an underlying metabolic defect. Presentations include mental confusion, hysteria, delirium, dizziness, aggressiveness, anxiety, bizarre behavior, agitation, agony, hallucinations or schizophrenic-like behavior, frank psychosis, and finally coma (see also Chap. B3.7). Especially dramatic are acute attacks of hyperammonemia, i.e., *urea cycle disorders* [e.g., ornithine transcarbamylase (OTC) deficiency and *organic acidurias or*

G. F. Hoffmann et al. (eds.), *Inherited Metabolic Diseases*,
DOI: 10.1007/978-3-540-74723-9_C7, © Springer-Verlag Berlin Heidelberg 2010

177

Table C7.1 Psychiatric symptoms suggestive of inherited metabolic diseases

Association with organic symptoms (organomegaly, neurological features, etc.)
Cognitive decline
Confusion
Visual hallucinations
Catatonia
Aggravation with therapy

Table C7.2 Investigations for the differential diagnosis of psychiatric manifestations of inherited metabolic diseases

Plasma/serum
Ammonia
Lactate
Amino acids
Homocysteine
Very long-chain fatty acids
Ceruloplasmin
Copper
Sterols
Urine
Amino acids
Organic acids
Mucopolysaccharides (electrophoresis)
Porphyrins (especially porphobilinogen)
Purines and pyrimidines
Oligosaccharides
N-Acetylneuraminic acid
Copper (24-h collection)
Histology including electron microscopy (skin biopsy, bone marrow, lymphocytes)
Biogenic amines and pterins in cerebrospinal fluid
Enzyme studies (lysosomal enzymes, respiratory chain enzymes)
Mitochondrial DNA
Brain MR spectroscopy

maple syrup urine disease]. All these are in principle treatable disorders, especially the late-onset variants. However, if the appropriate metabolic investigations are not initiated, disease courses will become chronic leading to permanent handicap and early death. Topping the list of investigations in any patient presenting with acute encephalopathy including psychiatric presentation has to be ammonia. All too often acute psychosis after pregnancy or drunkenness were fatal misdiagnoses in patients suffering from urea cycle disorders, especially hemizygous females with OTC deficiency.

Psychiatric manifestations are classically found in *acute intermittent porphyria* (AIP) or *hereditary coproporphyria*. In AIP, a disorder of heme bio synthesis leading to intermittent elevations in porphobilinogen and related porphyrins, psychiatric manifestations of acute attacks comprise anxiety, depression, psychosis, or altered mental status. AIP is often mistaken for schizophrenia or hysteria. Before an initial attack there is also a high frequency of histrionic personality traits in many patients with AIP. An even higher incidence of anxiety disorder is observed in otherwise asymptomatic carriers. For patients with AIP, it is essential to get the correct diagnosis early because many psychotropic drugs may induce or exacerbate an acute attack of porphyria. The metabolic crisis may induce or aggravate psychiatric symptoms, leading to a long-term psychiatric career because of misinterpretation as treatment resistance. Diagnosis of porphyria requires the demonstration of pathological metabolites in urine (e.g., porphobilinogen).

Patients suffering from *methylene tetrahydrofolate reductase deficiency* are sometimes initially (mis-) diagnosed as suffering from schizophrenia or psychosis. In these patients, further symptoms often include strokes, peripheral neuropathy, and a progressive myelopathy. Similar psychiatric signs are also found in cobalamin metabolism defects (Cbl C and Cbl G). Besides symptoms like paraesthesias stroke events, patients with *Fabry disease* are at higher risk of depression and even suicide.

C7.3 Chronic Psychiatric Manifestations

Psychiatric symptoms are predominantly recognized in older children, adolescents, or adults suffering from neurometabolic diseases. The decisive manifestations in these disorders are mental deterioration and/or progressive neurological manifestations (see Chap. C5). However, these may be less obvious than psychiatric symptoms for some time. Psychiatric features can be the only presenting symptom before any significant neurological or extraneurological signs are recognized. These manifestations include behavior disturbances, changes of personality and character, mental regression, dementia, psychosis, depression, or schizophrenia. Such presentations are especially common in *X-linked adrenoleukodystrophy (cerebral form)*, *Hallervorden–Spatz disease*, *Huntington chorea*, *urea cycle disorders*, especially hemizygous OTC deficiency, and *Wilson disease*.

It is helpful to consider the relationship of psychiatric manifestations to the age of the patient.

C7.3.1 Infancy (1–12 months)

In infancy, autistic traits may be a leading feature of metabolic disease. They have been observed in untreated phenylketonuria (PKU) and inborn errors of biopterin metabolism. Autistic features may be also present in infants affected with late-onset subacute forms of disorders associated with hyperammonemia, especially in *urea cycle disorders*, as well as in infants with *succinic semialdehyde dehydrogenase deficiency*, *Smith–Lemli–Opitz syndrome*, *adenylosuccinase deficiency*, *dihydropyrimidine dehydrogenase deficiency*, *homocystinuria*, *nonketotic hyperglycinemia*, or *sulfite oxidase deficiency*. Children with the treatable pyrimidine nucleotide depletion disease due to *cytosolic 5'-nucleotidase superactivity* develop a pervasive developmental disorder. Patients with *Smith–Lemli–Opitz syndrome* often present severe sleeping problems as well as excessive screaming in early childhood.

C7.3.2 Early Childhood (1–5 years)

Episodes of psychotic behavior, depression, and mania are typical psychiatric signs of the late infantile form of GM_2 *gangliosidosis* (*Tay–Sachs* and *Sandhoff*). The disease is characterized mainly by developmental regression, spinocerebellar degeneration, ataxia, and spastic fright reaction. In this age group, it is important to be aware of other diseases with arrest or regression of cognitive function, most importantly *Rett syndrome*. In Rett syndrome, girls are affected and they present with characteristic behavior, regression of developmental achievements, and stereotyped movements of fingers and hands.

In *mucopolysaccharidosis type III (Sanfilippo)*, major clinical manifestations include regression of high-level achievements as well as loss of speech. Affected children often show agitation, autism, and disintegrative behavior. Mental retardation with episodes of psychosis, hyperactivity, or confusion may be seen in α- or β-mannosidosis.

C7.3.3 Childhood and Early Adolescence (5–15 years)

Progressive neurological and mental deterioration along with psychiatric manifestations can be found in a number of neurometabolic diseases such as *juvenile neuronal ceroid lipofuscinosis (Spielmeyer–Vogt)*. Intellectual deterioration and depression develops in addition to the loss of sight and retinitis. In patients with this disease alteration in behavior may be the presenting complaint and may be seen years before other manifestations are evident.

Dementia and deterioration are found alongside psychiatric manifestations in metabolic diseases with predominant cerebellar ataxia such as mitochondrial disorders, e.g., *MELAS*, and in *cerebrotendinous xanthomatosis*, GM_1 *gangliosidosis*, *Gaucher disease*, *Niemann–Pick disease type C*, the juvenile form of *Krabbe*, *Lafora disease*, and *metachromatic leukodystrophy (MLD)*. Psychiatric manifestations are most often present in the late juvenile and adult age group and are characterized by psychosis with disorganized thoughts, delusions, and auditory hallucinations. The subsequent rapid intellectual deterioration to dementia should be the clue to the suspicion of an underlying metabolic disease.

> **Remember**
>
> - In childhood psychotic behavior, depression, and mania are typically found in GM_2 gangliosidosis.

Severe behavioral problems in combination with mental retardation may be seen in creatine transporter deficiency, in monoamine oxidase A deficiency, as well as in maternal PKU.

C7.3.4 Late Adolescence and Adulthood (>15 years)

In late adolescence and adulthood, progressive neurologic and mental deterioration along with preponderant psychosis and dementia may be found in a variety of metabolic diseases discussed in the preceding section including *urea cycle disorders, MLD, Niemann–Pick disease type C, ceroid lipofuscinosis, cerebrotendinous xanthomatosis, Huntington chorea, and Lafora disease*. In adult, onset MLD psychotic changes may be those of schizophrenia. This is also true of Nieman–Pick type C disease. Paralysis of upward gaze is the characteristic give away sign, but it has been a missed in psychiatric evaluations.

In *Wilson disease*, toxic tissue levels of copper cause damage primarily the liver and basal ganglia (see also Chap. C2). Psychiatric manifestations may vary and include personality changes, depressive episodes, cognitive dysfunction, and psychosis. The overall prevalence of psychiatric symptoms in Wilson disease is >20%. In total, 10% of the patients present with psychiatric symptoms alone. Effective chelation treatment does improve the majority of psychiatric symptoms. However, initiation of chelation treatment in Wilson disease may precipitate an acute psychiatric crisis.

Psychiatric abnormalities have been reported in patients with homocystinuria due to *cystathionine β-synthase (CBS) deficiency*. Major diagnostic categories in patients with CBS deficiency include, in order of, decreasing incidence, personality disorders, chronic disorders of behavior, episodic depression, and chronic obsessive-compulsive disorder. Schizophrenia or psychotic episodes are uncommon in CBS-deficient patients.

PKU in late treated or untreated patients results not only in mental retardation but also varying degrees of psychiatric pathology especially (auto-) aggression. Some adult patients with early treated PKU have exhibited an atypical pattern of psychopathology with a variety of symptoms of anxiety and depression. PKU patients no longer observing dietary restriction have an increased risk of psychosocial difficulties; agoraphobia has been recognized as a common symptom. It is also possible that psychiatric disease, being common, simply coexists in some of these patients. Interestingly, psychiatric symptoms observed in PKU are not clearly related to phenylalanine levels.

Take Home Messages

> Many neurometabolic diseases manifest symptoms compatible with various psychiatric diagnoses. Psychiatric features may be a leading clinical correlate of certain metabolic diseases as well as an important sequel in long-term care. With improvements in treatment and prognosis, manifestations that affect long-term quality of life such as psychiatric problems become increasingly important in an older patient population.

> Recognition of metabolic diseases in the differential diagnosis of psychiatric manifestations is important since some metabolic diseases may be mistaken for diagnoses such as schizophrenia. In AIP, psychiatric symptoms may be at the forefront of clinical manifestations. Careful examination of mental and neurological status, psychiatric history, and recognition of psychotropic drugs or treatment regimens potentially exacerbating metabolic crises, e.g., in porphyrias or in Wilson disease, are mandatory.

Key References

Abbott MH, Folstein SE, Abbey H et al (1987) Psychiatric manifestations of homocystinuria due to cystathionine beta-synthase deficiency: prevalence, natural history, and relationship to neurologic impairment and vitamin B$_6$-responsiveness. Am J Med Genet 26:959–969

Argov Z, Navon R (1984) Clinical and genetic variations in the syndrome of adult GM2 gangliosidosis resulting from hexosaminidase A deficiency. Ann Neurol 16:14–20

Crimlisk HL (1997) The little imitator-porphyria: a neuropsychiatric disorder. J Neurol Neurosurg Psychiatry 62:319–328

Dening TR, Berrios GE (1989) Wilson's disease. Psychiatric symptoms in 195 cases. Arch Gen Psychiatry 46:1126–1134

Estrov Y, Scaglia F, Bodamer OAF (2000) Psychiatric symptoms of inherited metabolic diseases. J Inherit Metab Dis 23:2–6

Grewal RP (1993) Psychiatric disorders in patients with Fabry's disease. Int J Psychiatry Med 23:307–312

Rauschka H, Colsch B, Baumann N et al (2006) Late-onset metachromatic leukodystrophy: genotype strongly influences phenotype. Neurology 67:859–863

Sedel F, Lyon-Caen O, Saudubray JM (2007) Inborn errors of metabolism in adult neurology – a clinical approach focused on treatable diseases. Nat Clin Pract Neurol 3:279–290

Eye Disorders

C8

Alberto Burlina and Alessandro P. Burlina

Key Facts

> Eye involvement represents important and specific processes in the development of inherited metabolic disease.

> Ocular manifestations are common in inherited metabolic diseases. They result in characteristic signs, which are very useful in the diagnosis of the metabolic defect.

> Ophthalmological manifestations can occur early in life with bilateral symmetrical involvement. Monitoring of eye disease progression is necessary in many inherited metabolic diseases (i.e., for cataracts in galactosemia).

> Specific localized therapies are available (mainly surgical approaches) and, as for other organs, involved in inherited metabolic diseases, the main treatment consists of the primary therapy of the metabolic defect.

C8.1 General Remarks

The eye is the most highly specialized of the sensor organs and is often implicated in metabolic disorders that affect the senses. Moreover, the eye has important physiological links to the central nervous system and, thus, tends to be involved in diseases affecting the central nervous system. Because the eye is such a complex organ, one or more of its structural or functional components may be affected by a single disease.

Ophthalmological manifestations occur in various metabolic disorders. In some instances, the occurrence of eye abnormalities suggests that it might be induced by direct toxic mechanisms of abnormal metabolic products or accumulation of normal metabolites; by defects of synthetic pathways; or by deficient energy metabolism. In other diseases, it remains to be elucidated how the systemic metabolic abnormalities contribute to ocular defects.

Two situations may arise in clinical practice. Either the patient presents with a known metabolic disorder, and the ocular defect appears to be as expected manifestation of the disease, or the patient presents primarily with eye abnormalities and a metabolic disorder can be suspected. For many metabolic diseases, symmetrical bilateral involvement is the rule.

Severe visual impairment from birth is often not recognized until around 2 months of age, when normal sighted children have developed eye contact. Severe poor vision needs to be detected within the first weeks of life. In some conditions, anomalies of the eye can be more easily detected, such as cataracts in galactosemia. In other conditions, such as in some peroxisomal diseases, fundoscopic examination may still be normal in the neonatal period, whereas recordings of

A. Burlina (✉)
Department of Pediatrics, Division of Metabolic Disorders, University Hospital, Via Giustiniani 3, 35128 Padova, Italy
e-mail: burlina@pediatria.unipd.it

G. F. Hoffmann et al. (eds.), *Inherited Metabolic Diseases*,
DOI: 10.1007/978-3-540-74723-9_C8, © Springer-Verlag Berlin Heidelberg 2010

electroretinogram and visual evoked responses are already abnormal.

In inborn errors of metabolism, we can detect the following eye pathology:

- Corneal clouding
- Lens defects and dislocations
- Retinal degeneration
- Optic atrophy

C8.2 Corneal Clouding

The three components of corneal tissue are epithelium, stroma and Descemet's membrane. Corneal transparency depends, in part, on stromal constituents, i.e., collagen fibrils and proteoglycans. The composition of proteoglycans in the cornea is involved in the organization of the collagen fibrils including fibrillar ultrastructure, fibril packing, organization, stability of the corneal lamellae, fibril size, as well as corneal hydration. About 80% of the stromal dry weight is collagen, primarily type I, together with others such as type V and VI collagens. The collagen fibrils are arranged in lamellae with adjacent lamellae arranged at right angles, forming an orthogonal grid. Corneal clarity is maintained by a crystalline array of stromal fibers and multiple translucent endothelial layers. The three components of corneal tissue (epithelium, stroma, and Descemet's membrane) may be involved separately or simultaneously, depending on the disease.

> **Remember**
>
> The cornea is optically sensitive to abnormal storage products, which may accumulate as a result of a systemic disorder.

If the abnormal substrate is produced by the corneal tissue, it may be found throughout the cornea. If it is found in elevated amounts in the blood, it is more commonly accumulated in the corneal periphery. Lesions

are relatively easy to detect using simple instruments such as a hand light or the ophthalmoscope. More subtle changes can be seen by slit-lamp examination.

> **Remember**
>
> Corneal clouding is relatively easy to detect using instruments such as a hand light or the ophthalmoscope.

Inherited metabolic diseases that affect the cornea are numerous and severe (Table C8.1).

> **Remember**
>
> The most frequently inherited metabolic diseases which present corneal clouding are lysosomal disorders (including Anderson–Fabry disease), lipid disorders, and tyrosinemia type II.

Table C8.1 Corneal clouding

Lysosomal disorders
Mucopolysaccharidoses: types I, II, IV, VI, VII (severe form)
Mannosidosis
Sialidosis (severe infantile)
Galactosialidosis
Fabry's disease
Mucolipidosis I, II, IV
Fucosidosis type III
Multiple sulfatase deficiency
Farber's disease
Cystinosis
Lipid disorders
Homozygous familial hypercholesterolemia
Lecithin:cholesterol acyltransferase deficiency (Tangier disease)
Fish-eye disease
Amino acid disorders
Tyrosinemia type II
Alkaptonuria
Metal disorder
Wilson's disease

C8.2.1 Lysosomal Disorders

Disease Info: Mucopolysaccharidoses

In the mucopolysaccharidoses (MPS), some clinical manifestations such as coarse facial features, thickened skin, organomegaly, and eye lesions result from the reduction in activity of specific lysosomal enzymes involved in the breakdown of glycosaminoglycans (GAG).

Ocular pathology is common in all types of MPS and results in frequent impairment of vision. The ocular complications include corneal opacification, retinopathy and raised intraocular pressure. Ocular hypertension and glaucoma are often difficult to diagnose and monitor in patients with MPS because of coexistent corneal opacification and thickening, and the physical and intellectual problems of some individuals.

Progressive corneal opacification (characteristically described as having the appearance of ground glass) affects all patients with MPS types I, IV, and VI. Corneal opacification is mild in MPS IS (Scheie disease) and MPS II (Hunter syndrome), and rarely requires corneal transplantation, and is not a prominent feature of MPS III (Sanfilipo syndrome). Progressive corneal opacification is also seen in MPS VII (Sly syndrome). The lesion is due to dermatan sulfate deposition in the cornea that is not present in normal cornea. Corneal opacification in MPS IV (Morquio disease) is due to keratin sulfate deposition.

Glycosaminoglycan deposition in the corneal stroma has been suggested by some authors to cause progressive increase in corneal thickness.

In animals with systemic MPS, corneal clouding results from storage of GAG in stromal keratocytes. The corneal epithelium is normal (MPS VI and VII) or minimally affected (MPS I), and stromal edema is not a feature even though the corneal endothelium demonstrated variable pathology. The corneal clouding is the result of storage in stromal keratocytes rather than corneal edema from endothelial dysfunction.

Other ocular manifestations are also common in MPS. Glaucoma, cataracts, optic nerve swelling and subsequently optic atrophy, pigmentary retinopathy have been reported in patients, often masked by corneal problems.

In the past, the ocular management of many patients with MPS has been conservative due to their short life span and intellectual impairment. Now, new treatments such as bone marrow transplantation and enzyme replacement therapy are leading to a longer and better-quality life for many MPS patients, and these treatments appear to be beneficial in reducing, but not eliminating, the ocular manifestations.

Disease Info: Anderson–Fabry disease

Anderson–Fabry disease, commonly named Fabry's disease, is an X-linked lysosomal disease that results from a deficient activity of the hydrolase α-galactosidase. It is associated with severe multiorgan dysfunction. The subtle eye manifestations of Fabry's disease are visually insignificant to the patient. However, they may prove to be useful in the diagnosis, in understanding the natural history of the disease and in assessing the response to enzyme replacement therapy. In Fabry's disease, ophthalmological abnormalities occur mostly at the level of the conjunctival and retinal vessels, the cornea and the lens (Fig. C8.1). They result from a progressive deposition of glycosphingolipids in ocular structures.

A vortex keratopathy ("cornea verticillata") represents the ocular manifestation most commonly reported in Fabry's disease. They can be the only ocular sign present in Fabry patients. The prevalence of cornea verticillata is similar in different age groups. It can be detected in 70% of Fabry patients. Cornea verticillata is well recognized only by slit-lamp microscopy. The earliest lesion is a diffuse haziness in the subepithelial layer that later appears as fine, straight or curved lines radiating from the periphery toward the center of the cornea in a characteristic pattern. They usually do not affect vision. Indistinguishable drug-induced phenocopies of Fabry cornea verticillata have been reported in patients on long-term chloroquine or amiadarone therapy.

A small number of patients exhibit a characteristic lens opacity with a "spoke-like" pattern usually referred to as "Fabry cataract." It consists of two types, anterior and posterior subcapsular cataracts. The former, which only occurs in hemizygous males, appears as granular, radially arranged wedges. The latter has the appearance of nearly translucent spoke-like or dendritic projections; they may also occur in heterozygous female carriers. These signs can be detected by basic slit-lamp examination, a procedure that is noninvasive, inexpensive, and not time consuming.

Conjunctival and retinal vascular lesions are also common and represent part of the diffuse systemic vascular involvement. Conjunctival and retinal vessels are tortuous and may exhibit aneurysmal dilatations. Vessel tortuosity shows an association with both cornea verticillata and Fabry cataract; hence, the isolated presence of tortuous vessels (especially in the fundus), without any corneal or lens involvement, is not diagnostic of Fabry's disease. Till now, there are no studies in the literature that report any changes in cornea verticillata or conjuctival and retinal vessels appearance after enzymatic replacement therapy.

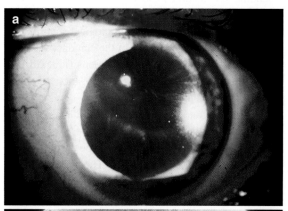

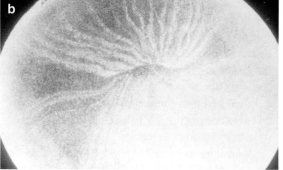

Fig. C8.1 Eye abnormalities associated with Fabry's disease: (**a**) cornea verticillata (vortex opacities located in the superficial corneal layers); (**b**) conjunctival vessel tortuosity

Other lysosomal defects may lead to corneal manifestations as the earliest indication of a metabolic disease. In *mucolipidosis type IV*, corneal clouding with major visual impairment is a prominent feature. Corneal clouding is one of the early symptoms; later, retinal degeneration and blindness may develop. Cytoplasmic membranous bodies are found in diverse tissues, including the conjunctiva, fibroblasts, liver, and spleen. Affected patients are usually mentally retarded. The late-onset form of *α-mannosidosis* also involves corneal clouding, in addition to cataracts, changes in bone and hearing loss. In *Farber's disease*, the severe form, presents with eye changes including a cherry-red spot, a paint gray ring around the cornea, modular corneal opacity and a pingueculum-like conjunctival lesion.

In the *juvenile/adult type of galactosialidosis*, corneal clouding with loss of visual acuity develops in the second decade of life. Additional ophtalmologic abnormalities include bilateral cherry-red spots, punctate lens opacities and color blindness. Other clinical symptoms include coarse face, growth disturbance, cardiac involvement, hernias, angiokeratomata, hearing loss, joint stiffness, vertebral changes and a progressive neurologic course with mental retardation, seizures, myoclonus and ataxia. In *steroid sulfatase deficiency*, corneal opacities are small punctate or filiform lesions located in the deep corneal stroma.

Disease Info: Cystinosis

The disease is a systemic metabolic disorder affecting the conjunctiva, cornea, iris, choroid and retinal pigment epithelium, as well as the kidney and other organs. It results from the accumulation of cystine within lysosomes. The disease is caused by mutations in the CTNS gene coding for cystonin, a lysosomal carrier protein. In the cornea, the crystals are located in the anterior stroma; they are iridescent and polychromatic, presenting first in the periphery and extending centrally. The corneal changes and associated photophobia are due to the anterior location of the crystal deposition. They may be present before nephropathy is severe; thus, they can be the first sign of the disease. The anterior location of the crystals can predispose the patient to recurrent erosions. Photophobia, watering and blepharospasm may become disabling; these symptoms are often related to erosions of the corneal epithelium, leading eventually to keratopathy.

Sight may be progressively reduced, leading to blindness in a severe form of the disease. Cataract and pigmentary retinopathy also develop.

Cysteamine eye drops are effective in reducing the deposits of crystals in the cornea and in improving the extreme photophobia. Corneal transplantation may be indicated for visual rehabilitation, as well as for recurrent erosions.

C8.2.2 Lipid Metabolism Disorders

Some disorders of high-density lipoproteins (HDL) metabolism, including Tangier disease, fish-eye disease, lecithin cholesterol acyltransferase deficiency and apoprotein A-1 (Apo A-I) deficiency must be included in the differential diagnosis of corneal opacity. The central corneal changes are gray dots occupying the full thickness of the stroma, mainly centrally, with peripheral condensation to form the arcus-like changes. Occasionally an arcus-like structure develops due to the deposition of a variety of phospholipids, low-density lipoproteins and triglycerides in the stroma of the peripheral cornea. Patients with these diseases have hypoalphalipoproteinemia with low HDL, low Apo A-I and elevated triglycerides. Those with Tangier disease have striking large yellow tonsils or pharyngeal plaques. They also have peripheral neuropathy manifested by weakness, paresthesias, autonomic dysregulation and ptosis. In addition, abnormal rectal mucosa, anemia, renal failure, and hepatosplenomegaly may occur. Corneal clouding is the only clinical manifestation in patients with fish-eye disease.

C8.2.3 Amino Acid Disorders

Disease Info: Tyrosinemia Type II

Tyrosinemia type II (oculocutaneous tyrosinemia, Richner–Hanhart syndrome) is due to a defect in cytosolic tyrosine aminotransferase. Photophobia, redness, watering eyes, and pain are often the presenting symptoms. At slit-lamp examination, central dendritic corneal erosions that stain poorly with fluorescein are present. The lesions are bilateral in contrast to herpetic ulcers that are unilateral. If not diagnosed and treated, ocular damage including corneal opacities, visual impairment, corneal plana, nystagmus, amblyopia and glaucoma are frequent complications.

Treatment consists of a phenylalanine and tyrosine restricted diet. There is no consensus as to the optimal blood level of tyrosine, but a level $<500\,\mu M$ is a reasonable goal. The eye symptoms resolve within a short period of treatment (few weeks). Treatment with systemic steroids should be avoided because the disease can worsen with such therapy.

Alkaptonuria is a rare autosomal recessive condition caused by deficient homogentisic acid oxidase. Homogentisic acid is excreted in excess in the urine, but its oxidized pigment derivatives (alkapton) also bind collagen, leading to pigment accumulation in connective tissue of the nose, sclera and ear lobes. Affected patients develop a degenerative arthropathy. Ocular changes occur in 70% of patients. Just inside the limbus, the cornea develops a black "oil-droplet" pigmentation that appears similar to spheroidal degeneration. Pigmentation gradually increases throughout adulthood.

Wilson's disease may be diagnosed by characteristic ocular findings. It is an autosomal recessive disorder that causes deposition of copper in the liver, corneas, kidneys and nervous system. The Kayser–Fleischer ring is the single most important diagnostic finding of the disease. When fully developed, it is seen with the naked eye, but subtle changes can be seen by slit-lamp examination (see Fig. 2 in Chap. C2). It consists of brownish–greenish deposit of copper in the Descemet's membrane just within the limbus of the cornea; it can be especially prominent at the upper pole, therefore it requires lifting of the eyelid for recognition. It is present in 60% of children at the stage of acute or subacute liver disease. It may be present in asymptomatic affected individual as well.

The ring is not absolutely pathognomonic of Wilson disease, because other causes of liver failure such as carotenemia and multiple myeloma may lead to similar rings. In Wilson's disease, another rare but characteristic abnormality is the "sunflower" subcapsular cataract. The rings improve with effective decoppering therapy or after liver transplantation, as does cataract.

Remember

The cornea verticillata and the Kayser–Fleischer ring are important diagnostic ocular findings for Fabry's disease and Wilson's disease, respectively.

C8.3 Lens Defects and Dislocations

C8.3.1 Cataracts

Cataract is defined as any opacity within the lens. Cataracts and dislocation of the lens are anomalies of the lens detectable in many inherited metabolic defects. At birth lens opacities, if not diagnosed or removed, are a major cause of blindness or amblyopia.

Remember

Early cataract investigation: look for the orange or red retinal reflex after a dilute dilating eye drop at the first pediatric examination after birth with an ophtalmoscope.

Often, the retinal reflex can be visualized with an ophtalmoscope alone. When cataracts are bilateral, they lead to irreversible nystagmus and amblyopia by 3 months of age. Thus, these cataracts must be quickly removed by surgery, preferably within the first few days or weeks of life.

Remember

The etiologic classification of congenital cataract is diverse and more then 90% remain unexplained. The most common etiologies include infections, metabolic disorders, and genetic syndromes.

A number of inherited metabolic diseases presents with cataracts (Table C8.2). It is a constant and early finding in neonates in defects of carbohydrate metabolism

Table C8.2 Cataracts according to age of presentation

Newborn period
Galactosemia (all defects)
Sorbitol dehydrogenase deficiency
Zellweger syndrome
Rhizomelic chondrodysplasia puntata
Lowe's syndrome
Childhood
Carbohydrate disorders
Galactosemias
Sorbitol dehydrogenase deficiency
Aldose reductase deficiency
Lysosomal disorders
Oligosaccharidoses: α-mannosidosis; sialidosis; galactosialidosis
Fabry's disease; neuronal ceroid lipofuscinosis (juvenile form)
Amino acid disorders
Delta1-Pyrroline-5-carboxylate synthase deficiency
Hyperornithinemia (ornithine aminotransferase deficiency)
Lysinuric protein intolerance
Lowe's syndrome
Lipid disorders
Sjögren–Larsson syndrome
Neutral lipid storage disorder
Cholesterol metabolism defects
Cerebrotendinous xanthomatosis (cholestanol lipidosis)
Mevalonate kinase deficiency (severe form)
Conradi–Hunermann syndrome
Smith–Lemli–Opitz syndrome
Peroxisomal disorders
Peroxisome biogenesis defects
Rhizomelic chondrodysplasia punctata
Mitochondrial oxidative phosphorylation disorders
Senger disease
Senger-like disease
β-Methylglutaconic aciduria
mitochondrial DNA mutations
Copper disordsers
Wilson's disease
Menkes disease

(galactose and polyol pathways), peroxisomal disorders (peroxisomal biogenesis) and Lowe syndrome. Cataracts develop later in life in lysosomal disorders (sialidosis, α-mannosidosis and Fabry's disease), Wilson's disease, Menkes disease, lipid disorders, some amino acid defects, and some mitochondrial disorders. Rarely, cataracts have been reported in metachromatic leukodystrophy, hypobetalipoproteinemia, vitamin E or D deficiencies and lactose intolerance. Hypoglycemic episodes of various origins during the perinatal period or in early infancy may result in lens opacities.

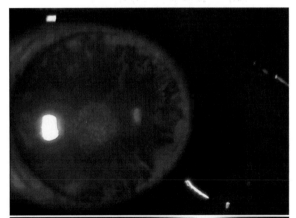

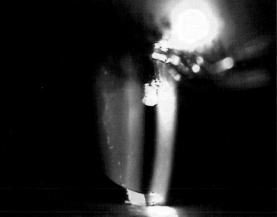

Fig. C8.2 Galactosemia: oil droplet cataract in untreated patient visible by slit-lamp examination

> **Remember**
>
> Cataracts are an early finding in defects of carbohydrate metabolism (galactose and polyol pathways), peroxisomal biogenesis, cholesterol biosynthesis and amino acid transport.

C8.3.2 Carbohydrate Metabolism

Disease Info: Galactosemia

The lens is avascular by nature, receiving its nutrients from the aqueous humor. Most of the glucose metabolized in the lens is handled by anaerobic glycolysis. The citric acid pathway produces about 20–30% of the total ATP in the lens, even though only about 3% of the glucose passes through the citric acid cycle. Three defects in galactose metabolism are known: galactose-1-phosphate uridyltransferase (GALT), galactose1-phosphate epimerase and galactokinase. At an early stage, "oil droplet" cataracts which are not true cataracts but refracture changes in the lens nucleus are present (Fig. C8.2). The lesion appears in retroillumination as a drop in the center of the lens like an oil droplet floating in the water. The accumulation in the lens of galactitol, a metabolite of galactose, creates a shift of water into the lens, due to the lack of permeability of galactitol, with ultimate disruption of the lenticular structure. In GALT deficiency, major manifestations include liver failure, jaundice, and tubulopathy. Demonstration of GALT deficiency establishes the diagnosis. This can be achieved using the fluorescent spot test used in neonatal screening (Beutler test) followed by quantitative tests for confirmation (enzyme activity in erythrocytes) and by mutation analysis. In epimerase deficiency, patients may have a symptomatology resembling transferase deficiency; enzyme activity is measured in erythrocytes and leukocytes. In galactokinase deficiency, cataracts may not be recognized until later because no other symptoms develop. The enzyme is measured in red blood cells. In all disorders, cataracts are usually reversible after the introduction of a galactose-free diet.

> **Remember**
>
> In all type of galactosemia, cataracts are usually reversible after the start of a galactose-free diet.

The polyol pathway consists of two enzymes: aldose reductase and sorbitol dehydrogenase. Aldose reductase reduces hexose sugars such as glucose and galactose to their respective polyols, sorbitol and galactitol. Polyol accumulation has been demonstrated to cause cataracts owing to increases in intracellular fluid resulting in lens swelling, increased membrane permeability, and electrolyte abnormalities. In *sorbitol dehydrogenase deficiency*, cataracts present at birth as the only sign. Patients with *glucose-6-phosphate dehydrogenase deficiency*, who usually come to the clinician's attention because of hemolytic anemia, may also develop cataracts.

C8.3.3 Lipid Metabolism Disorders

The lens membrane contains the highest cholesterol content of any known membrane, indicating the importance of normal cholesterol metabolism in lens maintenance. Disorders of *cholesterol biosynthesis* (*mevalonate kinase deficiency*, *Conradi–Hunermann syndrome* and *Smith–Lemli–Opitz syndrome*) present with a large and variable spectrum of morphogenic and congenital anomalies. Cataracts are present early in the very severe forms but due to the clinical and biochemical continuum of these defects may not develop in milder forms. In *cerebrotendinous xanthomatosis* bilateral, irregular, corticonuclear and anterior polar or posterior capsular cataracts can occur in the first decade. It may be associated with opacities of the crystalline lens. The lesion is associated with xanthomata and a progressive neurological syndrome of ataxia, pyramidal signs, cognitive impairment, epilepsy and peripheral neuropathy.

Patients with the *Sjögren–Larsson syndrome* have cataracts and it may also be present in another syndrome characterized by ichthyosis, the so-called neutral lipid storage disorder. This syndrome, whose etiology is still unknown, includes ataxia, myopathy, and hepatomegaly as further clinical features. Vacuolated lymphocytes are a frequent finding in the peripheral blood.

C8.3.4 Peroxisomal Disorders

Congenital cataracts in association with craniofacial dysmorphic features, hepatomegaly and renal cysts are frequently present in disorders of peroxisome biogenesis. To this group belong *Zellweger syndrome* and two allied conditions: *neonatal adrenoleukodystrophy* and *infantile Refsum disease*. Other ocular abnormalities include pigmentary degeneration of the retina, corneal opacities and glaucoma. Differences between these syndromes relate to the severity of the neurological abnormalities and modifications of clinical and pathological features. Measurement of plasma very long-chain fatty acids allows the diagnosis. *Chondrodysplasia punctata* and rhizomelic dwarfism combined with congenital cataracts lead to the diagnosis of chondrodysplasia punctata. Normal very long-chain fatty acids and low plasmalogens levels in tissues and red blood cells are the diagnostic abnormalities.

Cataracts are also present in the following forms of spastic paraplegias: SPG9 (autosomal dominant form), SPG21 and SPG25, both autosomal recessive disorders.

C8.3.5 Amino Acid Disorders

In *Lowe's oculo-cerebro-renal syndrome*, cataracts are a constant and hallmark finding. The lesion is already present prenatally as early as in the 24th week of gestation. Additional features are kidney pathology (Fanconi syndrome) and severe neurological impairments including muscular hypotonia, areflexia and mental retardation.

In other aminoacidopathies, including *ornithine aminotransferase* (OAT) *deficiency* (gyrate atrophy of the choroid and retina), *delta1-pyrroline-5-synthase deficiency* and *lysinuric protein intolerance,* cataracts can be a presenting sign.

C8.4 Lens Dislocations (Ectopia Lentis)

Remember

In the diagnostic work-up for patients with subluxation of the ocular lens, total plasma homocysteine must always be measured.

Dislocations of the ocular lens (ectopia lentis) are frequent, severe and characteristic sequels of both homocystinuria and Marfan syndrome. The probable mechanism for lenticular dislocation in Marfan syndrome is microfibril abnormalities of the lens capsule. The lens subluxation in homocystinuria most commonly occurs downwards, whereas in Marfan syndrome the lens usually subluxes upwards, although, it can occur in any direction in both the diseases. *Marfan syndrome* is due to alteration in microfibrils caused most commonly by mutations of the fibrillin-1 gene. The involvement of the ocular system includes a flat cornea, an increased axial length of the globe with hypoplastic iris, or hypoplastic ciliary muscle causing decreased miosis.

Disease Info: Homocystinuria

In patients with homocystinuria, subluxation of ocular lens is very characteristic and frequent ocular feature, estimated to occur in over 90% of patients (Fig. C8.3). The presence of the detached lens is often heralded by the clinical recognition of iridodonesis. It seldom occurs before 3 years of age and is usually present by 10 years of age. Prior patients usually develop rapidly worsening myopia, as well as astigmatism and sometimes glaucoma. Staphyloma may result from increased ocular pressure. Cataracts which can be congenital may occur in the lens. All these manifestations may be secondary to the ectopia lentis. The patient may also have retinal detachment and optic atrophy may follow central retinal artery occlusion.

Although the body habitus of patients with homocystinuria resembles that of Marfan syndrome, the etiology is different. Increased levels of plasma and urine homocysteine are found in all patients. Hypermethioninemia is an important finding. The diagnosis is confirmed by assays of the enzyme cystathionine β-synthetase in cultured fibroblasts, lynphoblasts, or mutation analysis. Prevention of the lens dislocation is possible in patients detected through neonatal screening and early treated with low methionine formulas or pyridoxine in the responsive disease variants.

In homocystinuria, due to 5,10-methylentetrahydrofolate reductase deficiency, ectopia lentis has never been reported.

Table C8.3 Ectopia lentis (dislocation of the lens)

Homocystinuria
Marfan syndrome
Molybdenum cofactor deficiency
Sulfite oxidase deficiency
Weill–Marchesani syndrome

Table C8.3 lists metabolic disorders in which ectopia lentis occurs.

C8.5 Degeneration of the Retina

Among the disorders that might be expected to affect the pigmented epithelium of the retina are diseases caused by storage of specific components or diseases in which the normal ability to synthesize pigment is absent. Included are disorders characterized by the presence of retinal pigmentation and a progressive red-corneal dystrophy as a prominent feature of retinal degeneration.

C8.5.1 Retinitis Pigmentosa (RP)

RP is a clinically and genetically heterogeneous group of hereditary disorders in which a progressive loss of photoreceptor and pigment epithelial function occurs. Diagnostic criteria include bilateral involvement, loss of peripheral vision, rod dysfunction and progressive loss of photoreception function. The history should include information regarding the nature of the earliest symptoms, the age at onset, and progression. The age at onset of RP varies but often begins in early childhood or infancy.

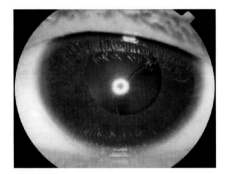

Fig. C8.3 The lens dislocation in homocystinuria is usually downward, while in Marfan syndrome it is upward

Remember

RP is characterized by progressive loss of photoreceptor function causing visual problems such as defective adaptation to the dark, or night blindness, visual field decrease, and reduction of visual activity.

In adults, careful questioning often elicits a history starting in childhood or adolescence when patients are asked to recall difficulties with outdoor activities at dusk or with indoor activities at night in minimal lighting. Patients rarely note a loss in peripheral vision as an early symptom, although they may be considered clumsy before constricted visual fields are detected. Other symptoms include pendular eye movements and nystagmus. Patients who present with initial symptoms of photophobia, sensations of flashing lights, abnormal central vision, abnormal color vision or marked asymmetry in ocular involvement may not have RP, but rather, another retinal disease.

Remember

The diagnosis of RP is typically made by seeing a pigmentary retinopathy on fundus examination. An electroretinogram is an important confirmatory test

The ocular examination should include measurements of the patient's best-corrected visual acuity, refraction, examination of the anterior segment, and measurement of intraocular pressure. Attention should be given to the lens, vitreous, optic disc, retinal vessels, macula and retinal periphery. The earliest ophtalmoscopic findings are a dull retinal reflex and a thread-like aspect of the retinal arteries. The electroretinogram is abnormal before gross fundoscopic evidence of RP is found.

Remember

The most frequent RP associated with metabolic defects are Sjögren–Larsson syndrome, neuronal ceroid lipofuscinoses, abetalipoproteinemia, 3-hydroxyacyl-CoA-dehydrogenase deficiency, Refsum disease, Kearns–Sayre syndrome and OAT deficiency.

The pigmented retinopathies can be divided into two groups: primary RP, in which the disease process is confined to the eyes and secondary RP, in which retinal degeneration is associated with involvement of additional organs. The first group includes gyrate atrophy of the choroid and retina caused by OAT deficiency.

Disease Info: OAT Deficiency

Patients come to the attention of the ophtalmologist in late childhood or puberty for evaluation of increasing myopia or decreased night vision. At this age, sharply demarcated, circular areas of chorioretinal degeneration are present in midperiphery of the ocular fundus (Fig. C8.4). In a few years, the retinal degeneration accelerates, the lesions enlarge, coalesce and extend toward the posterior pole of the fundus. Frequently, a posterior subcapsular cataract develops in the second decade. By the third decade, much of the fundus is involved and increased pigmentation is common in the macula area, while the optic disc remains pink and does not become atrophic. Visual acuity decreases gradually and visual fields are progressively and concentrically reduced.

OAT deficiency results in a 10–20-fold increase in ornithine in body fluids including aqueous humor and a lesion in photoreceptors rather than the retinal pigment epithelium. Therapeutic approaches include stimulation of residual OAT activity with pharmacological doses of pyridoxine, dietary reduction of ornithine through arginine reduction, increasing renal losses by administration of pharmacological doses of lysine and/or administration of creatine and proline. Because of slow disease progression, the evaluation of therapeutical approaches are difficult.

In hyperornithinemia–hyperammonemia–homocitrullinuria (HHH syndrome), the retina is not affected.

Secondary RP is most often associated with neurological disease, dysmorphic features, myopathy, nephropathy, deafness and skin abnormalities. Some of these conditions are well-defined inherited metabolic diseases (Table C8.4).

The *neuronal ceroid lipofuscinoses* (CLNs) are a group of progressive encephalopathies, which are characterized by neural and extraneural accumulation of ceroid and lipofuscin storage material (see also Chap. C5). Ceroid lipofuscinoses are among the most common neurodegenerative disorders. Three main types that cause RP have been distinguished on clinical,

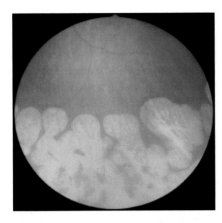

Fig. C8.4 Gyrate atrophy of choroid and retina in ornithine aminotransferase deficiency: the mid- and far-perphery show the typical atrophic areas in peripheral retina

neurophysiologic and genetic criteria: the infantile Santavuori–Haltia disease (CLN1), with onset between 6 and 18 months of age, regression of psychomotor development, myoclonic epilepsy, visual failure, microcephaly and "vanishing electroencephalogram (EEG)"; the late infantile Jansky–Bielschowski disease (CLN2), with onset between 2 and 4 years of age, epilepsy, regression of mental skills, ataxia, myoclonic jerks, pathologic EEG, electroretinogram and visual evoked potentials (VEP); and the juvenile Spielmeyer–Vogt–Batten disease (CLN3), with onset of visual impairment between the ages of 4 and 10 years, psychological disturbances, motor dysfunction and epilepsy, retinal degeneration and vacuolated lymphocytes.

Table C8.4 Secondary retinitis pigmentosa (RP)

Lysosomal disorders
   Neuronal ceroid lipofuscinoses
   Mucopolysaccharidoses: all except Morquio disease
   Mucolipidosis IV, Krabbe disease (late onset)
Lipid disorders
   Abetalipoproteinemia
   Peroxisomal disorders: peroxisome biogenesis disorders;
    Refsum disease
   β-Oxidation defects: long-chain hydroxyacyl-CoA
    dehydrogenase deficiency, mitochondrial trifunctional
    protein deficiency
   Sjögren-Larsson syndrome
Mitochondrial Disorders
   Kearns–Sayre syndrome
   NARP (neuropathy, ataxia, and RP)
   2-Methyl-3-hydroxybutyryl-CoA dehydrogenase
    deficiency

Different disorders of lipid metabolism present with RP. *Abetalipoproteinemia* is caused by the absence of apoprotein B and the malabsorption of fat and fat-soluble vitamins, especially vitamins A and E. The most common clinical manifestations are diarrhea and failure to thrive from early infancy. Other manifestations involve the nervous system, with signs of peripheral neuropathy, spinocerebellar ataxia and muscle weakness. Although the retinal dystrophy may occur at early age, it most commonly presents in late childhood. Fundus examination may be normal in the early stages, later there may be peripheral pigmentary retinopathy or a picture similar to retinitis punctata albescens with scattered white dots at the level of the retinal pigment epithelium. The electroretinogram may be normal initially but later becomes abnormal with scotopic responses first to be lost. The retinal and neurologic complications may be prevented or stabilized by early supplementation with vitamin E. Disorder of fatty acid oxidation, mostly 3-hydroxyacyl-C-A-dehydrogenase deficiency, present with a generalized red-cone dystrophy.

Disease Info: Sjögren–Larsson Syndrome

Sjögren–Larsson syndrome, caused by a deficiency of fatty aldehyde dehydrogenase, is characterized by a triad of intellectual disability, spastic diplegia or tetraplegia, and congenital ichthyosis with associated ocular features, which include pigmentary changes in the retina. Ocular features are characterized by a crystalline maculopathy and bilateral, glistening yellow–white dots involving the foveal and parafoveal area from the age of 1–2 years. The number of dots may increase with age, although the extent of macular involvement does not correlate with the severity of systemic features. Color vision, electroretinography and electrooculography have been shown to be normal. Most patients exhibit photophobia, subnormal visual acuity, myopia and astigmatism. It is unknown if reduced visual acuity is due to retinal deposits or due to demyelination of the optic pathways, the latter having been demonstrated by MRI in the affected patients.

Peroxisomal disorders are best diagnosed by determining plasma concentrations of very-long-chain fatty acids. Disorders with pigmentary retinopathy include Zellweger syndrome, neonatal adrenoleukodystrophy and isolated enzyme defects, such as acyl-CoA oxidase deficiency and peroxisomal thiolase deficiency. Nystagmus is common and ocular findings include retinal dystrophy, corneal clouding and cataract. Extensive photoreceptor degeneration and loss of ganglion cells with gliosis of nerve fibre layers have been reported.

Patients with *Refsum disease*, an inborn error caused by phytanic acid oxidase deficiency, present with RP (Fig. C8.5), peripheral polyneuropathy and elevated cerebrospinal fluid protein. Other symptoms include cerebellar ataxia, deafness, anemia, ichthyosis and skeletal and cardiac manifestations. Night blindness may be the first clinical symptom at school age.

Defects in the mitochondrial electron transport chain cause a variety of oculars manifestations. Chronic external ophtalmoplagia and retinal dystrophy similar to RP are often found. It is seen in several mitochondrial disorders. Electroretinogram shows evidence of rod and cone dysfunction with the rods being more severely affected. Retinal degeneration has been consistently reported only in the *Kearns–Sayre syndrome*, a progressive multisystem disorder, with onset usually before the age of 20 years. Clinical features include chronic progressive external ophtalmoplegia, ptosis, retinopathy, cardiac conduction defects and deafness. It is caused by deletion ± duplications of mitochondrial DNA (mtDNA).

Finally, several well-known autosomal recessive disorders comprise RP; these include pantothenate kimase - assosiated neurodegeneration, (*PKAN)*, (severe neurological regression, dystonia and acanthocytosis), *Laurence–Moon–Biedl* (obesity, polydactyly and mental retardation), *Usher type II* (deafness and severe mental retardation), *Joubert* (mental retardation, cerebellar vermis atrophy and attacks of hyperventilation), and *Cockayne* (dysmorphia, hypotonia, intacranial calcifications and deafness) syndromes.

C8.5.2 Pigment Retinopathies

Pigment retinopathies due to the storage of specific compounds include many lysosomal storage diseases. The cherry-red spot is due to ganglioside accumulation in the retinal ganglion cells. The absence of ganglion cells at the fovea gives rise to the red spot surrounded by white cells filled with storage material. As the ganglion cells die, the cherry-red spot fades, and optic atrophy becomes apparent.

The differential diagnosis mainly includes lysosomal disorders (Table C8.5). It is present at an early stage in most patients affected with *GM$_2$ gangliosidosis* (GM$_2$ type I, II, and III) and *GM$_1$ gangliosidosis* (type I). The electroretinogram is consistently normal, but the VEP are abnormal from the early stages of the disease, and the cortical response is generally abolished from the first months of age.

Niemann–Pick disease type A also leads to corneal opacification and dislocation of the anterior lens capsule.

In *sialidosis (mucolipicosis type I)*, formerly known as cherry-red spot myoclonus syndrome, the lesion presents in adulthood with a progressive myoclonus and normal intelligence. In *Farber's disease*, *metachromatic leucodystrophy* and *Gaucher disease type II*, a faint or irregular cherry-red spot can be present.

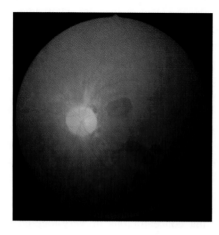

Fig. C8.5 Refsum's disease showing retinal pigment abnormality

Table C8.5 Metabolic diseases with cherry-red spots

Sialidosis type I and II
Galactosialidosis (early-infantile)
Tay–Sachs disease [*gangliosidosis* type 2 (GM$_2$), variant B, infantile]
Sandhoff disease (GM$_2$, variant O, infantile)
Gangliosidosis type 1-gangliosidosis (infantile)
Niemann–Pick disease type A
Gaucher disease type II
Farber disease
Metachromatic leukodystrophy

Retinal degeneration may occur in other defects of intermediary metabolism including defects of *intracellular cobalamin metabolism (Cbl C/D defects)* and *congenital disorders of glycosylation syndromes* (especially type Ia, phosphomannomutase deficiency).

C8.6 Optic Atrophy

Optic atrophy results from loss of ganglion cell axons that form the optic nerve, and/or a loss of the supporting microvascular tissue surrounding the optic nerve. Symptoms of optic atrophy include decreased visual acuity (ranging from no light perception to mild decreases in visual acuity), visual field defects and/or abnormalities in color vision and contrast sensitivity.

Remember

The hallmark clinical sign of optic atrophy is optic nerve pallor at fundoscopic examination.

Optic neuropathy is a more general term for optic nerve dysfunction and includes the early phase of the disease, before clinical signs of optic atrophy may be present.

Mostly no effective treatment exists, although correction of an underlying cause or elimination of an offending medication may halt progression.

Genetic defects are responsible for a substantial portion of optic atrophy. The lesion can be the only clinical feature (primary) or associated to various neurological and systemic symptoms (secondary).

C8.6.1 Primary Optic Atrophy

In primary optic atrophies, optic atrophy is often the only clinical feature of the disease. An example is Leber's hereditary optic nauropathy (LHON) or Costeff optic atrophy syndrome (OPA 3).

Disease Info: LHON

LHON is an inherited form of acute or subacute loss of central vision affecting predominantly young males. The disease is the paradigm of mitochondrial optic neuropathies where a primary role for mitochondrial dysfunction is certified by maternal inheritance and caused by missense mutations in different mtDNA genes, especially complex I subunits. The typical presentation is a rapid painless loss of central vision in one eye. Usually, fading of colors (dyschromatopsia) in one eye is followed by a similar involvement of the other eye, within days, months or rarely years. Visual acuity stabilizes at or below 20/200 within a few months. The accompanying visual field defect usually involves the central vision in the form of a large centrocecal absolute scotoma.

Fundus examination during the acute/subacute stage mostly reveals characteristic changes as follows.

(1) circumpapillary telangiectatic microangiopathy,
(2) swelling of the nerve fiber layer around the disc (pseudoedema), and
(3) absence of leakage on fluorescein angiography (in contrast to true edema).

Thus, the optic disc appears hyperemic, occasionally with peripapillar hemorrhages and the axonal loss rapidly leads to temporal atrophy of the optic disc. With time, the optic disc turns pale. The microangiopathy may be present in a number of asymptomatic at-risk family members along the maternal line, in whom it may remain stable over the years.

Optic atrophy with permanent severe loss of central vision but with relative preservation of pupillary light responses is the usual endpoint of the disease. However, spontaneous recovery of visual acuity has occasionally been reported even years after onset. Visual function may improve, sometimes suddenly, with contraction of the scotoma or reappearance of small islands of vision within it (fenestration). In long-lasting LHON, cupping of the optic disc has frequently been reported as a sign of the chronic stage of the pathological process.

LHON is due to homoplasmic mtDNA mutations, typically with wide variability in phenotypic penetrance. To date, LHON is the only human disease for which the influence of mtDNA background (haplogroups) has been solidly documented, particularly on the T14484C/ND6 and G11778A/ND4 LHON mutations. Recently, the association of LHON with a region of chromosome X suggests that one or more nuclear genes may act as modifiers, possibly explaining the male prevalence.

The recent identification of mutations in the nuclear gene OPA1 as the causative factor in dominant optic atrophy (DOA, Kjer's type) brought the unexpected finding that this gene encodes for a mitochondrial protein, suggesting that DOA and LHON may be linked by a similar pathogenesis.

Polymorphisms in this very same gene may be associated with normal tension glaucoma (NTG), which might be considered a genetically determined optic neuropathy that again shows similarities with both LHON and DOA.

Costeff optic atrophy syndrome or Type III 3-methylglutaconic aciduria (OPA 3) is a neuroophthalmologic disease that consists of early onset bilateral optic atrophy and late-onset spasticity, extrapyramidal dysfunction and cognitive deficits. Urinary excretion of 3-methylglutaconic acid and of 3-methylglutaric acid is increased. The disorder is mapping to chromosome 19q13.2–q13.3, and the causative gene has been identified in the FLJ22187-cDNA clone, which consists of two exons and encodes a peptide of 179 amino acid residues. Milder mutations in OPA3 should be sought in patients with optic atrophy with later onset, even in the absence of additional neurological abnormalities. *Behr syndrome* is clinically similar to Costeff syndrome, but it is distinguished by the absence of 3-methylglutaconic aciduria.

C8.6.2 Secondary Optic Atrophy

Secondary optic atrophy occurs often in inherited metabolic diseases and is due to accumulation or shortage of substrates or formation of harmful metabolites such as in mitochondrial defects, peroxisomal defects and lysosomal defects and occasionally in some other metabolic defects (Table C8.6).

C8.6.2.1 Mitochondrial Disorders

In addition to the relative selective involvement of the optic nerve in some disorders with mitochondrial

Table C8.6 Secondary optic atrophy

Mitochondrial disorders
MERRF (mitochondrial encephalopathy with ragged-red fibers and stroke-like episodes)
MELAS (mitochondrial encephalomyopathy, lactic acidosis, stroke-like episodes)
Kearns–Sayre syndrome
NARP(neuropathy, ataxia, retinitis pigmentosa)
Leigh syndrome
Peroxisomal disorders
Zellweger spectrum disorders
Adrenoleukodystrophy
Primary hyperoxaluria type I
Lysosomal disorders
Mucopolysaccharidoses
Oligosaccharidoses
Niemann–Pick type C
Niemann–Pick type A or B
GM_1 gangliosidosis
Sandhoff disease
Multiple sulfatase deficiency
Krabbe disease
Metachromatic leukodystrophy
Neuronal ceroid lipofucinoses
Cystinosis
Other metabolic disorders
2-Methyl-3-hydroxybutyryl-CoA dehydrogenase deficiency
Cobalamin C/D disorders
Propionic acidemia
Homocystinuria
Smith–Lemli–Opitz syndrome
Mevalonic aciduria
Canavan disease
Alexander disease
Pelizaeus–Merzbacher disease
Menkes disease

dysfunction, optic atrophy may occur in mitochondrial encephalomyopathies due to mtDNA point mutations in *tRNA* genes, such as *myoclonic epilepsy, ragged-red-fibres (MERRF)* and *mitochondrial encephalomyopathy, lactic acidosis, and stroke-like syndrome (MELAS)*, *NARP (neuropathy, ataxia and pigmentary retinopathy)* and *Leigh syndrome* (see also Chap. D1).

Although the visual system is not usually emphasized, optic atrophy is frequently reported in Leigh syndrome in addition to the bilateral necrotic lesions affecting the periventricular white matter, basal ganglia and brainstem. Given the early onset of Leigh syndrome, it is difficult to document visual loss, but according to the few histopathological reports of the visual system there is a typical loss of retinal ganglion cells and nerve fiber layer dropout in the papillomacular bundle. There is progressive deterioration of brainstem functions, ataxia, seizures, peripheral neuropathy, intellectual deterioration, impaired hearing and poor vision. Visual loss may be secondary to optic atrophy or retinal degeneration. A variety of molecular defects in both nuclear DNA (nDNA) and mtDNA have been identified. Leigh syndrome can be inherited, depending on the particular defect, maternally (mtDNA defects), as an X-linked recessive trait (pyruvate dehydrogenase complex, PDHC defect) or as an autosomal recessive disease (defects in complexes I and II nuclear genes; defects in *SURF1* gene for complex IV assembly).

Optic atrophy has also been reported in mitochondrial diseases caused by defects in nuclear genes such as hereditary spastic paraplegia due to mutations in the paraplegin gene, and in the deafness-dystonia-optic atrophy syndrome (*Mohr–Tranebjaerg syndrome*) due to mutations in the X-linked *DDP1* gene. In this disease patients manifest optic atrophy with severely constricted visual fields, a pattern opposite to LHON and the other optic neuropathies that affect primarily the central visual field due to predominant loss of the papillomacular bundle.

> **Remember**
>
> The most characteristic and primary manifestation of LHON is visual loss due to optic nerve dysfunction.

C8.6.2.2 Peroxisomal Disorders

> **Remember**
>
> Ocular findings in peroxisomal biogenesis disorders include profound demyelination of the optic nerve.

Ocular findings in all peroxisomal biogenesis disorders, such as *Zellweger syndrome, neonatal adrenoleukodystroph and infantile Refsum disease*, include profound demyelination of the optic nerve, reduced numbers of optic nerve fibres, and inclusion-bearing macrophages surrounding the optic nerve retinal

ganglion cells. Single peroxisomal enzyme defects that lead to optic atrophy are *X-linked adrenoleukodystrophy* and *primary hyperoxaluria type I*. Patients with X-linked adrenoleukodystrophy show loss of retinal ganglion cells and sporadic macrophages surrounding the optic nerve fibres. Patients with primary hyperoxaluria type I harbor oxalate crystals in various tissues, including the eye, due to a deficiency of the peroxisomal enzyme alanine:glyoxylate aminotransferase. Optic atrophies can occur secondary to increased intracranial pressure caused by impeded cerebrospinal fluid drainage due to oxalate crystals. Crystals within the retinal ganglion cells can also directly cause apoptosis.

C8.6.2.3 Lysosomal Disorders

Lysosomal storage diseases can cause optic atrophy. In the *MPS*, pathology is optic disc swelling. Secondary raised intracranial pressure must be excluded. In the absence of raised intracranial pressure, optic nerve swelling and consequently atrophy arises from compression of the nerve by a thickened dura and sclera, resulting in compression at the level of the lamina cribrosa. Also, accumulation of glucosaminoglycans within ganglion cells is thought to eventually lead to degeneration and optic atrophy.

Optic atrophies may also occur secondary to retinopathy or can be caused by glaucoma.

Among the *oligosaccharidoses*, the gangliosidoses (GM$_1$ gangliosidosis, Tay–Sachs, and Sandhoff disease) and, occasionally, Niemann–Pick A or B disease, present with distinct ocular findings and optic neuropathies. Causes of optic neuropathies in *sphingolipidoses* could be loss of myelinated nerve fibres or thickening of the pial septum of the optic nerve. Mostly, ocular pathology in sphingolipidoses relates to the damage of the retinal ganglion cells that form the optic nerve. Abnormal accumulation of lipid material and loss of retinal ganglion cells results in optic atrophy.

Another lysosomal storage disease with optic atrophy is *Krabbe disease* (globoid cell leukodystrophy). In this disease, the lesion is a consequence of the severe loss of myelin and oligodendroglia that is characteristic of this disorder. Although the optic atrophy occurs early, it is usually overshadowed by the neurological deterioration. Optic atrophy is also a frequent cause of severely impaired vision in metachromatic leukodystrophy.

In addition, some disorders of lysosomal membrane transport such as Niemann–Pick C disease and infantile sialic acid storage disease can present with marked ocular abnormalities and sporadic optic neuropathies. In cystinosis, benign intracranial hypertension has led to optic atrophy. In neuronal ceroid lipofuscinoses, neuro ophthalmological abnormalities like optic atrophy, maculopathy and RP have been reported. It is likely that lysosomal storage of metabolites indirectly affect the optic nerve and its supporting system.

C8.6.3 Other Secondary Metabolic Optic Atrophies

Optic atrophies are described in a variety of inherited metabolic disorders. It should be emphasized that, while optic atrophy has been noted in these disorders, it is not a constant finding. In some cases, it may be a secondary effect of a metabolic crisis. The first group includes disorders where critical metabolites are either deficient or accumulate within the retinal ganglion cells or the supporting cells. Disorders in this group include *biotinidase deficiency*, *Smith–Lemli–Opitz syndrome*, *Menkes disease* and a subset of disorders of amino acid metabolism such as *homocystinuria, cobalamin C disease* and *propionic acidemia*.

A second group involves myelination defects of the optic nerve. Disorders in this group include some *hereditary ataxias* such as Friedreich ataxia, certain forms of Charcot–Marie–Tooth disease, *Canavan disease, abetalipoproteinemia, Pelizaeus–Merzbacher disease, Alexander disease* and the spastic paraplegia form with peripheral polyneuropathy (spastic paraplegia, optic atrophy and neuropathy).

Take Home Messages

> Ocular manifestations occur frequently in various inherited metabolic disorders. Accurate examination of the eye by clinical means and with the help of the ophthalmoscope and slit lamps may detect the following pathognomonic abnormalities: corneal clouding, lens defects and dislocation, retinal degeneration and optic atrophy. Ophthalmology evaluation is a key twist in the diagnostic focus of many inherited metabolic diseases, e.g. cataracts in galactosemia, ectopia lentis in homocystinuria, cornea verticillata in Fabry's disease, macular cherry-red spot in a number of sphingolipidoses.

> For some inherited metabolic diseases, specific treatment can restore or prevent the ocular manifestation in a short period of time, e.g. tyrosinemia type II, galactosemia and homocystinurina.

Acknowledgements We thank Dr. L. Pinello and Dr. E. Zanin (Department of Paediatrics, University of Padova) for providing ophthalogical pictures reported in the chapter.

Key References

Fernandes J, Saudubray JM, van den Berghe G, Walter JH (eds) (2006) Inborn metabolic diseases – diagnosis and treatment, 4th edn. Springer, New York

Huizing M, Brooks BP, Anikster Y (2005) Optic atrophies in metabolic disorders. Mol Genet Metab 86:51–60

Nyhan WL, Barshop BA, Ozand PT (2005) Atlas of metabolic diseases, 2nd edn. Hodder Arnold, London

Poll-The BT, Maillette de Buy Wenniger-Prick LJ, Barth PG, Duran M (2003) The eye as a window to inborn errors of metabolism. J Inherit Metab Dis 26:229–244

Skin and Hair Disorders

C9

Carlo Dionisi-Vici, May El Hachem, and Enrico Bertini

Key Facts

> A correct classification of skin and hair signs as well as the knowledge of characteristic cutaneous symptoms is important to understand and diagnose inherited metabolic diseases.

> The profile of cutaneous signs, the age of the patient when manifestations initially occurred and the presence of associated symptoms, is of particular importance.

> Dermatological evaluation can help identify complications of the disease or side effects of treatments.

> Cutaneous signs of several types often occur in a single given disorder.

> The principal lesions can be grouped into the following main groups: vascular lesions, skin eruptions, ichthyosis, papular and nodular skin lesions, abnormal pigmentation, photosensitivity, hair disorders, and skin laxity.

C9.1 General Remarks

A correct classification of skin and hair signs as well as the knowledge of cutaneous symptoms of inherited metabolic diseases is an important prerequisite to help understand and diagnose these complex and heterogeneous diseases. The profile of cutaneous signs, the age of the patient when manifestations initially occurred and the presence of associated symptoms is of particular importance. Sometimes cutaneous signs may represent a hallmark for a specific metabolic disorder, while in other instances a careful dermatological evaluation can help identify complications of the disease or adverse side effects of (over-)treatment.

Remember

Skin lesions can be grouped in the following main categories: vascular lesions, skin eruptions, ichthyosis, papular and nodular skin lesions, abnormal pigmentation, photosensitivity, hair disorders, and skin laxity.

Cutaneous signs of several types often occur in a single given disorder, and the principal lesions can be grouped in the following main categories: vascular lesions, skin eruptions, ichthyosis, papular and nodular skin lesions, abnormal pigmentation, photosensitivity, hair disorders, and skin laxity. We have summarized in the tables, for simplicity, containing the list of disorders that frequently cluster for each skin or hair lesion. For most disorders, skin and hair abnormalities have been obtained from the clinical synopsis of Online Mendelian Inheritance in

C. Dionisi-Vici (✉)
Division of Metabolism, Bambino Gesu Hospital,
Piazza S. Onofrio 4, 00165 Rome, Italy
e-mail: dionisi@opbg.net

G. F. Hoffmann et al. (eds.), *Inherited Metabolic Diseases*,
DOI: 10.1007/978-3-540-74723-9_C9, © Springer-Verlag Berlin Heidelberg 2010

Man (OMIM), available at http://www.ncbi.nlm.nih.gov/sites/entrez.

As shown in Table C9.1, vascular lesion can be sub-classified in different forms.

C9.2 Vascular Lesions

C9.2.1 Angiokeratoma

The angiokeratomata are flat or raised vascular skin lesions, and they develop classically as clusters, punctuate, reddish or blue–black angiectases. They do not blanch with pressure and the largest lesions may appear hyperkeratotic.

In Fabry disease, a metabolic disorder in which the skin lesions are a dominant feature of the clinical

> **Remember**
>
> The main vascular abnormalities include angiokeratoma, hemangiomas, petechiae, acrocyanosis, and telangiectasia.

Table C9.1 Vascular skin lesions

Disease	MIM number	Type of vascular skin lesions	Additional dermatological manifestations	Hair
Fabry disease	301500	Angiokeratoma	Hypohidrosis	
Gangliosidosis GM1	230500	Angiokeratoma corporis diffusum	Dermal melanocytosis	Hypertrichosis
Fucosidosis	230000	Angiokeratoma	Thin, dry skin Anhidrosis	Heavy eyebrows
Aspartylglucosaminuria	208400	Angiokeratoma corporis diffusum	Acne	
Galactosialidosis	256540	Angiokeratoma Widespread hemangiomas		
Mannososidosis	248510	Angiokeratoma		
Schindler disease type II	609242	Angiokeratoma corporis diffusum	Hyperkeratosis	
			Dry skin	
		Telangiectasia on lips and oral mucosa	Maculopapular eruption	
Mucolipidosis II	252500	Cavernous hemangioma	Tight skin	
Ethylmalonic encephalopathy	602473	Petechiae		
		Orthostatic acrocyanosis		
Hyperoxaluria type I	259900	Livedo reticularis Acrocyanosis		
Neuraminidase deficiency	256540	Widespread hemangiomas		
Smith–Lemli–Opitz syndrome	270400	Facial capillary hemangioma	Severe photosensitivity Eczema	Blonde hair
Transaldolase deficiency	606003	Telangiectases of the skin	Cutis laxa	Hypertrichosis
CDG type Ie	608799	Telangiectasia Hemangiomas	Dysplastic nails	
CDG type IIa	212066	Midfrontal capillary hemangioma		
CDG type IIf	603585	Petechiae Ecchymoses		
Prolidase deficiency	170100	Diffuse telangiectases	Crusting erythematous dermatitis	
			Severe progressive ulceration of lower extremities	

picture, angiokeratomata also known as angiokeratomas corporis diffusum, may be the first manifestations of the disease, and in some heterozygous females, they may be the only sign of disease, but males with this X-linked disorder have usually a number of years of frequent excruciating and unexplained pains. Pain appears most commonly in the extremities, particularly in the lower extremities, but patients may present with unexplained pain in the abdomen or elsewhere. Affected boys may have been referred to a psychiatrist because it is so difficult to find why they are complaining so vehemently. The appearance of the skin lesions creates an entirely different scenario. They are dark red, and they do not blanch with pressure. They seek out pressure points such as buttocks or knees, but they are often profuse in distribution over the scrotum and penis. They increase in number with time. Older lesions also increase in size. They are usually flat at first, but may become slightly palpable. Lesions may be seen on the oral mucosa or on the conjunctiva. Skin signs may also include hypohidrosis.

> **Remember**
>
> Angiokeratomas corporis may be the first manifestations of Fabry disease.

Angiokeratoma may also occur in some other lysosomal storage disorders. One or two angiokeratomata and dermal melanocytosis may be seen in GM^1 gangliosidosis, but usually these patients will already have been diagnosed because of hepatosplenomegaly, developmental delay, coarse features, and dysostosis multiplex that occur very early in infancy, whereas the skin lesions are rare before the first year of age. Similarly, a patch of angiokeratomata with thin and dry skin may be seen in fucosidosis, but again not among the earliest features, although they may appear from 6 months to 4 years; organomegaly, bone changes and developmental delay are evident earlier. Similar lesions may be seen in childhood in aspartylglucosaminuria, but long after the patient is known to have coarse features, acne, cataracts, joint laxity, and neurodegeneration. They may be seen in the juvenile form of galactosialidosis together with corneal opacities, bone findings, neurological degeneration, and widespread hemangiomas that bring the patient to attention again usually before the skin lesions appear. Also in β-mannosidosis,

angiokeratomata have been reported to occur along with mental retardation, coarse facial features, dysostosis multiplex, and hepatosplenomegaly. Schindler disease type II, also known as Kanzaki disease, is an adult-onset disorder characterized by angiokeratoma corporis diffusum, hyperkeratosis, dry skin, maculopapular eruption, telangiectasia on lips, and oral mucosa and mild intellectual impairment.

C9.2.2 Acrocyanosis, Angiomas, and Telangiectasia

Acrocyanosis appears as a bilateral mottled discoloration of the entire feet or hands. In relation to a vasospasm of small arterioles and venules with secondary dilatation of capillaries, the skin's color becomes bright red, with no trophic changes and pain. Orthostatic acrocyanosis is one of the principal signs of ethylmalonic encephalopathy, a devastating mitochondrial disorder affecting the brain, gastrointestinal tract, and peripheral vessels (Fig. C9.1).

> **Remember**
>
> Orthostatic acrocyanosis is a key sing of ethylmalonic encephalopathy.

Acrocyanosis may also be observed in other mitochondrial disorders with onset in early infancy and multisystem involvement (Bodemer et al. 1999). Acrocyanosis and livedo reticularis may be observed in hyperoxaluria type I along with urolithiasis, nephrocalcinosis, renal failure, peripheral vascular insufficiency, arterial occlusion, and Raynaud phenomenon.

Capillary malformations appearing as light pink to deep-red angiomas or as telangectasias may occur in several metabolic diseases. Widespread hemangiomas, coarse facies, conjunctival telangiectases, severe developmental delay seizures, and skeletal abnormalities can be observed in neuraminidase deficiency. Facial capillary hemangioma, severe photosensitivity, eczema, and blond hair are typical features of the Smith–Lemli–Opitz syndrome, a disorder of cholesterol biosynthesis presenting with characteristic facial appearance, ambiguos genitalia, failure to thrive, syndactily, microcephaly, and intellectual impairment

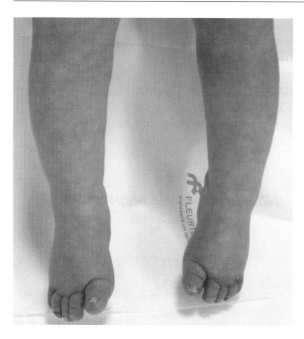

Fig. C9.1 Orthostatic acrocyanosis inethylmalonic encephalopathy

(see also paragraph on photosensitivity). In transaldolase deficiency, a newly recognized metabolic disease of pentose phosphate pathway reported in patients with liver failure and cirrhosis, dysmorphic facial features, renal, cardiac and hematological involvement, cutaneous signs include teleangectases, cutis laxa, and hypertrichosis (Valayannopoulos et al. 2006). More rarely, vascular signs have been observed in patients with congenital disorder of glycosylation type Ie, type IIa, and type IIf along with neurologic, facial and other multisystem abnormalities (Dyer et al. 2005). Prolidase deficiency, which also presents with diffuse teleangiectases, will be discussed in the skin eruption paragraph.

C9.3 Skin Eruptions (Table C9.2)

The main lesions discussed in this paragraph include seborrheic dermatitis, eczema, skin rashes, psoriasiform lesions (erythematous squamous lesions), lupus-like lesions, hyperkeratosis, vesiculo-bollus lesions, and ulcers of the skin. *Seborrheic dermatitis* is associated to increased sebum production and involves the

scalp, the skin folds, and the sebaceous follicle-rich areas of face and trunk. The lesions appear pink to erythematous, with or without edema, covered with greasy yellow–brown scales. The scaling on the scalp can vary from fine to thick and could be mild to moderate on the folds. The facial involvement is most prominent on the forehead, the eyebrows and around the nose. *Eczema* is an inflammatory dermatosis characterized by the appearance of erythema, edema, vesicles, scaling, and crusts. The lesions can be single, multiple or confluent and pruritus is generally present and intense. *Psoriasiform lesions* consist of erythemato-squamous papules, sharply demarcated with clear-cut borders. *Hyperkeratosis* is a horny thickening that firmly adheres to the skin that may be epidermal or follicular. *Vesico-bullous lesions* are circumscribed, translucent elevated lesions containing fluid arising from cleavage at various level of the skin. *Ulcer* is the result of loss of the entire epidermis and at least the upper dermis (papillary), which heals with scarring.

> **Remember**
>
> Skin eruptions include seborrheic dermatitis, eczema, skin rashes, psoriasiform lesions (erythematous squamous lesions), lupus-like lesions, hyperkeratosis, vesciculo-bollus lesions, and ulcers.

In multiple carboxylase deficiency, either due to holocarboxylase synthetase or to biotinidase deficiency, skin and hair abnormalities are prominent findings. The usual initial presentation is the classic organic aciduria emergency with massive ketosis and acidosis progressive to coma. Patients surviving the initial episode of metabolic decompensation often develop the dermatosis. Cutaneous signs consist in a bright red patchy or generalized body eruption, associated with alopecia. Lesions are often desquamative and typically periorificial. Complication by monilial infection is very common, especially around the mouth, the eyes and in the diaper area. Skin lesions become vesicular when they are complicated by mucocutaneous fungal infection. The clinical manifestations in holocarboxylase synthetase deficiency are more severe than in biotinidase deficiency, with an earlier age at onset and some patients unresponsive to biotine therapy. In biotinidase deficiency patients are less likely to develop life threatening

Table C9.2 Skin eruptions

Disease	MIM number	Type of skin eruptions	Additional dermatological manifestations	Hair
Biotinidase deficiency	253260	Skin rash	Cat odor	Alopecia
Holocarboxylase synthetase deficiency	253270	Seborrheic dermatitis		Loss of eyelashes
3-Methylcrotonyl-CoA carboxylase deficiency	210210	Skin infections		Loss of eyebrows
		Periorificial dermatitis		
Methylmalonic aciduria	251000	Scalded skin, superficial desquamation		Fine hair
Propionic aciduria	606954	Periorificial dermatitis		Alopecia
		Psoriasis-like lesions		
Mevalonic aciduria	610377	Skin Rash	Edema and arthralgia during crisis	
Hyper-IgD syndrome	260920	Morbilliform rash Erythematous macules or papules		
Acrodermatitis enteropatica	201100	Bullous, pustular dermatitis of extremities, oral, anal, and genital areas	Impaired would healing	Alopecia of scalp
			Paronychia	Alopecia of eyebrows
		Dermatitis, symmetric pattern		Alopecia of eyelashes
Hyperzynchemia with functional zinc depletion	601979	Skin rash		
Sulfite oxidase deficiency	272300	Mild eczema		Fine hair
Smith–Lemli–Opitz syndrome	270400	See Table C9.1		
Prolidase deficiency	170100	Diffuse telangiectases	Severe progressive ulceration of lower extremities	
		Crusting erythematous dermatitis		
Lysinuric protein intolerance	222700	Lupus-like erythematous squamous lesions	Hyperelastic skin	Fine sparse hair
Hyperzincaemia and hypercalprotectinaemia	194470	Inflammatory skin lesions	Pyoderma gangrenosum	
Tyrosinemia type II	276600	Painful punctate keratoses of digits, palms, and soles		

ketoacidosis. They may present with laryngeal stridor, convulsions and, if undiagnosed and untreated, all are hypotonic and most continue to become mentally retarded. In biotinidase deficiency, the effect of biotin treatment is spectacular with rapid and complete remission of skin, neurological and metabolic abnormalities. Visual and auditory impairment are often irreversible despite biotin therapy. More rarely, patients with the isolated defect of 3-methylcrotonyl-CoA carboxylase may present with skin signs similar to multiple carboxylase deficiency. The differential diagnosis includes acrodermatitis enteropathica. In fact the first patients described with biotinidase deficiency carried the diagnosis of acrodermatitis enteropathica. Patients with acrodermatitis enteropathica have diarrhea, are zinc deficient, and respond to treatment with zinc, but the diagnosis may be a wastebasket term, and any infant with this diagnosis should at the least have organic acid analysis of the urine and biotinidase of the plasma, as well as a work-up for immunodeficiency.

The typical skin lesions of methylmalonic aciduria and propionic aciduria usually occur in patients with the severe forms of these diseases, with no residual enzyme activity and subjected to a very severe natural protein-restricted diet (Fig. C9.2). Cutaneous manifestations could be divided into five categories: superficial scalded skin, superficial desquamation, bilateral and periorificial dermatitis, psoriasiform lesions, and alopecia (Bodemer et al. 1999). Different skin lesions can coexist in a given case and may be due to the enzyme deficiency itself or may be part of a multideficiency syndrome. Similar pictures, that strongly resemble to acrodermatitis enteropathica, may complicate any of the organic acidurias or disorders of amino acid metabolism that are overtreated with an excessive dietary restriction of natural protein and other essential nutrients. In patients with disorders related to branched-chain amino acid metabolism, skin lesions are often due to a selective deficiency of isoleucine and rapidly resolve when this essential amino acid is supplemented. As a presenting clinical manifestation of untreated disease, cheilitis and diffuse erythema with erosions and desquamation has been reported in two patients with methylmalonic aciduria with homocystinuria, cobalamin C type. In both the cases, skin lesions were already present prior to diagnosis, in the absence of iatrogenic nutritional restrictions or deficiency (Howard et al. 1997).

Recurrent morbilliform rashes and erythematous macules and papules can be frequently observed in mevalonic aciduria a disorder of cholesterol biosynthesis (Fig. C9.3). Patients have also facial dysmorphic features, global developmental delay, cataract, arthralgias with periarticular edema, recurrent febrile crises with lymphadenopathy, hepatosplenomegaly, vomiting, and diarrhea. Rash, edema, and arthralgia may occur during crisis. Similar skin signs can also be observed in hyper-IgD syndrome, the less severe allelic variant of mevalonic aciduria.

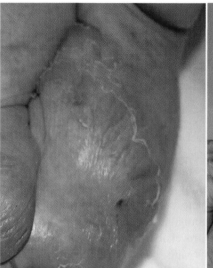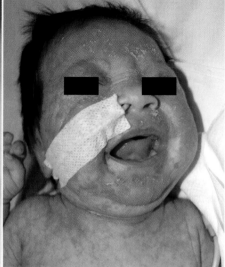

Fig. C9.2 Propionic aciduria with extensive skin lesions characterized by superficial scalded skin, desquamation and periorificial dermatitis

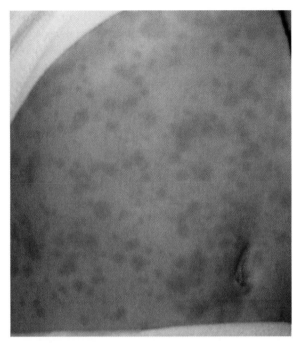

Fig. C9.3 Skin rash in mevalonic aciduria

Cutaneous ulcers, mainly severe progressive ulceration of lower extremities, can represent the hallmark finding of prolidase deficiency. The ulcers may be further complicated by secondary infection. Skin changes also include teleangiectases, purpuric ecchymoses, rashes, or crusting erythematous dermatitis. In addition, patients may have mental retardation, ophthalmoplegia, splenomegaly, dysmorphic features, and susceptibility to infections. Severe immunological abnormalities, fulfilling the criteria for diagnosis of systemic lupus erythematous, have been reported in prolidase deficiency (Shrinath et al. 1997). Interestingly, skin lupus-like lesions (Fig. C9.4) and immunological abnormalities have also been observed in lysinuric protein intolerance, a transport defect of dibasic aminoacid that usually presents with postprandial hyperammonemia, failure to thrive, severe renal, and pulmonary involvement (Dionisi-Vici et al. 1998).

Remember

Skin lesions and severe immunological abnormalities fulfilling the criteria for diagnosis of systemic lupus erythematous can be observed in prolidase deficiency and in lysinuric protein intolerance.

Ulcers in adolescence and adulthood may also develop in classical homocystinuria caused by cystathionine β-synthase deficiency; these ulcers result from the grounds of thromboembolic disease usually in the lower extremities.6pInflammatory skin lesions of various degree along with recurrent infections, growth failure, hepatosplenomegaly, arthritis, anemia, and persistently raised concentrations of C-reactive protein are the clinical features of hyperzincemia and hypercalprotectinemia, a newly described disorder of zinc metabolism, probably caused by dysregulation of calprotectin metabolism.

Hyperkeratotic lesions are a characteristic sign of oculocutaneous tyrosinemia or tyrosinemia type II. The combination of ocular and these lesions has also been called the Richner–Hanhart syndrome. The major manifestation of this disease is keratitis and corneal ulcers associated with skin lesions occurring on the palms and soles. The skin lesions that usually begin in

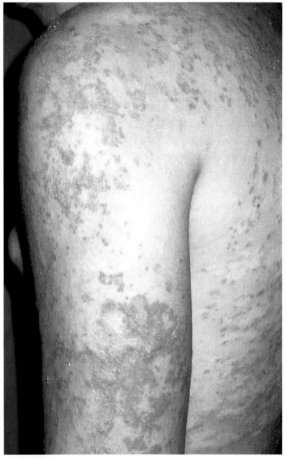

Fig. C9.4 Lupus-like skin lesions in lysinuric protein intolerance

early infancy, are painful, nonpruritic, and frequently associated with hyperhidrosis. Bullous lesions may occur and progress rapidly to erosions that become crusted and hyperkeratotic. Rarely, lesions have a subungueal localization.

C9.4 Ichthyosis (Table C9.3)

Ichthyosis is a very striking scaling dermatosis that results from overactive proliferation of skin cells. Extra skin piles up in scales, reminiscent of the skin of fish, and falls off. Dependent on the rate of the process, the scales may appear old and black or there may be the pronounced erythroderma of new skin. Ichthyosis is characterized by abnormal differentiation (cornification) of epidermis. Several features are useful to distinguish different forms of ichthyosis. They generally may appear with fine or thick scales, covering the skin red or normally colored, sometimes sparing the folds, palms and plantar-areas. In some forms, it can be observed superficial fissuring or blistering especially on the folds. The scales could be generalized or localized. In lamellar ichthyosis, they are accentuated on the extremities, large plate-like brown covering most of the body. Collodion baby is the most severe presentation of congenital ichthyosis (Fig. C9.5). The child is born encased in a translucent membrane which is taut and may impair ectropion, eclabion, ears deformities, and respiration and sucking. During the first 2 weeks of life, the membrane breaks up and peels off, often leaving fissures, with exposure to infection and water loss. This can lead to difficulties in thermal regulation and increased risk of infection and dehydratation. On the basis of a clinical classification, two major group of ichthyosis can be identified: (1) primary ichthyoses limited to the skin and (2) syndromic ichthyoses, in which associated features are present.

Remember

Ichthyoses can be classified in primary ichthyoses and syndromic ichthyoses, in which associated features are present. Ichthyoses, in inborn error of metabolism, usually belong to the group of syndromic ichthyoses.

Most ichthyoses are not part of an inborn error of metabolism, but in many metabolic diseases ichthyosis may be a very prominent presentation. As shown in the table, a large number of metabolic diseases – belonging to the group of syndromic ichthyoses – are listed. The purest form is X-linked ichthyosis resulting from defective activity of steroid sulfatase, which leads to deposition of cholesterol sulfate. These patients may have no other manifestations of the disease than dark, scaly skin. Mild corneal opacities, which do not interfere with vision, are found in about 25% of patients. Mental retardation, hypogonadism, shortness of stature and chondodysplasia punctata have been observed. Patients with multiple sulfatase deficiency are most debilitated by manifestations of metachromatic leukodystrophy and those of mucopolysaccharidosis. A patient with features of both and who also has ichthyosis doubtless has multiple sulfatase deficiency, also known as Austin disease.

In patients with Refsum disease, the skin may be the key to the diagnosis of this multisystem disease. Ataxia is an early manifestation. Deafness, peripheral neuropathy, and retinitis pigmentosa complete the syndrome.

Patients with Sjogren–Larsson syndrome in which the fatty alcohol oxidoreductase is defective have cataracts and ichthyosis (Fig. C9.6). In addition, they are mentally retarded and have spastic paraplegia. Retinitis pigmentosa may be evident on ophthalmoscopy; there may be glistening dots in the area of the macula.

Cataracts and ichthyosis are also seen in neutral lipid storage disorder, also known as Chanarin–Dorfman syndrome. There are vacuolated lymphocytes and, to distinguish it from Sjogren–Larrson disease, hepatomegaly. Patients also have muscle weakness ataxia and myopathy.

Ichthyosis is seen as an early, sometimes prenatal, congenital manifestation in neuronopathic Gaucher disease. There may even be a collodion baby appearance (Fig. C9.6). With time the skin may appear normal, but neurodegeneration is progressive. Ichthyotic lesions are also prominent in infants with CHILD syndrome, the acronym for congenital hemidysplasia with ichthyosiform.

Erythroderma and limb defects. Unilateral hypomelia (digital hypoplasia to complete limb absence), elbow and knee webbing, joint contractures, and ipsilateral epiphyseal stippling complete the clinical findings. The disorder is characterised by unilateral ichthyotic skin lesions with a sharp demarcation at the midline of the trunk with the facial area typically spared, although the

Table C9.3 Ichthyosis

Disease	MIM number	Skin	Hair
Steroid sulfatase deficiency	308100	Hypertrophic ichthyosis	
Multiple sulfatase deficiency – Austin disease	272200	Dark adherent skin scales	
		Ichthyosis	
Refsum disease	266500	Ichthyosis	
Sjogren–Larsson syndrome	270200	Ichthyosis	
Chanarin–Dorfman syndrome/neutral lipid storage disorder	275630	Nonbullous congenital ichthyosiform erythroderma	Diffuse alopecia
		Collodion baby	
Gaucher disease type II	608013	Erythematous skin ichthyosis, Collodion skin	
		Desquamation of skin soon after birth	
		Petechiae	
		Purpura	
Conradi–Huenermann syndrome	302960	Congenital ichthyosiform erythroderma	Coarse, sparse hair
		Follicular atrophoderma	Patchy areas of alopecia
		"Orange peel" skin	
		Ichthyosis	Sparse eyebrows
			Sparse eyelashes
CHILD syndrome	308050	Unilateral erythema and scaling	Unilateral alopecia
		Sharp midline demarcation	
		Hyperkeratosis	
		Onychorrhexis	
		Destruction of nails	
Rhizomelic chondrodysplasia punctata type I	215100	Ichthyosis	Alopecia
Chondrodysplasia punctata type 2	302960	Congenital ichthyosiform erythroderma	Coarse, sparse hair
		Follicular atrophoderma	Patchy areas of alopecia
		"Orange peel" skin	
		Ichthyosis	Sparse eyebrows
			Sparse eyelashes
CDG type If	609180	Ichthyosis	
CDG type Im	610768	Ichthyosis	Sparse eyebrows
			Sparse eyelashes
			Minimal hair growth
Serine deficiency		Ichthyosis	
Ichthyosis, split hairs, and aminoaciduria	242550	Lamellar ichthyosis	Split hair
		Collodion skin	

scalp may be involved. Studies of skin cell kinetics have indicated the lesions in this disease to be psoriasis. Punctate calcifications are present in the epiphyses and other cartilaginous structures of the affected side, which is usually the right side. The disease is inherited as an X-linked disorder and is thought to be lethal in males. Ichthyosis may also be seen in the Conradi–Huenermann or X-linked dominant chondrodysplasia punctata. Besides ichthyosis, Conradi–Huenermann syndrome is characterized by the typical calcifications and asymmetric rhizomelic limb shortness. Cataract and mental retardation have been found in a few affected females. The skin lesions may have a whorled pattern of hyperkeratotic, white adherent scales with underlying red skin and palmar and plantar hyperkeratosis and disappear by 3–6 months. Biochemically, Conradi–Huenermann syndrome

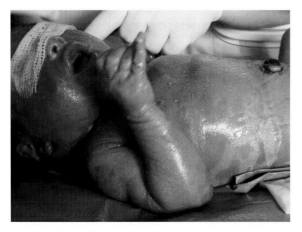

Fig. C9.5 Collodion skin in a neonate with Gaucher disease type II

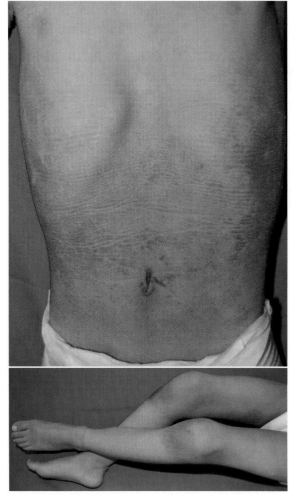

Fig. C9.6 Ichtyosis and spastic diplegia in a patient with Sjögren–Larrson syndrome

patients have normal or decreased cholesterol levels and elevated concentrations of 8-dehydrocholesterol and 8(9)-cholestenol in plasma and tissues due to a defect of 3-β-hydroxysteroid- Δ8, Δ7-isomerase. The sterol-4-demethylase, the enzymatic step just prior to sterol-8-isomerase is the underlying defect in CHILD syndrome.

Ichthyosis has recently been described along with psychomotor retardation, night blindness, and dwarfism in siblings with a distinct form (type 1f) carbohydrate deficient glycoprotein (CDG) syndrome. Sialotransferrin pattern in the serum was that of type 1. Activities of phosphomannose isomerase, phosphomannose mutase, and GDP-mannose synthase were normal. Another form of CDG syndrome (type 1m) causing hypoketotic hypoglycemia and death in early infancy can present with ichthyosis and hair abnormalities.

Ichthyosis has been observed in a girl with serine deficiency of unknown cause, presenting a progressive polyneuropathy, growth retardation, and delayed puberty. Despite no deficiency of any of the serine biosynthetic enzymes was detected, treatment with serine resulted in a clear improvement of neuromuscular and cutaneous signs (de Koning and Klomp 2004).

Differential diagnosis of syndromic ichthyosis include other rare conditions such as KID syndrome (keratitis, hepatitis, ichthyosis and deafness, MIM 148210), NISH syndrome (neonatal ichthyosis-sclerosing cholangitis syndrome MIM 697626), Netherton syndrome (MIM 256500), Rud syndrome (MIM 308200) and other related disorders, and ichthyosis with hepatomegaly and cerebellar ataxia (MIM 242520).

C9.5 Papular and Nodular Skin Lesions (Table C9.4)

Papules are small elevated lesions that may have a variety of shapes. Papules can be differentiated according to the color, margin, number, surface, and distribution. A nodule is a circumscribed, palpable, solid, round, or ellipsoidal lesion up to 1 cm in size. Depth of involvement distinguishes papule from nodule. Nodules can be located deep dermal, dermal-subdermal, or in the subcutaneous fat.

The clinical expression of Farber disease, resulting from deficiency of ceramidase, is striking and the diagnosis can be easily suspected with a careful clinical evaluation. The characteristic features are nodular lesions in the subcutaneous tissues around joints and pressure point areas and painful swelling of joints appearing in early infancy. Lesions are located in the interphalangeal and metacarpal regions as well as in the ankle, wrist, knee, and elbow. The patient complains of pain and stiffness of the joints and may be carrying a diagnosis of arthritis. Hoarseness is another feature. Development may be severely and progressively delayed. Deep tendon reflexes may be diminished or absent. Interstitial pneumonia is an infiltrative component of the disease. Infantile systemic hyalinosis (MIM 236490) presents with similar features and should be considered in the differential diagnosis.

In Hunter disease, uniquely among the mucopolysaccharidoses, there are localized nodular accumulations of mucopolysaccharide in the skin of the scapular area.

Mitochondrial disorders have long been regarded as diseases of the neuromuscular system and internal organs. However, since almost every tissue, including the skin, is dependent on mitochondrial energy supply, it is not surprising to observe dermatological signs in this extremely heterogeneous group of disorders. Reviewing the literature of skin disorders associated with mitochondrial encephalomyopathies the most recurring signs are lipomas (Birch-Machin 2000). Lipomas usually occurs in the adult forms of mitochondrial disorders in patients bearing mutations of mitochondrial DNA and appear as multiple and symmetrical

Table C9.4 Papular and nodular skin lesions

Disease	MIM number	Papular and nodular skin lesions	Additional dermatological manifestations	Hair
Farber lipogranulomatosis	228000	Lipogranulomatosis Periarticular subcutaneous nodules		
MPS type II	309900	Pebbly skin lesions on back, upper arms	Tight blue cutaneous pigmentation	Hypertrichosis
Mitochondrial diseases		Lipomas	Hyperpigmentation Hypopigmentation Acrocyanosis Skin rashes Erythema Keratoderma Anhidrosis Purpuric lesions	See Table C9.7
Familial hypercholesterolemia	143890	Xanthomatosis		
Sitosterolemia	210250	Tendinous and tuberous xanthoma		
Lipoprotein lipase deficiency Apolipoprotein E deficiency	238600 107741	Xanthomatosis		
Cerebrotendinous xanthomatosis	213700	Tuberous xanthoma Xantelasma		
Glycogenosis type I a/ b	232200 232220	Xanthoma		
Niemann–Pick disease type A	257200	Xanthoma		
CDG type Ia	212065	Abnormal subcutaneous fat tissue distribution Fat pads "Orange peel" skin Inverted nipples		Sparse hair Trichorrhexis nodosa Pili torti
CDG type IIc	266265	Localized cellulitis		

lesions. The mechanisms underlying the appearance of lipomas have not yet been fully understood. A recent study demonstrated that lipomatosis in a patient with tRNA(Lys) mutations was associated with a pattern of altered expression of master regulators of adipogenesis and with a distorted pattern of brown vs. white adipocyte differentiation (Guallar et al. 2006).

In lipoprotein disorders, lipoproteins can enter the skin, subcutaneous tissues, and tendons producing xantomata through lipid accumulation and infiltration. Different species of lipoproteins produce different types of xantomata and characteristic phenotypes associated with specific metabolic defects. According to the morphological characteristics, different types of lipid infiltrates can be distinguished: eruptive-, tuberoeruptive-, tuberous-, tendineous-, planar-, and subcutaneous-xantomata, xantelasma, corneal arcus, and tonsillar infiltration (Goldsmith 2003). Diffuse cutaneous xanthomata of tuberous and subcutaneous types are seen along with tendinous xanthomata, xantelasma, and corneal arcus in familial hypercholesterolemia homozygotes (Fig. C9.7). This disorder of low-density lipoprotein metabolism leads to early coronary artery disease and myocardial infarction; early adult myocardial infarction is seen in heterozygotes. In homozygotes the xanthomata are large, flat, and sometimes distinctly yellowish. A similar picture can occur in sitosterolemia, which, if untreated, also results in premature atherosclerosis and occasionally hemolysis. The xanthomata of

patients with lipoprotein lipase deficiency and with other forms of chylomicronemia are very different. Severe elevation of circulating triglyceride concentrations is associated with eruptive skin xantomata that appear as yellow papules on a slightly erythematous base. Typical locations are over the buttocks, shoulders, and extensor surfaces of the extremities. They occur when triglyceride levels are very high, and they disappear promptly on dietary reduction of triglycerides. These patients have chylomicronemia and do not develop vascular disease, whereas they are subject to recurrent attacks of pancreatitis. Diagnosis may be made by the appearance of the blood, which looks like milky tomato soup. In cerebrotendinous xantomatosis, accumulation of abnormal sterol derivates is responsible for the development of xantomata in the brain and tendons. Patients are at risk for myocardial infarction and also present with several neurologic signs and juvenile cataracts. Xantomata may be observed as a late event in glycogen storage disease type 1 with poor metabolic control in relation to increased serum levels of triglycerides and cholesterol. In Niemann–Pick disease type A, xantomata may also occur along with extreme hepatosplenomegaly, severe developmental delay and dystonia.

The enlarged fat pads of the patient with CDG syndrome type 1a are unique and absolutely diagnostic (Fig. C9.8A). The enlargement of fat pads is usually evident toward the end of the first year. They are

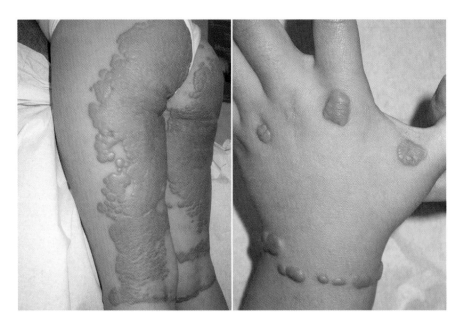

Fig. C9.7 Diffuse cutaneous xanthomata in homozygous hypercholesterolemia

typically located over the upper and outer areas of the buttocks or lower back, but they may be seen elsewhere including the lateral thighs and upper arms. The skin may feel thickened and later there may be lipoatrophy leaving streaks on the lower extremities. Hair changes, consisting of sparse appearance, slow growing, coarse texture and trichorrexis nodosa have also been observed (Silengo et al. 2003). These infants present with predominant neurological signs, dysmorphic facial features, failure to thrive, inverted nipples (Fig. C9.8B) associated with systemic manifestations affecting heart, kidneys, and gastrointestinal system.

> **Remember**
>
> The enlarged fat pads of the patient with CDG syndrome type 1a are unique and diagnostic.

C9.6 Abnormal Pigmentation
(Table C9.5)

C9.6.1 Hypopigmentation

Skin hypopigmentation is in most cases caused by an enzyme deficiency involving the production, metabolism, or distribution of melanin. Oculocutaneous albinism, not discussed in this chapter, is a group of inherited disorders characterized by a generalized reduction in pigmentation of hair, skin, and/or eyes.

Besides oculocutaneous albinism, differential diagnosis of skin hypopigmentation includes several genetically determined disorders often associated with immune dysfunctions [e.g., Hermansky–Pudlak syndrome (MIM 203300), Chediak–Higashi syndrome (MIM 214500), Griscelli syndrome type 1 (MIM 214450) type 2 (607624) and type 3 (609227), and the so called (Dionisi-) Vici syndrome (MIM 242840 immunodeficiency with cleft lip/palate, cataract, hypopigmentation and absent corpus callosum)] as well as some metabolic diseases.

> **Remember**
>
> Differential diagnosis of skin hypopigmentation includes some metabolic diseases and several genetically determined disorders often associated with immune dysfunctions.

Patients with phenylketonuria prior to the development of screening diagnosis and early treatment were fair of hair and skin and blue-eyed in the majority of cases. Early treatment has made it clear that it is not the gene, but the abnormal chemical environment in the untreated state that interferes with normal pigmentation. Also patients with cystinosis and some with homocystinuria have thin hypopigmented skin, and fine brittle hair. Moreover, skin hypopigmentation, along with early onset severe developmental delay, coarse facial features, hepatosplenomegaly, failure to thrive, and dysostosis multiplex is one of the characteristic signs of infantile sialic acid storage disease.

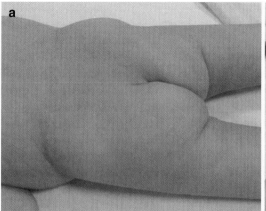 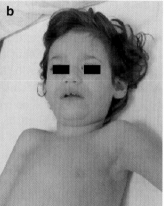

Fig. C9.8 Enlarged fat pads (**a**) and inverted nipples (**b**) in carbohydrate deficient glycoprotein syndrome type Ia

Table C9.5 Abnormal pigmentation

Disease	MIM number	Abnormal pigmentation	Additional dermatological manifestations	Hair
Phenylketonuria	261600	Pale pigmentation	Dry skin Eczema Scleroderma Mousy odor	Blond hair
Cystinosis	219800	Light skin pigmentation	Recurrent corneal erosions	Light hair pigmentation
Homocystinuria	236200	Hypopigmentation	Livedo Ulceration	Fine, brittle hair
Infantile sialic acid storage disease	269920	Hypopigmented skin		Fair hair
Methionine malabsorption syndrome	250900			White hair
Alkaptonuria	203500	Ochronosis		
Adrenoleukodystrophy/ adrenomyeloneuropathy	300100	Hyperpigmentation		Scarce and thin hair Alopecia
Glycerol kinase deficiency with adrenal insufficiency	307030	Hyperpigmentation		
Kearns–Sayre syndrome	530000	Hyperpigmentation		
Hemochromatosis	235200	Hyperpigmentation Telangiectases		Alopecia
Wilson disease	277900	Hyperpigmentation		
Gaucher disease type I	230800	Hyperpigmentation		

C9.6.2 Hyperpigmentation

In alkaptonuria, defective activity of homogentisic acid oxidase leads to the accumulation of homogentisic acid, which is then oxidized to form black insoluble pigment. Pigment deposition is greatest in cartilage; so it is prominent in the ears. It may also be seen early in the sclerae and in the nose, initially as salt and pepper spots, but later these may become confluent. In an older patient it may be widely distributed, especially distally on the fingers. Deposition in joint cartilage leads to debilitating early osteoarthritis. The skin may serve as an alerting clue to the diagnosis.

Skin hyperpigmentation is characteristic of adrenal insufficiency and this may be the first substantial clue in late childhood to the presence of adrenoleukodystrophy or, later in life, of adrenomyeloneuropathy, an X-linked recessive trait characterized by progressive demyelination of the nervous system, resulting in the accumulation of very-long chain fatty acids in the nervous system, adrenal gland, and testes, which disrupts normal activity.

> **Remember**
>
> Skin hyperpigmentation is characteristic of adrenal insufficiency and may be the first substantial clue in late childhood to the presence of adrenoleukodystrophy.

Adrenal insufficiency is also seen in those patients with glycokinase deficiency who have a contiguous gene deletion syndrome. Dependent on the size of the deletion, some also have Duchenne muscular dystrophy and/or ornithine transcarbamylase deficiency. Likewise, adrenal insufficiency can cause skin hyperpigmentation in Kearns–Sayre syndrome.

In hereditary hemochromatosis, bluish–gray hyperpigmentations are seen on the light exposed sebostatic scaling skin areas. Bronze diabetes with liver cirrhosis, hypogonadism, and loss of libido are found in more advanced cases. Hyperpigmentation of mucous membranes and conjunctival membranes occur in 15–20% of patients. There can be a loss of axillary and pubic hair because of hepatotesticular insufficiency. Besides skin signs, fully developed clinical manifestations of hereditary hemochromatosis include a multiorgan involvement affecting liver, heart, pancreas, endocrine organs, and joints. Patients with Wilson disease suffer from progressive severe dystonia, and skin manifestations are characterized by reticulated brownish hyperpigmentation of the lower legs, blue lunulae, and corneal pigmentation known as Kayser–Fleischer ring. There is additionally a premature graying of the hair and development of liver cirrhosis. Cutaneous hyperpigmentation can be observed in Gaucher type 1.

C9.7 Photosensitivity (Table C9.6)

The phenotypic expression of diseases with increased photosensitivity mainly depends on UV or light exposure. Early recognition and prompt diagnosis may prevent complications associated with prolonged unprotected exposure to sunlight allowing recognition of families at risk for rare heritable disorders associated with photosensitivity. Drugs and chemicals may interact with UV to induce photosensitivity, and recognition of the associated reaction patterns greatly assists clinical classification of these disorders, which include some metabolic diseases, the DNA repair deficient disorders, and other genodermatoses.

Photosensitive skin lesions characterize many of the porphyries, a clinically and genetically heterogeneous group of diseases arising from enzymatic defects along the pathway of porphyrin-heme biosynthesis. In erythropoietic protoporphyria, photosensitivity begins early in life. Skin signs can occur acutely with burning, stinging, and pruritus in sun-exposed areas accompanied by pain in the extremities. These are followed by erythema, edema, erosions, and scarring. The vesicular lesions in response to sun tend to be smaller and more

Table C9.6 Photosensitivity

Disease	MIM number	Photosensitivity	Additional dermatological manifestations	Hair
Erythropoietic protoporphyria	177000	Light-sensitive dermatitis Itching Burning Erythema	Edema Mild scarring	
Congenital erythropoietic porphyria	263700	Photosensitivity Blistering Scarring	Conjunctivitis Corneal scarring Red stained teeth Mutilating skin deformity Pseudoscleroderma Hyperpigmentation Hypopigmentation	Hypertrichosis Alopecia Loss of eyelashes Loss of eyebrows
Porphyria cutanea tarda type I	176090	Photosensitivity	Mechanically fragile skin	Facial hypertrichosis
Porphyria cutanea tarda type II	176100	Blisters in sun-exposed areas Hyperpigmentation in sun-exposed areas	Pseudoscleroderma Fingernail onycholysis	Alopecia
Porphyria variegata	176200	Photosensitivity		
Coproporphyria	121300	Photosensitivity		
Hartnup disorder	234500	Light-sensitive dermatitis	Atrophic glossitis	
Tryptophanuria with dwarfism	276100	Cutaneous photosensitivity		
Smith–Lemli–Opitz syndrome	270400	See Table C9.1		

patchy than in the other porphyrias of childhood. They leave tiny areas of flat depressed atrophy of skin that may be very subtle but are telltale markers of the disease. Unusual late complications include biliary tract stones and hepatic failure. The most dramatic and earliest in onset is congenital erythropoietic porphyria, the disease in which there is pink urine and red teeth. These patients may also have hemolytic anemia and splenomegaly. The skin lesions are vesicular and bullous. The skin appears quite fragile, and ulcers or erosions appear. There may be residual scarring and alternating hyperpigmentation and depigmentation. Mutilation of fingers, nasal tips, and ears may eventually occur. Patients with porphyria cutanea tarda type I, the heterozygous, autosomal dominant form of uroporphyrinogen decarboxylase-III deficiency, present first symptoms in adulthood. The skin is fragile and minor trauma leads to erosions. Patients also develop hepatic siderosis. In patients with hepatoerythropoietic porphyria (also called porphyria cutanea tarda type II), the homozygous form of uroporphyrinogen decarboxylase-III deficiency, onset is neonatal or shortly thereafter. Patients may also have hemolytic anemia and splenomegaly. The urine may be black or pink. The skin is fragile and develops vesicles and blisters in response to sun exposure. Hypertrichosis about the face is common. Liver disease is a complication. Patients with variegate porphyria have abdominal and neurological crises. Onset is from puberty to adulthood. Late changes in the skin may be pseudosclerodermatous. Patients with hereditary coproporphyria have hemolytic anemia and abdominal and neurological crises. Onset is in adulthood. Abdominal or psychiatric symptoms may be precipitated by drugs that increase hepatic cytochrome P450.

Hartnup disease is characterized by a pellagra-like light-sensitive rash, cerebellar ataxia, emotional instability, and aminoaciduria. Patients have a transport disorder involving the intestine and the renal tubule, and failure to absorb tryptophan leads to the dermatological picture of pellagra. Cutaneous manifestations of this disease have been rare in the U.S., presumably because most eat such a high-protein diet that deficiency is avoided. Tryptophanuria with dwarfism was described in three siblings with mental defect, cutaneous photosensitivity, and gait disturbance resembling cerebellar ataxia. The clinical features resembled Hartnup disease but the chemical findings were different and the defect was thought to concern the

conversion of tryptophane to kynurenine.6pThe differential diagnosis of photosensitive dermatoses includes the different forms of xeroderma pigmentosum and of Fanconi anemia, Cockayne syndrome type A (MIM 216400) and B (MIM 133540), Bloom syndrome (MIM 210900), and trichothiodystrophy (601675). All of these disorders of DNA repair are important to recognize because of their frequent complication by neoplasia.

> **Remember**
>
> The differential diagnosis of photosensitive dermatoses includes the different forms of DNA repair disorders.

C9.8 Hair Disorders

C9.8.1 Hair Shaft Abnormalities

Hair shaft abnormalities are highly heterogeneous and range from changes in color, density, length, and structure of the hair to absence of the hair (alopecia). The hair of patients with hair shaft diseases that may occur as localized or generalized disorders feels dry and looks lusterless. Alopecia may be universal (loss of scalp hair, eyebrows and eyelashes), total (loss of scalp hair), and partial.

Trichorrhexis nodosa is a characteristic sign in some patients with argininosuccinic aciduria. The patient is recognized for an appearance at a distance of alopecia, but on close examination it is clear that very short hairs are abundant. The hair shafts are fragile and break easily. A longer hair under the microscope displays the characteristic nodules. Abnormal appearance of the hair is also seen in Menkes disease. The typical appearance is that of pili torti, in which the hair shaft is twisted. These patients may also have trichorrhexis nodosa or monilethrix in which there is segmental narrowing of the hair shaft. These hairs tend to break readily too, but the patient never appears to have alopecia. As a consequence of reduced tyrosinase activity, hair and skin appear hypopigmented. In addition, patients show skin laxity. Menkes disease, also called kinky hair disease, is a devastating cerebral degenerative disease, with refractory seizures, bone lesions, skin and joint laxity, and tortuous cerebral arteries. In the occipital horn syndrome, the milder allelic variant of Menkes disease, the hair appears coarse (Fig. C9.9) and the skin is soft, mildly extensible and redundant with easy bruisability.

In some cases of congenital disorder of glycosylation type 1 hair aspects are unusual, they appear sparse, slow growing, lacking luster and coarse in texture. Enhanced fragility in the form of trichorrexis nodosa, torsion of the shaft along the longitudinal axis, and pili torti has also been observed (Silengo et al. 2003).

The classic presentation of sulfite oxidase deficiency involves neonatal seizures, progressive encephalopathy, dislocation of lenses, and death at an early age. Dermatological signs include mild eczema and fine hair.6pAlopecia totalis is the characteristic appearance of holocarboxylase synthetase (Fig. C9.10). Patients have no hair on the head, no eyebrows, eyelashes, or lanugo hair. Patients with biotinidase deficiency have patchy alopecia in the pattern of the patient with acrodermatitis enteropathica.

Patients with organic acidurias, such as methylmalonic aciduria, propionic aciduria, or maple syrup urine disease, all of whom must be treated with very strict restriction of the intake of protein, may have fine hair or develop alopecia when the protein restriction is too stringent or when intercurrent infection increases demand (see Sect. C9.4).

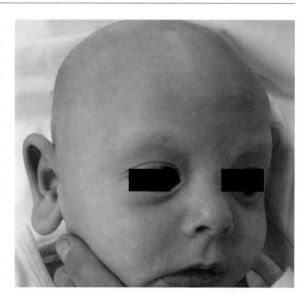

Fig. C9.10 Alopecia totalis with absence of eyebrows and eyelashes in a child with multiple carboxylase defect due to holocarboxylase synthetase deficiency

As shown in Table C9.7, in many other metabolic diseases already discussed in previous paragraphs of this chapter, patients may have hair shaft abnormalities or alopecia.

C9.8.2 Hypertrichosis *(Table C9.8)*

Hirsutism or hypetricosis is a common finding in several lysosomal storage diseases. In most cases, patients have a characteristic coarse facial features, neurological abnormalities, intellectual delay, dysostosis multiplex, and hepatosplenomegaly.

> **Remember**
>
> Hirsutism, hypetricosis, coarse facial features, neurological abnormalities, intellectual delay, dysostosis multiplex, and hepatosplenomegaly are common findings in several lysosomal storage diseases.

In the wide spectrum of clinical abnormalities of mitochondrial diseases, diffuse hypertichosis is a typical sign of the Leigh syndrome encephalomayopathy with

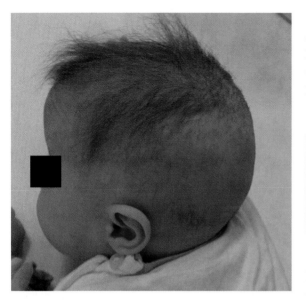

Fig. C9.9 Coarse, sparse, and fragile hair in Menkes disease

Table C9.7 Hair shaft abnormalities

Disease	MIM number	Skin	Hair
Argininosuccinic aciduria	207900		Trichorrhexis nodosa
			Dry brittle hair
Menkes disease	309400	Hypopigmentation, skin laxity	Steely, kinky, sparse hair
Occipital horn syndrome	304150	Soft, extensible and redundant skin	Coarse hair
		Easy bruisability	
CDG type Ia	212065	See Table C9.4	Sparse hair
			Trichorrhexis nodosa
			Pili torti
Sulfite oxidase deficiency	272300	Mild eczema	Fine hair
Mitochondrial diseases		See Table C9.4	Hypertrichosis
			Alopecia
			Thin, dry, brittle, sparse hair
			Trichothiodystrophy
			Trichorrexis nodosa
			Pili torti
Biotinidase deficiency	253260	See Table C9.2	Alopecia
Holocarboxylase synthetase deficiency	253270		Loss of eyelashes
3-Methylcrotonyl-CoA carboxylase deficiency	210210		Loss of eyebrows
Congenital erythropoietic porphyria	263700	See Table C9.6	Hypertrichosis
			Alopecia
			Loss of eyelashes
			Loss of eyebrows
Porphyria cutanea tarda type I	176090	See Table C9.6	Facial hypertrichosis
Porphyria cutanea tarda type II	176100		Alopecia
Hemochromatosis	235200	See Table C9.5	Alopecia
Adrenoleukodystrophy/ adrenomyeloneuropaty	300100	See Table C9.5	Scarce and thin hair
			Alopecia
Chanarin–Dorfman syndrome/ neutral lipid storage disorder	275630	See Table C9.3	Diffuse alopecia
Rhizomelic chondrodysplasia punctata type I	215100	See Table C9.3	Alopecia
CHILD syndrome	308050	See Table C9.3	Unilateral alopecia
Conradi–Huenermann syndrome	302960	See Table C9.3	Coarse, sparse hair
			Patchy areas of alopecia
			Sparse eyebrows
			Sparse eyelashes
Acrodermatitis enteropatica	201100	See Table C9.2	Alopecia of scalp
			Alopecia of eyebrows
			Alopecia of eyelashes

Table C9.8 Hypertrichosis

Disease	MIM number	Skin	Hair
MPS type I	607014	Skin thickening	Hypertrichosis
MPS type II	309900	Coarse facies	Synophrys
MPS type IIIA	252900	Pebbly skin lesions on back, upper arms	Hirsutism
MPS type IIIB	252920		Coarse hair
MPS type IIIC	252930	Thigh blue cutaneous pigmentation	
MPS type IIID	252940		
MPS type VI	253200		
MPS type VII	253220		
MPS type VIII	253230		
Mucolipidosis type IIIA	252600		
Gangliosidosis GM1	230500		
Mannosidosis	248500		
Sialuria	269921		
Transaldolase deficiency	606003	See Table C9.1	Hypertrichosis
Leigh syndrome – SURF1 mutations	256000		Hypertrichosis
Infantile lactic acidosis/ SUCLG1 mutations	611224		Hypertrichosis
Mitochondrial diseases		See Table C9.4	See Table C9.4

cytochome-c-oxidase deficiency and mutations in the *SURF1* gene (Fig. C9.11).

C9.9 Skin Laxity (Table C9.9)

Type II autosomal recessive cutis laxa (MIM 219200), characterized by loose skin with redundant folds, slow return on stretching and unaffected facial skin, is a recently discovered defect of *N*-glycosylation at the level of Golgi apparatus (Fig. C9.12, kindly provided by E. Morava). In addition to skin signs, patients present with widely persistent fontanelles, slight oxycephaly, dental caries, frontal bossing, downward slanted palpebral fissures, hip dislocation, scoliosis, and inguinal hernia. Isoelectrofocusing of serum transferring shows a type II CDG pattern and the disorder is caused by loss-of-function mutations in the ATP6V0A2 gene, which encodes the alpha-2 subunit of the V-type H + ATPase. The occurrence of mutations in the same gene in wrinkly skin syndrome (MIM 278250) indicates that autosomal recessive cutis laxa type II and some cases of wrinkly skin

Table C9.9 Skin laxity

Disease	MIM number	Skin	Hair
Type II autosomal recessive cutis laxa	219200	Loose skin with redundant folds	
Delta-1-pyrroline-5-carboxylate synthetase deficiency	138250	Skin hyperelasticity	
Menkes disease	309400	See Table C9.7	See Table C9.7
Occipital horn syndrome	304150	See Table C9.7	See Table C9.7
Transaldolase deficiency	606003	See Table C9.1	See Table C9.8
Lysinuric protein intolerance	222700	See Table C9.2	

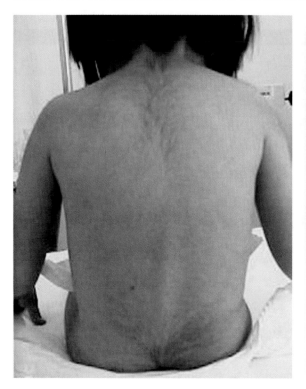

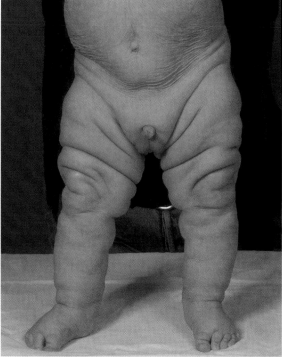

Fig. C9.11 Diffuse hypertichosis in a child with Leigh syndrome, cytochome-c-oxidase deficiency, and mutations in the *SURF1* gene

Fig. C9.12 Characteristic skin features in a child with type II autosomal recessive cutis laxa (kindly provided by Morava, Nimegen, The Netherlands)

syndrome may represent variable manifestations of the same genetic defect.

Skin hyperelasticity, lax joints, cataract, and mental retardation along with fasting hyperammonemia, hypoprolinemia, hypocitrullinemia, and hypoornithinemia are the characteristic findings of delta-1-pyrroline-5-carboxylate synthetase deficiency (MIM 138250)

In Menkes disease, the skin appears loose and redundant, particularly at the nape of the neck and on the trunk. In occipital horn syndrome, the less severe variant of Menkes disease, clinical findings include cutis laxa and joint hypermobility.. Skin laxity can also be observed in transaldolase deficiency and in lysinuric protein intolerance.

Differential diagnosis of skin laxity includes the subtypes of Ehler–Danlos syndrome, an umbrella term which encompasses a heterogeneous group of connective tissue disorders with distinct inheritance patterns, genetic defects, and prognostic implications.

Key References

Birch-Machin MA (2000) Mitochondria and skin disease. Clin Exp Dermatol 25:141–146

Bodemer C, Rötig A, Rustin P et al (1999) Hair and skin disorders as signs of mitochondrial disease. Pediatrics 103: 428–433

de Koning TJ, Klomp LW (2004) Serine-deficiency syndromes. Curr Opin Neurol 17:197–204

Dionisi-Vici C, De Felice L, el Hachem M et al (1998) Intravenous immune globulin in lysinuric protein intolerance. J Inherit Metab Dis 21:95–102

Dyer JA, Winters CJ, Chamlin SL (2005) Cutaneous findings in congenital disorders of glycosylation: the hanging fat sign. Pediatr Dermatol 22:457–460

Goldsmith LA (2003) Xanthomatoses and lipoprotein disorders. In: Eisen AZ, Wolf K et al (eds) Fitzpartick's dermatology in general medicine, McGraw-Hill, New York

Guallar JP, Vilà MR, López-Gallardo E et al (2006) Altered expression of master regulatory genes of adipogenesis in lipomas from patients bearing tRNA(Lys) point mutations in mitochondrial DNA. Mol Genet Metab 89: 283–285

Howard R, Frieden IJ, Crawford D et al (1997) Methylmalonic acidemia, cobalamin C type, presenting with cutaneous manifestations. Arch Dermatol 133:1563–1566

Online Mendelian Inheritance in Man. http://www.ncbi.nlm.nih.gov/sites/entrez

Shrinath M, Walter JH, Haeney M et al (1997) Prolidase deficiency and systemic lupus erythematosus. Arch Dis Child 76:441–444

Silengo M, Valenzise M, Pagliardini S. et al (2003) Hair changes in congenital disorders of glycosylation (CDG type 1). Eur J Pediatr 162:114–115

Valayannopoulos V, Verhoeven NM, Mention K et al (2006) Transaldolase deficiency: a new cause of hydrops fetalis and neonatal multi-organ disease. J Pediatr 149:713–717

Physical Abnormalities in Metabolic Diseases

C10

Ute Moog, Johannes Zschocke, and Stephanie Grünewald

Key Facts

› Inborn errors of metabolism have been delineated as important causes of syndromes with multiple congenital anomalies and/or dysmorphism, often in association with mental retardation.

› The most frequent are lysosomal storage disorders. Connective tissue, nervous tissue and, parenchymatous organs are primarily affected. It is, however, a misconception that all lysosomal storage disorders generally cause visceromegaly and characteristic skeletal changes.

› A substantial group affects predominantly or exclusively the central nervous system, causing chronic progressive neurologic and psychiatric dysfunction.

› Similarly, peroxisomal disorders present in many different ways, including dysmorphisms and relentless neural degeneration in infancy or early childhood, small stature, adrenal failure, spino-cerebellar degeneration or renal stones.

› Many disorders from the rapidly growing group of inherited glycosylation defects (CDG) present with multi-organ involvement, mostly accompanied by neurologic symptoms, while defects of cholesterol biosynthesis result in congenital malformation syndromes.

› Finally, physical abnormalities can also be characteristic features of mitochondrial disorders and homocystinuria.

C10.1 General Remarks

Over the last decades, the connection between physical (morphological) anomalies and inborn errors of metabolism has seen considerable re-evaluation. Traditionally, inherited metabolic disorders were presumed to be characterised primarily by abnormal function leading to abnormal laboratory parameters, an episodic or progressive disease course and sometimes multi-organ involvement. In contrast, primary genetic syndromes with multiple congenital anomalies (MCA) and/or dysmorphism, often in association with mental retardation (MR), were regarded to be caused by different groups of disorders. This apparently easy distinction changed most clearly in 1993 when Smith–Lemli–Opitz syndrome (SLOS), a classical MCA/MR syndrome without symptoms indicating a metabolic disease, was shown to be a disorder of cholesterol biosynthesis, thus bridging dysmorphology and metabolism. Subsequently, a variety of conditions with physical abnormalities such as dysmorphic signs, brain and other congenital malformations, as well as eye and skin abnormalities, were shown to be due to primary

U. Moog (✉)
Institute of Human Genetics, Ruprecht-Karls-University,
Im Neuenheimer Feld 366, D-69120 Heidelberg, Germany
e-mail: ute.moog@med.uni-heidelberg.de

G. F. Hoffmann et al. (eds.), *Inherited Metabolic Diseases*,
DOI: 10.1007/978-3-540-74723-9_C10, © Springer-Verlag Berlin Heidelberg 2010

enzyme deficiencies. In this chapter, we discuss which inborn errors of metabolism might present with physical abnormalities and which specific anomalies can be expected, relating them to the underlying pathogenetic mechanisms.

C10.2 Definitions

For this chapter, physical abnormalities are confined to those detectable by physical examination and exclude both structural brain and eye anomalies. They comprise congenital malformations which are disorders of blasto- and organo-genesis, and minor anomalies which result from disturbed phenogenesis. Metabolic diseases *sensu stricto* are defined as inborn disturbances of biosynthesis or degradation of substances within metabolic pathways; classical examples are genetic enzymopathies. Metabolic diseases in this sense are essentially different from primary disturbances of structural proteins and their modification, and from channelopathies and membrane diseases; consequently, these will not be considered. In addition, primary endocrinopathies or disorders of hormone syntheses are not brought into focus; they may be mediated by enzyme deficiencies, but the main pathogenetic mechanism is alteration of other effector molecules often involved in intercellular signalling or cellular regulation. Although arbitrary to some extent, these definitions help to narrow down the vast fields of physical anomalies and of diseases with biochemical abnormalities. In consequence, six subgroups and mechanisms can be identified which are presented in this chapter illustrated by prototypic examples.

C10.3 Lysosomal Storage Disorders: Disturbed Degradation of Macromolecules in Lysosomes

Genetic defects of lysosomal enzymes cause the accumulation of incompletely degraded macromolecules in lysosomes resulting in progressive impairment of the function of affected cell systems such as connective tissue, solid organs, cartilage, bone and, above all, the nervous system. The storage of macromolecules typically causes organomegaly and other morphological features. There are no acute metabolic crises, although some conditions, notably Fabry disease, may have acute presentations.

> **Remember**
>
> Cardinal clinical features of lysosomal disorders comprise:
>
> - Hydrops fetalis
> - Organomegaly and visceral disease
> - Dysostosis multiplex and dysmorphism
> - CNS disease – regression

In most cases, the typical clinical course is characterised by normal appearance at birth and normal development for a variable time span. However, the age of onset varies greatly depending on the underlying disorder and the amount of residual enzyme activity; non-immunologic hydrops fetalis is the most severe form and has the earliest (prenatal) onset. Severely affected children may show facial dysmorphism or cardiomyopathy at birth. More frequently, patients present with muscular hypotonia and developmental delay. Coarse facial features, typical skeletal changes (radiologically classified as dysostosis multiplex) or thickening of the skin in addition to hepatosplenomegaly and cardiomegaly are important physical signs. Lysosomal storage disorders with predominant central nervous system involvement frequently present with ataxia, hyperexcitability and spasticity; opthalmological examination may reveal a characteristic cherry-red spot in the macula region in some disorders. A differential diagnosis of typical findings in lysosomal storage diseases is given in Table C10.1; however, clinical presentation is generally variable.

Diagnostic work-up in children with suspected lysosomal storage disorders includes:

- Physical examination
- Ultrasound of parenchymatous organs
- Neurological examination, hearing tests, cranial MRI scan to consider
- X-ray examinations for dysostosis multiplex
- Cardiological examination (ECG, echocardiography)
- Opthalmological examinations (retina, macula, lens and cornea)

There are few general laboratory tests for lysosomal disorders. Several conditions are associated with increased concentrations of glycosaminoglycans (GAGs) or oligosaccharides in the urine. Microscopic examination of fresh leukocytes (bed-side blood smear, not from an EDTA tube), bone marrow cells or biopsies may show vacuoles in some conditions. Chiotriosidase, a chitinolytic enzyme and marker of monocyte/macrophage activation, is highly elevated in several lysosomal storage disorders including Gaucher and Niemann–Pick C diseases. It may be used for screening as well as monitoring of treatment; however, results may be false negative due to a common null allele of the *CHIT1* gene, and chitotriosidase activity is also increased in a large number of non-metabolic conditions including atherosclerosis, sarcoidosis, β-thalassemia or malaria. Reliable confirmation or exclusion of lysosomal storage disorders involves the measurement of specific enzyme activities in leukocytes or fibroblasts and/or molecular genetic analysis.

There has been considerable progress in the treatment of lysosomal storage disorders in the last years. Bone marrow transplantation has proven benefit in pre-symptomatic patients in some disorders (e.g. MPS I, late-onset Krabbe and metachromatic leukodystrophy), but not in others (MPS III, MPS IV). Enzyme replacement therapy is available for Gaucher diesease, Fabry disease and MPS I. For other disorders, treatment is largely symptomatic.

One of the most common lysosomal disorders, Pompe disease, a glycogen storage disease caused by the deficiency of acid maltase, usually shows no obvious morphological anomalies apart from sometimes an enlarged tongue. It is characterised by progressive muscle disease which in the severe infantile form presents in the neonatal period and leads to cardiac failure and death usually in the first year of life. There are also attenuated, juvenile and adult forms of the disease. The liver usually is not enlarged except in cardiac failure; CK is usually highly elevated. Enzyme replacement therapy is available.

Mucopolysaccharidoses (MPS) arise from the lack of specific lysosomal enzymes involved in the degradation of GAGs, long chains of sulphated or acetylated amino sugars attached to a protein skeleton. GAGs are major components of the viscous extracellular matrix. There are three major types of GAGs, and the clinical presentation of the different MPS types are linked to the tissue distribution of these subtypes. *Dermatan sulphate* is found in connective tissue and skin as well as bone, cartilage and tendons, internal organs, blood vessels, cornea and other tissues. Disorders affecting dermatan sulphate breakdown show typical progressive morphological changes as seen, for example, in Hurler's disease but are not necessarily associated with mental decline (intelligence is usually normal, e.g. in MPS type VI, Maroteaux–Lamy). In contrast, disorders affecting *heparan sulphate* (a ubiquitous constituent of glycoproteins and the basal membrane) are usually associated with mental retardation but, as in Sanfilippo's disease (MPS type III), do not always show the characteristic morphological changes. Similarly, in MPS type IV (Morquio), the deficient breakdown of *keratan sulphate*, a constituent of bone, cartilage and the cornea, causes a severe skeletal dysplasia but usually is not associated with mental retardation. Most patients are recognised by GAG analysis in the urine but results may be false negative particularly in MPS types III and IV requiring electrophoretic analysis; the different MPS types may be distinguished through the electrophoretic separation of the different GAGs. All MPS except the X-linked type II (Hunter) are inherited as autosomal recessive traits.

Disease Info: Hurler Disease, Scheie Disease

In *Hurler disease* (MPS IH,OMIM 607 014), the degradation of mucopolysaccharides, in particular of dermatan sulphate, is disturbed due to a deficiency of α-L-iduronidase. It is the classical form of MPS. Substrate accumulation takes place in both lysosomes and the extracellular matrix, in particular those of chondrocytes (causing disturbance of endochondral ossification), hepatocytes, dermis

Table C10.1 Typical clinical findings and relevant biochemical tests in lysosomal storage diseases

	Coarse facial features	Dysostosis multiplex	Organo megaly	Makrog lossia	Cardiac involvement	Hydrops fetalis	Angio keratoma	Neuro: Mental retardation
Mucopoly saccharidoses								
Hurler (MPS I)	++	++	+	++	+			++
Scheie (MPS I, atten.)	+	+	+	+				(+)
Hunter (MPS II)	++	(+)	+	+	+			++
Sanfilippo (MPS III)	(+)	(+)	(+)		(+)			++
Morquio (MPS IV)	+	(+)	+			+		
Maroteaux–Lamy (MPS VI)	+	+	+					
Oligosaccharidoses								
Fucosidosis	++	(+)	(+)		+		(+)	++
α-Mannosidosis	++	+	+				(+)	++
β-Mannosidosis	+						(+)	+
Aspartyl glucosaminuria	+	(+)	(+)		(+)		(+)	+
Schindler								+
Sialidose type I						+		
Sialidose type II	++	(+)	+		+	(+)	+	++
Sphingolipidoses								
GM$_1$ gangliosidosis	++	+	+	+	(+)	+	+	++
Tay-Sachs, Sandhoff		(+)						++
Metachromatic leukodystrophy								++
Krabbe								++
Niemann–Pick			++			+		+
Gaucher type I			++					
Gaucher type II			++			+		++
Fabry					+		+	

Angiokeratoma = red to dark blue lesions ((< 1 mm, slightly hyperkeratotic, do not blanche on pressure) mostly on buttocks, genitalia, lower trunk, thighs); *Cherry-red spot* = in the macula region; *Cardiac involvement* = cardiomyopathy, valve lesions, coronary artery disease; *Vacuolated lymphocytes* = typical vacuoles or evidence of storage in lymphocytes. *F* fibroblasts; *L* leukocytes; *S* serum; *M* muscle
++ prominent feature, + often present, (+) sometimes present

and subcutis and synovia. Inflammation and apoptosis in cartilage and synovial tissue is caused by stimulation of lipopolysaccharide signalling pathways. Somatic features affecting the skeleton, facies and internal organs, as well as neurologic features, evolve within the first year of life. Death occurs by age 1–10 years, with a mean age at death of 6 years. The craniofacial phenotype is characterised by progressive coarsening apparent at 3–6 months, a large scaphocephalic head with bulging frontal bones, depressed nasal bridge, broad tip of the nose, full cheek and lips, a large tongue, hypertrophy of the gums and a mouth held open. The patients are generally hirsute and have thick and abundant hair. A protuberant abdomen, recurrent (umbilical) hernias, corneal clouding, optic nerve head swelling and retinal degeneration, frequent ear, nose and throat infections, decreasing growth velocity by the age of 2 years with resulting short stature, short neck, and short, broad hands and feet, joint stiffness and cardiac disease are all frequent physical findings. Radiologically, a pattern of

Spasticity	Peripheral neuropathy	Myoclonic seizures	Eyes		Diagnosis				
			Corneal clouding	Cherry-red macular spot	Vacuolated lymphocytes	GAG (urine) elevated	Pathol. Oligosaccharides	Enzyme studies in:	OMIM
			++			+		L/F	607014
			+			+		L/F	607016
						+		S/L/F	309900
+			+			(+)		L/F	252920
			(+)			+		L/F	253000
			+			+		L/F	253200
+		+			+		+	L/F	230000
(+)			++		+		+	L/F	248500
+	+						+	L/F	248510
			(+)		(+)		+	L/F	208400
+		+					+	L/F	104170
+	+	++		++	+		+	F	256550
		(+)		++	+		+	F	256550
(+)			+	++			+	L/F	230500
+		+		++			+	L/F	272750
+	++			(+)				L/F	250200
+	++			(+)				L/F	245200
		(+)	(+)	(+)	+			F	257200
							+	L/F	230800
+		+					+	L/F	230900
								S/L/F	301500

skeletal changes called "dysostosis multiplex" may be seen. As in other lysosomal storage diseases, progressive dermal melanocytosis, e.g. extensive Mongolian spots, may be a clue to the diagnosis, particularly in infants with darker skin types. Dermal melanocytosis results from arrest of transdermal migration of melanocytes from the neural crest to the epidermis. Pathogenetically, abnormal increases in nerve growth factor (NGF) activity caused by the binding of accumulating metabolites to the tyrosine kinase-type receptors for NGF has been discussed as a primary cause. The attenuated form of α-L-iduronidase deficiency is denoted *Scheie disease* (MPS IS, OMIM 607 016); it has a much later onset, a milder course and symptoms restricted to milder somatic features; stature is normal. *Hurler–Scheie syndrome* (MPS IH/S, OMIM 607 015) has an intermediate phenotypic expression. Bone marrow transplantation has proven benefit in pre-symptomatic patients with MPS I. Enzyme replacement therapy is licensed and available but has no beneficial effect on brain manifestation as the intravenously applied enzyme does not cross the blood-brain barrier.

Dysostosis Multiplex

Dysostosis multiplex is the typical skeletal abnormality found in MPS I and other lysosomal disorders. In severe MPS I, defective ossification may not be evident until the characteristic gibbus deformity of the lumbar spine is apparent at 6–14 months of age. As vertebrae become progressively flattened and beaked, spinal deformities, including kyphosis, scoliosis and kyphoscoliosis, may develop. Hips may be affected, resulting in dysplasia or subluxation. Long-bone irregularities produce valgus and varus deformities, and genu valgum may occur in the knees. Phalangeal dysostosis and synovial thickening produce the characteristic claw deformity and trigger digits. Carpal tunnel syndrome and phalangeal involvement diminish hand function. By the time severely affected children are 2 years of age, joint stiffening and progressive arthropathy affect all joints. Radiographs obtained at birth can detect dysostosis in some patients with MPS I.

Patients with attenuated MPS I have progressive arthropathy, which ultimately leads to loss of joint range of motion. Patients present with mild to severe skeletal involvement and tend to have short stature. Kyphosis and/or scoliosis are frequent presenting symptoms, with attendant hip and back pain. Patients also may experience generalised pain and malaise, which may be attributable to osteopenia and microfractures. Patients with moderate to severe skeletal disease should be monitored by an orthopedic surgeon, preferably one who is familiar with MPS disorders. Early detection of skeletal abnormalities, such as kyphoscoliosis, before irreversible changes occur may provide more surgical options. Spine deformities may require fusion; acetabular hip dysplasia can be addressed with osteotomy and genu valgum with epiphyseal stapling. Flexor tendon or carpal tunnel release can provide relief and the return of some hand function. Premature cessation of skeletal growth may occur in MPS I and should be taken into account when surgical procedures are being planned. Physical therapists can assess the degree of joint restriction and develop interventions to maintain joint function and muscle strength. In patients with attenuated MPS I, joint stiffness and pain may be lessened through passive and active range-of-motion exercises and hydrotherapy. In severe MPS I, these interventions may stabilise but not improve joint function and stiffness. The benefit of physical therapy in patients with severe orthopedic compromise is controversial. Occupational therapists can improve the quality of life and functional independence; the most effective occupational therapies are those that patients can perform on their own.

(Bernhard Zabel, University Children's Hospital, Freiburg i. Brsg., Germany)

Oligosaccharidoses are disorders in the breakdown of complex carbohydrate side-chains of glycosylated proteins (glycoproteins), leading to increased concentration of oligosaccharides in the urine. They are less common than MPS which they resemble clinically with variable coarsening of the face, skeletal deformities, hepatomegaly and sometimes corneal clouding. Psychomotor development is usually delayed; progressive neurological symptoms and seizures are common. Early presentation with hydrops fetalis or neonatal cardiomegaly is more frequent than in patients with MPS. Elevation of urinary oligosaccharides is also found in several sphingolipidoses such as GM1 and GM2 gangliosidoses and galactosialidosis.

Sphingolipidoses are disorders in the breakdown of membrane lipids that are found throughout the body but are of special importance in the nervous tissue. Some sphingolipids are essential components of myelin sheaths; others are prevalent particularly in the grey matter of the brain. Sphingolipidoses thus usually present with primary disturbances of the central or peripheral nervous system; in addition, sphingolipids frequently accumulate in the reticuloendothelial system or other cells. Typical clinical features include progressive psychomotor retardation and neurological problems such as epilepsy, ataxia and/or spasticity. Hepatosplenomegaly is not uncommon. Progressive facial coarsening and dysostosis multiplex are found in GM1 gangliosidosis; liver disease is a characteristic feature of Niemann–Pick disease; a lysosomal leukodystrophy is found in Krabbe disease and metachromatic leukodystrophy. Several sphingolipidoses show a cherry-red macula spot, there may be foam cells in the bone marrow or vacuolated lymphocytes. Neurological and neuroradiological findings are not always specific. The diagnosis is made by enzyme or molecular analyses. All sphingolipidoses except Fabry disease are inherited as autosomal recessive traits.

Disease Info: Gaucher Disease, Fabry Disease

The most common form of Gaucher disease (OMIM 230800), the non-neuronopathic type I, is characterised by accumulation of sphingolipds in cells of the reticuloendothelial system leading to massive (hepato-) splenomegaly and anaemia, thrombocytopenia and hematomas. Progressive bone changes may be associated with acute "bone crises" (pain, fever) as well as with osteonecrosis, arthrosis and osteopenia. Long-term complications include growth retardation and lung fibrosis. The diagnosis of Gaucher disease is supported by highly elevated chitotriosidase activity in serum and the presence of characteristic Gaucher cells, for example, in bone marrow, and is confirmed by enzyme analysis. Enzyme replacement therapy is available but again has no effect on brain manifestation in the neuronopathic type II of Gaucher disease (10% of cases).

Fabry disease (OMIM 301 500) typically presents in the first decade of life with episodes of acute painful acroparesthesias in arms or legs triggered, for example, by physical exertion or temperature changes and lasting for hours or days. There may be hypohidrosis and episodic fever; 80% of patients show typical angiokeratoma skin lesions. Corneal and lenticular opacities as well as proteinuria are common. In middle age, deterioration of renal function usually leads to renal failure and cardiovascular disease may occur. Intelligence is normal; there is no hepatosplenomegaly or facial dysmorphy. Fabry disease is inherited as an X-linked trait but carrier females frequently show complications in adulthood including progressive renal failure, hypertrophic cardiomyopathy and stroke. The diagnosis is confirmed by α-galactosidase analysis or mutation testing. Enzyme replacement therapy is available.

C10.4 Peroxisomal Disorders: Disturbance of Generalised Biogenesis or of Modification of Substrates

Many oxygen-dependent reactions take place in the peroxisomes to protect the cell against oxygen radicals; the produced H_2O_2 is metabolised by a catalase. Important peroxisomal functions include β-oxidation of very long-chain fatty acids (VLCFA) and related substances, α-oxidation of 3-methyl fatty acids, and biosynthesis of etherlipids, and bile acids. Peroxisomal disorders are classified into generalised defects of peroxisome biogenesis and single peroxisomal enzyme deficiencies, but clinical phenotypes are variable and overlapping. Generalised peroxisomal disorders are multi-system diseases that cause dysmorphic features and skeletal changes (specifically proximal shortening of the limbs) as well as neurological and opthalmological abnormalities and hepatointestinal dysfunction. Morphological abnormalities such as rhizomelic chondrodysplasia punctata are generally related to a deficiency in biosynthetic functions and may be caused both by single enzyme deficiencies in this pathway as well as generalised peroxisomal disorders. Variant, milder phenotypes are dominated by neurological manifestations. Patients may follow a neurodegenerative course after a period of normal development. An important clue may be white matter abnormalities consistent with the pathologic appearance of sudanophilic leukodystrophy. Peroxisomal disorders should therefore be included in the differential diagnosis of infants and young children with severe hypotonia and seizure disorders, but not in patients with mental retardation alone.

Children with peroxisomal disorders may show elevated transaminases and a tendency to hypoglycemia, as well as hypocholesterolemia and increased serum concentrations of iron and transferrin. Organic acid analysis may reveal dicarboxylic aciduria, in particular elevated 2-hydroxysebacic acid reflecting impaired peroxisomal β-oxidation. The specific laboratory finding in peroxisomal disorders (with the exception of rhizomelic chondrodysplasia punctata) is an elevation of VLCFA in serum or cultured fibroblasts, usually determined by GC-MS. VLCFAs are found consistently and reliably elevated in all disorders of peroxisome biogenesis as well as in single defects of VLCFA transport or β-oxidation. The ratio of C26/C22 is the most sensitive index. The analysis of plasmalogens in erythrocytes is indicated in suspected rhizomelic chondrodysplasia punctata. If levels are decreased, the analysis of phytanic acid in plasma will distinguish classical rhizomelic chondrodysplasia punctata, in which phytanic acid is increased (at least after the first months of life), from single enzyme defects that may produce the same clinical and radiologic features. If plasmalogens are normal, other disorders with punctate calcifications such as Warfarin embryopathy (should be evident from the prenatal history) or X-linked chondrodysplasia punctata (due to a defect in of sterol biosynthesis) must be considered.

Remember

The decisive marker for peroxisomal diseases, with the exception of rhizomelic chondrodysplasia punctata, is the elevation of VLCFA. Additional biochemical investigations for peroxisomal disorders are not usually warranted.

Disease Info: Zellweger Syndrome

The prototypic disorder of disturbed peroxisomal biogenesis with multiple enzyme abnormalities is *Zellweger syndrome* (ZS, OMIM 214 100). It is caused by defects in a number of *PEX* genes which encode peroxins, proteins necessary for peroxisomal biogenesis and for the import of proteins. Children with ZS typically present in the neonatal period with severe hypotonia, no or little psychomotor development, seizures and other neurologic disturbances. MRI of the brain often shows gross abnormalities reflecting defects of early brain development. The craniofacial features in ZS are characteristic with macrocephaly, large fontanels and wide sutures, a high forehead, flat and square face, shallow supraorbital ridges, telecanthus, epicanthic folds, broad and depressed nasal bridge, anteverted nares, dysplastic ears and redundant skin in the neck. The limbs show variable contractures; calcified stippling of the patella and other bones is seen in about half of the patients. Hepatomegaly, hepatic fibrosis and renal cysts are additional characteristic findings. Eye anomalies include cataracts, nystagmus, optic atrophy and retinal changes. Most patients with severe ZS die within the first year of life; survivors often show severely impaired development, post-natal growth failure, blindness or severe visual handicap and significant sensorineural hearing impairment, Facial dysmorphy in these cases may be less marked with a high forehead and, typically, attached ear lobules.

C10.5 Disorders of Catabolism of Small Molecules: Substrate Accumulation Can Affect Macromolecular Functions

Disorders of biosynthesis and catabolism of small molecules, e.g. amino acids, organic acids, lipids, vitamins and cofactors usually are not associated with physical abnormalities. There are, however, exceptions, in particular when accumulating substrates or their metabolites affect macromolecules. A well-known example is *homocystinuria* (OMIM 236 200).

The principal cause of homocystinuria is cystathionine β-synthase deficiency leading to accumulation of homocystine which is the dimeric form of the amino acid homocysteine. The major clinical features of homocystinuria consist of MR, a characteristic marfanoid habitus but with joint limitations and generalised osteoporosis, eye features such as ectopia lentis and myopia, and vascular problems complicated by thromboembolic events. However, clinical variability is high. Homocystinuria may present as unspecific MR, but about one-third of the patients have normal intelligence. Psychiatric problems are seen in about 50% of patients. Physical findings in homocystinuria are partly due to the effects of the accumulating homocystine on collagen, fibrillin and other elements of the connective tissue. Lens dislocation results from disruption of disulphide bonds of fibrous proteins. The diagnosis is made through the identification of highly elevated concentrations of total homocysteine in plasma, or even a pathological sulphite test in urine. About half of the patients respond well to substitution of the cofactor pyridoxine (vitamin B_6), sometimes in combination with folic acid and betaine. In all other patients including partial responders, a diet restricted in methionine, and intake of betaine must be initiated.

C10.6 Disorders of Cholesterol Biosynthesis: Disorders Affecting Developmental Signalling Pathways

Sterol synthesis defects present clinically as multisystem disorders with dysmorphic features and variable skeletal dysplasias; they should be considered in cases of otherwise unexplained recurrent abortions and fetal dysmorphy. The biochemical diagnosis is not always straightforward: serum cholesterol is usually normal in all disorders except (sometimes) Smith–Lemli–Opitz syndrome (SLOS, OMIM 270 400), and even specific sterol analysis may yield normal results. In these instances, the diagnosis can be reached by mutation analysis or functional studies (fibroblasts cultured in sterol-free media).

The identification of SLOS as a disorder of cholesterol biosynthesis proofed that enzymopathies within metabolic pathways can have a major impact on developmental signalling pathways and lead to MCA/MR syndromes. Other disorders of post-sequalene cholesterol biosynthesis include desmosterolosis (OMIM 602 398), X-linked dominant chondrodysplasia punctata (CDPX2; OMIM 302 960), CHILD syndrome (OMIM 308 050), lathosterolosis (607 330) and hydrops-ectopic calcification-moth-eaten skeletal dysplasia (HEM; 215 140). They are all associated with congenital malformations. A summary of clinical features in primary deficiencies of sterol-biosynthetic enzymes is given in Table C10.2. Antley–Bixler syndrome or lanosterolosis, a multiple malformation syndrome with craniofacial dysmorphy, limb anomalies and, in some patients, ambiguous genitalia, is caused by the deficiency of POR, a flavoprotein that donates electrons to all P_{450} oxidoreductases including 3β-hydroxysterol 14α-demethylase.

Mevalonic aciduria is caused by a deficiency of mevalonate kinase, which catalyses an early (pre-squalen) step in sterol biosynthesis. Affected children show facial dysmorphism and severe neurological abnormalities including progressive ataxia due to cerebellar atrophy, psychomotor retardation and retinitis pigmentosa. In addition, there may be dystrophy and recurrent crises with fever, skin rash, lymphadenopathy and hepatosplenomegaly. Hyper-IgD syndrome with recurrent febrile attacks represents an attenuated form of the disease, with residual enzyme function.

Disease Info: Smith–Lemli–Opitz Syndrome (SLOS)

SLOS is the most common defect of the cholesterol pathway. It is caused by the deficiency of 7-dehydrocholesterol reductase, the last step of cholesterol synthesis, leading to elevated levels of 7- and 8-dehydrocholesterol and (often) reduced levels of cholesterol. As diagnostic markers, 7-and 8-dehydrocholesterol are measured by GC-MS in serum or

Table C10.2 Clincial features in disorders of distal (post-sequalene) sterol biosynthesis

	Clinical features	Enzyme	OMIM
SLOS	Psychomotor retardation, growth retardation, microcephaly, facial dysmorphism, cleft palate, genital anomalies in males, postaxial polydactyly, syndactyly of toes 2/3, photosensitivity	7-dehydrocholesterol reductase	270 400
Desmosterolosis	Psychomotor retardation, facial dysmorphy, cleft palate, multiple malformations, ambiguous genitalia, short limbs, osteosclerosis	3β-Hydroxysterol Δ^{24}-reductase	602 398
CHILD syndrome	Unilateral ichthyotic skin lesions with a sharp demarcation at the midline of the trunk, stippled epiphyses on the affected side, limb defects; X-linked inheritance, lethal in males	Sterol-4-demethylase	308 050
Greenberg dysplasia	Non-immune hydrops fetalis, severe chondrodysplasia punctata, prenatally lethal	3β-Hydroxysterol Δ^{14}-reductase (lamin B receptor; *LBR* gene)	215140
Pelger–Huët anomaly	Psychomotor retardation, epilepsy (heterozygous mutations; additional skeletal abnormalities when homozygous for specific mutations)	3β-Hydroxysterol Δ^{14}-reductase (lamin B receptor; *LBR* gene)	169400
Chondrodysplasia punctata Conradi–Hünermann	Psychomotor retardation, rhizomelic short stature with asymmetric shortening of proximal limbs, stippled epiphyses, cataracts, ichthyosis; X-linked inheritance, lethal in males	3β-Hydroxysterol Δ^8,Δ^7-isomerase	302 960
Lathosterolosis	Severe malformations, overlapping the spectrum of Smith–Lemli–Opitz syndrome; lipid storage	3β-Hydroxysterol Δ^5-desaturase	607330

tissues. SLOS is characterised clinically by recognisable craniofacial features in childhood with microcephaly and bitemporal narrowing, ptosis, broad nasal tip with anteverted nostrils, broad upper alveolar ridges (and later, broad upper secondary incisors) and micrognathia. In addition, children with SLOS show syndactyly of the second and third toes, genital anomalies in males, short stature, photosensitivity and mostly severe mental retardation. The phenotypic spectrum, however, is very broad. Facial appearances change with age and become less characteristic in adulthood. Also, genital anomalies may become less prominent or even disappear. Structural brain anomalies occur in 37%; not infrequently they belong to the holoprosencephaly spectrum, a failure of normal bilobar development of the forebrain. Malformations of the heart, lungs and the gastrointestinal system, may be associated. Dietary cholesterol supplementation may have benefits especially on the behavioural problems in some SLOS patients. Trials combining high cholesterol diets with statin treatment so far have given inconclusive results.

Given the multiple biological functions of cholesterol, the link between abnormal cholesterol metabolism and abnormal morphogenesis in SLOS is complex and only partly unravelled. Some of the malformations relate to impairment of Sonic hedgehog (SHH) functioning, one of the major embryonic signalling pathways. Genetic disorders in this pathway cause holoprosencephaly, and mutations in *GLI3,* one of the downstream effectors of *SHH,* cause Pallister–Hall syndrome (PHS, 146 510) with clinical features overlapping those of SLOS. The different conditions may thus be grouped to one syndrome family that share the same pathway and part of their phenotypic characteristics. Other SLOS features may relate to deficient total sterols and alteration of cellular membrane properties, and to possible toxic effects of cholesterol precursors.

C10.7 Energy Defects: Mitochondrial Defects Potentially Affecting Morphogenesis

Mitochondrial disorders in a strict sense are disorders of enzymes or enzyme complexes directly involved in the generation of ATP by oxidative phosphorylation, discussed in detail in Chap. D6. They are often multi-system disorders affecting neuromuscular and other systems and as such may also affect morphogenesis. Whilst mitochondrial dysfunction caused by mtDNA mutations is not usually associated with physical abnormalities, mitochondrial energy deficiency resulting from mutations in nuclear encoded genes may occasionally result in congenital malformations and (various) dysmorphism. An important disorder to consider is glutaric aciduria type II, also known as multiple acyl CoA dehydrogenase deficiency.

Multiple acyl CoA dehydrogenase deficiency is a defect in the mitochondrial transfer of electrons from fatty acids to the electron transport chain, by genetic defects of the electron transfer flavoprotein (ETF) or ETF:ubiquinone oxidoreductase (ETFQO). Attenuated forms of the disease are characterised by predominant muscle and hepatic disease, but severe multiple acyl CoA dehydrogenase deficiency results in the virtual absence of fatty acid oxidation with significant physical abnormalities, overwhelming metabolic decompensation hence poor prognosis. Malformations are predominantly found in the brain, kidneys, e.g. renal cysts and genitals. Craniofacial dysmorphism may be reminiscent of Zellweger syndrome, as it is characterised by macrocephaly, large anterior fontanel, high forehead, flat nasal bridge, increased inner canthal distance and malformed ears. An unpleasant acrid body odour may be noted. Acidosis, cardiomyopathy, liver dysfunction and epileptic encephalopathy all contribute to an early fatal course. The diagnosis is made through the identification of a wide variety of abnormal metabolites in urinary organic acid analysis.

C10.8 Glycosylation Defects: Disorders of Protein Modification

Glycosylation, i.e. the transfer of glycans to proteins or lipids, is the most complex post-translational modification of molecules in humans. Human disorders in glycosylation pathways are mainly known for N-linked (attached to the amide group of an asparagine of the protein) or O-linked glycans (to the hydroxyl group of serine or threonine). *N*-glycosylation requires assembly of glycans in the cytosol and ER, transfer to the protein and a subsequent processing pathway mainly located in the Golgi apparatus. Multiple enzymes, transporters and transferases are involved in that pathway. Type I disorders of *N*-glycosylation affect the early assembly pathway; in type II disorders, the processing pathway is disturbed. *O*-glycosylation, mainly confined to the Golgi apparatus is a much shorter – however, more variable – pathway, consisting of assembly and transfer of the glycans to a protein. The diversity of *O*-glycosylation is due to variable sugars in the first position of the glycans, such like mannose in the *O*-mannosylation pathway. However, in view of the multitude of enzymes involved it has recently been suggested to discontinue this system of classification and describe the individual disorders by their enzymatic deficiency.

The clinical features of congenital disorders of glycosylation (CDG) are as diverse as the numerous functions of glycoproteins which can be enzymes, transporter proteins, membrane components or hormones. CDGs may present as single organ diseases, but are often multi-system disorders, comprising structural malformations and abnormal function, occurring in various combinations and covering a spectrum of severity. Symptoms comprise psychomotor retardation and neurological abnormalities, multiple function deficits like bleeding diathesis, endocrine or gastrointestinal disturbances, organ manifestations (e.g. heart or kidney), skeletal manifestations (e.g. short stature, contractures and osteopenia), as well as other physical abnormalities. Many CDG patients already display symptoms at birth; this is also the case in the most common primary glycosylation disorder, phosphomannomutase deficiency (CDG-Ia).

Most *N*-glycosylation disorders are readily detected by isoelectric focusing (IEF) of serum transferrin, although results may be false negative in some disorders, and abnormal results may be caused by a variety of other conditions. Abnormal *O*-glycosylation involving the so-called core 1 *O*-glycans with the first sugar being *N*-acetylgalactosamine (the most commonly observed *O*-glycosylation type) can be detected by IEF of apolipoprotein CIII in serum. For other *O*-glycosylation defects, such like *O*-mannosylation defects (Walker–Warburg syndrome or muscle–eye–brain disease), particular staining of the α-dystroglycan complex in a muscle

Disease Info: Phosphomannomutase (PMM) Deficiency

By far the most common and prototypic CDG is PMM deficiency (OMIM 212065), previously denoted CDG 1a, caused by mutations in the *PMM2* gene. The phenotypic spectrum is very broad. Commonly, the central nervous system is involved and children show psychomotor retardation, hypotonia, hyporeflexia, ataxia and seizures. Dysmorphic features include a prominent forehead, large ears and a thin upper lip. Fat distribution is abnormal with fat pads at the buttocks or other sites and lipoatrophic changes. The nipples are typically inverted. Retinitis pigmentosa, strabismus and myopia are the most common ophthalmologic signs. Skeletal manifestations consist of growth retardation, osteopenia, contractures, spine anomalies, "bone-in-bone" appearance and other changes. In the multivisceral form of PMM deficiency, multiple other manifestations may exist, and include liver, cardiac, renal and gastrointestinal involvements.

biopsy will show abnormal *O*-mannosylation. For the majority of CDG subtypes identified so far, mutational analysis can be performed to confirm the diagnosis.

The group of CDGs is rapidly growing. At the time of writing, nearly 40 CDGs have been characterised, 14 of which affect *N*-glycosylation of proteins, 11 are linked to *O*-glycosylation pathways and in 15 others both or other pathways are affected. Recently, not only dystroglycanopathies but also several malformation syndromes have been recognised as glycosylation defects, e.g. the autosomal recessive Peters' Plus syndrome which is caused by mutations in B3GALTL resulting in an *O*-fucosylation defect.

As so far only very few patients have been identified for many of the CDGs, it is impossible to describe characteristic dysmorphic features. Major clinical signs and symptoms of different CDGs as reported in the literature have been listed in Table C10.3.

As there are many more glycosylation pathways, it is to be expected that far more glycosylation disorders will be identified in the middle-term future and one needs to be open for any possible clinical presentation. Certainly, the book of CDGs is not closed, and will have to be updated rapidly.

Table C10.3 Human genetic disorders of glycosylation

Relevant gene	Deficient protein	OMIM	Clinical features
Disorders of protein N-glycosylation			
PMM2 (*CDG-Ia*)	Phosphomannomutase 2	601785	MR, cerebellar hypoplasia, abnormal fat pads, hypotonia, failure to thrive, multi-organ involvement, stroke-like episodes, seizures, cardiomyopathy, nephrotic syndrome, hyperinsulinemic hypoglycemia, coagulopathy, hypergonadotropic hypogonadism
MPI (*CDG-Ib*)	Phosphomannose isomerase	602579	Protein-loosing enteropathy, hepatic fibrosis, coagulopathy, hyperinsulinemic hypoglycemia
ALG6 (*CDG-Ic*)	Glucosyltransferase 1	603147	MR, hypotonia, epilepsy, coagulopathy, strabismus
NOT56L (*CDG-Id*)	Mannosyltransferase 6	601110	MR, optic atrophy, iris coloboma, secondary microcephaly, arthrogryposis multiplex, epilepsy
ALG 12 (*CDG-Ig*)	Mannosyltransferase 8	607143	MR, genital hypoplasia, microcephaly, undetectable IgF1 and IgFB3, cardiomegaly
ALG 8 (*CDG-Ih*)	Glucosyltransferase 2	608104	Protein-loosing enteropathy, renal failure, hepatic failure, cataracts, osteopenia, MR
ALG2 (*CDG-Ii*)	Mannosyltransferase 2	607906	Intractable seizures, iris coloboma, hepatomegaly, poor vision
DPAGT1 (*CDG-Ij*)	UDP-GlcNAc:Dol-P-GlcNAc-P transferase	608093	MR, seizures, esotropia, microcephaly
HMT1 (*CDG-Ik*)	Mannosyltransferase 1	608540	MR, secondary microcephaly, nephrotic syndrome, early death
DIBD1 (*CDG-Il*)	Mannosyltransferase 7–9	608776	Severe microcephaly, seizures, hepatomegaly, renal cysts, early death
RFT1 (*CDG-In*)	Flippase of Man5GlcNAc2-PP-Dol	611633	Intrauterine growth retardation, arthrogryposis, failure to thrive, impaired vision, drug resistant epilepsy, abnormal coagulation
MGAT2 (*CDG-IIa*)	N-acetylglucosaminyltransferase 2	602616	MR, facial dysmorphism, stereotypic behaviour, seizures, dysmorphy, liver disease
GLS1 (*CDG-IIb*)	Glucosidase 1	606056	Seizures, liver disease, early death
TUSC3	Oligosaccharyltransferase subunit	601385	Non-dysmorphic, mental retardation
Disorders of protein O-glycosylation			
O-xylosylglycan synthesis			
EXT1/EXT2 (multiple cartilaginous exotoses)	Glucuronyltransferase/N-acetylglucosaminyltransferase	608177/608210	MR, multiple exostosis, hypertrichosis
B4GALT7 (progeroid type of Ehlers–Danlos syndrome)	β-1,4-galactosyltransferase 7	604327	MR, short stature, macrocephaly, abnormal bones, loose skin
O-N-acetylgalactosaminylglycan synthesis			
GALNT3 (familial tumoral calcinosis)	Polypeptide N-acetylgalactosaminyltransferase 3	601756	Massive calcium deposits in skin and tissue
O-xylosyl/N-acetylgalactosaminylglycan synthesis			
SLC35D1 (Schneckenbecken dysplasia)	Solute carrier family 35	610804	Micromelic dwarfism, macrocephaly, abnormal bones, precocious ossified bones
O-mannosylglycan synthesis			
POMT1/POMT2	Protein-O-mannosyltransferase 1 and 2	607423	Type II lissencephaly, cerebellar malformation, ventriculomegaly, anterior chamber malformations, severe muscular hypotonia, severe MR, death in infancy

Gene	Protein/Enzyme	OMIM	Clinical features
POMGNT1	Protein-*O*-mannose β-1,2-*N*-acetylglucosaminyltransferase	606822	Congenital muscular dystrophy, ocular abnormalities, lissencephaly
FKTN	Fukutin	607440	Fukuyama congenital muscular dystrophy
FKRP	Fukutin-related protein	606596	Limb-girdle muscular dystrophy type
LARGE	*N*-acetylglucosaminyltransferase-like protein	603590	Congenital muscular dystrophy, brain abnormalities
O-fucosylglycan synthesis			
SCDO3 (spondylocostal dysostosis type 3)	*O*-fucose-specific β-1,3-*N*-acetylglucosaminyltransferase	602576	Spondylocostal dysostosis
B3GALTL (Peters plus syndrome)	*O*-fucose-specific β-1,3-glucosyltransferase	610308	MR, anterior eye chamber defects, disproportionate short stature, cleft palate
Disorders of glycosphingolipid and glycosylphosphatidylinositol anchor glycosylation			
SIAT9 (Amish infantile epilepsy)	Lactosylceramide α-2,3 sialyltransferase (GM3 synthase)	609056	Amish infantile epilepsy
PIGM (glycosylphosphatidylinositol deficiency)	Phosphatidylinositolglycan, class M	610273	Portal venous thrombosis, absence seizures
Disorders of multiple glycosylation functions and other pathways			
DPM1 (*CDG-Ie*)	GDP-Man:Dol-P-mannosyltransferase (Dol-P-Man synthase 1)	603503	MR, microcephaly, epilepsy, blindness
MPDU1 (*CDG-If*)	Lec35 (Man-P-Dol utilisation 1)	608799	MR, growth retardation, ichthyosis, ataxia, pigmentary retinopathy
B4GALT1 (*CDG-IId*)	β-1,4-galactosyltransferase 1	607091	MR, myopathy, Dandy–Walker-malformation, macrocephaly
GNE (hereditary inclusion body myopathy)	UDP-GlcNAc epimerase/kinase	600737	Ascending muscle weakness, "Rimmed vacuoles" on biopsy
SLC35A1 (*CDG-IIf*) (CMP-sialic acid transporter deficiency)	CMP-sialic acid transporter	605634	Thrombocytopenia, haemorrhages, respiratory distress syndrome, opportunistic infections
SLC35C1 (*CDG-IIc*) (GDP-fucose transporter deficiency)	GDP-fucose transporter	605881	MR, growth retardation, microcephaly, persistent neutrophilia, recurrent fever
Dolichol pathway			
DK1 (*CDG-Im*)	Dolichol kinase	610768	Seizures, ichtyosis, dilated cardiomyopathy, early death
COG complex			
COG7 defect (*CDG-IIe*)	Component of conserved oligomeric Golgi complex 7	606978	MR, progressive microcephaly, dysmorphy, growth retardation, hypotonia, adducted thumbs, cardiac defects, wrinkled skin, hyperthermia, early death
COG1 defect (*CDG-IIg*)	Component of conserved oligomeric Golgi complex 1	606973	MR, growth retardation, progressive microcephaly, hypotonia
COG8 defect	Component of conserved oligomeric Golgi complex 8	606979	Severe psychomotor retardation, seizures, failure to thrive
V-ATPase			
ATP6VOA2 defect (cutis laxa type II)	V0 subunit A2 of vesicular H(+)-ATPase	611716	MR, wrinkled skin/cutis laxa, pachygyria, seizures, late closure of the fontanelle

Key References

Brown GK (2005) Congenital brain malformations in mitochondrial disease. J Inherit Metab Dis 28:393–401

Clayton PT, Thompson E (1988) Dysmorphic syndromes with demonstrable biochemical abnormalities. J Med Genet 25:463–472

de Lonlay P, Seta N, Barrot S et al (2001) A broad spectrum of clinical presentations in congenital disorders of glycosylation I: a series of 26 cases. J Med Genet 38:14–19

Epstein CJ, Erickson RP, Wynshaw-Boris A (eds) (2008) Inborn errors of development, 2nd edn. Oxford University Press, Oxford, New York

Faust PL, Banka D, Siriratsivawong R et al (2005) Peroxisome biogenesis disorders: the role of peroxisomes and metabolic dysfunction in developing brain. J Inherit Metab Dis 28:369–383

Gorlin RJ, Cohen MM, Hennekam RCM (2001) Syndromes of the head and neck, 4th edn. Oxford University Press, Oxford, New York

Grünewald S (2007) Congenital disorders of glycosylation: rapidly enlarging group of (neuro)metabolic disorders. Early Hum Dev 83:825–830

Hennekam RC (2005) Congenital brain anomalies in distal cholesterol biosynthesis defects. J Inherit Metab Dis 28: 385–392

Herman GE (2003) Disorders of cholesterol biosynthesis: prototypic metabolic malformation syndromes. Hum Mol Genet 12 R75–88

Jaeken J, Matthijs G (2001) Congenital disorders of glycosylation. Annu Rev Genomics Hum Genet 2:129–151

Mudd SH, Skovby F, Levy HL et al (1985) The natural history of homocystinuria due to cystathionine beta-synthase deficiency. Am J Hum Genet 37:1–31

Porter FD (2008) Smith-Lemli-Opitz syndrome: pathogenesis, diagnosis and management. Eur J Hum Genet 16: 535–541

Wanders RJ (2004) Metabolic and molecular basis of peroxisomal disorders: a review. Am J Med Genet 126A: 355–375

Hematological Disorders

C11

Ellen Crushell and Joe T R Clarke

Key Facts

> Complete blood count and blood film are indicated in all metabolic diagnostic work-ups.

> Hematological disorders may be the lead symptom or a secondary finding in many metabolic disorders.

> Hemolytic anemia may be the only sign of an inherited disorder of red cell energy metabolism.

> Macrocytic anemia is an important pointer to many metabolic disorders.

> Hematological abnormalities due to metabolic disease are rarely seen in isolation.

Abbreviations

ACE	Angiotensin converting enzyme
AD	Autosomal dominant
ALAS	5-Aminolevulinic acid synthase
AR	Autosomal recessive
ASAT	Anemia, sideroblastic, and spinocerebellar ataxia
CBC	Complete blood count
CDG	Congenital disoders of glycosylation
GSD	Glycogen storage disease
HDL	High-density lipoprotein

HPRT	Hypoxanthine guanine phosphoribosyltransferase
IRT	Immunoreactive trypsin
IVA	Isovaleric aciduria
LCAT	Lecithin:cholesterol acyltransferase
MCV	Mean corpuscular volume
ML	Mucolipidosis
MLASA	Mitochondrial myopathy and sideroblastic anemia
MMA	Methylmalonic aciduria
MPS	Mucopolysaccharides/oses
NCL	Neuronal ceroid-lipofuscinosis
NP	Niemann–Pick
OA	Organic acid analysis
PA	Propionic acidemia
RBC	Red blood cell
TG	Triglycerides
TPI	Triose phosphate isomerase
UMP	Uridine monophosphate
XLR	X-linked recessive

C11.1 General Remarks

Hematologic abnormalities are common features of inherited metabolic diseases. Many of these have other major manifestations, including neurological features. On the other hand, in some inherited metabolic diseases, particularly those involving red cell energy metabolism, the hematological abnormalities may be the only manifestation of disease. The identification of a hematological abnormality, along with documentation of any nonhematological problems, often leads to the diagnosis of a specific inherited metabolic disease. A complete blood count and blood film may provide

E. Crushell (✉)
26 Wainsfort Grove, Terenure, Dublin 6 W, Ireland
e-mail: ellen.crushell@gmail.com

G. F. Hoffmann et al. (eds.), *Inherited Metabolic Diseases*,
DOI: 10.1007/978-3-540-74723-9_C11, © Springer-Verlag Berlin Heidelberg 2010

diagnostic clues and should be included in the work-up of all patients with a suspected metabolic disorder.

While many metabolic disorders are associated with secondary hematological findings [e.g., hypersplenism in Gaucher disease, neutropenia in propionic academia (PA)], sometimes the hematological disorder is the lead feature, as in Pearson marrow pancreas syndrome or the macrocytic anemia of inherited disorders of cobalamin metabolism. In many instances, the hematological abnormalities involve all the formed elements of the blood. In this chapter, these are discussed in the context of the most common or the most prominent abnormality. For example, type 1 Gaucher disease often presents as thrombocytopenia; however, neutropenia and anemia are almost always present, though rarely as prominent as the decrease in platelet counts.

C11.2 Abnormal Cell Morphology

Abnormal cell morphology on blood film or bone marrow aspirate may be the first pointer toward a metabolic diagnosis. See Table C11.1 for various abnormal cell morphologies found in metabolic disease. It is important to be aware that various primary hematological disorders (including malignancies) may produce similar morphological findings. Also, a "normal" blood film does not rule out a metabolic diagnosis such as a mucopolysaccharidosis where vacuolated lymphocytes may be few and far between.

C11.3 Hemolytic Anemia

Hemolytic anemia may be caused by factors within the red cell (intrinsic) or in the environment of the cell (extrinsic) (Table C11.2). Mature red cells contain no mitochondria and are totally dependent upon anaerobic glycolysis and the hexose monophosphate shunt to meet their energy needs and requirements for NADPH. Deficiencies of any of the enzymes involved may be associated with hemolytic anemia as a result of a deficiency of ATP or of reducing equivalents.

By far, the most common of the hereditary intrinsic defects causing hemolytic anemia is glucose-6-phosphate dehydrogenase deficiency. It is an X-linked recessive (XLR) condition that occurs with very high frequency in Mediterranean, African, and Asian populations. In some regions of Greece, one in three males is affected; in West Africa and some parts of India, the prevalence is up to 20–25%; in China, including Hong Kong, 3–5% of males are affected. Acute hemolysis is usually associated with exposure to oxidizing chemicals or drugs or ingestion of certain foods, such as fava beans, hence the historical name for the disease: favism (Table C11.3). Some parts of the world have introduced mass programs of newborn screening for the condition in an attempt to prevent the development of acute hemolysis, severe hyperbilirubinemia, and kernicterus.

Chronic isolated hemolytic anemia, characterized by jaundice, gallstones, indirect hyperbilirubinemia, and splenomegaly, is also seen in patients with inherited deficiencies of pyruvate kinase, 2,3 diphosphoglyceromutase, glucose phosphate isomerase, or hexokinase. The diagnosis may be suspected from the red cell morphology; however, confirmation generally requires analysis of the specific red cell enzymes; pyruvate kinase deficiency is the most common of this group of nonspherocytic hemolytic anemias (Table C11.2).

Deficiencies of other enzymes involved in anaerobic glycolysis also lead to hemolytic anemia with significant non-hematological problems, such as mental retardation, myopathy, ataxia, chronic metabolic acidosis, or stroke (Table C11.4).

The extrinsic hemolytic anemias may be caused by any inborn error that produces severe liver disease in infancy, such as galactosemia and neonatal hemochromatosis. Erythropoietic protoporphyria and Wilson disease also lead to hemolytic anemia. Skin changes such as photosensitivity, ulcers, or abnormal pigmentation, should prompt a porphyria screen in neonates and young children. Hemolytic anemia is often not the lead sign, but an associated finding, along with poor growth, poor feeding, vomiting, and hypotonia in methylmalonic aciduria, PA, and isovaleric aciduria, abetalipoproteinemia, and Wolman disease in the first year of life.

Early onset xanthomas and hypercholesterolemia (and elevated phytosterols) are seen in phytosterolemia. Lecithin:cholesterol acyltransferase deficiency is associated with corneal opacities and proteinuria.

Table C11.1 Abnormal blood cell morphology

Cell type	Morphology	Disorder
Red cells	Target cells	Liver disease
		Lecithin:cholesterol acyltransferase deficiency
		Abetalipoproteinaemia
	Spherocytes	Hypersplenism
		Liver disease
	Spiculated red cells – echinocytes ("burr") or acanthocytes ("spur")	Renal failure
		Vitamin E deficiency
		Abetalipoproteinaemia
		Wolman disease
		Cbl C defects
		Hallervorden–Spatz (panthothenate kinase) syndrome
		Pyruvate kinase deficiency
White cells	Basophilic stippling	Lead poisoning
		Iron deficiency
		Hemolytic anemias
		Pyrimidine-5' nucleotidase deficiency
	Vacuolated lymphocytes	Aspartylglucosaminuria
		Multiple sulfatase deficiency
		Ceroid lipofuscinoses
		Mucolipidosis II
		GM_1 gangliosidosis
		Mucopolysaccharidoses
		Niemann–Pick disease types A, C
		Pompe
		Sialidosis
		Wolman
	(Alder) Reilly bodies	Mucopolysaccharidoses
	"Sea blue" histiocytes	Niemann–Pick disease
		Ceroid lipofuscinoses
		Adult cholesterol ester storage disease
		GM_1 gangliosidosis
Bone Marrow	Foam cells	Niemann–Pick disease types A, B, C, D
		Gaucher disease types 1, 2, 3
		Gangliosidosis – GM_1 and GM_2
		Sialidosis I, II (late infantile)
		Mucolipidosis II, III, IV
		Fucosidosis
		Mannosidosis
		Ceroid lipofuscinoses
		Farber disease
		Wolman disease
		Cholesterol ester storage disease
		Cerebrotendinous xanthomatosis
		Chronic hyperlipidemia

Adapted from Lanzkowsky (2005)

Table C11.2 Hemolytic anemias

Intrinsic defects	Disorder/enzyme deficiency	Associated abnormalities and diagnosis
Anaerobic glycolytic enzyme deficiencies		
Isolated hemolytic anemia	Pyruvate kinase	Nonspherocytic hemolytic anemia, red cell enzyme assay
	Glucose phosphate isomerase	Nonspherocytic hemolytic anemia, red cell enzyme assay
	Hexokinase	Nonspherocytic hemolytic anemia, red cell enzyme assay
	2,3-diphosphoglyceromutase	Nonspherocytic hemolytic anemia, red cell enzyme assay
+ Neurological abnormalities	Phosphofructokinase	Prominent myopathy, cardiomyopathy in infants with severe disease. Diagnosis by enzyme assay or *PFKM* mutation analysis
	Triosephosphate isomerase	Autosomal dominant, early onset, neurodegenerative disease. Diagnosis by red cell enzyme assay or *TPI* mutation analysis
	Phosphoglycerate kinase	X-linked recessive (XLR) myopathy with chronic progressive encephalopathy. Diagnosis by red cell enzyme assay or *PGK1* mutation analysis
Hexose monophosphate shunt defects		
	Glucose-6-phosphate dehydrogenase	XLR hemolytic anemia. Diagnosis by red cell enzyme assay
	Glutathione synthetase	Autosomal recessive, metabolic acidosis, pyroglutamic aciduria (5-oxoprolinuria). Diagnosis by *GSS* mutation analysis
	Glutathione reductase	Nonspherocytic hemolytic anemia. Progressive neurological abnormalities in severe form. Diagnosis by red cell enzyme assay
Abnormal erythrocyte nucleotide metabolism		
	Adenosine triphosphatase	Red cell enzyme assay
	Adenylate kinase	*AK1* mutation analysis
	Pyrimidine 5-nucleotidase	Accumulation of pyrimidine nucleotides in red cells, most common disorder of nucleotide metabolism causing hemolytic anemia. Red cell assay
Extrinsic causes of hemolysis		
Hypersplenism	Gaucher disease	Leukocyte or fibroblast β-glucosidase, *GBA* mutation analysis
	Niemann–Pick disease	Leukocyte or fibroblast acid sphingomyelinase, *SMPD1* mutation analysis
Defects of porphyrin metabolism	Congenital erythropoietic porphyria	Autosomal recessive photosensitivity of the skin with blistering and scarring, red coloring of teeth and urine. Diagnosis by urinary porphyrin analysis, measurement of enzyme (uroporphyrinogen III cosynthetase), *UROS* mutation analysis
Disorders of lipid metabolism	Lecithin:cholesterol acyltransferase (LCAT)	Corneal opacities, "target cell" anemia, proteinuria, progressive renal impairment, low plasma esterified cholesterol. Diagnosis by plasma LCAT assay and by *LCAT* mutation analysis
	Abetalipoproteinemia	Steatorrhea, ataxia, 'burr' cells (acanthocytes), hypocholesterolemia. Diagnosis by plasma apolipoprotein analysis, *MTP* mutation analysis
Defects of sterol metabolism	Phytosterolemia (sitosterolemia)	Premature coronary artery disease. Diagnosis by plasma sterol analysis
Intoxications	Wilson disease	Hepatocellular dysfunction, neurological abnormalities, Kayser–Fleischer rings. Diagnosis by plasma ceruloplasmin analysis, urinary copper excretion, *ATP7B* mutation analysis

Table C11.3 Partial list of agents inducing hemolytic anemia in glucose-6-phosphate dehydrogenase deficiency

Antimalarials	*Antipyretics/analgesics*	*Others*
Primaquine	Acetylsalicylic acid	Chloramphenical
Pamaquine	Acetanilide	Isoniazid
Sulfonamides	*Infections*	*p*-Aminosalicylic acid
Sulfadiazine	Viral respiratory infections	Phenytoin
Sulfisoxazole	Viral hepatitis	Vitamin K (water soluble)
Nitrofurans	Typhoid	Naphthalene (moth balls)
Nitrofurantoin		Nalidixic acid

Table C11.4 Hemolytic anemia + neurological abnormalities

Disorder/enzyme deficiency	Gene	Inheritance	Diagnostic tests
Triosephosphate isomerase	*TPI1*	Autosomal dominant (AD)	Red cell enzyme assay, *TPI* mutation analysis
Phosphoglycerate kinase	*PGK1*	XLR	Red cell enzyme assay, *PGK* mutation analysis
Phosphofructokinase[a]	*PFKM*	AR	Ischemic exercise test, enzyme assay, in muscle, *PFK* mutation analysis
Abetalipoproteinemia	*MTP*	AR	Plasma apolipoprotein analysis, *MTP* mutation analysis
Hypobetalipoproteinemi[a]	*APOB*	AD	Plasma apolipoprotein analysis, *APOB* mutation analysis
Glutathione synthetase	*GSS*	AR	Red cell GSS assay, urinary organic acids showing pyroglutamic aciduria, mutation analysis
Wilson disease	*ATP7B*	AR	Plasma ceruloplasmin, urinary copper excretion, mutation analysis

[a]Myopathy

C11.4 Macrocytic Anemia

Inherited disorders of absorption, transport, or metabolism of vitamin B$_{12}$ (cobalamin) and folate may present with macrocytic anemia as the leading sign (Table C11.5). Elevated homocysteine with low methionine points toward a remethylation defect of homocysteine to methionine (Table C11.6).

Remember

- Over 95% of patients with macrocytic anemia in childhood are secondary to acquired deficiencies of folate or cobalamin.
- Macrocytosis may be masked by iron deficiency and thalassemia.
- High homocysteine and low methionine suggests inborn errors of cobalamin metabolism.
- Intermittent orotic aciduria may be seen in congenital folate deficiency.
- Absence of methylmalonic aciduria does not rule out a cobalamin defect.

Congenital (or acquired) disorders of nucleotide metabolism may also present with macrocytic anemia. In orotic aciduria caused by uridine monophosphate synthase deficiency, pyrimidine biosynthesis is interrupted, while in Lesch–Nyhan (hypoxanthine guanine phosphoribosyltransferase deficiency) disease, purine nucleotide regeneration is impaired (the resulting macrocytic anemia is usually a late feature). Thiamine-responsive megaloblastic anemia is associated with diabetes and sensorineural deafness (in some, the full DIDMOAD spectrum – diabetes insipidus, diabetes mellitus, optic atrophy and deafness – is present) only the anemia, however, will respond to high-dose thiamine treatment; the underlying defect is in thiamine transport.

The sideroblastic anemia in Pearson marrow pancreas syndrome associated with mitochondrial DNA deletions is macrocytic and associated with exocrine pancreatic dysfunction, growth failure, and lactic acidosis. The clinical phenotype may be or evolve into that of Kearns–Sayre syndrome.

Table C11.5 Macrocytosis[a]

Disorder	Disorder/enzyme deficiency	Associated abnormalities and diagnosis
Disorders of nucleotide metabolism		
Orotic aciduria	Uridine monophosphate (UMP) synthase deficiency	Autosomal recessive megaloblastic anemia and marked orotic aciduria responsive to treatment with uridine. Confirmation of diagnosis by *UMPS* mutation analysis
Thiamine-responsive megaloblastic anemia	Thiamine transporter protein	Autosomal recessive anemia responsive to high-dose thiamine treatment. Diagnosis confirmed by *SLC19A2* mutation analysis
Lesch–Nyhan disease	Hypoxanthine guanine phosphoribosyltransferase deficiency	X-linked recessive spasticity, variable psychomotor retardation, self-mutilation, with high plasma, and urinary urate. Diagnosis confirmed by enzyme assay and mutation analysis
Coblamin disorders		
Malabsorption	Imerslund–Grasbeck syndrome	Autosomal recessive megaloblastic anemia, with low plasma vitamin B_{12} levels
	Intrinsic factor deficiency	Low plasma vitamin B_{12} analysis; Schilling test – corrected by intrinsic factor
Transport	Transcobalamin II deficiency with normal serum cobalamin levels	Variable psychomotor retardation, hypotonia, methylmalonic aciduria (MMA), hyperhomocysteinemia, low methionine, normal plasma vitamin B_{12} levels. Diagnosis confirmed by measurement of plasma TC II
Metabolism	Defective synthesis of methylcobalamin – *cbl*E, *cbl*G	Variable psychomotor retardation, associated with hyperhomocysteinemia with low methionine and without MMA, normal plasma folate and vitamin B_{12}. Diagnosis by complementation studies in fibroblasts
	Defective synthesis of both adenosylcobalamin and methylcobalamin – *cbl*C, *cbl*D, *cbl*F	Psychomotor retardation, variable retinal dystrophy, associated with MMA and hyperhomocysteinemia with low methionine, normal plasma folate and vitamin B_{12}. Diagnosis by complementation studies in fibroblasts
Folate disorders		
Malabsorption	Congenital folate malabsorption	Chronic encaphalopathy, movement disorder, psychomotor retardation, pancytopenia, hypomethioninemia, low plasma folate
Metabolism	Methylene-tetrahydrofolate reductase (MTHFR) deficiency	Psychiatric disturbances, psychomotor retardation, movement disorder, with hyperhomocysteinemia, and low methionine. Diagnosis confirmed by enzyme assay or *MTHFR* mutation analysis
	Glutamate formiminotransferase deficiency	Variable psychomotor retardation, marked increase in urinary FIGLU excretion
	Dihydrofolate reductase deficiency	Phenotype unclear, mild psychomotor retardation? Features of folic acid deficiency that respond to treatment with N(5)-formyltetrahydrofolate but not to folic acid. Confirmation by *DHFR* mutation analysis
Others		
Mevalonic aciduria	Mevalonic acid kinase deficiency	Developmental delay, failure to thrive, hepatosplenomegaly, dysmorphic facies, recurrent fever with lymphadenopathy, with urinary excretion of mevalonic acid. Diagnosis confirmed by enzyme assay or *MVK* mutation analysis

[a]MCV > 85 fL and megaloblasts in bone marrow

Table C11.6 Key metabolic investigations of macrocytic anemia

Plasma cobalamin, plasma and red cell folate levels
Plasma total homocysteine, amino acids, lactate, urate
Urinary organic acids
Urinary orotic acid
Urine amino acids

Results from these initial investigations will determine further testing – e.g., Schilling test, folate challenge, mutation analysis, specific enzyme, or complementation studies

C11.5 Sideroblastic Anemia

Sideroblasts are red cell precursors with iron-loaded (Prussian blue staining) mitochondria clustered in a ring around the nucleus. Sideroblastic anemia is caused by mitochondrial dysfunction that may be primary or acquired. The acquired forms far outnumber the congenital forms; however, a hereditary form should be particularly sought in the young and in those without a history to suggest acquired forms (e.g., alcohol ingestion) (Table C11.7). Four of the eight enzymes necessary for the biosynthesis of heme are located in mitochondria (the other four are cytoplasmic and deficiencies do not result in sideroblasts, e.g., the porphyrias). Defective mitochondrial heme synthesis causes iron accumulation within the mitochondria resulting in oxidative mitochondrial damage and the formation of sideroblasts. Sideroblastic anemia is usually microcytic or normocytic with hypochromia; megaloblastic sideroblastic anemia suggests Pearson syndrome or thiamine-responsive megaloblastic anemia.

The acquired sideroblastic anemias are caused by inhibitors of 5-aminolevulinate synthase, such as isoniazid, cylcoserine, and lead. Chloramphenicol and ethanol also inhibit mitochondrial function resulting in sideroblastic anemia.

Partial response to pyridoxine treatment has been seen in some of the congenital and acquired sideroblastic anemias.

C11.6 Cytopenias

Decreased numbers of the formed elements of blood may occur as a result of defects in production or increased destruction. Pancytopenia is virtually a constant finding with propionate intoxication, which is a feature of some of the organic acidurias during acute decompensation. The mechanism is not understood, and there is no specific treatment other than restoration of metabolic control in these disorders. During periods of good metabolic control, the hematological picture generally normalizes.

Neutropenia is a chronic finding seen in glycogen storage disease 1b/c; patients often develop inflammatory bowel disease later in the course of the disease. The neutropenia responds to granulocyte-colony stimulating factor treatment. The neutropenia in Barth syndrome (XLR inheritance) may have a cyclical pattern associated with intermittent ulcers of the mouth.

Table C11.7 Sideroblastic anemias

Disorder	Gene	Inheritance	Diagnostic tests
Pearson marrow-pancrease syndrome[a]	mtDNA	Maternal/sporadic	Plasma immunoreactive trypsin (IRT), stool trypsin, analysis of mtDNA for deletions
Mitochondrial myopathy and sideroblastic anemia [b]	PUS1	Autosomal recessive	Mutation analysis
Anemia, sideroblastic, and spinocerebellar ataxia	ABC7	X-linked recessive (XLR)	Mutation analysis
Pyridoxine-responsive megaloblastic anemia	ALAS2	XLR	Response to high-dose pyridoxine treatment, mutation analysis

[a]Pancreatic insufficiency often precedes development of anemia
[b]With lactic acidosis

C11.6.1 Pancytopenia *(Table C11.8)*

Table C11.8 Pancytopenia

Associated finding	Disorder	Diagostic tests
Splenomegaly	Gaucher disease types 1 and 3	Leukocyte or fibroblast β-glucosidase, *GBA* mutation analysis
	Niemann–Pick disease type B	Leukocyte or fibroblast acid sphingomyelinase, *SMPD1* mutation analysis
+ Neurological abnormalities	Gaucher disease type 3	Leukocyte or fibroblast β-glucosidase, *GBA* mutation analysis
	Niemann–Pick disease type A	Leukocyte or fibroblast acid sphingomyelinase, *ASM* mutation analysis
Ketoacidosis, hyperammonemia, hypotonia	Propionic acidemia, methylmalonic aciduria, and isovaleric aciduria	Urinary organic acids, plasma acylcarnitine profile
Failure to thrive, diarrhea	Folate malabsorption	Plasma and red cell folate, plasma vitamin B_{12}, folate challenge test
	Transcobalamin II deficiency	Plasma transcobalamin II level, plasma vitamin B_{12} (normal)

C11.6.2 Neutropenia *(Table C11.9)*

Table C11.9 Neutropenia

Associated findings	Disorder	Diagnostic tests
Hepatomegaly, hypoglycemia, short stature, inflammatory bowel disease (late)	Glycogen storage disease 1b	Glucose challenge. Analysis of glucose-6-phosphatase in fresh (unfrozen) liver and liver that has been frozen and thawed for demonstration of latency. *G6PT* mutation analysis.
Hyperammonemia, failure to thrive, interstitial pneumonia, diarrhea	Lysinuric protein intolerance	Plasma and urine amino acids
Ketoacidosis, hypotonia, failure to thrive, developmental delay	Propionic acidemia, methylmalonic aciduria, isovaleric aciduria	Urinary organic acids, blood acylcarnitine profile
Cardiomyopathy and skeletal myopathy, short stature in a male	Barth syndrome	Urinary organic acids, cardiolipin electrophoresis, *TAZ* mutation analysis
Macrocytic anemia, developmental delay, and failure to thrive	Orotic aciduria	Urinary orotic acid, uridine monophosphates synthase (*UMPS*) enzyme assay or *UMPS* mutation analysis
Coarse facies, developmental delay, hepatomegaly, skeletal abnormalities	Aspartylglucosaminuria	Urine oligosaccharides, enzyme studies, *AGA* mutation analysis

C11.6.3 Thrombocytopenia *(Table C11.10)*

Table C11.10 Thrombocytopenia

Associated finding	Disorder	Diagnostic tests
Splenomegaly	Gaucher disease type 1	Leukocyte or fibroblast β-glucosidase, *GBA* mutation analysis
	Niemann–Pick disease type B	Leukocyte or fibroblast acid sphingomyelinase, *SMPD1* mutation analysis
Ketoacidosis, hypotonia, failure to thrive, developmental delay	Methylmalonic aciduria, Propionic acidemia, Isovaleric aciduria	Urinary organic acids, plasma acylcarnitine profile
Cardiomyopathy, ketoacidosis, macrocytic anemia	Cobalamin defects	Plasma homocysteine, amino acids, urinary organic acids, plasma cobalamin, complementation studies on cultured skin fibroblasts, specific mutation analysis
Lactic acidosis, hypotonia, dermatosis, alopecia	Holocarboxylase synthetase deficiency	Plasma lactate, ammonia, urinary organic acids, enzyme assay on fibroblasts

C11.7 Others

C11.7.1 Bleeding Tendency

Coagulopathy may be seen in any metabolic disorder associated with severe liver disease, such as galactosemia, fructosemia, tyrosinemia type I, and neonatal hemochromatosis. Because of deficient glycosylation, coagulation factors (especially XI) may be deficient in congenital disoders of glycosylation (CDG). Bleeding tendency associated with (hepato)splenomegaly, but without significant hepatic dysfunction, is found in Gaucher disease type 1 and glycogen storage disease type Ia and Ib/c.

C11.7.2 Hypercoagulability

The classic disorder associated with hypercoagulable states is homocystinuria. It has been shown that good metabolic control through dietary and medical intervention reduces the number of vascular events in classical homocystinuria. CDG is also associated with hypercoagulable states.

C11.7.3 Hyperleukocytosis

Hyperleukocytosis >100,000/mm^3 has been described in CDG IIc (GDP fucose transporter 1) or leukocyte adhesion deficiency S.

C11.7.4 Hemophagocytosis

Hemophagocytosis is encountered occasionally in patients with carnitine palmitoyltransferase I deficiency, propionic aciduria, hemochromatosis, lysinuric protein intolerance, Gaucher disease, and Niemann–Pick disease.

C11.7.5 Methemoglobinemia

Methemoglobinemia is the result of the failure of reduction of oxidized circulating hemoglobin, either as the result of exposure to strong oxidizing agents, such as nitrites or failure of the normal enzymatic reduction of heme. Congenital methemoglobinemia may occur as a result of deficiency of NADH-cytochrome b5 reductase that is limited to red cells (type I) or a generalized deficiency of the enzyme (type II), both are caused by mutations of the *CYB5R3* (formerly *DIA1*) gene. In type I, the only clinical abnormality is chronic persistent cyanosis resulting from methemoglobin accumulation and in type II, the methemoglobiemia is associated with a chronic progressive encephalopathy.

Key References

Cappellini MD, Fiorelli G (2008) Glucose-6-phosphate dehydrogenase deficiency. Lancet 371:64–74

Chiarelli LR, Fermo E, Zanella A et al (2006) Hereditary erythrocyte pyrimidine 5'-nucleotidase deficiency: a biochemical, genetic and clinical overview. Hematology 11:67–72

Finsterer J (2007) Hematological manifestations of primary mitochondrial disorders. Acta Haematol 118:88–98

Lanzkowsky, P (2005) Manual of pediatric hematology and oncology, 4th edn. Burlington, MA, Elsevier Academic Press.

Merle U, Schaefer M, Ferenci P et al (2007) Clinical presentation, diagnosis and long-term outcome of Wilson's disease: a cohort study. Gut 56:154

Ogier de Baulny H, Saudubray JM (2002) Branched-chain organic acidurias. Semin Neonatol 7:65–74

Rampoldi L, Danek A, Monaco AP (2002) Clinical features and molecular bases of neuroacanthocytosis. J Mol Med 80:475–491

Rosenblatt DS, Whitehead VM (1999) Cobalamin and folate deficiency: acquired and hereditary disorders in children. Semin Hematol 36:19–34

Sassa S (2000) Hematologic aspects of the porphyrias. Int J Hematol 71:1–17

Zanella A, Fermo E, Bianchi P et al (2005) Red cell pyruvate kinase deficiency: molecular and clinical aspects. Br J Haematol 130:11–25

Zimran A, Altarescu G, Rudensky B et al (2005) Survey of the hematological aspects of Gaucher disease. Hematology 10: 151–156

Immunological Problems

C12

Ertan Mayatepek

Key Facts

> Immunological problems can develop as permanent key manifestations of a metabolic disease (e.g., adenosine deaminase deficiency) or can occur inconstantly in individual patients.

> Inherited metabolic diseases associated with T cell immunodeficiency mainly feature purine nucleoside phosphorylase deficiency. This disease is characterized by severe viral, bacterial, or fungal infections. Milder impaired T cell function is sometimes seen in lysinuric protein intolerance, Menkes disease or Zellweger syndrome.

> B cell immunodeficiency has been observed in patients with transcobalamin II deficiency or propionic acidemia.

> Adenosine deaminase deficiency represents the best characterized inherited metabolic disease with combined T and B cell immunodeficiencies. Recurrent infections caused by a broad variety of microorganisms often become life-threatening. Bone marrow transplantation has been successful in some patients.

> Besides adenosine deaminase deficiency, immunological dysfunction affecting both the B and T cell lines has been reported in acrodermatitis enteropathica, biotinidase and holocarboxylase synthetase deficiencies, hereditary orotic aciduria, deficiency of intestinal folic acid absorption, α-mannosidosis, and in some patients with methylmalonic aciduria.

> Phagocytic dysfunction and neutropenia are characteristic findings in glycogen storage disease type I non-a. Dysfunction of phagocytes or neutropenia is also frequently observed in classical galactosemia, X-linked cardioskeletal myopathy (Barth syndrome), glutathione synthetase deficiency, or Pearson syndrome.

> NK cell immunodeficiency is very rarely associated with inborn errors of metabolism. In single cases, this immunological dysfunction has been reported in lysinuric protein intolerance.

C12.1 General Remarks

A wide range of immunological problems has been identified in association with inherited metabolic diseases, sometimes in single case reports, and in others as a constant clinical manifestation. In clinical practice, two situations arise: (1) the patient presents with a known metabolic disorder and immunological problems appear as recognized manifestations of the disease or (2) the patient presents with immunological problems and an underlying metabolic disorder is sought. Some metabolic defects lead to symptoms such as chronic or recurrent infection, or infection with unusual agents. An example of an inherited metabolic disease linked to an inflammatory periodic fever syndrome is mevalonic aciduria. Mutations and consecutively reduced activity of mevalonate kinase have

E. Mayatepek

Department of General Pediatrics, University Children's Hospital, Moorenstrasse 5, 40225 Düsseldorf, Germany
e-mai: mayatepek@uni-duesseldorf.de

G. F. Hoffmann et al. (eds.), *Inherited Metabolic Diseases*,
DOI: 10.1007/978-3-540-74723-9_C12, © Springer-Verlag Berlin Heidelberg 2010

been found in mevalonic aciduria as well as in hyperimmunoglobinemia D syndrome. Besides congenital malformations, hepatosplenomegaly, failure to thrive, developmental retardation and others, the clinical course of mevalonic aciduria is characterized by recurrent crises of fever, vomiting, and diarrhea, suggesting an infectious or autoimmune disease.

Clinically significant immunodeficiency presents with both, an unusual history of infection and corresponding confirmatory laboratory tests. Other patients may have milder manifestations or sometimes only laboratory evidence of immunological abnormalities. One or several major components of the immune system can be affected in distinctive metabolic diseases, single or combined T or B cell immunodeficiencies, phagocyte immunodeficiency, or natural killer (NK) cell immunodeficiency (Table C12.1 and C12.2).

C12.2 Inherited Metabolic Diseases Associated with T Cell Immunodeficiency

Purine nucleoside phosphorylase is required for normal catabolism of purines. In *purine nucleoside phosphorylase deficiency*, substrates accumulate that affect the immune and nervous systems. This disease is the

Table C12.1 Diagnostic tests in patients with a known metabolic disorder and frequent infections

History
Physical examination
Differential blood count
Sedimentation rate
Urine analysis
Chest X-ray
Immune work-up
B cell disorders
Quantitative immunoglobulins
Isohemagglutinin
Specific antibody titers
T cell disorders
Skin tests for tetanus, mumps and monilia (>3 years of age)
Lymphocyte count/differentiation
Lymphocyte stimulation
Thymus on X-ray studies
Phagocyte disorders
Granulocyte count
Nitro blue tetrazolium test
Neutrophil function tests

Table C12.2 Investigations for differential diagnosis of inherited metabolic diseases in patients with immunological problems

Urine
Purines and pyrimidines
Organic acids
Amino acids
Orotic acid
Oligosaccharides
Plasma/Serum
Lactate
Copper
Zinc
Very long-chain fatty acids
Folic acid
Transcobalmin II
Enzyme studies
Galactose-1-phosphate uridyl transferase
Biotinidase
Lysosomal enzymes
Mutational analysis (e.g., GSD type I non-a or Pearson syndrome)

most important metabolic disease associated with clinically relevant isolated T cell immunodeficiency resulting in severe immunodeficiency. The number of T cells is greatly reduced leading to lymphopenia and cutaneous anergy. Recurrent infections are usually obvious at least by the end of the first year. There is an enhanced susceptibility to viral diseases, such as varicella, measles, cytomegalovirus, and vaccina. Severe pyogenic or fungal infections also occur. T cell dysfunction may worsen in the course of the disease. Affected patients may have autoantibodies and autoimmune hemolytic anemia. Neurological symptoms include abnormal motor development, ataxia, and spasticity. Bone marrow transplantation can be curative.

Lysinuric protein intolerance is characterized by defective transport of the dibasic amino acids lysine, arginine, and ornithine in the intestine and renal tubules. Biochemically, this defect leads to decreased levels of these amino acids in plasma and increased levels in urine interfering with the urea cycle and consecutively hyperammonemia. Intestinal protein intolerance, failure to thrive, hepatosplenomegaly, and osteoporosis as well as progressive encephalopathy develop. Decrease in CD4+ T cell number, lymphopenia, and leukopenia have been reported, as well as decreased leukocyte phagocytic activity. As in purine nucleoside phosphorylase deficiency, varicella infection may follow an especially severe course.

Impaired T cell function has been also described in *Menkes disease*. This disorder is caused by a defect in a membrane copper transport channel which interferes with the absorption of copper and its distribution to the cells, resulting in generalized copper deficiency. Clinical symptoms of classical Menkes disease include neonatal hypothermia, unconjugated hyperbilirubinemia, mental retardation, seizures, typical facies, "kinky" hair, and abnormalities of connective tissue and bone. Immunological problems or infections are rare, but pulmonary infection secondary to inhalation may prove lethal.

Thymic hypoplasia and defective T cell function has been noted in some patients with *Zellweger syndrome*, the most severe of the disorders of peroxisome biogenesis. Affected infants exhibit extreme muscular hypotonia, seizures, liver dysfunction, dysmorphic skeletal, and eye abnormalities, failure to thrive, and mostly early death due to the progressive encephalopathy. Immunological problems are not usually of high clinical relevance.

C12.3   Inherited Metabolic Diseases Associated with B Cell Immunodeficiency

Transcobalamin II is necessary for intestinal absorption of cobalamin and transport to tissues. *Deficiency of transcobalamin* II leads to severe megaloblastic anemia with hypocellular bone marrow, leukopenia, thrombocytopenia, vomiting, failure to thrive, diarrhea, and lethargy. A frequent finding in transcobalamin II deficiency is the presence of hypogammaglobulinemia, particularly IgG. Less often, levels of IgA and IgM are found decreased. Failure to produce specific antibodies against diphtheria or poliomyelitis has been demonstrated in several patients. Although phagocytic killing is usually normal, a specific impairment of neutrophils against *Staphylococcus aureus* has been reported in a single patient. Immunological abnormalities usually resolve after cobalamin supplementation.

Propionic acidemia is caused by deficiency of propionyl-CoA carboxylase, a biotin-dependent enzyme. In the long-term mental retardation, an extrapyramidal movement disorder and osteoporosis develop in most patients. Decreased levels of IgG and IgM as well as B cell lymphopenia have been observed during periods of metabolic decompensation.

C12.4   Inherited Metabolic Diseases Associated with Combined T and B Cell Immunodeficiencies

Adenosine deaminase deficiency represents the best characterized metabolic disease leading to combined immunodeficieny. Adenosine deaminase deficiency accounts for up to 50% of the patients with autosomal recessive severe combined immunodeficiency (SCID) disease. Adenosine deaminase converts adenosine and deoxyadenosine to inosine and deoxyinosine. The resulting accumulation of deoxyadenosine and adenosine exerts toxicity to lymphocytes. Obviously, the severity of the disease correlates with accumulation of toxic metabolites and inversely with residual adenosine deaminase expression. Multiple, recurrent infections are usually more severe than in purine nucleoside phosphorylase deficiency and become rapidly life threatening. Typical laboratory findings include lymphopenia (usually <500 total lymphocytes per cubic millimeter), involving both the B and T cells as well as hypogammaglobulinemia. While IgM deficiency may be detected early, IgG deficiency manifests only after the age of 3 months, when the maternal supply becomes exhausted. Further immunologic abnormalities include a deficiency of antibody formation following specific immunization, and absence or severe diminution of lymphocyte proliferation induced by mitogens. This condition is progressive, since residual B and T cell function that may be found at birth disappears later on. Only a few patients have been reported with delayed (up to 3 years of age) or late (up to 8 years of age) onset. Infections can be caused by a broad variety of microorganisms. Localization of infections are predominantly the skin, and the respiratory as well as the gastrointestinal tract, where they often lead to intractable diarrhea and malnutrition. In patients older than 6 months of age, hypoplasia or apparent absence of lymphoid tissue may constitute a diagnostic sign. In about half of the patients bony abnormalities include prominence of the costochondral junctions. In some patients neurologic abnormalities are found, including spasticity, head lag, movement disorders, and nystagmus. Injections of bovine adenosine deaminase conjugated to polyethylene glycol (PEG-ADA) results in normalization of T cell number and cellular and humoral responses. Bone marrow transplantation has been very successful in some patients.

The disturbance of zinc homeostasis in *acrodermatitis enteropathica* results from a partial block in intestinal absorption. Reduced zinc absorption leads to impairment of the function of many zinc metalloenzymes, which are involved in major metabolic pathways. Symptoms usually start in infancy. The most dramatic clinical feature is a characteristic skin rash. In patients with zinc deficiency states, impaired humoral and cell-mediated immune responses can usually be demonstrated. Secondary infections are common, mostly with Candida or Staphylococci. Mucosal lesions include gingivitis, stomatitis, and glossitis. Further symptoms include diarrhea, failure to thrive, alopecia, irritability, and mood changes. Zinc therapy leads to clinical remission.

Biotin is a cofactor for carboxylation of 3-methylcrotonyl-CoA, propionyl-CoA, acetyl-CoA, and pyruvate. *Biotinidase deficiency* and *holocarboxylase synthetase deficiency* result in multiple carboxylase deficiency. Symptoms include lactic acidosis, muscular hypotonia, seizures, ataxia, psychomotor retardation, skin rashes, hair loss, and immune defects. Immunologic dysfunction affecting both the B and T cell lines has been reported in several children with biotinidase deficiency. Symptoms include mucocutaneous candidiasis, absence of delayed hypersensitivity as assessed by skin testing and by in vitro lymphocyte responses to Candida challenge, decreased IgA levels, poor antibody formation to pneumococcal immunization, subnormal amounts of T lymphocytes, reduced leukocyte killing against Candida, lack of myeloperoxidase acitivity in neutrophils, impaired lymphocyte suppressor activity, and decreased prostaglandin E_2 production in vitro. One child with biotinidase deficiency was diagnosed initially as having SCID and was treated with bone marrow transplantation, but the symptoms were not ameliorated until biotin was given. In general, immunological findings in biotinidase deficiency are inconsistent. However, biotin treatment corrects the immunologic as well as the metabolic abnormalities.

Hereditary orotic aciduria is an inborn error of pyrimidine metabolism characterized by growth retardation, developmental delay, and megaloblastic anemia unresponsive to cobalamin and folic acid. Lymphopenia and increased susceptibility to infections, including candidiasis, bacterial meningitis, and fatal varicella have been observed. Immunologic abnormalities are variable and include low T cell number, impaired delayed-type hypersensitivity response, reduced T cell-mediated killing, and decreased levels of IgG and IgA.

Deficiency of intestinal folic acid absorption leads to megaloblastic anemia, pychomotor retardation, seizures,

and ataxia. Recurrent infections are an occasional clinical feature. Inconstantly found immunologic abnormalities include decreased levels of IgM, IgG, and IgA as well as decreased proliferation to phytohemagglutinin and pokeweed mitogen (PWM).

α-Mannosidosis caused by deficiency of α-mannosidase leads to the accumulation of mannose-rich oligosaccharides in neural and visceral tissues. This lysosomal storage disease is characterized by progressive mental retardation, deafness, cataracts, corneal clouding, dysostosis multiplex, progressive ataxia, hernias and hepatomegaly. Many patients with α-mannosidosis have recurrent infections. Immunologic abnormalities may include decreased IgG levels, impaired lymphoproliferation to phytohemagglutinin, defective chemotaxis, phagocytosis, and bactericidal killing. In one patient, pancytopenia resulting from antineutrophil antibodies has been reported.

Leukopenia occurs in about 50% of patients with *methylmalonic aciduria*, a classical organic aciduria affecting branched-chain amino acid metabolism. Immunologic abnormalities associated with methylmalonic aciduria may include neutropenia, pancytopenia, decreased B and T cell numbers, low IgG levels, and impaired phagocyte chemotaxis. Specific lack of responsiveness to Candida antigen has been observed resulting in extensive dermatosis. In addition, methylmalonic acid inhibits bone marrow stem-cell growth in vitro.

C12.5 Inherited Metabolic Diseases Associated with Phagocyte Immunodeficiency

Galactosemia results from galactose-1-phosphate uridyl transferase deficiency and is characterized by jaundice, hepatomegaly, nuclear cataracts, mental disability, and feeding difficulties. Neonates with galactosemia are at increased risk for life-threatening sepsis from *Escherichia coli*. Granulocyte chemotaxis is impaired, whereas bactericidal activity is usually not affected. In vitro exposure of neutrophils from affected neonates to galactose results in impaired function.

Glycogen storage disease (GSD) *type I non-a* presents with hepatomegaly, hypoglycemia acidosis, and growth failure. The condition is clearly distinguished from GSD type Ia by the occurrence of recurrent severe bacterial infections and immunologic abnormalities, resulting from neutropenia as well as defective function of leukocytes. Neutrophil function is variable, in most patients random movement, chemotaxis, microbial killing, and respiratory burst are diminished. In contrast, monocytes have decreased respiratory burst, but usually have normal random and directed motility. T cell, B cell, and NK-cell functions are normal. In most patients, recurrent or chronic bacterial infections become a major clinical problem. These infections are underlined by a decreased number of neutrophils (usually below 1500/μL) combined with defective neutrophil and monocyte functions. Bone marrow examination shows hypercellularity. GSD type I non-a is caused by mutations in the glucose-6-phosphate translocase gene. This gene encodes a microsomal transmembrane protein that is expressed in numerous tissues, including monocytes and neutrophils. Frequently observed symptoms, such as inflammatory bowel disease similar to Crohn disease, oral lesions, and perianal abscesses are presumably related to defective neutrophil function. Neutrophil cell counts and some but not all neutrophil functions improve after subcutaneous treatment with granulocyte colony-stimulating factor.

X-linked cardioskeletal myopathy (*Barth syndrome*) is characterized by a congenital dilated cardiomyopathy and mitochondrial myopathy with growth failure. In most patients, moderate to severe neutropenia is a persistent feature leading to recurrent serious bacterial infections.

Glutathione synthetase deficiency causes severe metabolic acidosis and hemolytic anemia. In the course of the disease progressive neurological symptoms may develop, including psychomotor retardation, seizures, ataxia, and spasticity. In about 10% of affected patients, recurrent bacterial infections have been reported resulting from impaired bacterial killing. The patient's neutrophils fail to assemble microtubules during phagocytosis leading to damage to membranous structures. However, the susceptibility to infections is relatively mild. Treatment with vitamins E and C can restore abnormal immunologic functions.

Pearson syndrome is caused by large deletions and duplications in the mitochondrial DNA and characterized by exocrine pancreatic and liver dysfunction, failure to thrive as well as neuromyopathy. In addition to anemia and thrombocytopenia, neutropenia is a frequent finding.

In *isovaleric aciduria*, as in propionic acidemia or methylmalonic aciduria, neutropenia, and pancytopenia can develop during periods of acidosis. Neonatal sepsis can lead to early death. The bone marrow contains large numbers of immature cells, suggesting an arrest of maturation. The underlying mechanism, however, is not clear but probably related to the accumulation of CoA esters of organic acids.

Other inborn errors of metabolism including *acrodermatitis enteropathica, methylmalonic aciduria, propionic acidemia, Gaucher disease, lysinuric protein intolerance, Niemann-Pick disease, or α-mannosidosis* are at least in some patients associated with phagocyte dysfunction or macrophage activating syndrome.

C 12.6. Inherited Metabolic Diseases Associated with NK Cell Immunodeficiency

Lysinuric protein intolerance is one of the very few inborn errors of metabolism in whom NK cell immunodeficiency has been reported at least in single instances. Other syndromes such as the Chediak–Higashi syndrome, Sutor syndrome, Griscelli syndrome, or xeroderma pigmentosum form this specific subgroup of immunodeficiency disorders.

Take Home Messages

> Patients with inherited metabolic diseases may have immunological problems resulting in increased susceptibility to infections. In addition, infections may be secondary to chronic disease, malnutrition, movement disorders, or poor control of swallowing and resulting aspiration. In most metabolic defects, immunological abnormalities are secondary to the metabolic derangement. Immune dysfunction can affect any of the major components of the immune system: T cells, B cells (including immunoglobulins), phagocytes, e.g., neutrophils, monocytes, macrophages, natural killer (NK) cells, and complement.

> Primary metabolic immunodeficiency diseases include adenosine deaminase deficiency or purine nucleoside phosphorylase deficiency. Other inherited diseases with often compromised immunity include, beside others, inborn errors of cobalamin and folate metabolism, organic acidurias, and disorders of carbohydrate metabolism. In most of them, correction of the metabolic defect restores normal immune function.

Key References

Carapella-de Lacua E, Aiuti F, Lucarelli P et al (1975) A patient with nucleoside phosporylaswe deficiency, selective T-cell deficiency and autoimmune hemolytic anemia. J Pediatr 93:1000–1003

Cowan MJ, Wara DW, Packman S et al (1979) Multiple biotin-dependent carboxylase deficiencies associated with defects in T-cell and B-cell immunity. Lancet 2:115–118

Desnick RJ, Sharp HL, Grabowski GA et al (1976) Mannosidosis: clinical, morphologic, immunologic, and biochemical studies. Pediatr Res 10:985–996

Dionisi-Vici C, de Felice L, el Hachem M et al (1998) Intravenous immunoglobulin in lysinuric protein intolerance. J Inherit Metab Dis 21:95–102

Gitzelmann R, Bosshard WU (1993) Defective neutrophil and monocyte function in glycogen storage disease type Ib: a literature review. Eur J Pediatr 152:33S–38S

Hirschhorn R (1993) Overview of biochemical abnormalities and molecular genetics of adenosine deaminase deficiency. Pediatr Res 33:35S–41S

Houten SM, Kuis W, Duran M et al (1999) Muations in MVK, encoding mevalonate kinase, cause hyperimmunoglobulinaemia D and periodic fever syndrome. Nature Genet 22:175–177

Kobayashi R, Blum P, Gard S et al (1980) Granulocyte function in patients with galactose-1-phosphate uridyl transferase deficiency (galactosemia). Clin Res 28:109A

Ming JE, Stiehm ER, Graham JM Jr (2003) Syndromic immunodeficienies: genetic syndromes associated with immune abnormalities. Crit Rev Clin Lab Sci 40:587–642

Spielberg SP, Boxer LA, Oliver JM et al (1979) Oxidative damage to neutrophils in glutathione synthetase deficiency. Br J Haematol 42:215–223

Newborn Screening for Inherited Metabolic Disease

D1

Piero Rinaldo and Dietrich Matern

Key Facts

> The classic presentation of inborn errors of metabolism is with a free period of apparent health that may last days or even years, but it is followed by overwhelming life threatening disease.

> The episode usually follows catabolism introduced usually by acute infection; sometimes after surgery.

> Initial laboratory evaluation needs only the routine clinical laboratory to establish acidosis or alkaoisis, hyperammonemia, ketosis, hypoclycimia, or latic acidemia.

D1.1 General Remarks

Routine screening of all newborns for inherited disorders began in the 1960s after Horst Bickel had established an effective dietary therapy for phenylketonuria (PKU), and Robert Guthrie introduced a simple bacterial inhibition assay to detect elevated concentrations of phenylalanine in dried blood spots, a type of specimen universally now known as the "Guthrie card." Over time, newborn screening was extended to several other treatable metabolic and endocrine disorders including galactosemia, maple syrup urine disease, biotinidase deficiency, hypothyroidism, congenital adrenal hyperplasia (CAH), and hemoglobinopathies. In recent years, the scope of newborn screening has leaped forward exponentially by the introduction of acylcarnitine and amino acid analysis in Guthrie cards by tandem mass spectrometry (MS/MS). This multiplex platform allows the concurrent detection of disorders of amino acid, organic acid, and fatty acid intermediary metabolism and thus several of the most prevalent treatable inborn errors of metabolism. Although the implementation of MS/MS is not pursued consistently in different countries, there is a notable trend toward overall screening expansion. For example, by July 2009, all babies born in the United States were screened for the metabolic conditions included in the uniform panel recommended by the American College of Medical Genetics (ACMG). This chapter contains information on how to proceed when the results of first tier newborn screening for certain disorders are reported to be abnormal.

P. Rinaldo (✉)
Biochemical Genetics Laboratory, Mayo Clinic College of Medicine, 200 First Street S. W., Rochester, MN 55905, USA
e-mail: rinaldo@mayo.edu

G. F. Hoffmann et al. (eds.), *Inherited Metabolic Diseases*,
DOI: 10.1007/978-3-540-74723-9_D1, © Springer-Verlag Berlin Heidelberg 2010

D1.2 Hyperphenylalaninemias

Newborn hyperphenylalanemia can be caused by a variety of conditions. The primary genetic deficiency is that of phenylalanine hydroxylase, the enzyme that catalyzes the conversion of phenylalanine to tyrosine. Missing phenylalanine hydroxylase activity is the cause of PKU. In addition, abnormalities in the biosynthesis or regeneration of tetrahydrobiopterin (BH$_4$), the cofactor of this enzyme, are also detected. Secondary causes of an elevated concentration of phenylalanine include parenteral nutrition, drugs (trimethoprim, chemotherapeutic agents), and liver disease. Persistent hyperphenylalaninemia above 360–600 µmol/L is harmful to the developing brain, leading to progressive mental retardation, epilepsy, spasticity, and psychiatric problems. It can be prevented by early diagnosis and dietary restriction of phenylalanine intake, ideally beginning as soon as possible after birth but not later than 14 days of age.

Most neonates with significant hyperphenylalaninemia suffer from phenylalanine hydroxylase deficiency; the incidence in most Caucasian populations is between 1:4,000 and 1:12,000. For practical purposes, two forms of phenylalanine hydroxylase deficiency are distinguished: PKU, which requires treatment, and mild hyperphenylalaninemia (phenylalanine levels <600 µmol/L), which does not. Flowchart 1 depicts the work-up of a neonate with hyperphenylalaninemia recognized through newborn screening, according to the ACT sheet established by ACMG (available online at http://www.acmg.net/). High phenylalanine values should be confirmed through quantitative analysis of plasma amino acids so that concentrations of tyrosine as well as phenylalanine are known. Analysis of urinary pterins and the activity of dihydropteridin reductase in blood should always be carried out to exclude BH$_4$ cofactor deficiency. A positive response of the BH$_4$ loading test is of immediate therapeutic relevance. Treatment of PKU should be started immediately with a phenylalanine restricted diet and supplementation of essential amino acids. Recommended therapeutic phenylalanine values differ between countries but should not be above 240–360 µmol/L in the first 6–10 years of life. Most diets are more liberal for teenagers. There is no consensus with regard to whether or not treatment is necessary in adulthood, with the exception of pregnancy, when plasma concentrations of phenylalanine must be kept below 360 µmol/L throughout gestation in order to minimize the potential teratogenic effects of phenylalanine on a developing fetus.

D1.3 Galactosemia

The activated 1-phosphate metabolites of both galactose and fructose are highly toxic, particularly for liver, kidneys, and brain. In classical galactosemia, galactose-1-phosphate (Gal-1-P) accumulates because of a defective synthesis of UDP-galactose catalyzed by galactose-1-phosphate uridyltransferase (GALT). Affected children show symptoms such as vomiting, diarrhea, and jaundice progressing after the start of milk (lactose) feedings, usually from the 3rd or 4th day of life onwards. Untreated, the disease usually progresses to hepatic and renal failure, and death; there may be progressive bilateral cataracts. The severe acute manifestations of galactosemia can be prevented by exclusion of galactose from the diet. Late complications such as ovarian failure and impaired speech and language development may occur despite good compliance with treatment. The preventive potential of newborn screening may not be fully realized if infants become symptomatic before the newborn screening results are available. The incidence of classic galactosemia in newborn screening programs in the United States has ranged from 1:55,000 to 1:80,000. False negative findings in newborn screening may be observed after blood transfusion.

Newborn screening is carried out either by measurement of the activity of GALT alone or (less frequently in the US) in combination with determination of the total galactose concentration. The combined approach allows identification not only of GALT deficiency, but also of galactokinase deficiency and epimerase deficiency. A positive screening result is followed up by measurement of GALT activity in red blood cells. When GALT activity is reduced, further diagnostic characterization is possible by isoelectric focusing of the GALT protein on a gel, which helps to determine either the classic GG variant, the other common variant Duarte (DD), compound heterozygotes (DG), or heterozygotes. A large number of different mutations have been identified in the GALT gene. The Duarte variant has an allele frequency of ca. 6% and is associated with a 50% reduction in enzyme activity, which does not usually require dietary intervention. Even in compound heterozygotes with a severe mutation on the other allele, diet may not be necessary. Therefore, a majority of children with elevated galactose concentrations found in newborn screening may have a mild form of GALT deficiency that does not require treatment. In these children, galactose and Gal-1-P concentrations on an ordinary diet often normalize within a few weeks or months.

When galactose is <20 mg/dL (1.1 mmol/L) it is sufficient to check the general condition (feeding, vomiting, weight gain, and liver size) and to send another blood spot sample for galactose measurements (preferentially taken 60 min after a milk feed) to the newborn screening laboratory.

When *galactose is between 20–50 mg/dL* (1.1–2.8 mmol/L) or when it has been determined that the infant has a GG or DG phenotype, determination of plasma galactose and erythrocyte Gal-1-P are carried out in 1–3 mL of EDTA blood shipped at ambient temperature. Molecular genetic testing of the GALT gene is also available to confirm the diagnosis. EDTA blood may be stored at room temperature for a couple of days, if necessary. Lactose-free milk feedings are recommended until final results are available.

Immediate hospital admission is necessary in the presence of *galactose concentrations above 50 mg/dL* (>2.8 mmol/L), laboratory signs of liver disease, or clinical distress. Lactose-free feedings should be commenced as soon as the appropriate blood and urine samples have been taken (amino acids and reducing substances in the urine, determination of plasma galactose and erythrocyte Gal-1-P, complete blood cell count). Coagulation studies and blood cultures (*Escherichia coli* sepsis is common) should be considered in all patients not clinically normal.

The indication for long-term therapy ultimately rests on degree of GALT deficiency and the concentration of Gal-1-P in erythrocytes, which is normally below 0.3 mg/dL (11 μmol/L) but may rise up to 100 mg/dL (~4 mmol/L) in classical galactosemia. It is impossible to obtain completely normal Gal-1-P levels in most GG patients because of a substantial endogenous production of galactose. Therapeutic target concentrations of 2–4 (at most five) mg/dL are realistic.

D1.4 Biotinidase Deficiency

The carboxylation of 3-methylcrotonyl-CoA, propionyl-CoA, acetyl-CoA, and pyruvate is biotin dependent. The individual apoenzymes need to be covalently bound to biotin in order to generate the active holoenzymes. This reaction is catalyzed by the enzyme holocarboxylase synthetase. A deficiency of this enzyme causes severe, multiple carboxylase deficiency, which usually presents in the newborn period. Affected children show severe metabolic decompensation typical for an organic aciduria and progressive neurological problems; in addition, there are usually skin rashes and alopecia. Another, milder but therefore often insidious form of multiple carboxylase deficiency is caused by an impaired release of covalently bound biotin from dietary and endogenous proteins, a reaction that is catalyzed by the enzyme biotinidase. The deficiency of biotinidase causes a depletion of free biotin and progressive neurological and dermatological symptoms usually starting in infancy. Symptomatology includes seizures, ataxia, hearing loss, optic atrophy, spastic diplegia, and developmental delay as well as skin rash and alopecia. These characteristic symptoms may occur in half of the affected patients, but less specific symptoms such as hypotonia, developmental delay, and seizures may occur in some cases. Because of the insidious onset of symptoms, the diagnosis is often delayed or even missed. This is a major concern since this form of multiple carboxylase deficiency can be effectively treated with biotin. A semiquantitative colorimetric or fluorometric measurement of biotinidase activity in dried blood spots has therefore been included in newborn screening programs in many countries.

False positive results may occur with improper handling of samples (e.g., exposure to excessive heat). On the other hand, false negative findings in newborn screening may be observed after blood transfusion or when the neonate received a catecholamine infusion during blood sampling. Residual biotinidase activity may vary, depending on the underlying mutations in the biotinidase gene. Mild forms of biotinidase deficiency with relatively high enzyme activity levels occur that do not cause disease and do not require treatment. Nevertheless, it is advisable to start biotin supplementation immediately after an abnormal newborn screening result has been reported, before confirmatory tests are completed. It is also advisable to collect samples for blood ammonia, plasma lactate, and urinary organic acids before commencing biotin supplementation to evaluate the baseline metabolic status. Treatment is simple and does not involve complicated dietary regimens as in some other disorders that are included in newborn screening programs. Temporary initiation of biotin supplementation does not interfere with breastfeeding and parent–child interaction. The recommended starting dose is 10 mg/day. If a reduced biotinidase activity is confirmed in the repeat blood spot screening test, biotinidase activity should be determined in serum. A residual activity of 0–10% indicates profound biotinidase deficiency. Long-term treatment with 5–20 mg biotin/day is usually adequate. Treatment can be reevaluated by determining the activity of carboxylases in lymphocytes. Biotinidase activity between 10 and 25% indicate partial deficiency which may not require long-term treatment. Many centers recommend treatment of these children with 10 mg/day for the first year of life. It is not yet clear what regimens are optimal for control of late complications, particularly to the optic and auditory nerves.

D1.5 Congenital Hypothyroidism

Congenital hypothyroidism occurs in infants who are born without the ability to produce adequate amounts of thyroid hormone. Thyroid hormone is essential for normal growth and brain development. If untreated, congenital deficiency of thyroid hormone results in mental retardation and stunted growth. Infants with untreated congenital hypothyroidism may appear clinically normal up to 3 months of age, by which time some brain damage will already have occurred. When symptoms or clinical signs are present, they may include prolonged newborn jaundice, constipation, lethargy, poor muscle tone, feeding problems, macroglossia, mottled and dry skin, distended abdomen, and umbilical hernia.

The most common causes are total or partial failure of the thyroid gland to develop (aplasia or hypoplasia) or its development in an abnormal location (an ectopic gland). These types of hypothyroidism rarely recur in siblings. Less commonly, the hypothyroidism results from a hereditary inability to manufacture thyroid hormones, maternal medications during gestation (iodine and antithyroid drugs), or maternal antibodies.

The initial screening test is the assay of thyroid stimulating hormone (TSH) to detect an elevated concentration (usually >20 μU/mL). However, in some laboratories the assay of thyroxine (T_4) is preferred, others measure both. Newborns with TSH >50 μU/mL are considered very likely to have congenital hypothyroidism, and, therefore, require immediate follow-up testing of plasma and treatment. Those having a less prominent elevation of TSH are evaluated by confirmatory serum tests (free T_4, T_3 resin uptake, and TSH).

Treatment includes oral L-T_4 at a dosage to maintain blood TSH concentration <4 μU/mL and T_3/T_4 in the age-related range. Dosage and follow-up should be coordinated in consultation with a pediatric endocrinologist.

D1.6 Congenital Adrenal Hypoplasia (CAH)

Infants with CAH have a deficiency of one of several adrenal enzymes involved in steroid biosynthesis resulting in limited cortisol production and, in some cases, limited aldosterone production. The pituitary gland senses the cortisol deficiency and produces increased amounts of ACTH. The adrenal glands enlarge but continue to produce inadequate amounts of cortisol. Some of the precursors of cortisol are virilizing hormones. As a result of cortisol deficiency, affected infants are unable to respond adequately to the stress of injury or illness. Because of aldosterone deficiency, sodium and water are lost in the urine resulting in dehydration. Potassium accumulates in the blood, causing irritability or lethargy, vomiting, and muscle weakness, including cardiac muscle irritability and weakness, leading to shock and death in a salt-wasting crisis.

Male infants with CAH usually appear normal at birth. Female infants usually show the effects of elevated virilizing hormones: an enlarged clitoris and fusion of the labia majora over the vaginal opening. Occasionally, the female infant may be virilized so as to appear to have a male penile structure with hypospadia. Such newborns should not have a palpable gonad in the labial/scrotal sac. Their ovaries, uterus, and Fallopian tubes are normal.

Several types of genetic defects cause the enzymatic deficiencies of CAH. All are autosomal recessive. The traditional newborn screening test is designed to detect the accumulation of 17-hydroxy progesterone (17-OHP), the result in most cases (>90%) of underlying 21-hydroxylase deficiency. In clinical practice, however, one should remember that an abnormal newborn screening test can also indicate rarer enzyme deficiencies which cause CAH, for example, 11-hydroxylase deficiency.

The screening test for CAH is an immunoassay for 17-OHP, a precursor of cortisol. Cross reactivity with other steroids is a frequent interference, in particular among premature newborns. If screening indicates the possibility of CAH, an emerging, cost-effective approach is to perform on the same blood spot a second tier test by LC-MS/MS for the determination of 17-OHP, androstenedione, and most importantly cortisol, the end product of the pathway (Lacey et al. 2004). This approach can eliminate more than 90% of potential false positive results of the primary screening (frequently >1% of all newborns, and a much greater proportion of premature babies), and could include additional informative markers such as 11-deoxy cortisol and 21-deoxy cortisol (Minutti et al. 2004). Overall, steroid profiling by LC-MS/MS achieves improved specificity, and could potentially evolve into a first tier screening with clinically validated cutoffs based on birth weight, gender, and comparison with disease ranges.

Effective treatment for CAH is hormone replacement. Decisions about hormonal treatment should be made in consultation with a pediatric endocrinologist and may include hydrocortisone and mineralocorticoids. Medications need to be adjusted as the child grows. Serum adrenal hormone levels and renin are monitored. Female infants who have virilization of the genitalia may need surgical correction. This is usually done in stages, with the first surgery before the age of 2 years. Infants with CAH, if detected early and treated with appropriate doses of medication, can have normal growth, development, and intellectual potential. In addition, fertility is usually normal.

D1.7 Expanded Newborn Screening of Metabolic Conditions by MS/MS

Tandem MS/MS has been used for the detection and analysis of acylcarnitines since the 1980s. This technique has been extended to newborn screening because of the development of automated, high-throughput techniques of sample preparation and injection into the instrument. In most laboratories, acylcarnitines and amino acids are derivatized as butyl esters.

Amino acids are of course the building block of proteins. Acylcarnitines are formed from free carnitine and acyl-CoA moieties derived from fatty acids and organic acids (which may have been derived from amino acids) through the action of one of several carnitine-acyl-CoA transferases. The concentration of acylcarnitine species increases in response to many possible metabolic defects, leading to complex profiles with as many as 18 informative markers, each of them requiring various degrees of differential diagnosis. In other words, the many progresses achieved at the analytical level have no remedy, or substitute, for the inevitable complexity of post-analytical interpretation (Rinaldo, Cowan, Matern 2008).

More than 60 metabolic conditions could be detected by multiplex analysis of acylcarnitine and amino acid. Forty-two of them have been included in the screening panel recommended by the American College of Medical Genetics ACMG in 2006, which includes a total of 29 primary targets (collectively described as the uniform panel) and 25 secondary targets (Watson 2006a & b). The metabolic conditions screened for by MS/MS are divided in 20 primary and 22 secondary targets, based on our understanding of the natural history and severity of the disorders and available evidence of effective modalities of treatment. However, it must be underscored that sorting, and "elimination," of conditions that are detected based on exactly the same markers is unrealistic and potentially dangerous. In reality, all but one of the secondary targets, 2–4 dienoyl-CoA reductase deficiency, are involved to some degree in the differential diagnosis of one or more primary targets.

Table D1.1 summarizes the main characteristics of the 42 metabolic conditions included in the ACMG recommended panel. In addition to basic disease information (MIM number, common name if applicable, and name of the deficiency enzyme or function), the table lists the analytes and major ratios relevant to the detection of each condition. This information is combined with an estimate of the likelihood of correct identification (sensitivity) and of detection of carriers. The latter situation is usually encountered when a newborn investigated for an abnormal result is found to be an obligate heterozygote born to an affected, possibly asymptomatic and therefore undiagnosed mother.

Table D1.2 focuses primarily on the analytes rather than the conditions. It also highlights the critical need

Table D1.1 Inborn errors included in the American College of Medical Genetics recommended panel

Group	MIM number	Common name	Code	Name of deficient enzyme or function	Biochemical markers		Likelihood of identification by NBS using cutoffs based on disease ranges	Detection of carriers by NBS
					Informative analytes	Informative ratios		
AA	261600	Phenylketonuria (PKU) (classic)	PKU	Phenylalanine hydroxylase	Phe	Phe/Tyr	High	Possible (maternal cases)
AA	261600	Hyper-phenylalaninemia	H-PHE	Phenylalanine hydroxylase	Phe	Phe/Tyr	Low if cutoff >150 μmol/L	–
AA	248600	Maple syrup urine disease	MSUD	Branched-chain α-keto acid dehydrogenase	Ile + Leu (Xle), Val	Xle/Phe Xle/Ala Val/Phe	High (with 2nd tier test)	–
AA	207900	Argininosuccinic acidemia	ASA	Argininosuccinate lyase	ASA, Cit	ASA/Arg Cit/Arg	Low if Asa not measured	–
AA	215700	Citrullinemia type I	CIT	Argininosuccinate synthetase	Cit	Cit/Arg	High	–
AA	605814 603472	Citrullinemia type II (newborn/adult)	CIT	Aspartate glutamate carrier (citrin)	Cit, Arg, Met, Thr	Cit/Arg	Unknown, but likely to be low at age <7 days	–
AA	236200	Homocystinuria	HCY	Cystathionine β-synthase	Met	Met/Phe	High (with 2nd tier test)	–
AA	180960 250850 606664	Hypermethioninemias	MET	Methionine adenosyltransferase I/III, S-adenosylhomocysteine hydrolase, Glycine N-methyltransferase deficiency	Met	Met/Phe	High	–
AA	276700	Tyrosinemia type I	TYR I	Fumarylacetoacetate hydrolase	Succinylacetone	–	Low if based on Tyr and succinylacetone is not measured (Turgeon et al. 2008)	–
AA	276600	Tyrosinemia type II	TYR II	Tyrosine transaminase	Tyr	–	High	–
AA	207800	Argininemia	ARG	Arginase	Arg	Cit/Arg	High	–
AA	276710	Tyrosinemia type III	TYR III	4-Hydroxyphenyl pyruvate acid oxidase (dioxygenase)	Tyr	–	Unknown, but likely to be high	–
AA	126090 261630	Disorders of biopterin regeneration	BIOPT (REG)	Dihydropteridine reductase, pterin-4α-carbinolamine dehydratase 2	Phe	Phe/Tyr	High	–
AA	600225 261640	Disorders of biopterin biosynthesis	BIOPT (BS)	GTP cyclohydrolase, 6-pyruvoil tetrahydropterin synthase	Phe	Phe/Tyr	High	–
FAO	212140	Carnitine uptake defect	CUD	Plasma membrane carnitine transporter	C0	AC/Cit	High	Possible (maternal cases)
FAO	201475	Very long-chain acyl-CoA dehydrogenase deficiency	VLCAD	Very long-chain acyl-CoA dehydrogenase	C14:2 C14:1 C14	C14:1/C2 C14:1/C16	Potential false negatives	Possible
FAO	609015	Trifunctional protein deficiency	TFP	Trifunctional protein (α, β subunit)	C16:1-OH C16-OH C18:1-OH C18-OH	C16-OH/C16	High	–
FAO	609016	Long-chain 3-OH acyl-CoA dehydrogenase deficiency	LCHAD	Long-chain L-3-hydroxy dehydrogenase	C16:1-OH C16-OH C18:1-OH C18-OH	C16-OH/C16	High	–

Class	OMIM	Disorder	Abbrev.	Selected species	Ratios	Detectability	Possible maternal cases
FAO	607008	Medium-chain acyl-CoA dehydrogenase deficiency / Medium-chain acyl-CoA dehydrogenase	MCAD	C6 C8 C10:1 C10	C8/C2 C8/C10	High	Possible (maternal cases)a
FAO	255110	Carnitine:acylcarnitine translocase deficiency / Carnitine:acylcarnitine translocase	CACT	C14 C16 C18		High	–
FAO	255110	Carnitine palmitoyl-transferase II deficiency / Carnitine palmitoyltransferase II	CPT II	C14 C16 C18	(C16 + C18:1)/C2	High	–
FAO	130410 231675 608053	Glutaric acidemia type II / α-ETF β-ETF ETF-QO	GA II	C4 C5 C8 C5DC C14 C16	All related ratios	High	–
FAO	255120	Carnitine palmitoyl-transferase Ia deficiency (L) / Carnitine palmitoyltransferase Ia	CPT I	C0 C16 C18	C0/(C16 + C18)	High	–
FAO	201470	Short-chain acyl-CoA dehydrogenase deficiency / Short-chain acyl-CoA dehydrogenase	SCAD	C4	C4/C2 C4/C3 C4/C8	High	–
FAO	602199	Medium-chain ketoacyl-CoA dehydrogenase deficiency / Medium-chain ketoacyl-CoA thiolase	MCKAT	C8 C8-OH		Unknown	–
FAO	601609	Medium/short-chain 3-OH acyl-CoA dehydrogenase deficiency / Short-chain L-3-hydroxy acyl-CoA dehydrogenase	M/SCHAD	C4-OH		Unknown	–
FAO	222745	2,4 Dienoyl reductase deficiency / 2,4-Dienoyl-CoA reductase	DE-RED	C10:2		Unknown	–
OA	251000	Methylmalonic acidemia (Mut) / Methylmalonyl-CoA mutase	MUT	C3	C3/C2 C3/C16	High (with 2nd tier test)	Possible (maternal cases)
OA	251100 251110	Methylmalonic acidemia (Cbl A, B) / Adenosylcobalamin synthesis	Cbl A Cbl B	C3	C3/C2 C3/C16	High (with 2nd tier test)	–
OA	277400 611935	Methylmalonic acidemia (Cbl C, D) / MMA mutase, Hcy:MTHFR methyl transferase, MMADHC protein (C2ORF25)	Cbl C Cbl D	C3	C3/C2 C3/C16	High (with 2nd tier test)	–
OA	606054	Propionic acidemia / Propionyl-CoA carboxylase	PA	C3	C3/C2 C3/C16	High (with 2nd tier test)	–
OA	253270	Multiple carboxylase deficiency / Holocarboxylase synthetase	MCD	C3 C5-OH	All related ratios	Uncertain	Possible (maternal cases)
OA	243500	Isovaleric acidemia / Isovaleryl-CoA dehydrogenase	IVA	C5	C5/C0 C5/C2 C5/C3	High	–
OA	231670	Glutaric acidemia type I / Glutaryl-CoA deydrogenase	GA I	C5DC (C0)	C5DC/C5-OH C5DC/C8 C5DC/C16	Potential false negatives	Possible (maternal cases)a
OA	210200	3-Methyl crotonyl-CoA carboxylase deficiency / 3-Methylcrotonyl-CoA carboxylase (α, β subunit)	3MCC	C5-OH (C0)	C5-OH/C8 C5-OH/C0	High	Possible (maternal cases)
OA	203750	β-Ketothiolase deficiency / β-Ketothiolase	BKT	C5-OH C5:1 C4-OH	C5-OH/C8	High	–
OA	246450	3-Hydroxy 3-methyl glutaric acidemia / 3-Hydroxy-3-methylglutaryl-CoA lyase	HMG	C5-OH C6DC	C5-OH/C8 C5-OH/C0	High	–
OA	600301	2-Methyl butyryl-CoA dehydrogenase deficiency / 2-Methylbutyryl-CoA dehydrogenase	2MBG	C5	C5/C0 C5/C2 C5/C3	High	–
OA	250950	3-Methyl glutaconic acidemia / 3-Methylglutaconyl-CoA hydratase	3MGA	C5-OH	C5-OH/C8	High	–
OA	611283	Isobutyryl-CoA dehydrogenase deficiency / Isobutyryl-CoA dehydrogenase	IBG	C4	C4/C2 C4/C3 C4/C8	High	–
OA	300256	2-Methyl 3-hydroxybutyryl-CoA dehydrogenase deficiency / 2-Methyl 3-hydroxybutyryl-CoA dehydrogenase	2M3HBA	C5-OH C5:1	C5-OH/C8	Uncertain	–
OA	248360	Malonic acidemia / Malonyl-CoA decarboxylase	MAL	C3DC	C3DC/C10	High	

For abbreviations of metabolites see Table D1.2. AC sum of selected species $(C_0 + C_2 + C_3 + C_{16} + C_{18} + C_{18:1})$

aDetection is possible due to secondary carnitine deficiency of the newborn

Table D1.2 Metabolites investigated by mass spectrometry screening

Informative marker	Molecular weight (butyl ester)	Differential diagnosis PRIMARY conditions	Differential diagnosis SECONDARY conditions	Differential diagnosis OTHER conditions	Critical ratio	2nd tier test	Initial confirmatory testing	Urgency of clinical action
Glycine (Gly)	132	–	–	NKHG	–	–	PAA, CSF GLY	Low
Alanine (Ala)	146	–	–	LA	–	–	PAA, L and P	Low
Proline (Pro)	172	–	–	PRO I, PRO II, LA	–	–	PAA	Low
Valine (Val)	174	MSUD	–	PDH (E3), VAL	–	Allo-Ile	PAA, UOA	High
Threonine (Thr)	176	–	CIT II	–	–	–	PAA	Low
Glutamine + Pyroglutamic acid (Gln + Pyrog)	186	–	—	OXO-PRO OTC CPS	Gln/Cit	Orotic acid	PAA, UOA	Uncertain
Leucine/Isoleucine/OH Proline (Xle)	188	MSUD	–	PDH (E3), OH-PRO	–	Allo-Ile	PAA, UOA	High
Ornithine + Asparagine (Orn + Asn)	189	–	–	H-ORN, HHH	–	–	PAA, UAA	Uncertain
Lysine (Lys)	203	–	RED	H-LYS	–	–	PAA, PAC	Low
Methionine (Met)	206	HCY	MET	MTHFR, Cbl E, Cbl G, Cbl D v1	Met/Phe	HCY	PAA, tHCY	High
Phenylalanine (Phe)	222	Phenylketonuria	H-PHE, BIOPT (BS), BIOPT (REG)	–	Phe/Tyr	–	PAA, UPTR	High
Arginine (Arg)	231	ARG	CIT II	–	–	–	PAA	Moderate
Citrulline (Cit)	(215) 232	CIT I, ASA	CIT II	PC OTC CPS	–	–	PAA, UOA	High
Tyrosine (Tyr)	238	TYR I	TYR II, TYR III	–	–	SUAC	PAA, UOA	Moderate
Glutamic acid (Glu)	260	ASA	–	OTC CPS	Glu/Cit	Orotic acid	PAA, UOA	Uncertain
Argininosuccinic acid (ASA)	459	CUD	–	–	ASA/Arg	–	PAA, UOA	High
Carnitine (C0)	218		CPT I	Maternal cases (CUD, GA I, 3MCC)	C0/(C16 + C18)	–	PC, PAC	Moderate
Propionylcarnitine (C3)	274	PA, MUT, CBL A,B	Cb C, D	SUCLA2, Vit B12 def (mat)	C3/C2	MMA MCA HCY	PC, PAC, UOA	High
Formiminoglutamic acid (FIGLU)	287	–	SCAD, IBG	FIGLU			PAC, UOA	Low
Butyryl-/Isobutyrylcarnitine (C4)	288	–	SCAD, IBG, GA II	EE, FIGLU		EMA	UAG, UOA, PAC, UAC	Low
Tiglylcarnitine (C5:1)	300	BKT	2M3HBA	–			see C5-OH	High
Isovaleryl-/2-methylbutyrylcarnitine (C5)	302	IVA	2MBG, GA II	EE			UAG, UOA, PAC	High
OH Butyrylcarnitine (C4-OH)	304	BKT	2M3HBA, S/MCHAD	–			UOA, PAC	Uncertain
Hexanoylcarnitine (C6)	316	MCAD	GA II	–			see C8	see C8

OH Isovalerylcarnitine (C5-OH)	318	3MCC, HMG, BKT, MCD	2M3HBA, 3MGA	BIOT (partial)	C5-OH/C0, C5-OH/C8	–	–	UOA, PAC, UAC	Low for 3MCC, high for other conditions
Octanoylcarnitine (C8)	344	MCAD	GA II, MCKAT	–	C8/C2	–	–	UAG, UOA, PAC	High
Malonyl-/OH Octanoylcarnitine (C3DC)	360	–	MAL, MCKAT	–	C3DC/C10	–	–	UOA, PAC	
Decadienoylcarnitine (C10:2)	368	–	DE-RED	–		–	–	PAC, PAA	Uncertain
Decenoylcarnitine (C10:1)	370	MCAD	GA II	–		–	–	*see C8*	*see C8*
Decanoylcarnitine (C10)	372	MCAD	GA II	–		–	–	*see C8*	*see C8*
Succinyl-/methylmalonylcarnitine (C4DC)	374	MUT, Cbl A,B	–	SUCLA2		MMA MCA HCY	–	UOA, PAC	Low
Glutaryl-/OH Decanoylcarnitine (C5DC)	388	GA I	GA II	–	C5DC/C5OH	–	–	UOA, PAC, UAC	High
Dodecenoylcarnitine (C12:1)	398	VLCAD	–	–		–	–	*see C14:1*	
Dodecanoylcarnitine (C12)	400	VLCAD	–	–		–	–	*see C14:2*	
Methylglutarylcarnitine (C6DC)	402	HMG	–	–		–	–	*see C5-OH*	
Tetradecanedioylcarnitine (C14:2)	424	VLCAD, LCHAD/TFP	GA II	–		–	–	*see C14:1*	
Tetradecenoylcarnitine (C14:1)	426	VLCAD, LCHAD/TFP	GA II	–	C4:1/C2, C14:1/C16	–	–	PAC, UOA, DNA	High
Tetradecanoylcarnitine (C14)	428	VLCAD, LCHAD/TFP	CACT, CPT II	–		–	–	*see C14:1*	
Palmitoylcarnitine (C16)	456	VLCAD	CPT I (low), CACT, CPT II	–		–	–	PC, PAC, UOA	High
OH Hexadecenoylcarnitine (C16:1-OH)	470	LCHAD/TFP	–	–		–	–	*see C16-OH*	
OH Palmitoylcarnitine (C16-OH)	472	LCHAD/TFP	–	–	C16-OH/C16	–	–	PC,PAC,UOA	High
Linoleylcarnitine (C18:2)	480	LCHAD/TFP	CPT II	–		–	–	*see C16*	
Oleylcarnitine (C18:1)	482	VLCAD, LCHAD/TFP	CPT I (low), CACT, CPT II, GA II	–		–	–	*see C16*	
Stearylcarnitine (C18)	484	VLCAD	CPT I (low), CACT, CPT II, GA II	–		–	–	*see C16*	
OH Oleylcarnitine (C18:1-OH)	498	LCHAD/TFP	–	–		–	–	*see C16-OH*	
OH Stearylcarnitine (C18-OH)	500	LCHAD/TFP	–	–		–	–	*see C16-OH*	

PAAs plasma amino acids; *PAC* plasma acylcarnitines; *PC* plasma carnitine; *tHCY* total homocysteine; *UOA* urinary organic acids

Fig D1.1 Short-term
follow-up algorithm for
elevated phenylalanine
detected by newborn
screening. Reproduced from
http://www.acmg.net, with
permission

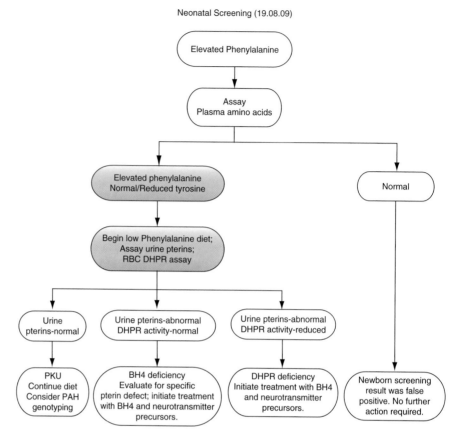

Neonatal Screening (19.08.09)

for differential diagnosis, the availability of particularly informative ratios, and the existence of second tier tests which, like in the case of CAH, could dramatically improve the overall performance of a screening program (Matern et al. 2007). Finally, the table mentions the confirmatory tests to be performed as first line of confirmatory evaluation, and a subjective assessment of the urgency of clinical action. Obviously, many factors may have a role in the timing of clinical intervention, and such estimates should be considered carefully on a case by case basis.

The inherent complexity of these tables should be sufficient to call attention to the need to carefully monitor the performance of a screening laboratory, and to assess it based on objective metrics (Rinaldo, Zafari 2006). A collaborative effort that involves more than 100 laboratories worldwide has set the following targets of adequate performance for newborn screening by MS/MS: (1) detection rate of at least 1:3,000 births (assuming testing for most of the 20 conditions included in the uniform panel); (2) False positive rate <0.3%; and (3) Positive predictive value >20%. To achieve these targets, the collaborative project collects data to

define evidence-based, clinically driven cutoff target ranges for all analytes detected by MS/MS, and calculated ratios. The cutoff target range could be either above (high) or below (low) the range of the normal population. Briefly, the high target range is defined as the interval between the cumulative 99%ile of the normal population and the lowest 5%ile of disease ranges, if the analyte is informative for multiple conditions. On the other hand, the low target range is defined as the interval between the highest 99%ile of disease ranges, if the analyte is informative for multiple conditions, and the 1%ile of the normal population. When the degree of overlap between normal population and disease range makes it inapplicable to use the criteria stated above, one or both limits are modified to give priority to the disease range, and may require the use of a second tier test to maintain adequate specificity (low false positive rate) (Matern et al. 2007 and Oglesbee et al. 2008). This effort is based on data from more than 7,500 true positive cases, 3–5 new cases are added daily. More information about this initiative can be found at the project website at: http://www.region4genetics.org.

Take Home Messages

> NBS is a universal public health program aimed to avoid mortality, morbidity and disabilities by early identification of treatable conditions and pre-symptomatic intervention

> Many biochemical markers detected by MS/MS require a careful differential diagnosis between multiple conditions

> Guidelines for clinical and laboratory follow up of an abnormal NBS result are available on line, see for example www.acmg.net.

Key References

Lacey JM, Minutti CZ, Magera MJ, Tausher AL, Casetta B, McCann M, Lymp J, Hahn SH, Rinaldo P, Matern D (2004) Improved specificity of newborn screening for congenital adrenal hyperplasia by second tier steroid profiling using tandem mass spectrometry. Clin Chem 50:621–625

Matern D, Tortorelli S, Oglesbee D, Gavrilov D, Rinaldo P (2007) Reduction of the false positive rate in newborn screening by implementation of MS/MS-based second tier tests: the Mayo Clinic experience (2004–2007). J Inherit Metab Dis 30:585–592

Minutti CZ, Lacey JM, Magera MJ, Hahn SH, McCann N, Schulge A, Cheillan D, Dorche C, Chace DH, Lymp JF, Limmerman D, Rinaldo P, Matern D (2004) Steroid profiling by tandem mass spectrometry improves the positive predictive value of newborn screening for congenital adrenal hyperplasia. J Clin Endocrinol Metab 89:3687–3693

Oglesbee D, Sanders KA, Lacey JM, Magera MJ, Casetta B, Strauss KA, Tertorelli S, Rinaldo P, Matern D (2008) 2nd-Tier test for quantification of alloisoleucine and branched-chain amino acids in dried blood spots to improve newborn screening for maple syrup urine disease (MSUD). Clin Chem 54:542–549

Rinaldo P, Zafari S, Tortorelli S, Matern D (2006) Making the case for objective performance metrics in newborn screening by tandem mass spectrometry. MRDD Res Rev 12:255–261

Rinaldo P, Cowan TM, Matern D (2008) Acylcarnitine profile analysis. Genet Med 10:151–156

Turgeon C, Magera MJ, Allard P, Torterelli S, Gavrilov D, O glesbee D, Raymond K,   Rinaldo P, Matern D (2008) Combined newborn screening for succinylacetone, amino acids, and acylcarnitines in dried blood spots. Clin Chem 54: 657–664

Watson MS, Lloyd-Puryear MA, Mann MY, Rinaldo P, Howell RR (eds) (2006a) Newborn screening: toward a uniform screening panel and system (main report). Genet Med 8(Supplement):12S-252S

Watson MS, Mann MY, Lloyd-Puryear MA, Rinaldo P, Howell RR (eds) (2006b) Newborn screening: toward a uniform screening panel and system (executive summary). Genet Med 8(Supplement):1S-11S

Biochemical Studies

D2

K. M. Gibson and C. Jakobs

Key Facts

> Evidence for the presence of an inherited metabolic disease may often be derived from detailed clinical evaluation of the patient and examination of the family history (Nyhan et al. 2005).

> Important stumbling blocks in identifying an inherited metabolic disease include the fact that signs and symptoms are often nonspecific, leading to initial testing to exclude routine childhood illnesses and delaying consideration of metabolic disorders.

> Even when appropriately suspected, ordering physicians may be unfamiliar with important biochemical interrelationships and the appropriate diagnostic tests to order, occasionally leading to inappropriate sample collection and storage.

> Absence of acute metabolic decompensation (e.g., hyperammonemia, hypoglycemia, overwhelming metabolic acidosis, and anion gap) does not necessarily rule out an inherited metabolic disease.

> Consultation and coordination with a licensed clinical biochemical genetics laboratory helps insure that appropriate tests are ordered, the correct samples are obtained, and the limitations of the testing scheme are clearly defined prior to metabolic work-up.

K. M. Gibson (✉)
Department of Biological Sciences, Michigan Technological University, Dow 740, ESE 1400, Townsend Drive, Houghton, MI 49931, USA
e-mail: kmgibson@mtu.edu

This chapter draws extensively on previously published work: Hoffmann et al. (2002). The authors acknowledge the use of that material.

D2.1 General Remarks

Most known inherited metabolic diseases are identified via biochemical analyses of various body fluids, predominantly blood and urine, but also cerebrospinal, vitreous, and even bile fluids. Concentrations of physiologically relevant metabolites[*] in plasma or serum are generally tightly controlled, and thus increases/decreases of specific intermediates may have diagnostic relevance. Normative data for many compounds of intermediary metabolism are highly dependent upon the metabolic state at sampling, and appropriate interpretation of assay results requires knowledge of intake and other physiological data, including fasting or postprandial status or postexercise status. Some disorders may only be identified through specific function tests (e.g., loading) that stress metabolic conditions or result in supraphysiological increases in metabolite load (see Chap. D8). Such tests have inherent risks and escalate the potential for metabolic overload and decompensation; accordingly, such tests should only be instituted by experienced clinicians in the appropriate hospital setting, and only when other diagnostic options that carry less patient risk have been exhausted (Table D2.1).

Many inherited metabolic disorders induce the accumulation of substrates, which are metabolized via alternative processes (alternate pathways, liver biotransformation) and/or removed via excretion in the urine. Studies carried out in urine for many such diseases may be more straightforward and sensitive than plasma/serum analyses. Differences in fluid intake and

G. F. Hoffmann et al. (eds.), *Inherited Metabolic Diseases*,
DOI: 10.1007/978-3-540-74723-9_D2, © Springer-Verlag Berlin Heidelberg 2010

Table D2.1 An overview of metabolic investigations described in this chapter

Simple colorimetric evaluations in urine
Amino and organic acids, carnitine, and acylcarnitines
Lactate, pyruvate, nonesterified fatty acids, and ketones
Congenital disorders of glycosylation
Purines and pyrimidines, orotic acid
Sugars and polyols
Glutathione
Mucopolysaccharides and oligosaccharides
Very long-chain fatty and pristanic acids (peroxisomal function)
Creatine and folate
Sterols, bile acids, and porphyrins
Biogenic amines and pterins

*see also Blau et al. 2003, 2005

urinary dilution, and their effect on metabolite concentrations, are usually accounted for by correcting urine metabolite levels with creatinine output. Urine analyses are generally less influenced by metabolic and nutritional changes, since the specimen is collected over a time period and often (but not always) there are significant differences between normal and pathological values that are readily recognized. As a general rule, a spot urine sample (morning void to enhance metabolite concentrations) is sufficient for most studies. Exceptions may occur, however, as in the case of some fatty acid oxidation disorders that frequently show urinary abnormalities only under fasting or loading conditions, or in the case of certain disorders (e.g., cystinuria, porphyrias, etc.) where a 24-h urine collection may be required.

Laboratory investigations for inherited metabolic diseases are complex and susceptible to technical problems. To maintain acceptable standards, laboratories performing biochemical investigations for inherited metabolic diseases should process a sufficiently high number of samples to maintain diagnostic acumen and should participate in quality assurance/quality control (QA/QC) processes.

Referring physicians should bear in mind that many analyses are often qualitative and not quantitative (although the expanding implementation of tandem mass spectrometry (MS–MS) is changing this paradigm), thereby leading to a certain level of subjective interpretation. Furthermore, the conditions examined are biochemically heterogeneous in their expression, which can complicate identification of subtle abnormalities. For these reasons, diagnostic

laboratories must adhere to the accepted practices of internal and external QC schemes, which insure ongoing education of laboratory staff and competence in analytical performance. External schema are particularly important, providing data on accuracy and bias of results. Participation in external QC schemes (and acceptable performance) is a requirement for external accreditation of the laboratory. In the USA, the College of American Pathologists (CAP) offers proficiency testing for urine and blood amino acids, urine organic acids, plasma acylcarnitines, and qualitative mucopolysaccharide analyses. European Research Network for Inherited Disorders of Metabolism offers these and a more extensive menu of special assays in urine and blood, proficiency testing for purine and pyrimidine analysis, and has recently instituted a pilot program for lysosomal enzyme analysis. Depending on the country or region, laboratory accreditation may be optional or mandatory, the latter being the case in the USA (CAP).

D2.2 Simple Colorimetric Evaluations of Urine

A number of simple tests are available that may be carried out in nonspecialized hospitals or at the bedside, and provide important first clues for the diagnosis of metabolic disorders.

D2.2.1 Dinitrophenylhydrazine (DNPH) Test

Method

Mix 1.0 mL urine with 1.0 mL 0.2% DNPH solution.

The DNPH assay detects urine α-keto acids via formation of hydrazones that precipitate out of solution. Several metabolic disorders may be detected, including phenylketonuria (PKU), maple syrup urine disease (MSUD), tyrosinemia type I, tyrosyluria, histidinemia, and methionine malabsorption syndrome. Acetone also yields a positive result and may suggest ketonuria associated with hyperglycinemia, branched-chain organic acidurias, and glycogen storage disorders. A 2 N HCl test is performed on all DNPH positives to determine the presence of false positive results. Substances with low acid solubility may cause interference. Mandelamine (methenamine mandelate), an antibacterial medication, and radiopaque contrast material will form a precipitate immediately upon the addition of DNPH. The color and immediacy of precipitate formation distinguishes it from the yellowish precipitate of α-keto acid hydrazones. Information on medications is critical prior to use of the DNPH test. The DNPH test may be carried out by caregivers and may be useful in the management of patients with MSUD living at some distance from the Metabolic Center.

D2.2.1.1 Reducing Substances in Urine

Method

Commercially available test tablets (e.g., Clinitest®, Bayer Corporation).

Numerous disorders lead to the urinary excretion of sugars and other reducing substances, some of which are described in Table D2.2. Urine reducing substances may be detected with commercially available test tablets which provide a color change in the presence of reducing substances. This test, in conjunction with the Multistix analysis described later, can assist in differentiating between glucose-related and nonglucose-related reducing substances.

Table D2.2 Urine reducing substances (with associated disorders or conditions)

Galactose (classical galactosemia, galactokinase deficiency, liver disease, secondary galactose intolerance)
Fructose (fructose intolerance, essential fructosuria)
4-Hydroxyphenylpyruvate (tyrosinemia types I/II, bacterial contamination of urine)
Homogentisic acid (alkaptonuria)
Xylose (pentosuria)
Glucose (diabetes mellitus, Fanconi syndrome)
Oxalate (hyperoxaluria)
Salicylates, ascorbic acid (drugs)
Uric acid (hyperuricosuria)
Hippurate (sodium benzoate treatment of hyperglycinemia and hyperammonemia)

D2.2.1.2 Rapid Urinalysis

Method

Commercially available reagent test strips (Multistix 10 SG/Multistix PRO 11®, Bayer Corporation).

Multistix 10 SG and Multistix PRO 11 provide qualitative colorimetric analysis of protein, blood, leukocytes, nitrite, glucose, ketones (acetoacetic acid), pH, specific gravity, creatinine, bilirubin, and urobilinogen in urine. Methodology, interpretation, and characteristics of the approximate linearity of these measurements are provided in the package insert. In addition, for each test expected values, limitations, and interfering substances are described. This screening procedure can provide insight into likelihood of bacterial infection/contamination, kidney and liver function, acid–base balance, and/or carbohydrate metabolism.

A number of interferences can occur for each metabolite estimated. Certain medications (e.g., riboflavin or drugs containing azo dyes, or nitrofurantoin) may lead to urine discoloration and test interference. False negatives for glucose may be encountered with ascorbate levels >50 mg/dL or in the presence of ketones. Ascorbate interferes with bilirubin estimation, as does indican (indoxyl sulfate). Estimation of ketones is hampered by the presence of highly pigmented samples, levodopa metabolites, and sulfhydryls. False positives for heme (blood) may arise from oxidizing contaminants (hypochlorite) or microbial peroxidase (urinary tract infection). Finally, protein in the urine may be overestimated in highly buffered or alkaline samples or in urine contaminated with quaternary ammonium compounds (antiseptics and detergents).

D2.2.2 Cyanide Nitroprusside Test (Brand Reaction)

Method

Add 0.4 mL of 5% NaCN to 1.0 mL urine. After 10 min add 0.2 mL of 0.5% Na-nitroprusside (Na-nitroferricyanide). Mix and immediately assess the color.

Table D2.3 Intermediates generating a positive nitroprusside reaction (and associated disorder or condition)

Cystine (cystinuria, hyperaminoaciduria)
Homocysteine (homocystinuria, cobalamin disorders, cystathioninuria, urinary tract infection)
Glutathione (disorders of the γ-glutamyl cycle)
Drugs (see text)

The Brand reaction identifies free sulfhydryl or disulfide compounds in urine. Cyanide reduces any disulfides to free sulfhydryls. In the subsequent reaction, a reddish color results when free sulfhydryl groups complex with nitroprusside. A positive result is usually due to cystine in the urine. Familial cystinuria is among the most common aminoacidurias. Disulfides are also excreted in other metabolic disorders such as homocystinuria and β-mercaptolactate-cysteine disulfiduria. Both will produce a positive result. The urine specimen should be at approximately neutral pH. If the sample has been preserved with acid, a false positive reaction may occur. Drugs such as N-acetylcysteine, 2-mercaptoethanesulfonate, 2-mercaptopropionylglycine, captopril, penicillamine, and large amounts of synthetic penicillin metabolites and acetoacetate will yield false positives; accordingly, a listing of medications must be obtained. Bacterial contamination may also generate a false positive. Cystathionine, methionine, and taurine are not detected (Table D2.3).

D2.2.3 Ehrlichs Aldehyde Reagent

Method

Add 1.0 mL of urine to 0.1 mL 2% p-dimethylaminobenzaldehyde in 2 N HCl. Mix and assess color formation after 10 min.

The Ehrlichs test detects porphobilinogen (PBG) or urobilinogen in urine. PBG yields a red color in urine for the patient with acute porphyria. Urobilinogen, a component of heme degradation, results when bilirubin analogs are secreted into the bile and further degraded by intestinal bacteria. In the normal patient, some urobilinogen is reabsorbed and transported to the kidneys where it is converted to urobilin (yellow) and excreted. However, the majority of urobilinogen is converted microbially to sterobilin (deep red-brown).

Urobilin is responsible for the characteristic color of urine, while sterobilin is a major pigment of feces. Indoles in the urine may also give a positive Ehrlich test.

Individuals with porphyria may present with acute attacks, skin lesions, or both, but rarely prior to the onset of puberty. An attack usually consists of severe abdominal pain and may be associated with neurological findings. Such attacks are associated with excessive amounts of δ-aminolevulinic acid (ALA) and PBG in the urine. PBG deaminase deficiency (acute intermittent porphyria) is the most common form of porphyria. A positive Ehrlich test, coupled with hepatosplenomegaly, indicates that evaluation of tyrosine metabolites in urine (nitrosonaphthol test) should be pursued.

D2.2.4 Nitrosonaphthol Test (Tyrosine Metabolites)

Method

Three drops of clear urine are sequentially treated with 1.0 mL 2.6 N nitric acid, 1 drop 2.5% sodium nitrite, and 0.2 mL 1 mg/mL 1-nitroso-2-naphthol. After 15 min, the color formation is recorded. As blank, water is substituted for urine; N-acetyl-L-tyrosine (0.04 mg/mL 1 M HCl) is employed to develop a qualitative standard curve.

4-Hydroxylated phenolic acids (and to a limited extent hydroxylated indoles derived from tryptophan) conjugate with 1-nitroso-2-naphthol in the presence of nitric acid to yield orange/red chromophores. The corresponding tyrosine analogs include 4-hydroxyphenylpyruvate, 4-hydroxyphenyllactate and 4-hydroxyphenylacetate, and tyrosine itself. A limitation of this method is transient newborn tyrosinemia, a common finding as the hepatic enzymes involved in tyrosine metabolism may develop slowly. 4-Hydroxyphenylacetate may be elevated as a result of intestinal bacterial metabolism, malabsorption and other disorders, and may lead to false positives. Some disorders of carbohydrate metabolism, and liver dysfunction, may also alter tyrosine metabolism and produce positives. Patients undergoing parenteral nutrition are often supplemented with tyrosine analogs, which can lead to difficulties in interpretation. Patients with adrenal tumors may excrete increased homovanillic acid (HVA) and/or 5-hydroxyindoleacetic acids (HIAA) (end products of dopamine and serotonin metabolism, respectively), which yield pink and purple chromophores with nitrosonaphthol. Any positive should be correlated with clinical history and/or followed-up with more specialized testing (blood amino acids/urine organic acids).

D2.2.5 Sulfite Test

Method

Commercially available dipstick (Merckoquant 10013, Merck Darmstadt, Germany); fresh urine.

The sulfite test recognizes increased concentrations of sulfite in the urine that may be a marker of primary deficiencies of the enzyme sulfite oxidase or molybdenum cofactor deficiency. Children affected with one of these disorders typically suffer from severe epileptic encephalopathy, which usually starts in the neonatal period or infancy. Testing for urinary sulfite should be part of baseline investigations in any child with unexplained psychomotor delay particularly in combination with severe epilepsy. The test may be falsely negative if old urine samples are used for testing. False positive results may be caused by various drugs and other conditions that cause increased urinary sulfite concentrations.

D2.3 Amino Acids

Physiological amino acids occupy essential positions in intermediary metabolism as the building blocks of proteins, but also are involved in numerous other metabolic processes including methylation reactions, neurotransmission, energy production, and others. A long list of inherited metabolic diseases either directly or indirectly affect amino acid metabolism (both catabolic and anabolic processes), and lend themselves to detection through careful analysis of the appropriate physiological fluid.

D2.3.1 Plasma

Sample

One to two milliliter heparinized blood, with plasma immediately separated. If shipped, the sample should be sent on dry ice.

Quantitative amino acid analysis in plasma (or serum) by ion-exchange chromatography or HPLC (ninhydrin or phenylisothiocyanate derivitization) provides pertinent information on alterations in amino acid homeostasis and is one of the first-line investigations performed in a patient with suspected inherited metabolic disease. It is also the confirmatory adjuvant for follow-up of positive newborn screening results (see Chap. E1). Analysis should be performed promptly in patients with hyperammonemia or with an acute presentation of a suspected amino acid disorder; the results should be available STAT. Routine (fasting) amino acid analysis is also necessary in patients that are protein restricted or receiving specific metabolic dietary therapy, in order to adjust amino acid intake and to identify any deficiencies of essential amino acids. Many amino acids (but not all as yet, especially the dibasic amino acids) can also be quantified reliably in dried blood spots (Guthrie cards) by electrospray tandem MS–MS or fast atom bombardment (FAB) MS (see later). For some disorders such as PKU this is a superior technology (throughput, time savings) to classical chromatographic methods (analysis time from 2 to 3 h) with less invasive approaches for the patient. The newest technological advance for amino acid analysis is the UPLC–MS/MS methodology. This system employs high flow rate (to 20,000 psi) and small resin particle size to enable extremely rapid analysis and resolution. Analysis of a sample from a suspected MSUD patient can be achieved in minutes with absolute quantification (stable isotope internal standards). An added advantage over current electrospray MS–MS is that stereoisomers (e.g., leucine/isoleucine) are separated on the UPLC system. This technology is rapidly developing, and may eventually replace older (yet still robust) ninhydrin-based amino acid analyzers widely in use.

Remember

Although amino acid analysis can be quantitatively performed, slight deviations in one (or even a few) intermediate(s) do not necessarily indicate a defect of amino acid metabolism. The entire pattern of physiologically relevant amino acids should be reviewed by an experienced biochemical geneticist whose training has included evaluation of numerous chromatograms over a number of years.

When looking at 20–30 physiologically relevant amino acids in plasma, artifacts are a common occurrence (Table D2.4), linked to other pathological states, infection, nutritional status, and a host of other variables. Plasma amino acid levels are dependent upon metabolic status, and routine sampling should occur 4–6h after the last meal. Furthermore, it may be useful to quantify amino acids in postprandial (and fasting) samples, particularly when disordered energy metabolism is suspected. For postprandial analyses it may be advisable to provide a defined meal to achieve standardized substrate intake (see Chap. D8 for more information). Postprandial samples may reveal significant elevations of essential amino acids. For example, an excessive alanine increase indicates impaired pyruvate handling and may suggest a mitochondrial disorder. Conversely, fasting results in a marked elevation of the branched-chain amino acids (leucine, isoleucine, and valine), while most other amino acids are low.

For optimal results in amino acid analysis, it is important to separate plasma or serum from cells as soon as possible. Hemolysis or transport of whole blood

Table D2.4 Facts and artifacts for selected plasma amino acid elevations (and associated conditions)

Glycine (organic acidurias, nonketotic hyperglycinemia, valproate treatment)

Serine (tracks with glycine as a result of metabolic interconversion; decreased in serine biosynthetic defects)

Phenylalanine (phenylketonuria and biopterin disorders, tyrosinemias, liver disease)

Tyrosine (tyrosinemia I, II, III; liver disease)

Arginine (argininemia; decreased in trauma, shock, hemolysis).

Methylhistidines, anserine, carnosine (consumption of fowl)

Methionine (homocystinuria, cobalamin disorders, pernicious anemia, liver disease)

Citrulline (argininosuccinic aciduria and citrullinemias, decreased in certain forms of pyruvate carboxylase deficiency and urea cycle disorders (ornithine transcarbamylase, carbamylphosphate synthetase, NAGS))

results in essentially useless values for some amino acids (e.g., arginine or taurine), either through the action of erythrocyte enzymes such as arginase (which converts arginine to ornithine) or through concentration gradients between cells and fluid (e.g., liberation of taurine from platelets). Exact arginine concentrations are essential for diagnosis and treatment monitoring of urea cycle defects. Even after prompt separation, shipment at ambient temperature results in questionable values for several amino acids, e.g., glutamate, aspartate (both artificially elevated), glutamine, asparagine, cysteine, and homocyst(e)ine (reduced). The concentrations of some amino acids (phenylalanine, tyrosine, valine, isoleucine, and leucine) are less affected by overnight shipment of room temperature plasma or serum, but frozen samples are optimal to avoid artifactual results.

Certain amino acids, notably homocysteine and tryptophan, require specific methods for exact quantification. Determination of total homocysteine is critical for the evaluation of hyperhomocysteinemias, due to both cystathionine-β-synthase deficiency and cobalamin disorders. For optimal results, immediately centrifuge the blood sample, order total homocysteine, and transport plasma to the laboratory (if short transit time, room temperature is acceptable; for longer transport times, freeze plasma and ship on dry ice). Analytically, homocysteine is released from disulfide conjugates by treatment with reducing agents, and the total homocysteine concentration is determined. Normative data for total homocysteine (fasting) in children <10 year approximates 3.5–9 μmol/L; >10 year, 4.5–11 μmol/L; women (premenopausal) 6–15 μmol/L; and postmenopausal 6–19 μmol/L; men 8–18 μmol/L. Reference ranges, however, must be established in the individual laboratories and include normal and pathological samples.

D2.3.2 Urine

Sample

Minimum 10 mL urine, preferably a morning void but a random sample is acceptable, without preservatives. If shipped, transport on dry ice.

Quantitation of urine amino acids is usually less revealing than comparable studies in plasma since amino acids are normally well reabsorbed in the renal tubules; accordingly, subtle to moderate changes in amino acid homeostasis cannot be recognized using urine analyses. Various methodologies are available, including standard quantitative analysis (above) and qualitative assessment by thin-layer or paper chromatography. The qualitative analysis is relatively inexpensive, provides insight into renal tubular function and has the capacity to identify several amino acidopathies/amino acidurias; it is therefore a key element of routine selective screening for inherited metabolic diseases. Quantitative urine amino acid analysis is appropriate in instances in which a renal tubular reabsorption defect such as cystinuria is suspected, and (in conjunction with plasma analysis) in hyperammonemia when increased urinary excretion of specific amino acids (e.g., argininosuccinate and citrulline) may be diagnostic for certain urea cycle defects and in lysinuric protein intolerance (Hommes 1991).

D2.3.3 Cerebrospinal Fluid

Sample

One milliliter cerebrospinal fluid (CSF), freeze immediately, in conjunction with a plasma sample obtained at the time of lumbar puncture. If shipped, always transport on dry ice.

Quantitation of amino acids in CSF may be pursued in patients with suspected neurometabolic disorders, in particular severe (neonatal) epileptic encephalopathy (see also Table D2.5). It is highly desirable to obtain a concurrent plasma sample for amino acid analysis as calculation of the plasma/CSF ratio of specific amino acids may be required for the diagnosis of nonketotic hyperglycinemia (glycine CSF/plasma ratio >0.06) and serine biosynthesis deficiency (3-phosphoglycerate dehydrogenase deficiency; serine CSF:plasma ratio <0.2). An increased glycine CSF/plasma ratio is only meaningful, however, in the presence of elevated plasma glycine. If plasma glycine is abnormally low, elevation of the CSF/plasma ratio in the face of a normal CSF glycine level is not consistent with nonketotic hyperglycinemia. Raised levels of alanine and threonine in CSF are indicators of mitochondriopathies. Again, interpretation of CSF amino acid values beyond normal limits is more reliable if concurrent plasma concentrations are available. Heavily bloodstained

Table D2.5 Inherited metabolic diseases requiring CSF investigations for diagnosis[a]

Disorder	Relevant parameter
Glucose transporter deficiency	Glucose ratio (cerebrospinal fluid (CSF)/blood)
Selected mitochondrial encephalomyopathies	CSF lactate, pyruvate, alanine, threonine
Nonketotic hyperglycinaemia	Glycine ratio (CSF/plasma)
Serine biosynthesis defects	CSF amino acids (low serine; serine CSF/plasma ratio)
Cohen syndrome	β-Alanine in CSF
Isolated pipecolic oxidase deficiency	Pipecolic acid
Defects of monoamine metabolism	CSF monoamines and metabolites
Autosomal dominant GTP cyclohydrolase I deficiency	CSF biogenic amines and pterins
Sepiapterine reductase deficiency	CSF biogenic amines and pterins
GABA transaminase deficiency	CSF GABA, β-alanine, homocarnosine
Folate-binding protein deficiency	CSF 5-methyltetrahydrofolate
Cerebral folate deficiency	CSF 5-methyltetrahydrofolate
Selected cases of glutaric aciduria I	CSF glutarate
Selected cases of leucine catabolic defects	CSF 3-hydroxyisovaleric acid

[a]Modified from Hoffmann et al (1998)

CSF samples are unusable; slightly blood contaminated specimens should be rapidly centrifuged and the supernatant frozen (notify the laboratory). Immediate deep-freezing and special analytical methods are required for the determination of numerous CSF metabolites (free and total GABA, homocarnosine, carnosine, biogenic amines, and pterins).

D2.4 Organic Acids

Samples

Urine

Minimum 10 mL random (morning) urine, without preservatives. If transported, send on dry ice.

Plasma, CSF, and vitreous fluid (only limited, specific indications)

Minimum 1 mL, freeze immediately and send on dry ice.

The major source of organic acids in mammals include the amino acids, lipids and carbohydrates, and to a limited extent nucleic acids and steroids. Urine organic acid analysis is most readily performed by gas chromatography-mass spectroscopy (GC-MS), which provides insight into a wide range of metabolic pathways and is accordingly a mainstay of selective metabolic screening. Urine organic acid by GC alone is not recommended, as slight elevations of metabolites are missed and confirmatory identification via fragmentation patterns is not possible. In addition to the classical organic acidurias, urine organic acid analysis is a key diagnostic component in the evaluation of patients with suspected amino acid disorders, fatty acid oxidation defects, or disorders of mitochondrial energy metabolism.

Organic acids may be extracted from urine following acidification with mineral acids and are then converted to derivatives (e.g., trimethylsilyl- or methyl esters) for analysis by GC-MS. One or more non-physiological internal standards are included in the analysis for internal QC and for retention time standardization (e.g., 2-phenylbutyrate, undecanoic acid). Organic acid analysis in urine is suggested in the patient with systemic intoxication, unexplained metabolic crisis, or unexplained laboratory findings of disturbed intermediary metabolism such as metabolic acidosis, elevated lactate, elevated anion gap, hypoglycemia, ketonemia, neonatal ketonuria, or hyperammonemia. Furthermore, organic acid analysis is indicated in children with unclear hepatopathy, neurological/neuromuscular symptoms including epileptic encephalopathy, and in children with multisystem disorders (particularly when symptoms fluctuate or progress).

Organic acids are optimally analyzed in urine as they are usually efficiently excreted via the kidneys (high water solubility) and show higher concentrations in urine than other body fluids. Nonetheless, exact quantification of specific organic acids in plasma or CSF with isotope dilution analysis (only in selected laboratories) may be useful in selected cases for exclusionary purposes or for therapeutic assessment. Examples (Table D2.5) include glutaric aciduria type I (glutaric acid and 3-hydroxyglutaric acid), cobalamin defects (methylmalonic acid), tyrosinemia type I (succinylacetone) and various cerebral organic acidurias such as succinic semialdehyde dehydrogenase deficiency (4-hydroxybutyric aciduria) and

Canavan disease (N-acetylaspartic acid). Stable isotope dilution assays (either by routine GC-MS or via liquid chromatography-tandem MS) are the methods of choice for prenatal diagnoses, when metabolite levels may be low and accurate quantification is required. For postmortem studies, urine should be obtained via bladder puncture; organic acid analysis in postmortem plasma, CSF or vitreous fluid is much less informative.

> **Remember**
>
> Organic acid analyses in urine are, for the most part, run in a qualitative or only semiquantitative fashion. Exact quantitation of the hundreds of normal (and abnormal) intermediates detected in a human urine sample is laborious, technically challenging, and time-consuming, but is offered in some laboratories. A key to diagnosis for qualitative analysis is pattern recognition, especially in those instances in which elevations may be only very slight. An experienced diagnostic laboratory, with ample involvement in internal/external QC/QA, is optimal for the best diagnostic outcome.

> **Remember**
>
> Organic acid analysis in plasma is almost never of diagnostic value. Urine is the fluid of choice for analysis. However, in selected instances of fatty acid oxidation defects, increases of C14:0 and C14:1 fatty acids can provide evidence for long-chain hydroxyacyl-CoA dehydrogenase deficiency. This disorder is readily detected by plasma acylcarnitine analysis (see later).

D2.5 Acylcarnitine Analysis

> **Sample**
>
> Three to six dried blood spots on filter paper (Guthrie card) or 1–2 cc EDTA blood (plasma rapidly separated). Plasma sent on dry ice, blood spots at room temperature.

Acylcarnitine analysis in dried blood spots by electro-spray tandem MS–MS or FAB MS–MS facilitates diagnosis of most organic acidurias and fatty acid oxidation defects. This method has enabled the massive growth of expanded newborn screening around the world, not only in North America and Europe but also in Australia, Saudi Arabia, Qatar, and many other countries. The rapidity of analysis (<2 min/sample for newborn screening) lends itself to high throughput analysis. For acylcarnitine analysis, the characteristic daughter ion of all acylcarnitines is m/z 85 (a fragment of the parent carnitine moiety), an ion selectively monitored for quantitation. Tandem MS–MS analysis of acylcarnitines in plasma is also a primary evaluation for selective screening of inherited metabolic diseases, with diagnostic relevance to organic acidurias, fatty acid oxidation defects, and amino acid disorders (when the appropriate amino acid ion fragment is quantified).

In selected laboratories, acylcarnitine analysis in cultured fibroblasts can provide important diagnostic information on the primary disorder. For example, fibroblasts may be cultured in the presence of [U–^{13}C] leucine, isoleucine, or valine with added L-carnitine. Isolation of cell culture medium and fibroblasts, followed by lysis, enables analysis for ^{13}C-carnitine esters of the corresponding acyl-CoA intermediates, which occur in amino acid degradation (L-carnitine transesterifies the acyl-CoA species). Accumulation of any one Acylcarnitine provides evidence for the site of the specific defect in the pathway. Acylcarnitine analysis by tandem MS–MS may also be employed in an emergency in children with acute metabolic crises or hypoglycemia; it is faster than the standard organic acid analysis for the diagnosis of organic acidurias, and provides more rapid and reliable identification of the fatty acid oxidation defects. The analysis of many (but not all) relevant amino acids, as well as orotic acid, which are required in the emergency of metabolic decompensation can be quantified simultaneously by MS–MS. Quantification of total and free carnitine by MS–MS using Guthrie cards is inaccurate and requires specific plasma/sera analysis (see later).

Remember

Acylcarnitine analysis in plasma has become a primary adjuvant for the routine analysis of inherited metabolic diseases. Its rapid throughput and sensitivity makes it the method of choice in emergency situations.

D2.6 Carnitine Status

Sample

One milliliter serum/plasma, ± 5 mL urine, shipped to the laboratory frozen.

Long-chain fatty acids are transported into the mitochondrion as their respective carnitine esters, a process that requires transesterification of acyl-CoA species at the inner and outer sides of the inner mitochondrial membrane. Similarly, acyl-CoA compounds that accumulate within the mitochondrial matrix may transesterify to L-carnitine esters, with transport of the mitochondrion and urinary excretion. This process of detoxification induces secondary carnitine depletion in disorders that alter the metabolism of mitochondrial CoA-activated carboxylic acids (e.g., organic acidurias, fatty acid oxidation defects, and respiratory chain abnormalities). In the work-up of a patient with a suspected inherited metabolic disease, reduced serum carnitine may be regarded as one potential indicator of these disorders. Quantification of total, free, and esterified carnitine in serum or plasma (carnitine status) using MS–MS is mandatory for recognizing carnitine deficiency and monitoring carnitine supplementation in these disorders, as well as identifying primary carnitine transporter deficiency. Many laboratories still successfully utilize spectrophotometric methods for carnitine analysis on the autoanalyzer.

Free carnitine is efficiently reabsorbed in the renal tubule, while filtered acylcarnitine species accumulate in the urine. Urine carnitine analyses should be performed in conjunction with plasma analyses, and may be indicated if plasma values are abnormal or for monitoring treatment. Increased urinary acylcarnitines are often detected in organic acidurias and fatty acid oxidation defects, and in the context of normal plasma carnitine values suggest good detoxification capacity. High urine concentrations of free carnitine and a reduced renal tubular reabsorption rate (<90%) may reveal renal tubular dysfunction as a cause of systemic carnitine depletion or primary carnitine transporter deficiency.

D2.7 Lactate, Pyruvate, Ketone Bodies, and Nonesterified Fatty Acids

Sample

One milliliter serum/plasma, ship on dry ice (to avoid lipolysis). If determinations of pyruvate and acetoacetate are requested, rapid deproteinization at the bedside (using perchloric acid) is fundamental for an accurate value.

Lactate, pyruvate, and the ketone bodies (primarily 3-hydroxybutyrate and acetoacetate, but also acetone) are intermediates in blood which provide key information on a number of metabolic processes, including pyruvate metabolism, the citric acid cycle, gluconeogenesis, hepatic glycogenolysis, oxidation of fatty acids, ketogenesis, and the respiratory chain. When quantified in blood in conjunction with glucose and nonesterified fatty acids (NEFA), a wealth of information may be gleaned concerning the function of intermediary metabolism in the patient. All of these intermediates may be determined employing spectrophotometric assays (commercial kits available), generally relying on NAD$^+$/NADH coupled systems. During fasting, lactate is employed in the liver for glucose production; in the fed state, lactate is a source of energy for muscle and heart. Pyruvate is a key product of carbohydrate, fat, and protein breakdown that enters the citric acid cycle as acetyl-CoA (catalyzed by pyruvate dehydrogenase). The concentration of ketone bodies in the circulation is regulated by the interplay between hepatic ketogenesis and peripheral consumption as fuel source. Especially during the fasting state, ketone bodies are critical for brain energy needs. Also in the fasting state, free fatty acids are oxidized in the mitochondrion to acetyl-CoA species, which are interconverted in the liver (hepatic 3-hydroxy-3-methylglutaryl-CoA lyase activity) to ketone bodies (acetoacetate primarily).

Remember

Lactate, pyruvate, and the ketone bodies may be quantified in plasma, urine, and cerebrospinal fluid. Nutritional status must be known (fasting, postprandial, or post-loading with triglyceride or other diet).

To accurately quantify the keto species (acetoacetate and pyruvate), blood should be immediately deproteinized with perchloric acid at the bedside.

The analysis of NEFA in plasma or serum, in addition to the studies outlined above, provides important information on lipid catabolism and ketogenesis and is essential for any patient with acute metabolic coma or hypoglycemia. NEFA quantification is a critical investigation at the end of a fasting test. Normal values vary greatly according to the metabolic state. High insulin levels in the fed state inhibit lipolysis, resulting in low concentrations of both NEFA (<300 μmol/L) and ketone bodies (<100 μmol/L). Conversely, increased lipolysis during fasting leads to a continuous rise of NEFA levels up to 2–3 mmol/L within 24 h and a corresponding increase of ketone bodies to concentrations that generally exceed those of NEFA. Interpretation of the results at an early stage of the fast may be inconclusive, since NEFA may exceed 1 mmol/L prior to elevations of ketone bodies. A molar concentration of ketone bodies is less than NEFA after a 24 h fast suggests a disorder of fatty acid oxidation or ketogenesis; a molar concentration of ketone bodies <50% of NEFA is strongly suggestive of such disorders. The determination of NEFA without simultaneous determination of ketone bodies has little diagnostic utility.

D2.8 Investigations for Congenital Disorders of Glycosylation (CDG)

Sample

One milliliter serum or plasma, shipped to the laboratory on dry ice.

In the discipline of inherited metabolic diseases, no other area has grown at such a staggering rate as that of the CDG disorders. To date, at least 12 different forms of CDG I and six forms of CDG II diseases have been described. The two main subcategories are differentiated by the pattern of serum transferrins following isoelectric focusing, the most common approach for the diagnosis of the CDG disorders. The phenotypic spectrum is broad and covers every system; many of the disorders have a neurological component, but some may have only visceral (gastrointestinal) involvement, while others may feature mainly immune dysfunction. One CDG disorder features accumulation of a specific tetrasaccharide in the urine of affected patients. Thus, evaluation of serum transferrins has become a common analysis in selective screening for inherited metabolic diseases.

Remember

Isoelectric focusing of serum transferrins, while an excellent screening tool to detect CDG, does not provide 100% detection.

In humans, the glycosylation process may involve more than 300 glycosyltransferases, glycosidases and sugar transporters, all residing in cytosolic as well as endoplasmic reticulum and Golgi compartments. More than 30 different enzymes are involved in the production of oligosaccharide side chains that may be either lipid- or protein-linked. Diagnosis and differentiation of several types of CDG involves the demonstration of pathological glycosylation patterns in the isoelectric focusing pattern of serum transferrins. This test does not, however, detect all forms of CDG, and notably in two forms of CDG II the serum isoelectric focusing pattern is normal. Once an abnormal transferrin pattern is detected, additional studies may include HPLC of the oligosaccharides, enzymology, immunocytochemistry, and mutational studies. An emerging approach for CDG identification is electrospray MS–MS for analysis of glycosylation patterns of serum transferrins. Secondary disturbances of glycosylation may be linked to chronic alcoholism, classic galactosemia, or fructose intolerance (deficient mannose-6-phosphate synthesis).

D2.9 Purines and Pyrimidines

Sample

Minimum 10 mL urine, preferably morning void or 24 h urine collection (refrigerate and avoid light). Sample must be sent refrigerated or on dry ice (especially for diagnosis of adenylosuccinase deficiency).

The spectrum of clinical features in the disorders of purine and pyrimidine metabolism is exceptionally broad, encompassing immunodeficiency, seizures, nephrolithiasis, developmental delay, autistic features, and growth abnormalities. Purine/pyrimidine nucleotides are involved in nucleic acid synthesis, formation of phospholipids and glycogen, and are critical for sialylation reactions involved in protein glycosylation. The HPLC analysis of purines and pyrimidines in urine may be particularly indicated in patients with renal calculi and related problems, neurological problems, or both. Other symptoms may include arthritis, muscle cramps, and muscle wasting. Purine and pyrimidine excretion is significantly influenced by diet and may vary considerably during the day; thus, a 24-h urine collection may be optimal for analysis, but purines are a favorite food for microorganisms, and thus 24 h collections are accurate only when each voided sample is added to a container in a freezer. For diagnostic work, a spot sample assayed promptly is preferable. Urinary tract infections result in a markedly reduced concentration of purines or pyrimidines in the urine. Foodstuffs such as coffee, black tea, cocoa, or licorice contain methylxanthines and should be avoided during urine collection and 24-h prior. Succinylaminoimidazole carboxamide ribonucleoside, the marker metabolite of

Remember

Patients with dihydropyrimidine dehydrogenase (DHPD) deficiency and other pyrimidine degradation defects can manifest a life-threatening response to treatment with the antitumor agent 5-fluorouracil, making DHPD deficiency one of the classical pharmacogenetic disorders.

adenylosuccinase deficiency, is very unstable at room temperature; thus, if this disorder is suspected, the urine specimen must be maintained frozen and shipped on dry ice. For the diagnosis of disorders of pyrimidine breakdown, urine needs to be examined for dihydropyrimidines via GC-MS (as in organic acid analysis), since these substances are not recognized by HPLC alone. Some groups have begun to extend screening for inherited metabolic diseases in bloodspots to the use of filter papers soaked with urine for analysis of purines and pyrimidines using HPLC coupled to electrospray MS–MS methodology.

D2.9.1 Orotic Acid

Sample

Minimum 10 mL urine, sent on dry ice.

Pyrimidine biosynthesis, in which orotic acid is a major intermediate, is regulated at the level of carbamylphosphate synthetase II (CPS II), the enzyme catalyzing the first reaction in this pathway. The isoenzyme CPS I (a mitochondrial enzyme) catalyzes the production of carbamylphosphate during the process of urea synthesis. Under conditions in which mitochondrial carbamylphosphate accumulates (e.g., urea cycle disorders), cytosolic carbamylphosphate levels rise, and urine orotic acid excretion increases. This may be recognized in organic acid analysis, but orotic acid is a charged nitrogen species which has very limited solubility in organic solvents, and the amount detected by routine GC-MS is a fraction of the actual concentration. Thus, accurate quantification of orotic acid requires HPLC or electrospray tandem MS–MS methodology. Urine orotic acid analysis is one of the key investigations in significant hyperammonemia for the diagnosis of ornithine transcarbamylase (OTC) deficiency. In the past, heterozygous female carriers for OTC deficiency have been detected via urine orotic acid quantification following ingestion of allopurinol, a compound that blocks the conversion of orotic acid to uridine monophosphate. However, the allopurinol loading test is no longer widely employed, because mutational analysis provides more accurate information. Too, the allopurinol test may be normal in the presence of some OTC variants. Increased urine orotic acid may be found in other disorders as well, including mitochondrial disease, Rett syndrome, and Lesch–Nyhan syndrome.

D2.10 Disorders of Galactose Metabolism

Samples

Screening (galactose, GALT (galactose-1-phosphate uridyltransferase) activity
Three to six dried blood spots on filter paper (Guthrie card), routine mail.

Specific analyses (galactose, galactose-1-phoshate, galactitol, enzyme studies, and mutation analysis)
EDTA whole blood (2 cc) preferably 30 min post milk feed, send at ambient temperature. Red blood cells (RBCs) are used for enzyme studies, plasma for metabolite determination; leukocytes may be employed for isolation of genomic DNA for mutation screening. Store only at room temperature (no refrigeration or freezing), since hemolysis leads to significant artifact and galactokinase is a membrane bound protein lost with RBC hemolysis).

Inherited metabolic defects of galactose metabolism are recognized through determination of galactose concentration and GALT activity in dried blood spots (Guthrie card), a core part of newborn screening in most countries. More specific analyses are needed for those newborns with pathological screening tests (Chap. B2). Several laboratories quantify galactose in plasma (normal <3 mg/dL). During intervention in patients with galactosemia (GALT deficiency), galactose-1-phosphate is measured in erythrocytes (normal <0.3 mg/dl). Furthermore, many laboratories quantify urine galactitol (a further metabolite of galactose) using HPLC or stable isotope dilution methodology with GC-MS (normal <100 mmol/mol creatinine, age 0–1 year; <25 mmol/mol creatinine, age >1 year).

D2.11 Sugars

Sample

Minimum 10 mL urine, which may be transported refrigerated or on dry ice.

The detection of pathological urinary excretion of sugars is routinely assessed by thin-layer chromatography, which although not technologically advanced is still sufficient. This methodology has utility for the characterization of renal tubular defects and to provide evidence for selected disorders of carbohydrate metabolism. These include (but are not limited to) galactokinase deficiency, GALT deficiency (see above), UDP galactose-4-epimerase deficiency (rare), fructoaldolase (aldolase A), fructose-1,6-bisphosphatase (aldolase B) deficiency, and essential fructosuria. The sugars routinely tested

Remember

Urinary accumulation of glycerol may suggest X-linked heritable glycerol kinase deficiency, fructose-1,6-bisphosphatase deficiency, and may also be an artifact from the use of glycerin gels/ointments.

using thin-layer methodology include glucose, galactose, fructose, and lactose (laboratory specific). The determination of liver glycogen (the key storage form of liver glucose), when a disorder of glycogen storage is suspected, is more complex and requires liver biopsy. Glycogen is quantified only in a limited number of specialized laboratories. GC (with and withoutMS) method by which a number of sugar and polyols have been measured (e.g., C4-polyols threitol and erythritol; C5-sugars/polyols arabinose, xylulose, ribose, xylose, ribulose, xylitol, arabitol, and ribitol; C6-sugars/polyols fucose, fructose, glucose, mannitol, sorbitol, and galactitol; and some C7-sugars/polyols including seduheptulose and sediheptitol) was crucial in the discovery of two new defects in the pentose phosphate pathway (see D2.11.1).

D2.11.1 Polyols

Sample

Minimum 10 mL urine, shipped on dry ice or refrigerated if transit time is not extensive.

As in the case of the CDG, defects in polyol (sugar alcohols) metabolism represent an expanding area of interest for screening of a patient with suspected inherited metabolic disease. The polyols include C4 (erythritol and threitol), C5 (ribitol, arabitol, and xylitol), C6 (galactitol, sorbitol, and mannitol), and the C7-polyols (e.g., sedoheptitol and perseitol). These intermediates may be quantified utilizing GC, GC-MS, or electrospray MS–MS with internal standards. Two recently discovered disorders in the pentose phosphate pathway

have driven the expansion of this area of screening. The first is transaldolase deficiency, which features primarily hepatic dysfunction and the elevated excretion of erythritol, arabitol, ribitol, and the C7 compounds sedoheptitol and sedoheptulose. The other defect, ribose-5-phosphate isomerase deficiency, is rare (a single case). In that patient, a progressive leukoencephalopathy was associated with considerably increased urine concentrations of arabitol and ribitol, with considerably higher concentrations of these species in CSF and brain.

D2.12 Glutathione (and Analogs)

Sample

Three milliliter EDTA whole blood. Centrifuge, remove, and freeze plasma immediately. Deproteinize erythrocyte fraction with 5% sulphosalicylic acid (ratio approx. 1:1), shake/vortex thoroughly (until homogenous brown color), centrifuge twice at 5000 × g, remove, and freeze clear supernatant. Send plasma and erythrocyte extract on dry ice.

Defects of the γ-glutamyl cycle lead to a range of clinical problems including neonatal metabolic acidosis, hemolytic anemia, electrolyte disturbances, and a progressive neurological syndrome. All four enzyme defects are inherited in autosomal-recessive fashion; glutathione synthetase deficiency is the most prevalent disorder of this group. Initial investigations include the analysis of organic acids (elevated 5-oxoproline, i.e., pyroglutamic acid), in conjunction with quantification of glutathione and its metabolites in urine, erythrocytes, leukocytes, and/or fibroblasts. Enzyme studies are performed in erythrocytes or other nucleated cells (leukocytes, fibroblasts), but erythrocytes lack γ-glutamyl transpeptidase and 5-oxoprolinase activities.

D2.13 Glycosaminoglycans (Mucopolysaccharides)

Sample

Ten milliliter urine, sent on dry ice or refrigerated if transit time is not extensive.

Glycosaminoglycans (GAGs; mucopolysaccharides) are protein-bound oligosaccharides. Mucopolysaccharidoses (MPS) are the result of defective metabolism of certain GAG which accumulate in the lysosomes and are excreted in the urine. All MPS represent progressive diseases with considerable variability in phenotypic presentation.

Remember

Only MPS II is an X-linked disorder (the remaining MPS disorders are transmitted as autosomal-recessive traits), which may often (but not always) be identified in relation to the creamy-colored skin lesions that are unique to this disease.

These disorders may be detected using quantitative analysis of total urinary GAG concentration (in relation to creatinine), usually through determination of total uronic acid via Alcian blue or the carbazole reaction. MPS disorders are more reliably detected through electrophoretic separation of different GAG species, usually on cellulose acetate plates. For example, increased dermatan sulfate (associated with skeletal and organ changes) is found in MPS types I, II, VI, and VII; elevated heparan sulfate (associated with mental retardation and, especially behavioral disturbances in MPS III (Sanfilippo syndromes) is detected in MPS types I, II, III, and VII. The increased presence of

Remember

Morquio syndrome cannot be identified by quantitation of urine GAGs, as the characteristic metabolite (keratan sulfate) does not react with reagents typically employed to quantify uronic acids.

keratan sulfate (primarily associated with skeletal changes, including scoliosis and/or kyphoscoliosis) is pathognomonic for MPS type IV (the Morquio syndrome). Increased chondroin sulfate is characteristically found in MPS type VII and less consistently in MPS type IV, but chondroitin sulfate is a normal constituent of urine. Quantification of total urinary GAGs may produce borderline or false normal results, particularly in MPS types III and IV. In those instances, electrophoretic GAG separation is the method of choice for identification. The determination of quantitative GAG levels is amenable to MS–MS methodology, and some laboratories are employing this platform.

D2.14 Oligosaccharides

Sample

Ten milliliter urine shipped refrigerated or on dry ice. When possible, 24 h urine collections are optimal, but not necessary.

Many lysosomal storage disorders result in accumulation of specific oligosaccharides that accumulate and are excreted in the urine. This is most readily recognized through separation of individual oligosaccharides by thin-layer chromatography. The chromatographic separation is generally on silica gel, and the plates are developed with solvent systems in a single dimension. For detection, oligosaccharides are reacted with the orcinol reagent followed by heating at 100°C. Quantitative analysis is available only for free neuraminic acid (sialic acid), which accumulates in sialic acid storage disease (Salla disease). Oligosaccharide analysis provides evidence for the following disorders: fucosidosis, α- and β-mannosidoses, aspartylglycosaminuria, Schindler disease, sialidosis, GM_1- and GM_2-gangliosidoses, galactosialidosis, Gaucher disease, Pompe disease, and Salla disease. However, pathological oligosaccharide patterns are often variable and may be a challenge to recognize. A laboratory with extensive experience in this analysis is preferable. A high degree of clinical suspicion may be developed on the basis of coarse facial features, dysostosis multiplex, and/or ocular involvement (also findings in the MPS disorders). If the phenotype is strongly suggestive of one of these disorders, it is preferable to perform enzyme studies even in the face of normal oligosaccharide findings. Other lysosomal storage disorders generally require enzyme analysis for definitive diagnosis.

D2.15 Peroxisomal Function – Very Long-Chain Fatty, Phytanic, and Pristanic Acids

Samples

One milliliter serum/plasma for very long-chain fatty acids (VLCFAs), shipped on dry ice to avoid lipolysis (hemolysis is to be avoided as RBCs contribute extensively to VLCFA levels, and the patient should be fasted at draw); 1 mL EDTA whole blood for the analysis of plasmalogens in erythrocytes, express delivery, room temperature.

As cellular organelles, the peroxisomes catalyze a number of important processes. These include β-oxidation of VLCFAs, bile acids, biosynthesis of ether phospholipids, and α-oxidation of branched fatty acids such as phytanic acid. The methodological procedure of choice is quantification of VLCFA, phytanic, and pristanic acids using isotope dilution

Remember

Combined analysis of VLCFA, pristanic, and phytanic acids has great utility in diagnosing peroxisomal disorders. However, diseases such as rhizomelic chondrodysplasia types II and III and hyperoxaluria type I require additional studies (e.g., erythrocyte plasmalogens, urine glyoxylate and oxalate, etc.).

GS-MS, with deuterium labeled internal standards. Quantification of VLCFA via GC alone relies on peak area and retention time, and is not highly recommended. Peroxisome biogenesis disorders manifest multisystem pathology in affected patients. Most diseases of peroxisomal biogenesis result in defective peroxisomal β-oxidation, and result in accumulation of VLCFA species in serum or plasma. Additional studies to pinpoint the exact biochemical defect may

Remember

Circulating VLCFA, phytanic acid, and pristanic acid are essentially present in esterified form. Accordingly, they are not filtered by the kidney and cannot be detected in urine.

include bile acid analysis, plasmalogens, and other species. An isolated elevation of serum phytanic acid is detected in adult Refsum disease. Disorders of etherphospholipid biosynthesis, such as rhizomelic chondrodysplasia punctata or its variants, entails erythrocyte plasmalogen determination in more specialized laboratories.

D2.16 Creatine Disorders

Samples

AGAT (arginine:glycine amidinotransferase) and GAMT (guanidinoacetate methyltransferase) deficiency.

10 cc urine (preferably morning void) and 1–2 cc heparinized plasma, for analysis of creatine and guanidinoacetate in both fluids.

SLC6A8 (creatine transporter) defect.

10 cc urine (preferably morning void), for creatine determination expressed in relation to creatinine.

Much like the CDG and polyol disorders, the defects in creatine biosynthesis and transport have become an additional emerging field in the selective screening for inherited metabolic disorders. The biosynthetic disorders include L- AGAT deficiency (featuring low guanidinoacetate in urine and plasma), guanidinoacetate methyltransferase (GAMT) deficiency (elevated guanidinoacetate in urine and plasma), and the X-linked creatine transporter (SLC6A8) defect (increased creatine in urine, expressed in relation to creatinine). The latter represents an emerging focus of research into X-linked mental retardation. The nonspecific clinical features in all disorders may include developmental delay, language and speech disorders, autistic behavior, and seizures, occasionally associated with an extrapyramidal movement disorder. A sensitive investigation for all disorders is in vivo proton MRS of the brain, which reveals a significant reduction of creatine.

Remember

X-linked mental retardation syndromes should give rise to a high clinical suspicion for fragile X syndrome as well as the creatine transporter (SLC6A8) defect.

The method of choice for determining guanidinoacetate and creatine in body fluids is isotope dilution GC-MS, although liquid chromatography (LC)/MS–MS methods are becoming more widely available.

D2.17 Folate Metabolites

Samples

1–2 cc EDTA plasma (hemolysis must be avoided, as it artificially increases 5-methyltetrahydrofolate (MTHF) levels). Plasma must be deep frozen immediately at −80°C. CSF (any blood must immediately be removed by centrifugation), 1 cc, also deep frozen immediately at −80°C.

The active and principle form of circulating folate is 5-MTHF, one-carbon donor in a number of reactions. Biochemical processes including serine and glycine interconversion, homocysteine, and methionine interconversion, as well as purine biosynthesis, depend heavily on 5-MTHF as co-substrate. Serum folate deficiency leads to megaloblastic anemia, hyperhomocysteinemia, and neural tube defects in the newborn. The recently recognized cerebral folate deficiency is a neurological disorder featuring psychomotor retardation, paraplegia, cerebellar ataxia, and dyskinesia. In the latter, 5-MTHF in CSF is low. Quantitation of 5-MTHF is readily achieved in a number of laboratories employing HPLC separation with electrochemical detection (see Table D2.5).

D2.18 Cholesterol Biosynthetic Defects

Sample

1–2 cc EDTA/heparin serum/plasma, sent on dry ice.

Cholesterol is a key membrane component, and the precursor for numerous intermediates such as oxysterols, hormones, vitamins, and bile acids. Cholesterol is fundamental for membrane fluidity, and with sphingomyelin forms the lipid rafts/caveolae, sites at which intracellular signaling molecules aggregate. The predominance of disorders of cholesterol formation occurs at the postsqualene step, a step at which isoprenes formed in the biosynthetic pathway diverge to form ubiquinone, dolichol, or cholesterol. Two disorders (severe mevalonic aciduria and hyper IgD syndrome) represent defects of pre-squalene synthesis and can be identified via routine urine organic acid analysis under most circumstances. However, mevalonate excretion in the hyper IgD syndrome can be low, and a high degree of clinical suspicion (periodic fever, rash) can lead to specific quantitation of mevalonic acid by stable isotope dilution assay or directly to enzyme analysis for mevalonate kinase activity (leukocytes and fibroblasts).

Remember

Immune dysfunction and skin abnormalities (rash, psoriasis) may, in conjunction with other clinical features, suggest a disorder of cholesterol synthesis.

With the exception of the Smith–Lemli–Opitz syndrome (SLOS), the remaining post-squalene disorders are exceedingly rare. Plasma analysis of 7-dehydrocholesterol and (in some laboratories) 8-dehydrocholesterol, employing stable isotope dilution GC-MS, is the first-line investigation for identification of SLOS. Other suspected cholesterol defects (e.g., lathosterolemia, 4-methylsterol oxidase deficiency, Antley–Bixler syndrome, Greenberg dysplasia, desmosterolosis, and Conradi–Hünerman–Happle syndrome) require detailed sterol profiling in specialized laboratories, generally employing GC with the appropriate internal standards. In all of these disorders, clinical suspicion is raised by patients with abnormalities in morphogenesis, such as hand/toe polydactyly, internal organ defects, skeletal and/or skin abnormalities.

D2.19 Bile Acids

Sample

Ten milliliter urine, 2 mL EDTA/heparin plasma, or 2 mL bile fluid, shipped express delivery on dry ice. Stool may also be evaluated by specialist laboratories.

The primary bile acids, cholic acid (CA) and chenodeoxycholic acid (CDCA), are the end products of cholesterol metabolism that conjugate with glycine or taurine to form the excreted bile salts. A large group of enzymes, located in the endoplasmic reticulum, mitochondria, and peroxisomes of hepatocytes is involved in the pathway of bile acid synthesis. Therefore, alterations in concentrations of specific bile acids may be observed in various peroxisomal disorders, and also as specific defects of bile acid biosynthesis. Defective side chain oxidation of cholesterol is detected in patients with cerebrotendinous xanthomatosis (CTX), characterized by mitochondrial 27-hydroxylase deficiency. CTX results in accumulation of cholestanol and

> **Remember**
>
> Serum bile acid levels in healthy (fasting) individuals are generally <2 µg/mL, but may climb artifactually in liver cirrhosis, obstructive jaundice, and viral hepatitis.

cholesterol in most tissues, whereas serum CA and CDCA acids are significantly decreased. Although a number of methodological approaches are utilized to quantify bile acids in different fluids, the most reliable include GC-MS, LC-MS–MS, and FAB-MS. Older methodologies, including HPLC, radioimmunoassay, enzymatic analysis, and/or GC alone are more time consuming, laborious, and less sensitive than MS or MS–MS methodologies.

D2.20 Porphyrins

> **Samples**
>
> Twenty milliliter urine (random sample), 5 mL feces, 5–10 mL heparinized whole blood; no additives; store cool and dark, may be sent overnight at ambient temperature. In many instances, a 24 h urine collection is desirable.

Porphyrias are inherited abnormalities in heme biosynthesis. Heme formation is highest in the erythrocyte progenitors of the marrow but is also high in hepatocytes. Accordingly, the heritable porphyrias manifest significant hepatic involvement. The clinical presentation of the porphyrias facilitates their subdivision into two broad categories, including the acute and nonacute porphyric syndromes. The acute disorders feature debilitating abdominal pain, nausea, vomiting, constipation, and psychiatric findings. Urine levels of the heme precursor δ- ALA and PBG are significantly elevated. Conversely, the nonacute disorders feature

dermatological findings primarily in sun-exposed body regions. Congenital erythropoetic porphyria (Günther disease) features discoloration of the urine (brown, red-fluorescent spots in the diapers). Generally, ALA and PBG are readily detected in urine. They may be separated from other contaminants by ion-exchange chromatography. ALA in urine may be derivatized to a pyrrole analogue, and both ALA and PBG may be derivatized as dimethylaminobenzaldehyde derivatives (seeD2.2.3), which, in the presence of mineral acids, yields strongly fluorescent analogs for both compounds (Ex = 405 nm; Em = 615 nm). Less polar porphyrins (e.g., coproporphyrin and protoporphyrin) are often only detected in bile secretions. Commercially available kits can be utilized for determination of ALA and PBG.

D2.21 Biogenic Amines and Pterins (Specialized CSF/Urine Analyses)

> **CSF**
>
> Collect several samples (age <1 year: 0.5 mL fractions, use fractions 2–4 for metabolic investigations; age >1 year: 1 mL fractions, use fractions 3–5). Freeze samples immediately at the bedside (dry ice or liquid nitrogen), store at −70°C. The analysis of pterins requires the addition of specific antioxidants (contact the referring laboratory for explicit instructions). If bloodstained: centrifuge before freezing. It is strongly recommended that two CSF samples (of approx. 1 mL each) remain in storage at −70°C for follow-up studies that may be indicated from preliminary studies.
>
> *Urinary pterins*
> Ten milliliter random urine sample, keep cool and dark (dark urine collection bag), ship on dry ice. Alternatively: 5 mL urine, add 6 M HCl to pH 1.0–1.5, add 100 mg MnO_2, shake for 5 min (ambient temperature), centrifuge for 5 min (4,000 rpm), send supernatant protected against light (aluminum foil) by express mail.

For a suspected neurometabolic disorder, a lumbar puncture should only be pursued after basic analyses have been performed in blood and urine, and following neuroimaging studies (see Chap. 5). The use of CSF is not warranted in selective screening, and there must be a high degree of clinical suspicion to suggest a lumbar puncture. Nonetheless, several neurometabolic disorders can only be diagnosed by specific CSF studies (Table D2.5), especially the disorders of monoamine metabolism. As a rule with any CSF investigation, the analysis should include quantitative determination of lactate, pyruvate, amino acids, cell count, glucose, protein, immunoglobulin classes, specific immunoglobulins, and an evaluation of the integrity of the blood–brain barrier.

> **Remember**
>
> The analysis of monoamines in CSF requires analysis in only well-skilled, specialized laboratories with the appropriately derived collection protocols and age-related control ranges necessary for correct evaluation of the findings.

> **Remember**
>
> CSF monoamine concentrations show diurnal variation and a rostrocaudal gradient of concentration. Exact collection protocols must be followed for collection of CSF to insure meaningful data are obtained.

> **Remember**
>
> Many specialized laboratories provide collection tubes for CSF samples, as well as detailed instructions. Selected tubes in the collection set will contain pertinent antioxidant compounds (e.g., for tetrahydrobiopterin (BH_4)) that will insure accurate measurements.

Generally speaking, the term biogenic amine is equivalent to monamines, but in the case of inherited metabolic disorders encompasses catecholamines (dopamine, noradrenaline) and serotonin. These derive from the amino acid precursors, tyrosine and tryptophan. The end products of dopamine and serotonin metabolism include HVA and 5- HIAA. Defects in these pathways have a significant component of neurological dysfunction. Species including HVA, 5-HIAA, dopamine, 3,4-dihydroxyphenylacetate, 5-hydroxytryptophan, and 3-O-methyldopa are quantified by HPLC with electrochemical detection. Normative data vary extensively with age and sex, and thus it is fundamentally important to only send samples to a highly experienced, specialized laboratory.

Quantifying pterins in all body fluids (urine, CSF, plasma, etc.) is the most common and reliable method for diagnosing the inborn errors of BH_4 metabolism. BH_4 is a mandatory cofactor in the phenylalanine hydroxylase reaction, and its intracellular level regulates tyrosine and tryptophan hydroxylases, and nitric oxide synthase. Pterin analysis should be included in any study quantifying monoamines in CSF as well. A number of defects have been demonstrated in the biosynthetic pathway of BH_4 synthesis, including GTP cyclohydrolase deficiency, 6-pyruvoyl-tetrahydropterin synthase deficiency, and sepiapterin reductase deficiency. Quantitation of pterin levels is a valuable tool for identification of these disorders. The analysis of neopterin, biopterin, 5-MTHF, 5-HIAA, and HVA serves to differentiate between mild and severe forms of BH_4 deficiencies. Because of its key role in phenylalanine metabolism, selected screening for BH_4 deficiency should be pursued in newborns whose plasma phenylalanine exceeds 120 µmol/L. Notably, neopterin is also employed as a marker of T helper cell-derived cellular immune activation. Pterin analogs are generally present in physiological fluids in reduced forms, but may be artificially oxidized to highly fluorescent species prior to HPLC analysis with fluorescent detection. Neopterin, biopterin, and primapterin are blue-fluorescing species, whereas sepiapterin is a yellow-fluorescing compound.

Take Home Pearls

> Screening for an inherited metabolic disease requires interaction of both physician and laboratory personnel. Testing must be ordered in the context of the clinical symptoms and findings.
>
> Physicians who suspect a metabolic disease are best served to discuss the clinical features and general laboratory findings with a specialist who is trained and/or Board-certified in Clinical Biochemical Genetics.
>
> Key stumbling blocks in diagnostic testing are not knowing which tests to order, the limitations of the test, and the care and handling of the appropriate body fluids. This further underscores the value of discussion and interaction with the Biochemical Genetics laboratory director.

Key References

Blau N, Duran M, Blaskovics ME, Gibson KM (eds) (2003) Physician's guide to the laboratory diagnosis of metabolic diseases, 2nd edn. Springer, Berlin

Blau N, Hoffmann GF, Leonard J, Clarke JTR (eds) (2005) Physician's guide to the treatment and follow-up of metabolic diseases. Springer, Berlin

Hoffmann GF, Surtees RAH, Wevers RA (1998) Investigations of cerebrospinal fluid for neurometabolic disorders. Neuropediatrics 29:59–71

Hoffmann GF, Nyhan WL, Zschocke J, Kahler SG, Mayatepek E (2002) Inherited metabolic diseases – biochemical studies. Core handbooks in pediatrics, Lippincott Williams & Wilkins, Philadelphia, pp 95–109

Hommes FA (ed) (1991) Techniques in diagnostic human biochemical laboratories: a laboratory manual. Wiley-Liss, New York

Nyhan WL, Barshop BA, Ozand PT (2005) Atlas of metabolic diseases, 2nd edn. Hodder Arnold, London

Enzymes, Metabolic Pathways, Flux Control Analysis, and the Enzymology of Specific Groups of Inherited Metabolic Diseases

Ronald J. A. Wanders, Ben J. H. M. Poorthuis, and Richard J. T. Rodenburg

Key Facts

> Enzyme functions in a particular metabolic pathway are best described by K_m and V_{max} values.

> The central parameter in metabolic flux analysis is that of control strength, alternatively called flux control coefficient. It is described by the flux control coefficient which is set between 0 and 1. A flux control coefficient of 1 means that the particular enzyme has full control of flux through the pathway, whereas a flux control coefficient of 0 implies that the particular enzyme exerts virtually no control of flux.

> In any patient with a Zellweger spectrum-like phenotype in which very long-chain fatty acids have been found abnormal, a full enzymatic study in fibroblasts is warranted in order to resolve whether the patient has a defect in the biogenesis of peroxisomes or is affected by a single peroxisomal enzyme deficiency.

> The introduction of tandem mass spectrometry has revolutionized the diagnosis of fatty acid oxidation (FAO) disorders. Acylcarnitine analysis is the first-line test in patients suspected to suffer from an FAO disorder. If abnormal, enzyme studies should be performed to resolve the underlying enzymatic defect.

> Biochemical diagnostics of mitochondrial disorders usually involves a broad screening of mitochondrial enzyme activities and analysis of fluxes through the citric acid cycle and oxidative phosphorylation system. The analysis of fluxes can only be performed in freshly obtained tissue samples (usually muscle).

> Determination of the activity of lysosomal enzymes in leukocytes, plasma or dried blood spots, or in fibroblasts is the core in the laboratory diagnosis of lysosomal storage disorders.

D3.1 General Remarks

D3.1.1 Enzymes

The key players of *metabolism* are the *enzymes*, which are the true catalysts of biological systems. These remarkable molecular devices convert a particular *substrate* into a specific *product*, a process called *catalysis*. Nearly all the known enzymes are proteins, although proteins do not have an absolute monopoly on catalysis, since the discovery of catalytically active RNA molecules (*ribozymes*).

A remarkable feature of enzymes is their high level of *specificity*. Indeed, an enzyme usually converts only one or at most a few substrates into the corresponding products. The underlying basis for this specificity is

R. J. A. Wanders (✉)
Laboratory of Genetic Metabolic Diseases, Academic Medical Center, University of Amsterdam, Meibergdreef 9, 1105 AZ Amsterdam, The Netherlands
e-mail: r.j.wanders@amc.uva.nl

G. F. Hoffmann et al. (eds.), *Inherited Metabolic Diseases*,
DOI: 10.1007/978-3-540-74723-9_D3, © Springer-Verlag Berlin Heidelberg 2010

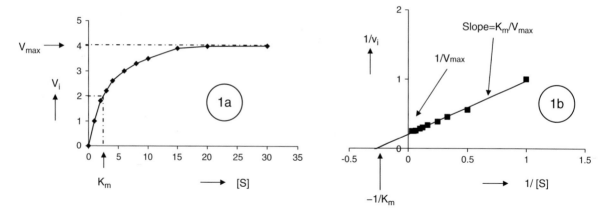

Fig. D3.1 Effect of the concentration of substrate S on the initial velocity (v_i) of an enzyme-catalyzed reaction represented in a V vs. [S] plot (**a**) or a double-reciprocal, Lineweaver–Burke plot of $1/v_i$ vs. $1/[S]$ (**b**)

that the *active site* at which catalysis takes place, generally takes the form of a three-dimensional *cleft* or *crevice* formed by steric groups that usually come from different parts of the amino acid sequence. Indeed, amino acid residues far apart in the primary amino acid sequence may interact more strongly than adjacent residues in the sequence, thus constituting the active site. For instance, in lysozyme, which is an enzyme that degrades the cell walls of some bacteria, the active site is formed by amino acids 35, 52, 62, 63, 101, and 108 in the sequence of 129 amino acids. The three-dimensional active site shields the substrate(s) from the solvent and creates a unique microenvironment, which allows catalysis to take place. What actually happens is that the active site of enzymes facilitates formation of the *transition state*, thereby providing the rate enhancement, which is so characteristic of enzymes.

Enzymes may accelerate reactions by factors of as much as a million or more. Indeed, most reactions in biological system do not take place at any perceptible rate in the absence of enzymes. Even a reaction as simple as the hydration of CO_2 is catalyzed by an enzyme, i.e., carbonic anhydrase. The transfer of CO_2 into the blood and then to the alveolar air would be less efficient in the absence of carbonic anhydrase.

In order to understand how a certain enzyme functions in a particular metabolic pathway it is important to know the properties of the enzyme in terms of its ability to convert a certain substrate [S] into a particular product [P]. These properties are best described in the K_m and V_{max} values of that particular enzyme for a certain substrate. The Michaelis constant (K_m) is defined

as the concentration of substrate at which the enzyme operates at 50% of its maximal velocity, whereas V_{max} is defined as the *turnover number* of an enzyme, which is the number of substrate molecules converted into product by an enzyme molecule in a unit time under conditions such that the enzyme is fully saturated with substrate. Figure D3.1a shows a plot of the reaction velocity (v_i) as a function of the substrate concentration [S] for an enzyme that obeys Michaelis–Menten kinetics, which clearly illustrates that the maximal velocity (V_{max}) is approached asymptotically. The Michaelis constant (K_m) can best be determined with the aid of a double-reciprocal or Lineweaver–Burke plot (Fig. D3.1b). A simple, direct measure describing the efficiency of a particular enzyme, is the *catalytic efficiency* of an enzyme defined as k_{cat}/K_m, or, alternatively, as V_{max}/K_m.

When localized within the cell, the activity of an enzyme may be changed by several distinct regulatory mechanisms. One key mechanism is *allosteric* control, in which the activity of an enzyme is stimulated or decreased by *effectors* of the enzyme, which bind at an allosteric site. Examples of allosteric *enzymes* are as follows: (1) carbamylphosphate synthase (allosteric effector (positive): N-acetyl glutamate), (2) pyruvate carboxylase (allosteric effector (positive): acetyl-CoA), (3) aspartate transcarbamylase (allosteric effector (negative): CTP), and (4) carnitine palmitoyltransferase 1 (CPT1) (allosteric effector (negative): malonyl-CoA).

A *second* level of control is exerted by the reversible covalent modification of enzymes. Many modifications are known at present, ranging from glycosylation, hydroxylation, acetylation, acylation, farnesylation, phosphorylation, ubiquitination, etc. Phosphorylation of proteins is again achieved by enzymes, so-called *protein kinases*, which catalyze the transfer of the terminal phosphoryl group of ATP to the hydroxyl groups of seryl, threonyl, or tyrosyl residues, thus forming *O*-phosphoseryl, *O*-phosphothreonyl, and/or *O*-phosphotyrosyl residues. Typical examples of mammalian enzymes undergoing phosphorylation/dephosphorylation are as follows: acetyl-CoA carboxylase, glycogen synthase, pyruvate dehydrogenase, and HMG-CoA reductase.

The activity of enzymes can also be regulated by changing its quantity. Indeed, some enzymes are constitutive in nature, which implies that the concentration remains essentially constant over time, whereas other enzymes are inducible. Examples of the latter category are as follows: (1) the enzymes of the urea cycle, as induced by a high-protein diet; (2) the enzymes of the mitochondrial fatty acid oxidation (FAO) system, as induced by a high-fat diet and prolonged fasting; and (3) HMG-CoA reductase and the other enzymes of the cholesterol biosynthesis pathway, as induced by low cholesterol.

D3.1.2   Control of Flux Through Metabolic Pathways

Many of the enzymes involved in the major metabolic pathways have been purified and their kinetic properties determined. Despite all this detailed knowledge, it has remained difficult to resolve the extent to which a particular enzyme contributes to the control of flux through the metabolic pathway in which the enzyme is involved. Quantitative studies of control mechanisms in metabolic pathways are hampered by the fact that the flux through a pathway cannot be described adequately by a rate equation analogous to that for a reaction catalyzed by a single enzyme. In order to circumvent this difficulty, computer simulations of metabolic pathways have been devised, although this approach has major drawbacks.

A breakthrough came in 1965 when Higgins (1965) introduced the concept of *control strength* as a quantitative measure to describe the contribution of a particular enzyme to the control of flux through a metabolic pathway. This concept was later reformulated and

extended by the groups of Kacser and Burns (1979) and Heinrich et al. (1977). The central parameter in metabolic flux analysis is that of control strength, alternatively called *flux control coefficient*, as defined by the *fractional* change in flux through a pathway, induced by a fractional change in activity of the enzyme catalyzing a particular step in the pathway involved. The value of a flux control coefficient is usually between 0 and 1. A flux control coefficient of 1 means that the particular enzyme has full control of flux through the pathway. In the old nomenclature, such an enzyme would be classified as "rate-controlling," "rate-limiting," or "pacemaker enzyme." On the other hand, a flux control coefficient of 0 means that the particular enzyme exerts virtually no control of flux.

Several methods are available for the determination of flux control coefficients. The *first* method makes use of specific inhibitors of particular enzymes. In practice, this means that the effect of adding increasing concentrations of a certain inhibitor on pathway flux is measured. From such plots the flux control coefficient of that enzyme can be calculated, especially if irreversible or noncompetitive inhibitors are available. This approach has been used successfully for instance by Groen et al. (1982a) who used a variety of different inhibitors to resolve the importance of the ATP/ADP-carrier as well as other steps in the control of the rate of mitochondrial oxidative phosphorylation (OXPHOS). These studies revealed that the control of flux of mitochondrial OXPHOS is distributed among different steps and furthermore that the value of the different flux control coefficients is very much dependent on the relative rate at which mitochondria respire between state 4 (resting state) and state 3 (maximal rate of respiration) (Groen et al. 1982a). The same inhibitor-based approach, which makes use of inhibitors, was also used to determine the flux control of other metabolic pathways including citrulline synthesis in mitochondria (Wanders et al. 1984), fatty acid β-oxidation in mitochondria (Eaton 2002), and gluconeogenesis in hepatocytes (Groen et al. 1982b, 1986). Another means of determining flux control coefficients is to measure the so-called elasticity coefficients described later.

Measurement of the flux control coefficient of a particular enzyme in a certain pathway provides considerable information and quantitatively describes how much control is exerted by that particular enzyme. It does not, however, reveal how this "control" is actually brought about. This issue has been resolved by Kacser and Burns (1979, 1981) when they formulated their *connectivity theorem*, which links the kinetic properties of individual enzymes in the pathway to the control exerted by these enzymes. The theorem states that there is a reciprocal relationship between the flux control coefficients of adjacent enzymes in a pathway and the so-called elasticity coefficients of the two enzymes toward their common intermediate whereby the *elasticity coefficient* is defined as the fractional change in the rate through an enzyme ($\delta v_i/v_i$) induced by a fractional change in substrate or product concentration ($\delta S_i/S_i$) while keeping all other factors able to influence the rate of the enzyme reaction constant. The elasticity coefficient is thus a quantitative expression for the *responsiveness* or *sensitivity* of an enzyme toward a change in substrate of product concentration.

A simple example may be helpful here. Let us take a simple two-enzyme pathway(S→I→P) in which the initial substrate [S] is converted into the intermediate product [I], which is then converted to the final product [P] by enzyme 2 (Fig. D3.2). Let us further assume that enzyme 2 has a high affinity for its substrate [I] ($K_m = 1.0$ mM) and enzyme 1 a low affinity for [I] as reflected in an inhibitor constant (K_i) of 100 mM for enzyme 1. Let us also assume that the concentration of [I] during the experiment would be 1.0 mM. What will happen now if we take away a little bit of enzyme 1, say 1%? At a constant concentration of [S], this will immediately lead to a decrease in the concentration of [I]. Since the concentration of [I] was in the same range as the K_m of enzyme 2 toward [I], the drop in [I] will lead to an immediate drop in the formation of [P]. Since enzyme 1 is practically insensitive to [I] due to the K_i of 100 mM, the drop in [I] will not affect enzyme 1 so that in the new steady state, pathway flux will be decreased by about 1%. This means that in this example, enzyme 1 exerts almost full control on flux through the pathway and this is explained by the low sensitivity of the enzyme toward its product [I] in combination with the high sensitivity of enzyme 2 toward [I].

In general, enzymes in metabolic pathways that show little product inhibition like enzyme 1 in the example of Fig. D3.2 exert major control on pathway flux. A good example of such an enzyme is carbamoyl-phosphate synthase, which shows minimal product

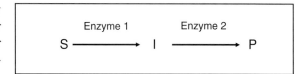

Fig. D3.2 Simplified scheme of a metabolic pathway consisting of two enzymes which convert the substrate S into product P with I as intermediate

inhibition by carbamoyl phosphate (high K_i-value for carbamoyl phosphate), whereas the next enzyme in line, which is ornithine transcarbamylase, has a high affinity for carbamoyl phosphate (low K_i-value). This implies that flux through the urea cycle is predominantly controlled by carbamoyl phosphate synthase with little control exerted by any of the subsequent steps, including ornithine transcarbamylase, argininosuccinate synthetase, argininosuccinate lyase, and arginase. Another example is HMG-CoA reductase, which converts HMG-CoA into mevalonate with mevalonate being a poor product inhibitor of HMG-CoA reductase.

Important to know is that the elasticity coefficients of enzymes in metabolic pathway can be determined experimentally and can be used to subsequently calculate the flux control coefficients (see Groen et al. (1982b) for detailed information).

The importance of certain enzymes for the overall flux through a metabolic pathway as reflected in their flux control coefficients is also important for inherited metabolic diseases, although this concept has not been widely introduced in the field. Indeed, the concept of flux control analysis gives a logical explanation for generally known facts, which are often intuitive. In the field of inherited metabolic diseases, it is, for instance, generally accepted that the effect of a particular residual activity of an enzyme in a patient is very much dependent on the enzyme involved. It is clear that a similar residual activity of for instance 5% has a markedly different effect on pathway flux if the enzyme has a flux control coefficient of 1.0 as compared to a flux control coefficient of 0.01.

Flux control analysis also provides a logical basis for the known fact that heterozygosity for some enzyme deficiencies is associated with clinical signs and symptoms, whereas in most other cases heterozygotes show no abnormalities whatsoever. In addition, flux control analysis provides a logical framework for the concept of *synergistic heterozygosity* as advanced by Vockley (2008).

D3.2 Peroxisomal Disorders

D3.2.1 Background

The peroxisomal disorders (PDs) represent a group of inherited diseases in man in which there is an impairment in either the biogenesis of peroxisomes or one of the metabolic functions of peroxisomes (Wanders 2004; Weller et al. 2003). Accordingly, the PDs are usually subdivided into two subgroups: (1) the peroxisome biogenesis disorders (PBDs) and (2) the single peroxisomal enzyme deficiencies. The group of PBDs is again subdivided into two categories, including the following: (1) the Zellweger spectrum disorders (ZSDs) with Zellweger syndrome, neonatal adrenoleukodystrophy, and infantile Refsum disease as representatives and (2) rhizomelic chondrodysplasia punctata type 1.

The principle features of the biogenesis of peroxisomes have been elucidated in recent years. In many respects, the biogenesis of peroxisomes resembles that of mitochondria, although peroxisomes do not possess their own DNA, like mitochondria do, which implies that the genetic information for *all* peroxisomal proteins, irrespective of their localization in the peroxisomal membrane or the peroxisomal matrix, is nuclear DNA encoded (Platta and Erdmann 2007).

Peroxisomal proteins are targeted to peroxisomes by virtue of distinct targeting signals (PTS), which are recognized by the peroxisomal protein uptake machinery, followed by their incorporation into either the peroxisomal membrane or the peroxisomal matrix. Multiple so-called peroxins encoded by PEX genes are involved in this process. This immediately explains why the group of PBDs, notably the ZSDs, is genetically heterogeneous. Indeed, the molecular basis of the ZSDs is remarkably diverse and involves mutations in 12 different PEX genes, including PEX 1, 2, 3, 5, 6, 10, 12, 13, 14, 16, 19, and 26 (Ebberink et al. 2009). Interestingly, mutations in *PEX7*, which codes for a specific peroxin, involved in the import of a distinct set of peroxisomal proteins, carrying the so-called PTS2 signal, are only found in patients with rhizomelic chondrodysplasia punctata, but not in patients having a ZSD-like phenotype.

With respect to the metabolic role of peroxisomes, peroxisomes are known to be involved in various metabolic processes, including (1) fatty acid β-oxidation, (2) etherphospholipid biosynthesis, (3) fatty acid α-oxidation, and (4) glyoxylate metabolism as most important peroxisomal functions, at least from the perspective of human disease (Wanders and Waterham 2006). Accordingly, the group of single peroxisomal enzyme deficiencies can be subdivided into subgroups based on whether the enzyme defect affects β-oxidation, α-oxidation, etherphospholipid biosynthesis, or glyoxylate metabolism. Table D3.1 lists the PDs as identified until now with details on the mutated gene and dysfunctional enzyme/transporter protein in each of the diseases.

D3.2.2 Laboratory Diagnosis

Once a patient is suspected to suffer from one of the PDs listed in Table D3.1 on clinical grounds, metabolite analysis of specific (sets of) metabolites should be initiated, which differs for each of the PDs (see Table D3.1). In general, most of the PDs known can be screened for reliably by analysis in plasma and/or erythrocytes. This is true for the ZSDs plus acyl-CoA oxidase deficiency and D-bifunctional protein deficiency by performing plasma very long-chain fatty acid (VLCFA) analysis. This is also true for the different forms of rhizomelic chondrodysplasia punctata if plasmalogen analysis is done in erythrocytes and also for Refsum disease if plasma phytanic acid is measured. The same applies to 2-methylacylCoA racemase (AMACR) and SCPx deficiency if plasma phytanic acid and/or the bile acid intermediates are measured. Alternatively, the latter can also be determined in urine. Finally, plasma VLCFA analysis is also very reliable for the identification of X-linked adrenoleukodystrophy, especially for hemizygote detection. Identification of the true defect in each of these cases warrants detailed enzymatic studies in fibroblasts as described later.

Remember

Most PDs known can be screened for reliably by analysis in plasma and/or erythrocytes (analysis of VLCFA, phytanic acid, and the bile acid intermediates in plasma, plasmalogen analysis in erythrocytes).

Table D3.1 Peroxisomal disorders plus information on the enzyme and gene defects, biochemical abnormalities and first-line tests

		Enzyme defect	Gene defect	Plasma					Erythrocytes
				VLCFA	BA	Ph	Pr	Pi	Plasmalogens
Peroxisome biogenesis disorders	Zellweger spectrum disorders	Generalized	PEX1,2,3,5, 6,10,12,13, 14,16,19, 26 + DLP1	⇑	↑	↑	↑	↑	↓
	Rhizomelic chondrodys- plasis punctata type 1	PTS2-proteins	PEX7	N	N	⇑	N	N	⇓
Single peroxi- somal enzyme deficien- cies	*Peroxisomal β-oxidation defects*								
	X-linked adrenoleu- kodystrophy	ALDP	ABCD1	⇑	N	N	N	N	N
	Acyl-CoA oxidase deficiency	ACOX1	ACOX1	⇑	N	N	N	N	N
	D-bifunctional protein deficiency	DBP	HSD17B4	⇑	↑	↑	↑	N	N
	SCPx-deficiency	SCPx	SCP2	N	⇑	⇑	⇑	N	N
	Methylacyl-CoA racemase (AMACR) deficiency	AMACR	AMACR	N	⇑	⇑	⇑	N	N
	Plasmalogen biosynthesis defects								
	RCDP type 2	Dihydroxyacetone phosphate acyltransferase	GNPAT	N	N	N	N	N	⇓
	RCDP type 3	ADHAPS	AGPS	N	N	N	N	N	⇓
	Phytanic acid α-oxidation defects								
	Refsum disease	PhyH/Phax	PHYH	N	N	⇑	N	N	N
	Glyoxylate metabolism defects								
	Hyperoxaluria type 1	Alanine glyoxylate aminotransferase	AGXT	N	N	N	N	N	

BA bile acid intermediates; *Ph* phytanic acid; *Pi* pipecolic acid; *Pr* pristanic acid; *VLCFA* very-long-chain fatty acids
The first-line test for each individual disorder is a double arrow (⇑/⇓)
Explanation of symbols: ⇑ = increased; N = normal; ⇓ = decreased.

D3.2.3 Enzymology of the PDs

Following the analysis of metabolites as described earlier, enzymatic studies are required for most of the PDs with some exceptions as described later in order to identify the ultimate genetic defect. The latter is especially important if prenatal diagnosis is required in the future. We describe the enzymology of the different groups of PDs:

1. In any patient with a ZSD-like phenotype in which VLCFAs have been found abnormal in plasma plus or minus abnormalities in any of the other peroxisomal parameters measured, including the bile acid intermediates, phytanic acid, pipecolic acid, and erythrocyte plasmalogens, a full enzymatic study in fibroblasts is warranted in order to resolve whether the patient has a defect in the biogenesis of peroxisomes or is affected by a single peroxisomal enzyme deficiency, notably at the level of acyl-CoA oxidase (Ferdinandusse et al. 2007) or D-bifunctional protein (Ferdinandusse et al. 2006a). Such a study includes: (1) measurement of C26:0 and pristanic acid β-oxidation, (2) plasmalogen biosynthesis, (3)

phytanic acid α-oxidation, and (4) immunofluorescence microscopy analysis of peroxisomes using antibodies raised against catalase. If all parameters including immunofluorescence microscopy analysis are abnormal, a PBD is very likely and subsequent complementation analysis, followed by molecular analysis of the relevant PEX gene, is necessary to identify the gene that is defective (see Wanders (2004)). If the abnormalities as observed in fibroblasts are restricted to the peroxisomal β-oxidation system only, one is probably dealing with either acyl-CoA oxidase (Ferdinandusse et al. 2007) or D-bifunctional protein deficiency, which can be resolved by direct measurement of the activity of these enzymes in fibroblasts, followed by analysis of either *ACOX1* or *HSD17B4* (see Wanders (2004)).

2. In any patient with a rhizomelic chondrodysplasia punctata-like phenotype, plasmalogens should be analyzed in erythrocytes and, if abnormal, it is fully sure that one is dealing with one of the peroxisomal forms of rhizomelic chondrodysplasia punctata, be it type 1, 2, or 3, as caused by mutations in either *PEX7*, *GNPAT* or *AGPS*. The latter two genes code for the two peroxisomal enzymes involved in etherphospholipid biosynthesis, i.e., dihydroxyacetone phosphate acyltransferase (DHAPAT) and alkyl-DHAP synthase. Resolution between these three forms of rhizomelic chondrodysplasia can be done via enzymatic studies in fibroblasts, which includes direct measurement of DHAPAT and alkyl-DHAP synthase, followed by molecular analysis of the different genes. Importantly, erythrocyte plasmalogen analysis has turned out to be an extremely powerful initial screening method since all the patients with RCDP, who have been analyzed by us, have shown clearly deficient plasmalogen levels in erythrocytes independent whether it was RCDP type 1, 2, or 3, with only one exception, which concerns a patient with a very mild Refsum-like phenotype (Horn et al. 2007).

3. In patients with a Refsum-like phenotype in whom plasma phytanic acid levels are elevated, fibroblast studies should be done with prime emphasis on phytanic acid α-oxidation, which, if abnormal, should be followed up by measurement of phytanoyl-CoA hydroxylase activity and molecular analysis of the *PHYH* genes. In some atypical patients, these studies have failed to show mutations in the *PHYH* gene. Subsequent studies have shown that in these patients it is the *PEX7* gene that is defective (van

den Brink et al. 2003). Apparently, mutations in the PEX7 gene can give rise to two different phenotypes including a Refsum-like phenotype in case of mild mutations (van den Brink et al. 2003), and rhizomelic chondrodysplasia punctata in case of severe mutations (Motley et al. 2002).

4. In a few other patients with some signs and symptoms reminiscent of Refsum disease, but, in addition, showing signs and symptoms not found in Refsum disease, the defect has turned out to be at some other level including SCPx (Ferdinandusse et al. 2006b) and AMACR (Ferdinandusse et al. 2006a).

5. Analysis of plasma VLCFA is also the first line of testing for the identification of X-ALD. Especially for hemizygote detection, plasma VLCFA analysis has turned out to be fully conclusive (Bezman et al. 2001). For X-linked ALD, detailed enzymatic studies in fibroblasts may not be warranted and instead molecular analysis of the X-ALD gene, i.e., *ABCD1*, might be initiated right away. At present, >700 different mutations have been identified (see www.XALD.nl).

6. Heterozygote detection is much less straightforward, especially if the patient is from a family having no family history of X-linked adrenoleukodystrophy. In such cases, a full study should be done: (1) in plasma including VLCFA analysis (which is only abnormal in 80% of obligate heterozygotes) and (2) fibroblasts, which should include immunofluorescence microscopy analysis of ALD protein. If the presumed mutation affects, the stability of ALD protein as is the case in about 65% of the mutations found in the *ABCD1* gene until now, one will see a *mosaic* pattern upon immunofluorescence microscopy analysis, using an antibody raised against ALD protein with some cells showing a punctuate fluorescence pattern, whereas other cells are lacking this.

7. Hyperoxaluria type 1 is also a peroxisomal disorder as it is caused by a functional deficiency of the peroxisomal enzyme alanine glyoxylate aminotransferase (AGT) encoded by the *AGXT* gene. Interestingly, a functional deficiency of AGT can be caused either by a deficient activity of the enzyme or by the mistargeting of the enzyme to the wrong organelle, i.e., the mitochondrion (Danpure et al. 1993). This leads to the bizarre situation that the detoxification of glyoxylate in the peroxisome is impaired thus leading to hyperoxaluria, not because the AGT enzyme is catalytically inactive, but because of a functionally active

AGT enzyme, which is not able to detoxify glyoxylate in the peroxisome, due to its aberrant localization in the mitochondrion. This immediately suggests that there is no place for enzymatic analysis of AGT in liver biopsies in the absence of parallel studies to determine the subcellular localization of AGT. For this reason, direct analysis of the AGXT gene by sequence analysis of all exons and flanking introns is the method of choice now for the identification of hyperoxaluria type 1 in any patient suspected to suffer from hyperoxaluria type 1, based on clinical grounds and/or laboratory findings including elevated oxalic acid, glycolic acid, and/or glyoxylic acid in urine (van Woerden et al. 2004).

D3.3 Mitochondrial FAO Disorders

D3.3.1 Background

Fatty acids (FAs) are an important source of energy for human beings. Most organs are able to oxidize FAs with some exceptions, notably erythrocytes and the brain. On the other hand, the heart is very much dependent on mitochondrial FAO with 60–90% of the energy equivalents being generated by means of mitochondrial fatty acid β-oxidation. Although both mitochondria and peroxisomes are able to oxidize fatty acids, mitochondria are responsible for the oxidation of the bulk of fatty acids, derived from our daily diet. FAs destined for mitochondria enter the cell via a mechanism which has remained ill-defined until now. Inside the cell, the FAs are rapidly esterified with coenzyme A (CoA) by one of several acyl-CoA synthetases to generate the corresponding acyl-CoA esters. Acyl-CoA esters cannot traverse the mitochondrial membrane and first need to be converted into the corresponding acylcarnitine esters by the enzyme CPT1, whereby the carnitine required for this reaction enters the cell via a coupled carnitine/Na^+-importer called OCTN2. The acylcarnitine generated in the CPT1 reaction then enters mitochondria via the mitochondrial carnitine acylcarnitine translocase (CACT), which exchanges acylcarnitines for free carnitine. Once inside the mitochondrion the acylcarnitine ester is reconverted into the corresponding acyl-CoA ester via the enzyme carnitine palmitoyltransferase 2 (CPT2). The acyl-CoA ester can then be broken down via subsequent rounds of β-oxidation and the acetyl-CoA units generated in each cycle of β-oxidation can subsequently be degraded to CO_2 and H_2O in the Krebs cycle or used for the synthesis of the ketone bodies acetoacetate and 3-hydroxybutyrate, which occurs primarily in the liver (Rinaldo et al. 2002).

D3.3.2 Laboratory Diagnosis of FAO Disorders

The introduction of tandem mass spectrometry (MS) in laboratories dealing with the diagnosis of inherited metabolic diseases in general and FAO disorders in particular, has revolutionized the diagnosis of FAO disorders. This is due to the fact that acylcarnitine species, which previously were notoriously difficult to measure, are relatively easy to quantify by means of tandem MS techniques. For this reason, acylcarnitine analysis is a first-line test in patients suspected to suffer from an FAO disorder. In fact, the same technique is also used in neonatal screening programs designed to identify neonates affected by a certain FAO disorder. If abnormal, enzyme studies should be done to resolve the underlying enzymatic defect as specified later.

D3.3.3 Enzymatic Analysis of FAO Disorders

In principle, there are two scenarios for the enzymatic work-up of patients suspected to suffer from an FAO disorder. The first scenario is that plasma or blood spot acylcarnitine analysis has been done and has shown a characteristic abnormal profile, which immediately suggests a specific defect in the FAO system. Figure D3.3 reveals that many of the currently known FAO disorders may show characteristic acylcarnitine profiles. This is true for (1) OCTN2 deficiency (primary carnitine deficiency), (2) CPT1 deficiency, (3) CPT2/CACT deficiency, (4) VLCAD deficiency, (5) MCAD deficiency, (6) SCAD deficiency, (7) LCHAD/MTP deficiency, and (8) SCHAD deficiency. In case of such a diagnostic acylcarnitine profile, the enzyme that is supposed to be deficient should be measured right away, preferably in lymphocytes, in order to identify the enzyme defect as soon as possible. The activities of

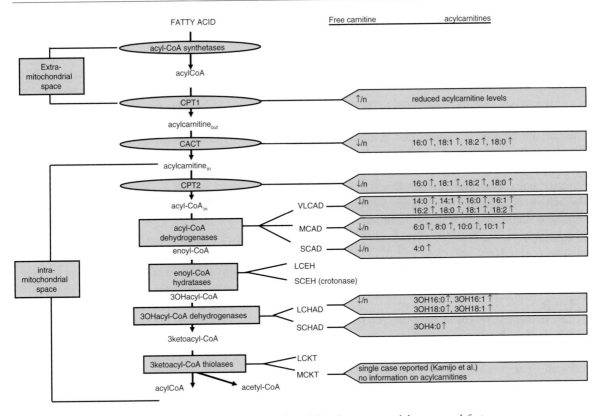

Fig. D3.3 Plasma acylcarnitine profiling and its importance for guiding the way toward the enzyme defect

Table D3.2 Mitochondrial fatty acid β-oxidation disorders plus information on the enzyme defect and enzyme tests

	Mitochondrial FAD disorders	Deficient enzyme	Mutated gene	Enzyme assay in fibroblasts	Enzyme assay in lymphocytes
1.	Primary carnitine deficiency	OCTN2	OCTN2	+	+[a]
2.	Carnitine palmitoyl transferase 1 deficiency	CPT1	CPT1	+	+[a]
3.	Carnitine acylcarnitine translocase deficiency	CACT	CACT	+	+[a]
4.	Carnitine palmitoyltransferase 2 deficiency	CPT2	CPT2	+	+
5.	VLCAD deficiency	VLCAD	ACADVL	+	+
6.	MCAD deficiency	MCAD	ACADM	+	+
7.	SCAD deficiency	SCAD	ACADS	+	+
8.	LCHAD/MTP deficiency	LCHAD/MTP	HADHA/HADHB	+	+
9.	SCHAD deficiency	SCHAD	HADH	+	+

[a]In principle feasible, but not yet validated in our laboratory

CPT2, VLCAD, MCAD, SCAD, LCHAD/MTP, and SCHAD can all be measured reliably and reproducibly in peripheral blood mononuclear cells. Although, OCTN2 and CPT1 are also expressed in lymphocytes, the activity of these two gene products is relatively low as compared to fibroblasts so that fibroblasts remain the best material for enzymatic analysis of OCTN2 and CPT1 (see Table D3.2).

In contrast to the clear-cut situation described earlier in which patients exhibit a characteristically abnormal acylcarnitine profiles, patients may show up with a less abnormal acylcarnitine profile. In addition, there are patients with signs and symptoms suggestive for an FAO defect such as hypoketotic hypoglycemia, cardiomyopathy, and/or muscle weakness, in the absence of any characteristic plasma acylcarnitine abnormalities. In such cases, a full enzymatic study should be done in cultured skin fibroblasts, which first involves whole cell β-oxidation analysis, to establish whether flux through the mitochondrial β-oxidation machinery is defective or not. Two different tests are advisable here. The first test is the tritium release assay in which intact fibroblasts are incubated with one of different tritium labeled fatty acids, notably myristic acid (C14:0), palmitic acid (C16:0), and oleic acid (C18:0). Use of such FAs has proven very helpful in the identification of disturbances in the mitochondrial FAO system (Olpin et al. 1997).

The second test, originally developed by Nada et al. (1995) involves loading of intact fibroblasts with deuterated fatty acids, notable deuterated palmitic acid, followed by acylcarnitine analysis of the suspending medium (Ventura et al. 1999). If one of the two different tests is abnormal, additional enzymatic analysis must be done to identify the underlying defect. In the Amsterdam laboratory, we have methods available for the measurement of all individual enzyme activities and also molecular analysis of all the different genes involved has been established in our laboratory.

D3.4 Mitochondrial Disorders

D3.4.1 Background

Mitochondrial disorders can be defined as disorders caused by a defect in the mitochondrial energy generating system. In "classical" mitochondrial disorders, the primary defect leading to a reduced mitochondrial energy generating capacity is located in the OXPHOS system, the citric acid cycle, or pyruvate dehydrogenase. In addition, there is a growing number of mitochondrial disorders in which the reduced mitochondrial energy generating capacity is caused by other defects, for example, in mitochondrial metabolite transporters (Mayr et al. 2007; Molinari et al. 2005). A major substrate for mitochondrial energy production is pyruvate,

which is transported into the mitochondria and subsequently converted into acetyl-CoA by the pyruvate dehydrogenase complex (PDHc), a key enzyme in energy metabolism. The activity of PDHc is regulated allosterically by its products acetyl-CoA and NADH, and by specific kinases and phosphatases, which are activated depending on the energy demands of the cell. Acetyl-CoA formed by PDHc and from other sources (e.g., oxidation of fatty acids) is taken up by the tricarboxylic acid (TCA) cycle. In the TCA cycle, the reduction equivalents NADH and $FADH_2$ are formed, which are the substrates for the OXPHOS system. The TCA cycle is a dynamic cycle of enzyme reactions, and metabolites can enter or leave at various steps within the cycle. Levels of intermediates of the TCA cycle can increase due to defects in subsequent steps of the mitochondrial energy generating system and can often be detected in urine of mitochondrial patients. The products of the TCA cycle, NADH, and $FADH_2$, are oxidized by respiratory chain complexes I and II, respectively, and electrons are transferred via coenzyme Q, complexes III, cytochrome c, and IV to molecular oxygen. The electron transfer is accompanied by proton translocation by respiratory chain complexes I, III, and IV. In this way, a mitochondrial inner-membrane potential is maintained, which provides the energy for complex V to convert ADP into the final product ATP. The five enzyme complexes of the OXPHOS system are multi-subunit assemblies of proteins, iron–sulfur clusters, flavins, copper ions, and heme groups. The largest OXPHOS enzyme is complex I, consisting of 45 different subunits, of which 7 are encoded by the mtDNA and 38 by the nuclear genome. There is evidence for a higher degree of organization of respiratory chain enzymes into supercomplexes, containing different combinations of respiratory chain enzyme complexes. Some of these can function as respirasomes with $NADH:O_2$ oxidoreductase activity (Acin-Perez et al. 2008). It has been suggested that supercomplexes can form even larger structures, the so-called respiratory strings (Wittig et al. 2006), although this remains to be established.

The clinical spectrum of mitochondrial disorders is very broad, and moreover, the genotype–phenotype correlation of mitochondrial disorders can be very poor. It seems likely that the complexity of the mitochondrial energy generating system, as described earlier, is one of the reasons for this. There are hundreds of proteins involved, and it can be envisioned that the effect of a mutation in one gene can be modulated, or enhanced, by polymorphisms in genes encoding other proteins involved in the mitochondrial energy generating system. For mtDNA mutations, evidence has been found for a role of the mtDNA haplotype in the pathogenicity of mtDNA mutations (Pulkes et al. 2000). Striking examples of clinical heterogeneity due to mutations in a single gene are disorders caused by mutations in POLG1, a gene encoding a subunit of the mtDNA polymerase. Originally described as a gene involved in progressive external ophthalmoplegia, and later in Alpers syndrome, which seem quite different clinical phenotypes, it is now recognized that the phenotype associated with POLG1 mutations is extremely diverse (Chinnery and Zeviani 2008).

Remember

It is worthwhile to include POLG1 mutation analysis in an early stage of the diagnostic work-up of mitochondrial patients.

D3.4.2 Laboratory Diagnosis of Mitochondrial Disorders

Given the complexity of the system, reaching a diagnosis is not always straightforward and often an in depth evaluation of clinical, biochemical, and genetic information is necessary. Biochemical diagnostics usually involves a broad screening of mitochondrial enzyme activities and analysis of fluxes through the citric acid cycle and OXPHOS system. The analysis of fluxes can only be performed in freshly obtained tissue samples (usually muscle), although assays for cultured fibroblasts have also been described. There are three types of assays to determine fluxes through the mitochondrial energy generating system, namely the analysis of the (1) ATP production rate, (2) substrate oxidation rate, and (3) oxygen consumption rate. A reduced rate of any of these parameters can be indicative of a defect in mitochondrial energy generating system. Moreover, by using different combinations of substrates, indications for the localization of the defect within the system can be obtained. For example, a reduced oxidation rate of pyruvate in the presence of malate, and a normal oxidation rate of pyruvate in the

presence of carnitine is indicative of an OXPHOS defect (Janssen et al. 2006). Also defects in the citric acid cycle and in a number of mitochondrial carriers can be detected in this way (Mayr et al. 2007). In addition to the analysis of fluxes, individual enzymes can be examined. Often muscle is the tissue of choice, but in certain cases a liver or heart biopsy should be considered. All of the enzymes mentioned earlier can be determined by spectrophotometric assays. Although for pyruvate dehydrogenase spectrophotometric analysis is possible, a more sensitive radiochemical assay with ^{14}C-labeled pyruvate is the preferred method of enzymatic analysis.

Remember

Assays of individual enzyme activities are available for pyruvate dehydrogenase, citric acid cycle enzymes, respiratory chain enzymes, and complex V. They can be performed both in freshly obtained tissue samples but also in frozen tissue samples, cultured cells, and blood cells. Given the tissue specific character of part of the mitochondrial disorder spectrum, it is very important to examine enzyme activities in clinically affected tissues.

Once flux as well as individual enzyme assays have been performed in a patient's muscle biopsy, there are a number of possible outcomes: (1) all parameters are normal, (2) mitochondrial energy generating system capacity is reduced and one or more enzymes are deficient, and (3) mitochondrial energy generating system capacity is reduced, but no enzyme deficiency is observed. In case all parameters are normal, a mitochondrial disorder is unlikely, especially if both enzyme activities and fluxes through the mitochondrial energy generating system have been examined in the affected tissue. However, if this is not the case, e.g., in patients with central nervous system impairment, a mitochondrial disorder cannot be completely excluded. In those cases, additional diagnostic tests may still be worthwhile, such as examination of the mtDNA, as tissue specific expression of the disease may be due to differences in heteroplasmy levels in different tissues. When only the mitochondrial energy generating system capacity is reduced, there are several possible explanations. First, it could be a primary mitochondrial dysfunctioning due to a defect in a mitochondrial protein/enzyme that was not examined. Examples of previously unidentified mitochondrial protein defects other than the classical mitochondrial defects are substrate carriers such as the glutamate, phosphate, or pyruvate carrier (Brivet et al. 2003; Mayr et al. 2007; Molinari et al. 2005). In these cases, detailed analysis in muscle and in cultured cells provided important biochemical clues for the identification of the primary defect. Second, as it has been shown that assays of the capacity of the mitochondrial energy generating system are more sensitive to detect certain mitochondrial defects, e.g., mutations in the mtDNA (Janssen et al. 2008), in such a constellation sequence analysis of the mtDNA should always be considered. Third, it could be a reflection of secondary mitochondrial dysfunctioning, e.g., due to a muscle dystrophy, a very poor clinical status of the patient, or other reasons.

In case of a reduced capacity of the mitochondrial energy generating system and a deficiency of one or more enzymes, several possibilities for subsequent diagnostic analysis are possible. In many cases, biochemical analysis of fibroblasts is useful. Both positive and negative results are informative. In case of normal enzyme activities in fibroblasts, in particular in cases with reduced activities of complex I, III, and/or IV in muscle, analysis of the mtDNA and of genes involved in mtDNA maintenance are indicated. In case of clearly reduced activities in fibroblasts, mtDNA depletion is less likely, and defects in either mtDNA or in nuclear genes encoding either structural components of the respiratory chain or assembly factors should be considered. A BN-PAGE analysis can be informative as well, as certain defects give a characteristic pattern in (2-dimensional) BN-PAGE.

As the number of genes in which defects have been described is already approaching 100 and still increases each year, it is not possible to routinely screen all the candidate genes with current technologies, although technical developments may allow for this in the near future. Cell model systems, such as patient-derived fibroblasts and myoblasts can be invaluable to establish the pathogenicity of newly identified mutations, e.g., by viral complementation studies (Hoefs et al. 2008). Also at the final stage of the diagnostic examination, functional assays, such as enzyme assays and assays for mitochondrial fluxes, provide important information to establish the diagnosis mitochondrial disorder at the molecular genetic level.

Remember

Once a mutation has been found, it is important to verify the functional implications of the presumed genetic defect in functional assays.

D3.5 Lysosomal Storage Disorders

D3.5.1 Background

Lysosomes play a very important role in the turnover of the cell. Turnover is the constant state of breakdown and resynthesis of macromolecules leading to renewal of these molecules, while their concentration remains constant. The main function of lysosomes is the breakdown of complex macromolecules by lysosomal enzymes to simple monomers and the transport of these monomers by specific membrane transporters out of the lysosomal compartment into the cytosol, where they can be reutilized for biosynthesis. This function is achieved by the presence of a large set of hydrolytic enzymes with an acidic pH optimum capable of hydrolyzing all cellular components including DNA, RNA, complex carbohydrates like glycolipids, glycoproteins, and glycosaminoglycans as well as proteins, neutral lipids, and phospholipids. With few exceptions, the reactions catalyzed by lysosomal hydrolases are irreversible.

The pH within the lysosome is maintained around five by an ATP-driven proton pump. Most lysosomal enzymes are glycoproteins and are present in the matrix of the lysosome. They are synthesized as larger precursors (pre-proenzymes) and glycosylated during transport in the endoplasmic reticulum and the Golgi apparatus. Some of the free mannose groups on the lysosomal precursor enzymes are phosphorylated to mannose-6-phosphate groups in the trans-Golgi, which are recognized by the mannose-6-phosphate receptors present in acidic endosomes. These mannose-6-phosphate receptors are essential for the lysosomal targeting of matrix enzymes to the lysosomes and are also present on the plasma membrane. After dissociation of the lysosomal precursor enzymes from the mannose-6-phosphate receptor in the acidic environment, they finally reach the endosomal/lysosomal compartment (Kornfeld 1987). Once, they have reached the endosomal/lysosomal compartments the precursor enzymes may be further processed by proteolytic cleavage to smaller molecular weight mature enzymes. Lysosomal enzymes can be active as monomers, homodimers (e.g., α-galactosidase and α-galactosaminidase and β-hexosaminidase B), or heterodimers (β-hexosaminidase A) and are mostly present as soluble enzymes. Like all other proteins lysosomal enzymes are also degraded in the lysosome and have a finite half-life. In most cell types, the lysosomal enzymes appear to be constitutively expressed.

Besides glycosylation, which is essential for the activity of all soluble lysosomal enzymes, another posttranslational modification is necessary for all sulfatases including the lysosomal sulfatases. This modification involves the oxidation of an essential cysteine residue to a formylglycine group by the formylglycine generating enzyme, which is present in the endoplasmic reticulum (Dierks et al. 2005). There is no evidence that the activity of lysosomal enzymes is regulated by covalent modifications once they are in their mature form.

The enzymes β-galactosidase and α-neuraminidase are present in an enzyme complex that also contains a third protein, the so-called "protective protein," which is actually an enzyme, cathepsin A, with proteolytic activity. The presence of this protein is essential for the stability of both β-galactosidase and neuraminidase.

In general, lysosomal enzymes have to work in concert in order to efficiently catalyze the stepwise breakdown of macromolecules like glycosaminoglycans, glycoproteins, and glycolipids. However, with the exception of the example discussed earlier there is no evidence that they are actually organized in enzyme complexes.

When the substrate is not water soluble as is the case with lipid molecules destined for degradation, which are present in internal membranes within the endosomal/lysosomal compartments, the lipid hydrolyzing enzymes may need an activator protein for full activity (Kolter and Sandhoff 2005). Examples are the GM_2-activator protein, which is specifically needed for the breakdown of GM_2-ganglioside by β-hexosaminidase A and the saposins A–D. The latter activator proteins are proteolytic cleavage products of the precursor protein prosaposin and are needed for the hydrolysis of complex glycolipids like sulfatide, globotriaosylceramide, galactosylceramide, glucosylceramide, and ceramide.

Substrates for lysosomal hydrolysis usually do not enter the lysosome by diffusion or transport of single molecules, but are delivered to the lysosome by endocytosis when their origin is outside the cell or phagocytosis when they are of intracellular origin. They may be taken up as single molecules or may be part of a larger molecular complex like a lipoprotein or even an organelle or a microorganism. In some cases, the uptake by endocytosis is a very efficient process catalyzed by the presence of a receptor such as the uptake of low-density lipoprotein (LDL), which is catalyzed by the presence of the LDL receptor. Also lysosomal enzymes carrying a mannose-6-phosphate group can be very efficiently taken up by most cell types because of the presence of a mannose-6-phosphate receptor on the plasma membrane.

Lysosomal storage disorders are characterized by the presence of nondegraded material in endosomal/lysosomal compartments. Any process that interferes with the lysosomal degradation or endosomal/lysosomal transport of molecules can give rise to storage. The cause may be environmental – for example, in drug-induced lipidoses or caused by the presence of undegradable materials- or genetic in nature. Here, we will discuss the genetic lysosomal storage disorders.

D3.5.2 Genetic Causes of Lysosomal Storage Diseases

D3.5.2.1 Single Enzyme Deficiencies

The majority of the inherited lysosomal storage disorders are caused by mutations in the genes coding for a lysosomal enzyme (see Table D3.3). These mutations may give rise to the complete absence or a severe reduction in activity of the lysosomal enzyme. Since most lysosomal enzymes are exohydrolases the stepwise breakdown of macromolecules stops at the step which is normally catalyzed by the enzyme that is now deficient. These deficiencies give rise to the storage of specific macromolecules, which causes disease. The storage is a slow, but continuous process, which explains why lysosomal storage disorders are chronic, progressive diseases. Most lysosomal storage diseases are autosomal recessive disorders with the exception of Fabry disease and mucopolysaccharidosis type II (Hunter's disease), which are X-linked. Since carriers are not affected, enzyme levels of 50% of normal are sufficient for normal lysosomal functioning. In fact, a

Table D3.3 Lysosomal storage disorders as classified in distinct subgroups

Disease	Eponyme	OMIM	Locus Gene	Gene product	Storage product
Sphingolipidoses/lipidoses (single enzyme defects and activator protein deficiencies)					
Farber disease	Lipogranulomatosis	228000	8p22 ASAH	Acid ceramidase	Cer
Fabry disease	Anderson–Fabry	301500	Xq22 GLA	α-Galactosidase A	Gb3
Gaucher disease	Glucosylceramidosis	606463 230900 231000 230800	1q21 GBA	β-Glucocerebrosidase	GlcCer
GM$_1$-gangliosidosis		230500 230600	3p21 GLB1	β-Galactosidase	GM$_1$
GM$_2$-gangliosidosis B	Tay–Sachs	272800	15q23 HEXA	β-Hexosaminidase α-subunit	GM$_2$
GM$_2$-gangliosidosis O	Sandhoff	268800	5q13 HEXB	β-Hexosaminidase β-subunit	GM$_2$
GM$_2$ gangliosidosis AB	Tay–Sachs AB variant	272750	5q32 GM2A	GM$_2$ activator protein	GM$_2$
Krabbe disease	Globoid cell leukodystrophy	245200	14q31 GALC	β-Galactocerebrosidase	GalCer
Metachromatic leukodystrophy	Arylsulfatase A deficiency	250100	22q13 ARSA	Arylsulfatase A	Sulfatide
Niemann–Pick types A and B		257200 607616	11p15 SPMPD1	Acid sphingomyelinase	SM
Wolman disease	Cholesteryl ester storage disease	278000	10q23.2 LIPA	Acid lipase	Cholesterolester, triglycerides
Prosaposin deficiency		176801	10q22 PSAP	Prosaposin	Multiple lipids
Saposin B deficiency	Metachromatic leukodystrophy variant	249900	10q22 PSAP	Saposin B	Sulfatide
Saposin C deficiency	Gaucher variant	610539	10q22 PSAP	Saposin C	GlcCer
Glycogen storage disease (single enzyme deficiency)					
Pompe disease	Glycogen storage disease type II	232300	17q25 GAA	α-Glucosidase	Glycogen
Mucopolysaccharidoses (MPS, single enzyme deficiencies)					
MPS I	Hurler Hurler/Scheie Scheie	607015 607015 607016	4p16 IDUA	α-Iduronidase	DS, HS
MPS II	Hunter	309900	Xq28 IDS	Iduronate sulfatase	DS, HS
MPS IIIA	Sanfilippo A	252900	17q25 SGS	Heparan N-sulfatase	HS
MPS IIIB	Sanfilippo B	252910	17q21 NAGLU	N-acetyl-α-glucosaminidase	HS
MPS IIIC	Sanfilippo C	252930	8p11 TMEM76 HGSNAT	α-Glucosaminide-acetyl-CoA transferase	HS
MPS IIID	Sanfilippo D	252940	12q14 GNS	N-acetylglucosamine-6-sulfatase	HS

Table D3.3 (continued)

Disease	Eponyme	OMIM	Locus Gene	Gene product	Storage product
MPS IVA	Morquio A	253000	16q24 GALNS	*N*-acetylgalactos-amine-6-sulfatase	KS, CS
MPS IVB	Morquio B	253010	3p21 GLB1	Acid β-galactosidase	KS
MPS VI	Maroteaux–Lamy	253200	5q12 ARSB	Arylsulfatase B	DS
MPS VII	Sly	253220	7q21 GUSB	β-Glucuronidase	DS, HS, CS
MPS IX	Hyaluronidase deficiency	601492	3p21 HYAL1	Hyaluronidase 1	HA
Glycoproteinoses (single enzyme deficiencies)					
Aspartylglucosaminuria		208400	4q32 AGA	Aspartylglucosaminidase	Aspartylglucosamine Oligosaccharides
Fucosidosis		230000	1p34 FUCA	α-Fucosidase	Oligosaccharides
α-Mannosidosis		248500	19q12 MAN2B1	α-Mannosidase	Oligosaccharides
β-Mannosidosis		248510	4q22 MANBA	β-Mannosidase	Oligosaccharides
Sialidosis	Sialidase deficiency Mucolipidosis type I	256550	6p21 NEU1	Sialidase, α-neuraminidase-1	Oligosaccharides
N-acetyl-α-glucosaminidase deficiency	Schindler disease Kanzaki disease	609241 609242	22q13 NAGA	*N*-acetyl-α-glucosaminidase	Oligosaccharides
Multiple enzyme deficiencies					
Mucolipidosis type II	I-cell disease	252500	12q23 GNPTAB	UDP-GlcNac phosphotrans-ferase, α/β subunits	Lipids and oligosaccharides
Mucolipidosis type IIIA	Pseudo-Hurler polydystrophy	252600	12q23 GNPTAB	UDP-GlcNac phosphotrans-ferase, α/β subunits	See above
Mucolipidosis type IIIB	Pseudo-Hurler polydystrophy	352605	16p GNPTG	UDP-GlcNac phosphotrans-ferase, γ-subunit	See above
Multiple sulfatase deficiency	Austin disease	272200	3p26 SUMF1	Formyl-glycine generating enzyme	Sulfatide, mucopolysaccha-rides
Galactosialidosis		256540	20q13 PPCA	Protective protein, cathepsin A	Glycosphingolipids, oligosaccharides
Lysosomal transport defects					
Cystinosis		219800 219900 219750	17p13 CTNS	Cystinosin	Cystine
Sialic acid storage disease	Salla disease	604322	6q14 SLC17A5	Sialin	Sialic acid
Methylmalonic aciduria	Vitamin B_{12} lysosomal release defect	277380	Unknown	Vitamin B_{12} carrier (CbIF)	Vitamin B_{12}
Lysosomal/endosomal trafficking defects, defects in fusion/fission of vesicles					
Niemann–Pick type C1		257220	18q11 NPC1	NPC1	Cholesterol, phospho-lipids, glycosphingolipids

(continued)

Table D3.3 (continued)

Disease	Eponyme	OMIM	Locus Gene	Gene product	Storage product
Niemann–Pick type C2		607625	14q24 NPC2	NPC2	Cholesterol, phospholipids, glycosphingolipids
Mucolipidosis type IV		252650	19p13 MCOLN1	Mucolipin-1	Phospholipids, glycosphingolipids, mucopolysaccharides
Danon disease	Pseudoglycogenosis II	300257	Xq24 LAMP2	LAMP2	Glycogen
Neuronal ceroid lipofuscinoses (NCL) (single enzyme deficiencies and other defects)					
CLN1	Haltia–Santavuori, infantile NCL	256730	1p32 CLN1	PPT1, palmitoyl protein thioesterase 1	SAPs
CLN2	Janský–Bielschowsky, late-infantile NCL	204500	11p15 CLN2	TPP1, tripeptidyl peptidase I	SCMAS
CLN3	Spielmeyer–Sjögren Batten, juvenile NCL	204200	16p12 CLN3	CLN3	SCMAS
CLN4A	Kufs	204300	Unknown	Unknown	SCMAS
CLN4B	Parry disease	162350	Unknown	Unknown	SAPs
CLN5	Variant Finnish late-infantile NCL	256731	13q22 CLN5	CLN5	SCMAS
CLN6	Variant Indian or Czech late infantile	601780	15q23 CLN6	CLN6	SCMAS
CLN7	Variant Turkish late infantile	610951	Unknown	Unknown	SCMAS
CLN8	Northern epilepsy	600143	8p32 CLN8	CLN8	SCMAS
CLN9	Variant Batten disease	609055	Unknown	Regulator of dihydroceramide synthase	SCMAS
CLN10	Congenital NCL	610127	11p15 CTSD	Cathepsin D	SAPs

Cer ceramide; CS chondroitin sulfate; DS dermatan sulfate; Gb3 globotriaosylceramide, gangliosides GM1 and GM2; GlcCer glucosylceramide; HA hyaluronan; HS heparansulfate; KS keratansulfate; SAPs sphingolipid activator proteins; SCMAS subunit c mitochondrial ATP synthase; SM sphingomyelin

reduction of enzyme activity to <10% of normal is usually necessary to cause disease.

A wide spectrum of disease expression is usually found and it is customary to classify the individual lysosomal storage disorders according to age of onset in a (late) infantile, juvenile, and adult form. In practice, there is often a continuum of clinical phenotypes varying from very severe to relatively mild. In several lysosomal disorders, the residual activity expressed by the mutant enzyme correlates with the severity of the disease (phenotype). Examples are metachromatic leukodystrophy caused by the deficiency of the lysosomal enzyme arylsulfatase A, and GM_2-gangliosidosis type Tay–Sachs caused by a deficiency of β-hexosaminidase A. A theoretical correlation between the residual enzyme activity and the steady-state concentration and turnover rates of its substrate was derived and a good correlation was found in patients with severe and attenuated phenotypes of GM_2-gangliosidosis and metachromatic leukodystrophy between the residual enzyme activities and the clinical phenotype (Leinekugel et al. 1992).

Although lysosomal enzymes are present in all cell types except red blood cells, cells and tissues may be differentially affected depending on the enzyme deficiency involved. It is the flux of substrate through the endosomal/lysosomal system that determines which cells and tissues will be affected and the clinical phenotype that emerges. Thus, it can be understood that the deficiency of α-glucosidase in Pompe disease will primarily affect the skeletal muscle, the heart, and the liver, which are most active in glycogen metabolism. Similarly, the defect in the turnover of sulfatide – an important component of myelin – due to the deficiency of arylsulfatase A will affect normal myelin function and white matter disease in metachromatic leukodystrophy, and a defect in the turnover of gangliosides due to deficiencies in β-hexosaminidase A and GM_2- and GM_1-gangliosidosis will lead to severe neuronal dysfunction. In reality, the pathophysiology is usually more complex, but these are important considerations.

D3.5.2.2 Activator Protein Deficiencies
(see Table D3.3)

Mutations in the genes encoding for the activator proteins give rise to a functional deficiency of glycolipid hydrolases, while the enzymes themselves are normally present. The phenotypes are similar to the phenotypes caused by the enzyme deficiencies. Examples are metachromatic leukodystrophy caused by saposin B deficiency, Gaucher disease caused by saposin C deficiency, and GM_2-gangliosidosis caused by GM_2-activator protein deficiency.

D3.5.2.3 Multiple Enzyme Deficiencies
(see Table D3.3)

A deficiency of the enzyme UDP-*N*-acetylglucosamine: lysosomal enzyme *N*-Acetylglucosamine-1-phospho transferase leads to mistargeting of lysosomal enzymes, which cannot be delivered to lysosomes, but are instead excreted into the plasma because they lack the mannose-6-phosphate targeting signal. Interestingly, although the phosphotransferase deficiency is present in all cells only cells of mesenchymal origin appear to be affected, suggesting that alternative routes of delivering lysosomal enzymes to lysosomes must exist in other cell types. The phosphotransferase enzyme consists of three subunits ($\alpha_2\beta_2\gamma_2$) encoded by two genes, one for the α and β subunits and the other one for the γ subunit.

Mutations in the gene for the α and β subunits give rise to mucolipidosis II (I-cell disease) and its attenuated form mucolipidosis III (pseudo-Hurler polydystrophy), while mutations in the γ subunit only lead to mucolipidosis III.

A defect in the formylglycine generating enzyme leads to a disease called multiple sulfatase deficiency in which all sulfatases including at least seven lysosomal sulfatases are deficient. In its most severe form the disease has Niemann–Pick features of a mucopolysaccharidosis, metachromatic leukodystrophy, and ichtyosis (due to steroid sulfatase deficiency), but the clinical presentation is very variable. A defect in the protective protein/cathepsin A leads to a deficiency of both β-galactosidase and α-neuraminidase and the lysosomal storage disorder galactosialidosis.

D3.5.2.4 Lysosomal/Endosomal Trafficking
Defects (see Table D3.3)

Lysosomal storage diseases can also be caused by abnormalities in lysosomal/endosomal trafficking or vesicle fusion (Walkley 2001).

Niemann–Pick type C is caused by two different gene defects *NPC1* and *NPC2*. NPC1 is a membrane protein with 13 transmembrane domains and a cholesterol sensing domain and is present in late endosomes, whereas NPC2 is a soluble lysosomal protein that is targeted to lysosomes by the mannose-6-phosphate receptor pathway. Despite numerous studies, the function of NPC1 is still poorly understood. It may function as a transmembrane efflux pump. NPC2 serves probably as a lysosomal lipid transfer protein with a high specificity for cholesterol. Both defects give rise to a similar clinical phenotype. Biochemically, both defects lead to a perturbed flow of substrate (primarily lipids) through the endosomal/lysosomal pathway and to a complex pattern of lipid storage consisting of cholesterol, glycosphingolipids, sphingoid bases, and phospholipids. Mucolipidosis IV is a lysosomal storage disease with a heterogeneous storage pattern consisting of phospholipids, glycosphingolipids, and mucopolysaccharides.

The disease is caused by a mutation in the MCOLN1 gene encoding the mucolipin1 protein, a lysosomal membrane protein with six transmembrane domains. There is evidence that this protein functions as a cation channel. This defect may lead to a reduced capacity in the fusion and fission of lysosomal membranes with endosomal and plasma membranes.

Danon disease is an X-linked glycogen storage disorder caused by a defect in the endosomal/lysosomal membrane protein LAMP-2. There is a failure of autophagic vacuoles to fuse with endosomes/lysosomes or of autophagolysosomes to mature into digestive organelles.

D3.5.2.5 Transport Defects (see Table D3.3)

Lysosomal storage diseases due to a defect in the transport of small molecules out of the lysosome are cystinosis caused by a defect in the cystine transport protein cystinosin, and sialic acid storage disease is due to a defect in the lysosomal sialic acid transporter sialin.

D3.5.2.6 Laboratory Diagnosis

The technical aspects of the laboratory diagnosis of lysosomal storage disorders have been reviewed in detail recently and for the practical details the reader is referred to these reviews (Lukacs 2008; Poorthuis and Aerts 2008; Sewell 2008; Verheijen 2008).

The laboratory diagnosis of lysosomal storage diseases consists of four different approaches, histology, metabolite analysis, enzymatic analysis, and mutation analysis that are complementary to each other.

D3.5.2.7 Histology

Lysosomal storage can be demonstrated by light or electron microscopy in easily accessible cells like white blood cells or in skin biopsies (see Chap. D5). In some diseases, biopsies are taken from affected organs such as bone marrow in Gaucher disease and a kidney biopsy in Fabry disease to establish a diagnosis. However, it is recommended to perform enzyme analysis first. Abnormal findings in the biopsy should always be confirmed by enzyme analysis. In some cases, histology is the first choice to obtain evidence for a lysosomal storage disorder, for example, when mucolipidosis IV or a neuronal ceroid lipofuscinosis is suspected.

D3.5.2.7 Metabolite Analysis

Lysosomal storage can be demonstrated by analysis of plasma and urine for storage products such as glycosaminoglycans, oligosaccharides, and glycosphingolipids. The combined quanlitative and quantitative analyses of glycosaminoglycans gives important information on the type of mucopolysaccharidosis involved and limits the number of enzymes that need to be tested to definitively establish the diagnosis (see Table D3.3). The same holds true for the analysis of oligosaccharides, which is usually only qualitative. Each lysosomal defect in the degradation of oligosaccharides shows a specific pattern of oligosaccharides in urine (see Table D3.3). Glycosphingolipid analyses in plasma and urine can be performed to obtain evidence for a sphingolipidosis. In the case of the sphingolipidoses, enzymatic tests are usually performed first based on the clinical information. The analysis of the specific storage product in plasma or urine serves to confirm the diagnosis and to exclude pseudodeficiencies, for example, in metachromatic leukodystrophy or in cases with normal results of the enzyme determination and strong clinical suspicion for Gaucher disease, metachromatic leukodystophy, or Krabbe disease to obtain evidence for an activator protein deficiency (see Table D3.3).

D3.5.3 Enzyme Analysis

D3.5.3.1 Single Enzyme Deficiencies
(see Table D3.3)

Determination of the activity of lysosomal enzymes in leukocytes, plasma, or dried blood spots prepared from whole blood or in fibroblasts is the core in the laboratory diagnosis of lysosomal storage disorders. Most lysosomal storage disorders due to single enzyme deficiencies can be diagnosed reliably and definitively by enzyme assays using artificial fluorescent substrates. Although the K_m of the enzymes measured with these substrates is usually much higher than with the natural substrate, the specificity of the substrates is sufficiently high to allow reliable diagnostic performance.

D3.5.4 Multiple Enzyme Deficiencies
(see Table D3.3)

Mucolipidoses II and III are diagnosed by the strongly increased levels of multiple lysosomal enzymes in plasma and their deficiency in fibroblasts. Multiple sulfatase deficiency is diagnosed by the deficiency of several lysosomal sulfatases in leukocytes and/or fibroblasts. Galactosialidosis is diagnosed by the deficiency of both β-galactosidase and α-neuraminidase in leukocytes and/or fibroblasts. Confirmation can be obtained by measuring cathepsin A in leukocytes or fibroblasts.

D3.5.5 Lysosomal Transport Defects (see Table D3.3)

Cystinosis is diagnosed by measuring increased cystine levels in leukocytes or granulocytes. The sialic acid storage disorders are diagnosed by the increased excretion of sialic acid in urine or increased levels of sialic acid in fibroblasts. A very rare defect in the release of Vitamin B_{12} from lysosomes gives rise to methylmalonic aciduria. The initial diagnosis can be established by organic acid analysis in urine.

D3.5.3.2 Lysosomal/Endosomal Trafficking Defects (see Table D3.3)

Niemann–Pick type C disease is diagnosed by showing cholesterol storage in fibroblasts followed by mutation analysis to discriminate between NPC1 and NPC2. Mutation analysis has superseded the laborious biochemical test used to show decreased cholesterol esterification in fibroblasts. Mucolipidosis IV may be diagnosed by a combination of electron microscopy of the skin and mutation analysis. Danon disease may be diagnosed by electron microscopy cardiac biopsies and mutation analysis.

D3.5.3.3 Neuronal Ceroid Lipofuscinosis

Three of the neuronal ceroid lipofuscinosis (CLN1, CLN2, and CLN10, see Table D3.3) are single lysosomal enzyme defects and can be diagnosed by lysosomal enzyme assays with artificial fluorescent substrates. For the remaining NCLs, a combination of electron microscopy of blood cells or skin biopsy and mutation analysis is recommended.

D3.5.6 Mutation Analysis

The molecular basis of most of the lysosomal storage diseases is known (see Table D3.3) and many mutations have been characterized. However, with few exceptions mutation analysis is rarely used as the initial step in the diagnostic work-up of patients suspected of suffering from a lysosomal storage disorder. Rather mutation analysis is complementary to enzymatic analysis. It is employed when enzyme determinations cannot be used to reach a diagnosis (see the examples

discussed earlier), for carrier testing, which is not possible with certainty by enzyme analysis and – increasingly – in prenatal diagnosis, especially in cases where enzymatic analysis is difficult. Sometimes, there is a relation between the genotype and the phenotype and mutation analysis can help in making a prognosis about the course of the disease.

Take Home Messages

> Enzymes are the key players of metabolism, converting a specific substrate into a specific product, a process called catalysis.

> The flux through a metabolic pathway under certain conditions is determined by the concerted action of all enzymes in the pathway, although the extent to which each particular enzyme contributes to the control of flux may vary widely as defined by each enzyme's flux control coefficient.

> Most peroxisomal disorders can be screened for by analysis in plasma (very long-chain fatty acids) and erythrocytes (plasmalogens) but subsequent detailed enzymatic and molecular studies in fibroblasts are necessary to pinpoint the true underlying enzymatic and subsequent genetic defect.

> Disorders of mitochondria energy production represent a group of clinically and genetically diverse diseases caused by mutations in either mitochondrial or nuclear DNA. Since metabolite abnormalities, including lactate may vary from (grossly) elevated to normal, correct diagnosis of patients may be problematic which requires a multiple approach, including measurement of enzyme activities in clinically affected tissues.

> Acylcarnitine analysis is a powerful first-line test in patients suspected to suffer from a FAO disorder, subsequently followed by enzymatic analysis, preferably lymphocytes, followed by molecular analysis in case the enzyme defect has been established.

> The inherited lysosomal storage disorders are a diverse group of diseases whose correct diagnosis involves a multiple approach involving histology, metabolite analysis, enzyme activity measurements and molecular analysis.

Key References

Acin-Perez R, Fernandez-Silva P, Peleato ML et al (2008) Respiratory active mitochondrial supercomplexes. Mol Cell 32:529–539

Bezman L, Moser AB, Raymond GV et al (2001) Adrenoleukodystrophy: incidence, new mutation rate, and results of extended family screening. Ann Neurol 49:512–517

Brivet M, Garcia-Cazorla A, Lyonnet S et al (2003) Impaired mitochondrial pyruvate importation in a patient and a fetus at risk. Mol Genet Metab 78:186–192

Chinnery PF, Zeviani M (2008) Polymerase gamma and disorders of mitochondrial DNA synthesis. Neuromuscul Disord 18:259–267

Danpure CJ, Purdue PE, Fryer P et al (1993) Enzymological and mutational analysis of a complex primary hyperoxaluria type 1 phenotype involving alanine:glyoxylate aminotransferase peroxisome-to-mitochondrion mistargeting and intraperoxisomal aggregation. Am J Hum Genet 53:417–432

Dierks T, Dickmanns A, Preusser-Kunze A et al (2005) Molecular basis for multiple sulfatase deficiency and mechanism for formylglycine generation of the human formylglycine-generating enzyme. Cell 121:541–552

Eaton S (2002) Control of mitochondrial beta-oxidation flux. Prog Lipid Res 41:197–239

Ebberink MS, Mooyer PA, Koster J et al (2009) Genotypephenotype correlation in PEX5-deficient peroxisome biogenesis defective cell lines. Hum Mutat 30:93–98

Ferdinandusse S, Denis S, Hogenhout EM et al (2007) Clinical, biochemical, and mutational spectrum of peroxisomal acylcoenzyme A oxidase deficiency. Hum Mutat 28:904–912

Ferdinandusse S, Denis S, Mooyer PA et al (2006a) Clinical and biochemical spectrum of D-bifunctional protein deficiency. Ann Neurol 59:92–104

Ferdinandusse S, Kostopoulos P, Denis S et al (2006b) Mutations in the gene encoding peroxisomal sterol carrier protein X (SCPx) cause leukencephalopathy with dystonia and motor neuropathy. Am J Hum Genet 78:1046–1052

Groen AK, Van der Meer R, Westerhoff HV et al (1982b) Control of metabolic fluxes. In: Sies H (ed) Metabolic compartmentation. Academic Press, New York, London

Groen AK, van Roermund CWT, Vervoorn RC, Tager JM (1986) Control of gluconeogenesis in rat liver cells. Flux control coefficients of the enzymes in the gluconeogenic pathway in the absence and presence of glucagon. Biochem J 237:379–389

Groen AK, Wanders RJA, Westerhoff HV et al (1982a) Quantification of the contribution of various steps to the control of mitochondrial respiration. J Biol Chem 257:2754–2757

Heinrich R, Rapoport SM, Rapoport TA (1977) Metabolic regulation and mathematical models. Prog Biophys Mol Biol 32:1–82

Higgins JJ (1965) Metabolic flux analysis. In: Chance B, Estabrook RW, Williamson JR (eds) Control of energy metabolism. Academic Press, New York, London

Hoefs SJ, Dieteren CE, Distelmaier F et al (2008) NDUFA2 complex I mutation leads to Leigh disease. Am J Hum Genet 82:1306–1315

Horn MA, van den Brink DM, Wanders RJA et al (2007) Phenotype of adult Refsum disease due to a defect in peroxin 7. Neurology 68:698–700

Janssen AJ, Schuelke M, Smeitink JAM et al (2008) Muscle 3243A–>G mutation load and capacity of the mitochondrial energy-generating system. Ann Neurol 63:473–481

Janssen AJ, Trijbels FJ, Sengers RC et al (2006) Measurement of the energy-generating capacity of human muscle mitochondria: diagnostic procedure and application to human pathology. Clin Chem 52:860–871

Kacser H, Burns JA (1979) Molecular democracy: who shares the controls? Biochem Soc Trans 7:1149–1160

Kacser H, Burns JA (1981) The molecular basis of dominance. Genetics 97:639–666

Kolter T, Sandhoff K (2005) Principles of lysosomal membrane digestion: stimulation of sphingolipid degradation by sphingolipid activator proteins and anionic lysosomal lipids. Annu Rev Cell Dev Biol 21:81–103

Kornfeld S (1987) Trafficking of lysosomal enzymes. FASEB J 1:462–468

Leinekugel P, Michel S, Conzelmann E, Sandhoff K (1992) Quantitative correlation between the residual activity of betahexosaminidase A and arylsulfatase A and the severity of the resulting lysosomal storage disease. Hum Genet 88:513–523

Lukacs Z (2008) Mucopolysaccharides. In: Blau N, Duran M, Gibson KM (eds) Laboratory guide to the methods in biochemical genetics. Springer, Berlin

Mayr JA, Merkel O, Kohlwein SD et al (2007) Mitochondrial phosphate-carrier deficiency: a novel disorder of oxidative phosphorylation. Am J Hum Genet 80:478–484

Molinari F, Raas-Rothschild A, Rio M et al (2005) Impaired mitochondrial glutamate transport in autosomal recessiveneonatal myoclonic epilepsy. Am J Hum Genet 76:334–339

Motley AM, Brites P, Gerez L et al (2002) Mutational spectrum in the PEX7 gene and functional analysis of mutant alleles in 78 patients with rhizomelic chondrodysplasia punctata type 1. Am J Hum Genet 70:612–624

Nada MA, Rhead WJ, Sprecher H Clark S (1995) Evidence for intermediate channeling in mitochondrial beta-oxidation. J Biol Chem 270:530–535

Olpin SE, Manning NJ, Pollitt RJ, Clarke S (1997) Improved detection of long-chain fatty acid oxidation defects in intact cells using [9,10-3H]oleic acid. J Inherit Metab Dis 20:415–419

Platta HW, Erdmann R (2007) The peroxisomal protein import machinery. FEBS Lett 581:2811–2819

Poorthuis BJHM, Aerts JMFG (2008) Glycosphingolipids. In: Blau N, Duran M, Gibson MK (eds) Laboratory guide to the methods in biochemical genetics. Springer, Berlin

Pulkes T, Sweeney MG, Hanna MG (2000) Increased risk of stroke in patients with the A12308G polymorphism in mitochondria. Lancet 356:2068–2069

Rinaldo P, Matern D, Bennett MJ (2002) Fatty acid oxidation disorders. Annu Rev Physiol 64:477–502

Sewell A (2008) Oligosaccharides. In: Blau N (ed) Laboratory guide to the methods in biochemical genetics. Springer, Berlin

van den Brink DM, Brites P, Haasjes J et al (2003) Identification of PEX7 as the second gene involved in Refsum disease. Am J Hum Genet 72:471–477

van Woerden CS, Groothoff JW, Wijburg FA et al (2004) Clinical implications of mutation analysis in primary hyperoxaluria type 1. Kidney Int 66:746–752

Ventura FV, Costa CG, Struys EA et al (1999) Quantitative acylcarnitine profiling in fibroblasts using [U-13C] palmitic acid: an improved tool for the diagnosis of fatty acid oxidation defects. Clin Chim Acta 281:1–17

Verheijen FW (2008) Sialic acid. In: Blau N, Duran M, Gibson KM (eds) Laboratory guide to the methods in biochemical genetics. Springer, Berlin

Vockley J (2008) Metabolism as a complex genetic trait, a systems biology approach: implications for inborn errors of metabolism and clinical diseases. J Inherit Metab Dis 31:619–629

Walkley SU (2001) New proteins from old diseases provide novel insights in cell biology. Curr Opin Neurol 14:805–810

Wanders RJA (2004) Metabolic and molecular basis of peroxisomal disorders: a review. Am J Med Genet 126A: 355–375

Wanders RJA, van Roermund CWT, Meijer AJ (1984) Analysis of the control of citrulline synthesis in isolated rat-liver mitochondria. Eur J Biochem 142:247–254

Wanders RJA, Waterham HR (2006) Biochemistry of mammalian peroxisomes revisited. Annu Rev Biochem 75: 295–332

Weller S, Gould SJ, Valle D (2003) Peroxisome biogenesis disorders. Annu Rev Genomics Hum Genet 4:165–211

Wittig I, Carrozzo R, Santorelli FM, Schagger (2006) Supercomplexes and subcomplexes of mitochondrial oxidative phosphorylation. Biochim Biophys Acta 1757:1066–1072

DNA Studies

D4

Johannes Zschocke

Key Facts

> Mutation studies have become an important component in the diagnostic work-up of patients, but their use should be balanced with other (phenotypic) diagnostic methods.

> Molecular analyses have a limited sensitivity as some disease-causing mutations are usually missed by standard methods, and failure to identify a diagnostic genotype may not necessarily exclude a diagnosis. Sensitivity depends on both genetic characteristics and the method employed.

> Identification of disease-causing mutations confirms the diagnosis, may provide prognostic information, and allows simple testing of other family members including prenatal diagnosis.

> The functional impact of novel genetic variants identified in a patient should be assessed with great care. They should be denoted "unclassified variants" unless they are likely to cause disease.

> Mutation analyses (like all specialized tests) are prone to errors. Confirmatory repeat analyses (either on a new sample or by analysis at a second independent laboratory) may be considered when the results of molecular studies are important for patient management but do not seem to fit the clinician's assessment of the case.

J. Zschocke
Divisions of Human Genetics and Clinical Genetics, Medical University Innsbruck, Schöpfstr. 41,6020 Innsbruck, Austria
e-mail: johannes.zschocke@i-med.ac.at

The last two decades have seen remarkable progress in the molecular understanding of inborn errors of metabolism. The localization and structure of most genes involved in monogenic metabolic disorders have been characterized, and information gained through the human genome project and reverse genetics has allowed the detection or confirmation of many "new" metabolic disorders. The identification of various disease-causing mutations in the individual conditions has not only greatly enhanced the diagnostic options but also led to an improved understanding of molecular disease mechanisms and sometimes new therapeutic options.

Mutation analyses are now frequently used for clinical purposes including confirmation of diagnosis and prediction of disease severity. Nevertheless, there is still uncertainty about how molecular analyses can complement or replace other diagnostic methods. Many metabolic disorders are reliably diagnosed and confirmed through biochemical and enzymatic investigations rather than through mutation analyses. Molecular analyses have a limited sensitivity as some disease-causing mutations are usually missed by standard methods, and failure to identify a diagnostic genotype may not necessarily exclude a diagnosis. Also, technical and interpretative difficulties may be underestimated both by clinicians and laboratories, and quality assessment schemes even for a common condition such as phenylketonuria have given rather disconcerting results. Nevertheless, there is an increasing number of disorders in which molecular studies are indicated at an early stage in the diagnostic process, usually because the disease is caused by prevalent mutations in particular populations or because invasive procedures are necessary to obtain samples for specific enzyme studies, e.g., liver biopsies. A collation of useful Internet resources that provide molecular or

G. F. Hoffmann et al. (eds.), *Inherited Metabolic Diseases*,
DOI: 10.1007/978-3-540-74723-9_D4, © Springer-Verlag Berlin Heidelberg 2010

metabolic information is given in Chap. E3. Laboratories that offer diagnostic mutation analyses may be found through the databases GeneTests (www.genetests.org, mostly North America), Orphanet (www.orpha.net), and EDDNAL (http://www.eddnal.com, both mostly European).

> **Remember**
>
> Mutation analyses in children may only be performed if there is an important medical consequence in childhood. Carrier analyses in healthy siblings of children with metabolic disorders are not indicated and should not usually be performed even when requested by the parents.

D4.1 Samples

> **Remember**
>
> *Sample for most applications*
>
> 5–10 ml EDTA full blood, shipped at ambient temperature. For long distances it may be preferable to extract the DNA and send that.

Mutation analysis can be performed in any human sample that contains cellular nuclei. The exact sample depends on the type of DNA that needs to be investigated. Routine diagnostic mutation analyses are usually performed in genomic DNA which is most conveniently extracted from 5 to 10 ml of anticoagulated full blood (usually EDTA blood). Smaller amounts of blood down to a few 100 µl may be acceptable but less satisfactory as DNA extraction from small samples is less reliable, less DNA is available, and the extraction method may be more expensive (discuss with laboratory). The sample should not be centrifuged but shipped as native full blood by normal (overnight) mail at ambient temperature. DNA is quite stable, and the sample may be stored at room temperature or in the refrigerator for 1–2 days if necessary (e.g., on weekends). Alternatively, whole blood may be stored frozen for several weeks or may be sent on dry ice; enquire with the molecular laboratory whether frozen blood is accepted. If EDTA blood is not available, other materials including dried blood spots on filter paper cards, coagulated blood, hair roots, buccal swabs, or even serum, urine, or feces may be used for extraction of genomic DNA or for polymerase chain reaction (PCR)-amplification of specific sequences, but these methods are less reliable and may be considerably more expensive.

An alternative template for genetic analysis is mRNA obtained from cells in which the target gene is expressed. As a single-stranded molecule, mRNA is quite unstable and in the laboratory is converted into double-stranded complementary DNA (cDNA) which can be stored indefinitely. cDNA analysis has certain advantages over genomic DNA. It does not have an intron–exon structure but contains the uninterrupted sequence that is translated into protein. The detection of unknown mutations may be more convenient from cDNA since fewer fragments are required for PCR-based analysis methods. Splicing mutations that cause the removal of whole exons from the translated sequence are easily recognized, thus confirming the pathological relevance of DNA variants in the introns. On the other hand, splicing variants that are observed under physiological or cell culture conditions are sometimes not likely to cause disease and may be difficult to interpret; RNA fragments that contain premature stop codons may be eliminated by nonsense-mediated decay, and the preparation of cDNA is more tedious than that of genomic DNA. While cDNA analysis may be the method of choice in conjunction with enzyme studies if organ tissue such as liver or skin fibroblasts is available for investigation, genomic DNA analysis remains the method of choice for most applications.

D4.2 Indications

> **Remember**
>
> It is a long way from the genotype to the phenotype in metabolic disorders, and a diagnosis may be made on all levels
>
> - Genotype = genetic information, may or may not determine disease manifestation.
> - Enzymatic phenotype = measurable protein function, mostly independent from external factors but often restricted to specific organs.

- Metabolic phenotype = concentration of metabolites, e.g., in body fluids, may vary considerably depending on the external factors including treatment.
- Clinical phenotype = result of genetic and external factors, key to diagnosis.

Remember

It is often difficult to predict the functional effects of mutations, and the impact of novel genetic variants identified in a patient should be discussed with great care.

Biochemical and enzymatic analyses, when available, are often preferable for the diagnosis of metabolic disorders as they reflect phenotypical parameters ("enzymatic" or "metabolic phenotype") and are therefore closer to the patient's clinical phenotype and disease expression. Nevertheless, there are various circumstances in which molecular studies are cheaper, faster, more convenient, or the only reliable method for diagnosis or confirmation of diagnosis of an inherited disorder. Many metabolic defects involve enzymes that are only expressed in specific organs such as the liver or the brain, necessitating invasive procedures (if at all possible) for enzymatic confirmation. Other disorders involving structural, receptor, or membrane proteins that do not cause metabolic alterations are not open for enzyme testing and therefore may be difficult to confirm by traditional methods. Molecular studies may be fast and efficient and therefore the method of choice for the confirmation of disorders that are caused by single prevalent mutations in the patient's population, e.g., the prevalent Caucasian medium-chain acyl-CoA dehydrogenase mutation c.985A>G (p.K329E). The identification of well-characterized mutations may provide information on disease severity, prognosis, or other clinical parameters in disorders with good genotype–phenotype correlations. Common genetic variants that potentially influence disease course or treatment may be easily detected through specific analyses, e.g., the factor-V-Leiden mutation or the methyltetrahydrofolate reductase variant p.A222V. Identification of disease-causing mutations in a particular patient allows rapid, cost-efficient and reliable testing of other family members including prenatal diagnosis. In any case, laboratories that offer molecular analyses for clinical purposes need to have good knowledge of the tested disorder, genotype–phenotype correlations, alternative diagnostic approaches, as well as the sensitivity and specificity of mutation analysis in the individual patient.

D4.3 Methods

A wide range of molecular methods is available for the identification of mutations and other DNA variants, most of which are based on the PCR. Different methods are used to screen for specific known variants or to examine the gene for unknown mutations. There is no uniform strategy that is suitable for all applications, and a combination of methods is often used. The exact approach depends on gene characteristics, type and frequency of mutations, and the sensitivity required to answer the clinical question. For adequate requesting of tests and interpretation of results, it is important that the clinician is familiar with the sensitivity, specificity, and indication of the most frequently used mutation detection strategies. In this chapter, we concentrate on PCR-based methods for the detection of point mutations or small deletions/insertions as these are by far the most frequent causes of inborn errors of metabolism.

There are several widely used *mutation screening methods* for the specific identification of selected DNA variants. Most methods are relatively inexpensive; commercial kits that test for several common mutations are available for some disorders such as cystic fibrosis. However, the sensitivity of these mutation-specific screening methods for the detection of relevant DNA changes is limited and will remain so by definition since rare and new mutations are not identified. Homozygosity or compound heterozygosity of disease-causing mutations is diagnostic in the investigated patients, but failure to identify a mutation does not exclude the disorder. Screened mutations are usually well characterized and their clinical relevance is well known. Mutation-specific screening methods are especially useful for the detection of common DNA polymorphisms that may influence multifactorial disorders such as atherosclerosis as well as for the confirmation of inherited disorders that are caused by specific prevalent mutations in a particular population.

DNA sequencing of the whole coding region of relevant genes is more demanding with regard to both the detection and the interpretation of DNA variants but is now regarded as method of choice for the majority of conditions. Current technology involves semi-automated DNA sequencers that detect fluorescently labeled DNA fragments with specific laser systems. In the standard approach, the genomic target region is first amplified by PCR. Fluorescently labeled base-specific fragments are then generated through cycle sequencing with unidirectional primers and ddNTP nucleotides, either of which is labeled with a fluorescent marker dye. These fragments are then separated on conventional acrylamide gels or through capillary electrophoresis. There is as yet no 100% reliable system for the automatic evaluation of the DNA sequences generated in this fashion, and skilled interpretation of the results is required particularly for the detection or exclusion of heterozygous mutations. It is also important to note that direct sequencing of coding exons detects neither large genomic rearrangements (deletions, duplications) nor intronic mutations outside splicing regions.

Some laboratories continue to use *mutation scanning methods* for rapid, cost-efficient mutation analysis particularly in large genes. These methods identify regions in which a mutation or other genetic variant is located and which are subsequently sequenced for characterization of the exact base change. Scanning methods considerably reduce sequencing load but are sometimes difficult to interpret and differ in their sensitivity, i.e., the reliability with which mutations are found. Failure to detect mutations in a patient by one of the less sensitive scanning methods such as single-strand configuration polymorphism analysis does not exclude the disorder in question, albeit making it more unlikely. Other methods such as denaturing gradient gel electrophoresis or denaturing high-performance liquid chromatography, when well designed, have a sensitivity that equals direct sequencing.

The capacity for mutation detection for common conditions will be greatly expanded through the introduction of *DNA arrays* probably within the next decade. DNA arrays are already used for the exclusion of candidate gene loci for autosomal recessive disorders in consanguineous families or families with several affected siblings. In these circumstances, DNA arrays may also allow the identification of novel disease genes on a research basis.

D4.4 Pitfalls

Remember

Mutation analysis, like any laboratory technique, has a certain error rate, which is difficult to eliminate completely.

Incorrect results or interpretations may be generated either through analytical or sampling errors, methodological limitations, insufficient knowledge of the types of mutations causing a particular disease, or inadequate consideration of family or population information. The following factors should be considered in the choice of mutation analysis methods and the interpretation of the results:

- What type of mutation usually causes the disease? Different approaches need to be chosen for different mutations such as point mutations, trinucleotide repeats, or large deletions.
- Are there certain prevalent disease-causing mutations in particular populations? Screening for such mutations may be a cost-efficient method for confirming the disease or reducing the likelihood of its presence in a patient. It is essential to take the ethnic origin of a patient into consideration when such an approach is chosen.
- What is the sensitivity of comprehensive mutation analysis with PCR-based methods such as DNA sequencing? For some disorders, this may approach 100%, while for others, only a proportion of mutations is recognized. PCR-based methods are usually restricted to coding exons and adjacent intron sequences of the particular gene and may fail to detect, e.g., large gene deletions spanning several exons.
- Could there be more than one mutation on the same chromosomal strand? Double mutants have been identified in many genes. It is not justified to conclude that there is compound heterozygosity when two mutations are identified in a patient with a recessive disease. This constellation is only one of the reasons why inheritance of mutations on separate chromosomes should be confirmed in samples from parents or other relatives. In addition, identification of common missense mutations through selective

screening may not be sufficient for predicting the phenotype in a particular patient as additional mutations affecting protein structure may be missed.

- What is the diagnostic specificity of mutation identification? Only a proportion of variants in a gene affect protein function and cause disease. Criteria that may be used to estimate pathogenetic relevance include type of mutation (missense or nonsense, predicted impact on amino acid sequence), extent of DNA analyzed, segregation with the disease in a family, prevalence of the mutation in the general population, and functional assessment through expression analysis.

- How important are nongenetic factors of pathogenesis? Disease penetrance may vary considerably even within single families. Strict genotype–phenotype correlations are observed only in a proportion of metabolic disorders, and the clinical picture in a patient may be insufficiently explained by the mutations in a single gene.

Clinicians who request mutation analyses should treat the results with care, just like all other laboratory tests. Quality assessment schemes, available only for very few conditions anyway, show that significant errors occur even in laboratories with good technical facilities and accreditation for diagnostic molecular genetic services. Confirmatory repeat analyses (either on a new sample or by analysis at a second independent laboratory) may be considered when the results of molecular studies are important for patient management but do not seem to fit the clinician's assessment of the case. Adequate interpretation of the results requires good knowledge of the respective disease and the underlying mutations that determine its pathogenicity. It is prudent to request molecular diagnostic services only from laboratories that are familiar with the respective disorders and the underlying genotype–phenotype correlations.

Key References

Zschocke J, Janssen B (2008) Molecular genetics: mutation analysis in the diagnosis of metabolic disorders. In: Blau N, Duran M, Gibson KM (eds) Laboratory guide to the methods in biochemical genetics. Springer, Heidelberg, pp 805–829

Zschocke J, Aulehla-Scholz C, Patton S (2008) Quality of diagnostic mutation analyses for phenylketonuria. J Inherit Metab Dis 31:697–702

Pathology – Biopsy

Hans H. Goebel

Key Facts

> Neurometabolic single organelle-multiorgan disorders, i.e., lysosomal, peroxisomal, polyglucosan, and mitochondrial disorders warrant biopsies for morphological (and often biochemical by direct tissue and/or indirect fibroblast culture) studies.

> Tissues suitable for biopsies are lymphocytes, skin, conjunctiva, skeletal muscle, rectum, and liver.

> Different neurometabolic disorders show different patterns of morphological expression in different tissues.

> Brain and peripheral nerves need not be biopsied because any neurometabolic disease morphologically expressed in the nervous system may also be encountered in any of the other tissues. Only rectum, among noncerebral tissues, may show exclusive lysosomal neuronal storage.

> Accessibility and morphological manifestation determine the target of biopsy in an individually suspected neurometabolic disorder.

> Preferential sites of biopsy are lymphocytes in vacuolar and certain nonvacuolar lysosomal diseases, skin in many lysosomal and Lafora diseases; skeletal muscle in many lysosomal, polyglucosan, and mitochondrial diseases; and liver in peroxisomal and lysosomal diseases.

H. H. Goebel
Department of Neuropathology, Mainz University Medical Center, Langenbeckstrabe 1, 55131 Mainz, Germany
e-mail: goebel@neuropatho.klinik.uni-mainz.de

D5.1 General Remarks

Pathology, i.e., pathomorphology concerning individual groups of metabolic diseases, as summarized in Chaps. A1–A3, may be divided into disease-specific or pathognomonic pathology. Recognition allows precise nosological diagnosis. Examples are lysosomal inclusions in certain lysosomal diseases or group-specific pathological features, e.g., lysosomal vacuoles in certain lysosomal diseases, or abnormally structured mitochondria in mitochondrial diseases. Lesions nonspecific for any disease may be characteristic of a particular class of metabolic diseases, e.g., sponginess of cerebral tissue in amino acid disorders. Secondary pathological phenomena may also be encountered, for instance, reactive cellular and fibrillar astrocytosis or demyelination in the brain following loss of nerve and glial cells, and fibrosis in liver or heart following atrophy or loss of hepatocytes or cardiomyocytes.

Inherited metabolic diseases are defined by biochemical and molecular criteria, while morphological investigations of tissues express pathomorphology (Table D5.1). While not always disease-specific, the pathological picture may pave the way for relevant biochemical and molecular studies. Postbiochemical and postmolecular morphological investigations may confirm findings.

The methodological spectrum of the anatomic pathologist, the neuropathologist, and the paidopathologist may encompass histological studies with a wide range of structural and histochemical stains, enzyme histochemical preparations requiring unfixed frozen tissue, of lysosomal, mitochondrial and peroxisomal enzymes, and electron microscopy. When antibodies against enzyme substrates or enzyme proteins are available, immunohistochemistry is employed.

Table D5.1 Neurometabolic diseases, morphologically expressed in various tissues

Frequently biopsied
  Lymphocytes
  Skeletal muscle
  Skin
Infrequently biopsied
  Bone marrow
  Brain
  Conjunctiva
  Intestine
  Kidney
  Liver
  Lymph nodes
  Peripheral nerves
  Tonsils

Table D5.2 Metabolic diseases with morphological pathology in various tissues suitable for biopsy (single organelle-multi organ disorders)

Lysosomal diseases
  Lymphocytes
  Bone marrow
  Brain
  Liver
  Rectum
  Skeletal muscle
  Skin
Mitochondrial diseases
  Brain
  Liver
  Skeletal muscle
Peroxisomal diseases
  Kidney
  Liver
  Adrenal glands
  Peripheral nerves
Polyglucosan diseases
  Brain
  Liver
  Skeletal muscle
  Skin

These techniques require different approaches, immediately after having obtained the biopsied tissue, e.g., fixation in formalin for regular histological studies and frozen unfixed tissue for certain histochemical and enzyme histochemical methods. Immunohistochemical preparations depend on the suitability of antibodies for fixed, paraffin-embedded or frozen tissues. Immediate proper fixation, i.e., of small tissue fragments in the specific fixative glutaraldehyde, is required for electron microscopy.

Biopsy obtains tissues of living patients, while autopsies may confirm a diagnosis and document the distribution of the disease and the intensity of the pathology. Clinico-pathological and clinico-radiological correlations allow for tissue-specific biochemical studies, e.g., muscle tissue in postinfantile type-II glycogenosis or in mitochondrial diseases. In many fatal inherited metabolic diseases, the diagnosis has been established by the time of autopsy.

Biopsies in patients with metabolic diseases are invasive, diagnostic surgical procedures. Skin, conjunctiva, rectum, and skeletal muscle may be investigated by open biopsy, allowing proper orientation and removal of tissue as well as tissue for different morphological preparations. Tissues of visceral organs and sometimes skeletal muscle may also be obtained by needle biopsies. A limited number of lysosomal disorders may morphologically be recognized in blood lymphocytes, requiring only venipuncture. It is essential to know that the biopsied organ will contain pathology of the disease, which is suspected or already ascertained by the clinician. Many inherited

metabolic diseases are multi-organ diseases, and respective pathology may be recognized in more than one tissue or organ, allowing biospy of variously available tissue, such as lymphocytes, skin, or conjunctiva (Table D5.2).

With the enormous expansion of biochemical and molecular assays in metabolic diseases, significance of a diagnostic biopsy or morphological study has considerably decreased. The number of biopsies is shrinking as is knowledge of postsurgical morphological findings. Hence, earlier comprehensive reviews are important (Goebel 1997, 1999; Goebel and Jänisch 1995; Goebel and Warlo 1990a, b).

Biopsies of extracerebral tissues in patients with metabolic diseases while often pathognomonic may be considered optional, whereas an earlier category of "essential" biopsies (Goebel 1999) has lost its value. Considering the diversity of tissues involved in metabolic diseases, each condition or group of conditions may require different approaches to different tissues or possibly a "sequential" order, such as in the neuronal ceroid-lipofuscinoses (NCL) commencing with lymphocytes and, if unyielding or equivocal, proceeding to skin and other tissues such as muscle and rectum.

Disease-specific morphological evaluation and advice as to respective biopsy procedures will therefore be provided according to tissues and organs.

Remember

Biopsies are rewarding for morphological diagnosis when disease-typical lesions are present in the tissue. Metabolic single organelle-multi-organ disorders are such conditions. Lesions may be identified by electron microscopy. The tissue target of biopsy is dictated by the morphological manifestation of the disease and the accessibility of the tissues.

D5.2 Circulating Blood Cells

In certain metabolic disorders, particularly lysosomal diseases (Table D5.3), the easiest cells to obtain are circulating white blood cells. A blood smear may show vacuolated lymphocytes in certain lysosomal disorders marked by lysosomal vacuoles, e.g., mucopolysaccharidoses, oligosaccharidoses, GM_1-gangliosidosis. However, the procedure may only be considered supportive rather than proving since swollen mitochondria may give the spurious light microscopic impression of lysosomal vacuoles. A PAS stain may show carbohydrate-containing intralysosomal contents. The

Table D5.3 Lysosomal pathology in lymphocytes

Vacuoles
  Aspartylglucosaminuria
  GM_1-gangliosidosis
  Mannosidosis
  Fucosidosis
  Juvenile neuronal ceroid-lipofuscinosis (NCL)
  Mucolipidosis I and II
  Mucopolysaccharidoses I–VII
  Salla disease
  Type-II glycogenosis
Solid non-vacuolar
  Infantile NCL
  Late-infantile NCL
  Late-infantile variant of NCL
  Mucolipidosis IV
  Niemann-Pick disease
  Type-II glycogenosis (when glycogen is well preserved)

lysosomal nature of vacuoles may be further confirmed by enzyme histochemical demonstration of increased activity of acid phosphatase, the marker enzyme for lysosomes. In most lysosomal diseases vacuoles only appear in lymphocytes, but in certain mucopolysaccharidoses there are granules in polymorphonuclear leukocytes known as Alder bodies.

At the electron microscopic level, non-vacuolar lysosomal residual bodies may be ascertained. Although lymphocytes are present in the buffy coat, numerical predominance of granulocytes may impede careful electron microscopic studies of such a specimen. Therefore, isolation of circulating lymphocytes, using the Ficoll technique, greatly facilitates ultrastructural investigation. For this reason, heparinised blood requires immediate isolation of the lymphocytes before fixation as a pellet in buffered glutaraldehyde and, then, routine embedding in resin for regular electron microscopic workup. Only at the electron microscopic level, may swollen mitochondria be distinguished from membrane-bound lysosomal vacuoles; the mitochondrial double membrane and marginal remnants of ruptured cristae provide clear distinction.

When disease-specific lysosomal inclusions of vacuolar or non-vacuolar nature are present, they should be photographed for permanent documentation. When absent, one may safely count in the electron microscope 200 consecutive properly identified lymphocytes to be sure that lysosomal storage is not present in the preparation.

Among metabolic diseases, lysosomal storage or residual bodies are vacuolar in mucopolysaccharidoses, oligosaccharidoses, mucolipidoses, GM_1-gangliosidosis (Fig. D5.1) and in juvenile or CLN3 NCL. In the latter vacuoles may occasionally contain fingerprint profiles, but their number is considerably lower than the number of vacuoles. Thus, empty lysosomal vacuoles usually predominate in juvenile NCL. On the other hand, non-vacuolar, i.e., granular or lamellar inclusions, often of disease-specific nature, are seen in type-II glycogenosis, Niemann-Pick disease, and Fabry disease. They are granular in infantile NCL/CLN1, curvilinear bodies in classical late-infantile NCL/CLN2 and ususally few but regularly shaped solid non-vacuolar lipopigments with a granular component and fingerprint profiles in late-infantile variants of NCL, i.e., CLN5, CLN6, CLN7, and CLN8.

Fig. D5.1 Electron microscopic abundant lysosomal membrane-bound vacuoles in a blood lymphocyte, GM$_1$ gangliosidosis

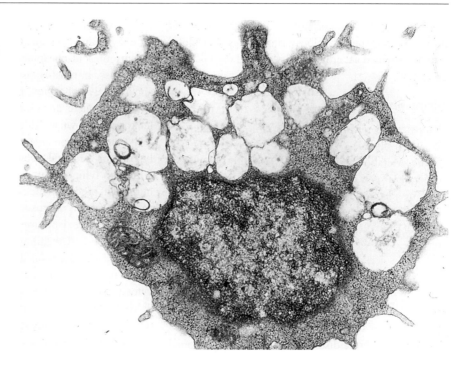

Remember

Lymphocytes are only suitable for morphological investigations in lysosomal diseases, not in mitochondrial or peroxisomal disorders. Electron microscopy – not light microscopy – may show lysosomal vacuoles or compact lysosomal inclusions which vary in ultratructure, according to the type of lysosomal disease.

D5.3 Skin

Skin is widely used for morphological investigations (Table D5.4). It offers easy accessibility by punch biopsy; a large diversity of cell types, i.e., epithelial, mesenchymal, and neuroectodermal, allowing metabolic conditions to be differently expressed in these cell types. In addition, fibroblast cultures may be obtained from separate biopsies of skin.

A prerequisite for gainful skin biopsy is that the clinically suspected disease manifests itself morphologically in the skin or in cultured fibroblasts. A rewarding biopsy requires a full-thickness skin biopsy, as diagnostically crucial eccrine sweat gland epithelial

complexes are often located in the cutis–subcutis region, while epidermis is of limited reward (Kaesgen and Goebel 1989).

The catalogue of morphologically diagnosable metabolic diseases affecting the skin in children includes lysosomal and peroxisomal diseases as well as Lafora disease (Table D5.4). Mitochondrial disorders – even those associated with abnormally structured mitochondria are seen predominantly in skeletal muscle fibers – and are not

Table D5.4 Pathology of metabolic diseases in skin

Vacuolar lysosomal diseases
MPS, ML, oligosaccharidosis
Avacuolar lysosomal disorders
Globoid cell leukodystrophy
GM$_1$ gangliosidosis
GM$_2$ gangliosidosis (Sandhoff type)
Farber disease
Fabry disease
Metachromatic leukodystrophy (when nerves are present)
Neuronal ceroid-lipofuscinosis
Niemann-Pick disease
Type-II glycogenosis
Peroxisomal diseases
Adrenoleukodystrophy
Polyglucosan diseases
Lafora disease

convincingly expressed in skin. Amino acid and other small-molecule disorders do not display meaningful pathomorphological data in skin.

In skin obtained by diagnostic biopsy, morphological investigations are largely to be performed with the electron microscope because it is only at the ultrastructural level that lesions appear distinct and sometimes disease-specific. Light microscopic studies may give spurious results even when employing special techniques, such as enzyme histochemistry, immunohistochemistry, or fluorescence microscopy. However, Lafora disease may be recognized at the light microscopic level by strongly PAS-positive diastase-resistant polyglucosan bodies in ductal cells of eccrine sweat glands. Lysosomal vacuolation may be excessive in respective lysosomal disorders, such as mucopolysaccharidoses, but confirmatory electron microscopy remains desirable. Another hint at electron microscopic lysosomal lesions may be increased enzyme histochemical activity of acid phosphatase at unusual sites, e.g., smooth muscle cells of arrectores pilorum muscle or mural cells of vessels. The secretory granules in secretory cells of eccrine sweat glands are PAS-positive, a nonspecific physiological feature, which is not to be taken as evidence of pathological lysosomal storage of glycolipids, glycoproteins, or glycosaminoglycans. Even semi-thin, 1 μm-thick, plastic sections stained with toluidine or methylene blue serve to identify various cytological components in the skin specimen for subsequent electron microscopic examination rather than to ascertain unequivocal pathology.

Among the biochemically heterogeneous lysosomal disorders, different entities are morphologically expressed in different cytological components of the skin. Some, like purely in particular neuronal forms, Tay-Sachs disease, or Gaucher disease do not express any pathology in the skin.

As in lymphocytes, dermal cells in lysosomal disorders may be characterized by lysosomal vacuolation or by the formation of non-vacuolar compact lysosomal residual bodies. Hence, known lysosomal disorders marked by lysosomal vacuolation, such as mucopolysaccharidoses, mucolipidoses, and oligosaccharidoses, show lysosomal vacuoles in mesenchymal cells, such as fibroblasts and mural cells of vessels. Certain lysosomal disorders, such as sialidosis and mucolipidosis IV, may show both lysosomal vacuolation and compact lysosomal residual bodies of lamellar type in different cell types of the skin.

Of the lysosomal diseases, type-II glycogenosis, and the NCL show ubiquitous lysosomal pathology affecting epithelial, mesenchymal, and neuroectodermal cells. In type-II glycogenosis, there is intralysosomal glycogen accretion and a lysosomal vacuolar appearance when glycogen is badly preserved in tissue handling after biopsy. In NCL, there are ultrastructurally distinct lipopigments. Granular lipopigments without any lipid droplets, the latter a conspicuous component of regular lipofuscin, may be encountered in genetic CLN1 or its infantile, late-infantile, juvenile, and adult clinical forms; curvilinear bodies are found in genetic CLN2 or classical late-infantile form, while other late infantile variant forms, genetic CLN5, CLN6, CLN7, and CLN8 types show a mixture of curvilinear profiles and fingerprint patterns. In genetic CLN3 or classic juvenile NCL, fingerprint profiles or fingerprint bodies prevail while, occasionally, vacuolation of lysosomes is also encountered – as in CLN3 in lymphocytes.

Dermal nerves contain myelinated and unmyelinated nerve fibers, covered by Schwann cells and, when still situated in fascicles, surrounded by perineurium or perineurial cells. Schwann cells of both myelinated and unmyelinated axons and perineurial cells may contain pathological lysosomes of different lamellar types, such as in mucolipidosis IV, sialidosis, Niemann-Pick disease, Sandhoff disease, and foremost the lysosomal leukodystrophies with involvement of the peripheral nervous system, such as metachromatic (MLD) and globoid cell (GCL) leukodystrophies. When myelinated nerves are encountered in the skin specimen, metachromasia of stored sulfatides in MLD may be demonstrated as brownish material in acid cresyl violet-stained fixed frozen sections and brownish material in toluidine blue-stained semi-thin sections. Disease-specific lysosomal residual bodies accrue in Schwann cells, particularly of myelinated nerve fibers, including prismatic or tufaceous bodies in MLD and needle-like inclusions in GCL. In addition, similar compact lysosomal residual bodies may be encountered in macrophages within the endoneurium, derived from damage to and breakdown of myelinated nerve fibers. The ultrastructure of lysosomal inclusions in GCL differs in the infantile and non-infantile forms in that needle-like structures are largely seen in infantile GCL and rather vacuolar lysosomes filled with indistinct lamellae are seen in non-infantile GCL (Goebel et al. 1990). A remarkable distinction in dermal morphological manifestation between MLD and GCL is the involvement of secretory cells of eccrine sweat glands with similar needle-like inclusions in GCL, but no abnormal lysosomal storage in MLD.

While mural cells of vessels are affected by lysosomal storage in a large number of lysosomal diseases, they are particularly involved in Fabry disease. They are even demonstrable in manifesting carriers of this X-linked inherited disorder.

Important tissue components of skin are the eccrine sweat glands, the secretory cells of which display a wide variety of lysosomal residual bodies both vacuolar and non-vacuolar in different disease. These lysosomal residual bodies can often be distinguished from secretory granules, both compact or electron-lucent. Sometimes, there is a disturbingly large number of membrane-bound vacuoles in secretory eccrine sweat gland epithelial cells, not associated with any lysosomal disorder, a nonspecific morphological feature of unknown connotation. While the ductal cells of eccrine sweat glands are not affected by lysosomal storage in lysosomal disorders, they are the main cell type involved in formation of polyglucosan bodies, not limited by a unit membrane, in Lafora disease (Fig. D5.2) (Goebel and Bönnemann 2004). Similarly, polyglucosan bodies may be encountered in apocrine sweat gland epithelial cells of the axilla.

> **Remember**
>
> Skin biopsy in the axillar region is not advisable when suspecting a lysosomal disorder because there are physiological inclusions.

Both, epithelial cells of apocrine sweat glands and ductal cells of eccrine sweat glands may contain nonspecific normal inclusions, the former rather uniform and compact, the latter of a lamellar ultrastructure. These cytoplasmic inclusions should not be confused with pathological storage bodies. Melanin- and melanosome-containing cells as well as mast cells also harbor cell type-specific inclusions, which should not be confused with true pathological lysosomal inclusions.

Not infrequently, axons, usually unmyelinated and in their terminal course, are nonspecifically enlarged by mitochondria and dense bodies, the latter possibly degenerating mitochondria (Dolman et al. 1977; Walter and Goebel 1988), but hardly ever by disease-specific lysosomal residual bodies. These have only been seen in the gangliosidoses and in mucolipidosis IV. When encountering such enlarged axons, a lysosomal disorder may be suspected. The enlargement of the axons may result from impaired axoplasmic transport as a result of lysosomal storage in respective neuronal perikarya.

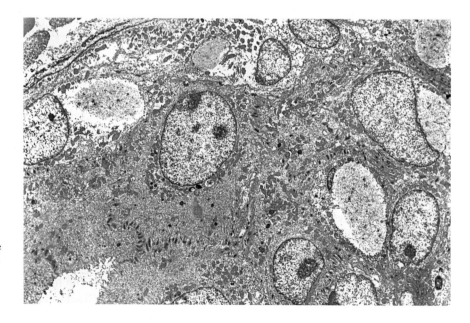

Fig. D5.2 Several electron microscopic non-membrane bound polyglucosan bodies in ductal sweat gland epithelial cells of the skin, Lafora disease

Cultures of dermal fibroblasts provide valuable sources of biochemical and molecular investigations, while morphological studies of cultured fibroblasts are largely unrewarding, except in mucolipidosis II or I-cell (inclusion cell) disease. Nonspecific lysosomal residual bodies may accrue over time in cultured fibroblasts giving rise to erroneous interpretations. Hence, performing a skin biopsy solely to produce tissue cultures may be considered incomplete in disorders in which meaningful morphological investigations may be made.

> **Remember**
>
> Skin is an important biopsy target in lysosomal diseases both of vacuolar and nonvacuolar forms because of the diverse cell types and accessibility. Electron microscopy is required for proper morphological diagnosis. When nerves are present, electron microscopy may permit the recognition of lysosomal leukodystrophies (metachromatic and globoid cell forms) and peroxisomal disorders (adrenoleukodystrophies and infantile Refsum disease). Mitochondrial diseases are not morphologically reliably expressed in skin.

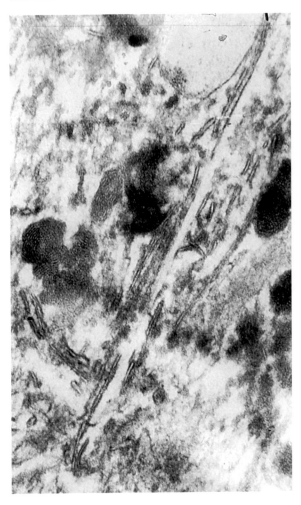

Fig. D5.3 Electron microscopic appearance of needle-like structures in Schwann cells in adrenoleukodystrophy

D5.4 Conjunctiva

Conjunctiva has occasionally been biopsied in children as a target alternative to skin. This may reflect a preference of the clinician, e.g., an ophthalmologist. It is seldom preferred by the pathologist. Sweat glands are absent from conjunctiva; vessels and nerves are, however, more abundant than in skin and are informative. Mural cells of vessels and Schwann cells of both myelinated and unmyelinated axons may harbor disease-specific lysosomal residual bodies, both vacuolar and nonvacuolar. Axons usually do not show any pathology in metabolic disorders except for nonspecific loss or regeneration. When axons are myelinated, their Schwann cells may harbor very typical disease-specific lysosomal bodies in lysosomal leukodystrophies, so-called prismatic or herring-bone inclusions in MLD. Examples are the needle-like inclusions in GCL or Krabbe leukodystrophy, and similar but not identical needle-like inclusions in peroxisomal adrenoleukodystrophies.

Diagnostically informative cytological components in skin are often widely spaced and scarce, and there is an abundance of noninformative collagen fibril aggregates. Disease-specific lesions in affected patients may not be present in the individual skin specimen biopsied. A second skin biopsy or biopsy of another tissue may be required. This may occasionally happen in the NCL.

Among the peroxisomal disorders, those forms marked by needle-like inclusions (Fig. D5.3) in Schwann cells, such as adrenoleukodystrophy, and infantile Refsum disease, may show group-specific pathology while other cell types, such as epithelial and mesenchymal cells do not seem to be involved in morphological pathology.

Fig. D5.4 An electron microscopic aggregate of membrane-bound lysosomal lamellar bodies in the Schwann cell cytoplasm of a myelinated peripheral nerve fibre of a patient with metachromatic leukodystrophy

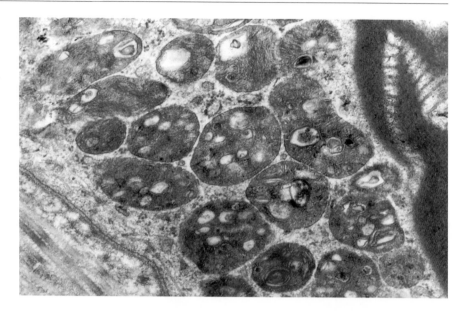

D5.5 Peripheral Nervous System

Because peripheral nerves are often encountered in dermal and conjunctival biopsy specimens, the biopsy of peripheral nerves as an invasive, purely diagnostic procedure will seldom provide more information on metabolic diseases than skin and conjunctiva may yield. In mitochondrial disorders, peripheral nerves are equally unsuitable as biopsy targets since they may give ambiguous and, thus, unreliable results. However, in specific constellations biopsy of nerves can yield useful information (Fig. D5.4) (Table D5.5). Polyglucosan bodies within axons may be an occasional nonspecific finding, but they may be increased in number in conditions associated with polygluco san body formation, polyglucosan diseases, such as type IV glycogenosis.

D5.6 Rectum

Neuronal perikarya or nerve cell bodies of the peripheral nervous system, largely situated in the rectum (Table D5.6), may serve as biopsy substitutes for neurons of the brain, because both are affected by lysosomal storage in many lysosomal diseases. Certain neuronal lysosomal disorders, e.g., mucolipidosis IV or

Sandhoff disease, may also involve non-neuronal cell types and tissues as well, while GM$_2$ gangliosidosis of Tay-Sachs type, as a purely neuronal lysosomal disease, can safely be ascertained by morphological studies on nerve cells only, i.e., neurons of the rectum and other tissues. Other nerve cell-containing regions of the peripheral nervous system located in dorsal root and autonomic ganglia are hardly ever a target of biopsy. In GM$_2$ gangliosidosis of all biochemical and molecular forms and in GM$_1$ gangliosidosis membraneous cytoplasmic bodies are the characteristic intraneuronal lysosomal inclusions.

Table D5.5 Morphological expression of neurometabolic diseases in peripheral nerves

Lysosomal diseases
Vacuolar forms
MPS, ML, oligosaccharidoses
Non-vacuolar forms
Fabry disease
Globoid cell leukodystrophy
Glycogenosis type-II
GM$_1$ gangliosidosis
Metachromatic leukodystrophy
Neuronal ceroid-lipofuscinosis
Peroxisomal disorders
Adrenoleukodystrophies
Infantile Refsum disease
Polyglucosan diseases
Polyglucosan body myopathy

Table D5.6 Morphological expression of neurometabolic diseases in rectum

Lysosomal diseases
Vacuolar forms
    MPS, ML, oligosaccharidoses
Non-vacuolar forms
    Fabry disease
    Farber disease
    Gaucher disease
    Globoid cell leukodystrophy
    Glycogenosis type-II
    GM_1 gangliosidosis
    GM_2 gangliosidosis
    Mucolipidosis IV
    Neuronal ceroid-lipofuscinoses (NCL)
    Niemann-Pick disease
Peroxisomal disorders
    Adrenoleukodystrophies
    Infantile Refsum disease
Polyglucosan diseases
    Lafora disease
    Type-IV glycogenosis

Remember

As nerves are wide-spread in skin and conjunctiva, peripheral nerve biopsies in metabolic disorders, especially in lysosomal diseases, are unnecessary. Likewise, when peroxisomal disorders affect peripheral nerves in skin and conjunctiva as seen in the adrenoleukodystrophies and infantile Refsum disease, nerve biopsies may be replaced by biopsies of skin and conjunctiva.

D5.7 Brain

In metabolic diseases, premortem morphological studies of brain tissue for diagnostic purposes have become rather obsolete. Among the metabolic disorders, there are hardly any which display disease-specific morphological findings confined to the brain and not encountered in extracerebral tissues. Conversely, pathology of those metabolic disorders clinically predominant in the brain does not appear disease-specific, such as in amino acid disorders or neurotransmitter defects. Moreover, brain biopsy is largely confined to the cortex and subcortical white matter, and this would fail to identify subcortical pathology and respective diseases as seen in Wilson disease or those mitochondrial encephalomyopathies which do not show mitochondrial pathology in biopsied muscle, such as Leigh syndrome.

In addition, the vast achievements in biochemical and molecular data affecting the brain have deplorably been insufficiently correlated with postmortem brain pathology.

Remember

Brain biopsy can now be considered an obsolete diagnostic procedure to procure pathomorphology of metabolic disorders, but autopsies of the brain are still important to confirm in vivo diagnosis and secure morphological information in newly defined metabolic conditions.

D5.8 Liver

For morphological studies (Table D5.7), a liver biopsy may be a very rare procedure because its pathology in numerous neurometabolic diseases is equally well expressed in other tissues more easily accessible, such as skin or skeletal muscle. Only in peroxisomal disorders (Powers 2004), which may be divided into those with abnormal or absent peroxisomes and those with

Table D5.7 Morphological expression of neurometabolic diseases in liver

Peroxisomal diseases
    Infantile Refsum disease
    Neonatal adrenoleukodystrophy
    Zellweger disease
Lysosomal diseases
Vacuolar forms
    MPS, ML, oligosaccharidoses
Non-vacuolar forms
    Fabry disease
    Gaucher disease
    Glycogenosis type-II
    GM_1 gangliosidosis
    NCL
    Niemann-Pick disease
Polyglucosan diseases
    Lafora disease
    Type IV glycogenosis

Fig. D5.5 Electron microscopic membrane-bound lysosomal vacuoles with some electron-dense dark amorphous material in hepatocytes of liver in Niemann-Pick disease type B

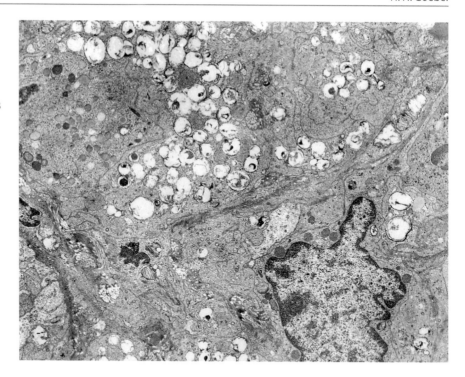

regular peroxisomes, liver as biopsy target may be the best choice, before or after respective biochemical and molecular investigations. Peroxisomes are absent in Zellweger syndrome, neonatal adrenoleukodystrophy and infantile Refsum disease. At the light microscopic level, the absence of the marker enzyme for peroxisomes, catalase, may suggest absence of peroxisomes which may then be confirmed by electron microscopic examination. In other peroxisomal conditions, peroxisomes may be present, but enlarged or abnormally structured, and "angulate lysosomes" may be encountered.

Among lysosomal disorders, Gaucher disease may be recognized morphologically in liver but not in skin or skeletal muscle. It is of course recognized in bone marrow. Many other lysosomal diseases are morphologically evident in liver (Fig. D5.5). Although the liver may be affected in mitochondrial diseases and even contain abnormally structured mitochondria, an advantage of liver biopsy over skeletal muscle biopsy exists among the mitochondrial disorders only in those

smallness of peroxisomes and those defined by individual enzyme deficiencies when peroxisomes are present in hepatocytes. Although lysosomal diseases widely affect the liver, there are more easily accessible tissues, such as lymphocytes and skin. In non-neuronopathic Gaucher and Niemann-Pick diseases, the liver is a warranted biopsy target.

affecting liver but not skeletal muscle, such as the mitochondrial DNA depletion syndromes.

D5.9 Skeletal Muscle

The main cytological components of skeletal muscle are the multinucleated striated muscle fibers (Table D5.8). They may show a remarkable gamut of abnormal mitochondria, i.e., increase in number, increase in size, abnormal shape, and pathological solid inclusions. Abnormal mitochondria are seen in a large number but not all mitochondrial diseases. However, individual mitochondrial myopathies do not show different ultrastructural patterns of mitochondria. In light microscopic specimens, accumulation of abnormal mitochondria in

Remember

Liver is the most important biopsy target in peroxisomal disorders to distinguish between those with defective biogenesis resulting in absence or

Table D5.8 Morphological manifestation of neurometabolic diseases in skeletal muscle

Mitochondrial diseases
Lysosomal diseases
Vacuolar forms
   MPS, ML, oligosaccharidoses
Non-vacuolar forms
   Fabry disease
   Glycogenosis type-II
   GM$_1$ gangliosidosis
   Mucolipidosis IV
   Neuronal ceroid-lipofuscinoses
   Niemann-Pick disease
Polyglucosan diseases
   Lafora disease
   Type IV glycogenosis
   Polyglucosan myopathy

muscle fibers may give rise to "ragged red fibers" when employing the modified Gomori trichrome stain, to "ragged blue fibers" in oxidative enzyme histochemical preparations, such as NADH tetrazolium reductase and succinic dehydrogenase (SDH) or "ragged brown fibres" in cytochrome-C oxidase preparations. Many times, however, ragged red fibers may lack enzyme histochemical activity of cytochrome-C oxidase, being so-called COX-negative muscle fibers, while SDH in ragged blue fibers is well expressed, an observation which is quite conspicuous in a combined COX-SDH enzyme histochemical preparation (Vogel 2001).

Among the lysosomal diseases, type-II glycogenosis, in both the infantile and non-infantile types, is best studied in skeletal muscle (Fig. D5.6). Lysosomal glycogen storage is not confined to striated muscle fibers but is apparent in other tissue components of skeletal muscle, such as satellite cells, mural cells of vessels, and fibroblasts. Mucolipidosis IV may show lysosomal lamellar bodies in muscle fibers and lysosomal vacuoles in interstitial cells. Niemann-Pick disease, especially type-C, may affect compartments of both striated and non-striated cells with the formation of typical lysosomal inclusions. On the other hand, vacuolar lysosomal disorders, such as mucopolysaccharidoses, may readily be recognized in interstitial cells within skeletal muscle but not in striated muscle fibers. The presence of nerve fascicles may provide evidence of lysosomal leukodystrophies, such as metachromatic and globoid cell forms. In Lafora disease, membrane-bound glycogen and debris displaying increased activity of acid phosphatase suggest lysosomal involvement, together with fibrillar glycogen which may be more apparent as polyglucosan bodies in type IV glycogenosis and its non-infantile variants. The formation of lysosomal glycogen in type-II glycogenosis is ubiquitous. Type-specific lipopigments of different genetic (CLN) forms of NCL are encountered in striated muscle fibers and interstitial cells, largely granular lipopigments (so-called granular osmiophilic deposits (GROD)) in the genetic CLN1 form. Curvilinear/

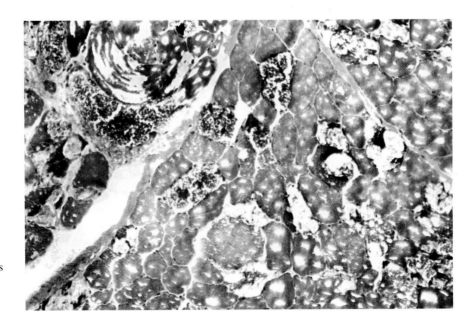

Fig. D5.6 Light microscopic deposition of lysosomal glycogen in and destruction of muscle fibres of skeletal muscle, type-II glycogenosis, modified Gomori trichrome stain

rectilinear, but not fingerprint profiles are encountered in the genetic forms CLN2, CLN3, CLN5, CLN6, CLN7, and CLN8. Finely granular lipopigments also accrue in skeletal muscle and peripheral nerve in vitamin-E deficiency, both the hereditary and acquired forms. This group includes abeta-lipoproteinemia or Bassen–Kornzweig syndrome.

Biopsied unfixed frozen muscle may also be a suitable organ for biochemical studies, such as the muscle-specific biochemical abnormalities seen in mitochondrial DNA-related, organ-defined mitochondrial disorders and in non-infantile type-II glycogenosis. The latter condition may show normal acid maltase levels in circulating blood cells, often the source for biochemical investigation of type-II glycogenosis, but absent or reduced activities in skeletal muscle (Sharma et al. 2005).

Other glycogenoses, such as types III, V, and VII, displaying increased storage of sarcoplasmic non-membrane-bound glycogen in skeletal muscle fibres, are associated with enzyme histochemical deficiency of the respective two enzymes myophosphorylase and phosphofructokinase in glycogenoses V and VII. The sarcoplasmic glycogen is strongly PAS-positive but liable to digestion by diastase; it may fade during prolonged postsurgical tissue-handling rendering the myopathology that of vacuolar myopathies. Increased amounts of sarcoplasmic lipid droplets, often confluent and then appearing as larger droplets at the light microscopic level, suggest a lipid myopathy, so-called neutral lipid storage disease with or without associated mitochondrial defects, while lysosomal lipid accumulation is evidence of a rare lysosomal disorder, the lipase-deficient Wolman disease.

Since cardiomyocytes, though uninuclear cells, show a similar constitution as skeletal muscle fibres, they may also be affected in metabolic disorders; thus skeletal muscle biopsy may serve as a substitute for cardiac biopsy.

Remember

Skeletal muscle is the primary and most important target for biopsy in mitochondrial diseases, in muscle-affecting glycogenoses, and in neutral lipid storage diseases. For proper diagnosis in skeletal muscle tissue, it is essential not only to perform a light and electron microscopic study but also to provide tissue for important biochemical and mitochondrial genomic investigations (mitochondrial diseases, glycogenoses, and lipid disorders). Preservation of unfixed frozen muscle tissue and archival storage is a diagnostic prerequisite.

D5.10 Other Tissues

Morphologically non-systematic observations concern biopsies of rather unusual tissues such as kidney, lymph nodes, spleen, appendix, or even urinary sediment. The latter contains lysosomal residual bodies derived from degenerated sloughed-off renal tubular cells. Bone marrow is particularly useful in Gaucher and Niemann-Pick diseases.

Take Home Messages

> Certain neurometabolic disorders are marked by cerebral and extracerebral morphological manifestations of individual, i.e. lysosomal, peroxisomal, mitochondrial, and polyglucosan diseases, these being single-organelle/multi-organ disorders. The extracerebral biopsy facilitates and corroborates the diagnostic armamentarium in these conditions, according to selective tissue manifestation and accessibility by biopsy. The preferential sites for biopsy are blood lymphocytes, skin, and rectum in lysosomal diseases, skeletal muscle in mitochondrial diseases, liver in peroxisomal disorders, and skin and skeletal muscle in polyglucosan diseases. Electron microscopy is the most rewarding diagnostic technique requiring immediate post-bioptic fixation of the tissues, especially in lysosomal and peroxisomal diseases. Many mitochondrial diseases are also recognised in skeletal muscle by light microscopy including mitochondria-related enzyme histochemial preparations.

Key References

Dolman CL, MacLeod PM, Chang E (1977) Fine structure of cutaneous nerves in ganglioside storage disease. J Neurol Neurosurg Psychiatry 40:588–594

Goebel HH (1997) Neurodegenerative diseases: biopsy diagnosis in children (Chapt. 14). In: Garcia JH, Budka H, McKeever PE, Sarnat HB, Sima AAF (eds) Neuropathology. The diagnostic approach. Mosby, St. Louis, pp 581–635

Goebel HH (1999) Extracerebral biopsies in neurodegenerative diseases of childhood. Brain Dev 21:435–443

Goebel HH, Bönnemann C (2004) Disorders of carbohydrate metabolism. Polyglucosan disorders (Chapter 27.2). In: Golden JA, Harding BN (eds) Pathology and genetics: developmental neuropathology. International Society of Neuropathology (ISN), Basel, pp 221–225

Goebel HH, Harzer K, Ernst JP et al (1990) Late-onset globoid cell leukodystrophy: Unusual ultrastructural pathology and subtotal β-galactocerebrosidase deficiency. J Child Neurol 5:299–307

Goebel HH, Jänisch W (1995) The neuropathology of metabolic encephalopathies and neurodegenerative diseases in children. In: Cruz-Sánchez FF et al (eds) Neuropathological diagnostic criteria for brain banking. IOS Press, Amsterdam, pp 136–147

Goebel HH, Warlo I (1990a) Biopsy studies in neurodegenerative diseases of childhood: part I. BNI Q 6:19–27

Goebel HH, Warlo I (1990b) Biospy studies in neurodegenerative diseases of childhood: part II. BNI Q 6:24–30

Kaesgen U, Goebel HH (1989) Intraepidermal morphologic manifestations in lysosomal diseases. Brain Dev 11:338–341

Powers JM (2004) Peroxisomal disorders (Chapter 31). In: Golden JA, Harding BN (eds) Pathology and genetics: developmental neuropathology. International Society of Neuropathology (ISN), Basel, pp 287–295

Sharma MC, Schultze C, von Moers A et al (2005) Delayed or late-onset type II glycogenosis with globular inclusions. Acta Neuropathol (Berl) 110:151–157

Vogel H (2001) Mitochondrial myopathies and the role of the pathologist in the molecular era. J Neuropathol Exp Neurol 60:217–227

Walter S, Goebel HH (1988) Ultrastructural pathology of dermal axons and Schwann cells in lysosomal diseases. Acta Neuropathol (Berl) 76:489–495

Suspected Mitochondrial Disorder

Nicole I. Wolf

Key Facts

> Lactate elevations in blood, CSF, or urine or frank lactic acidosis are a hallmark of disorders of energy metabolism, more specifically respiratory chain disorders, disorders of oxidative phosphorylation, mitochondrial disorders, or mitochondriopathies. These can involve any organ at any age.

> Organs commonly affected include muscle, brain, retina, extraocular muscles, heart, liver, kidney, pancreas, gut, and bone marrow (Table D6.1). Systemic growth may be impaired. It is sometimes said that the greater the number of organ systems involved, the greater the likelihood of a mitochondrial disorder.

Within a cell, mitochondria and the mitochondrial respiratory chain are at the center of all energy-related processes. Secondary respiratory chain dysfunction is common in many disorders – not only in disorders affecting intermediate metabolism, e.g., organic acidurias or fatty acid oxidation defects, but also in many other inherited diseases not primarily affecting metabolic pathways. Primary respiratory chain defects are disorders that directly involve oxidative phosphorylation and the electron transfer chain. Inheritance can be maternal or Mendelian, and a myriad of genes is involved, making the specific genetic diagnosis of a mitochondrial disorder still a challenge.

N. I. Wolf
Department of Child Neurology, VU Medisch Centrum,
1007 MB Amsterdam, The Netherlands
e-mail: n.wolf@vumc.nl

Mendelian inheritance is caused by mutations in nuclear DNA and follows dominant, recessive, or X-linked modes of inheritance. The mitochondrial DNA (mtDNA) is a circular structure of 16,569 bp, which codes for two ribosomal RNAs and 22 tRNAs needed for protein synthesis within the mitochondria, and 13 additional peptides as components of the respiratory chain. MtDNA is maternally inherited; the result of maternal inheritance is that familial mitochondrial disorders typically affect all the children of the affected women, but not children of the affected men. Paternal inheritance has shown to be possible in one case but is exceedingly rare and not relevant for genetic counseling.

Every cell in the human body, besides erythrocytes, contains thousands of mtDNA molecules. Usually, their sequence is identical (homoplasmy). If there are mutations, usually not every mtDNA molecule in the body will be affected, and wild type and mutated mtDNA will be present together even within one cell or tissue (heteroplasmy). Levels of mutant mtDNA may be very different from one oocyte to another and from one organ to another, depending on random segregation of mutant mtDNA during oogenesis, oocyte division, and blastocyst development. Only, the mildest mutations can be tolerated in homoplasmic mode. Heteroplasmic mutations may be devastating to the function of an individual mitochondrion in high numbers, but if present in a small percentage of mitochondria, or cells, they can be tolerated. The threshold proportion for symptoms differs widely for different mutations and tissues. Whether levels of mutant mtDNA are important for disease severity in mtDNA disorders remains still unclear for most mutations. Mitochondria proliferate throughout life, so there is an opportunity for the proportion of normal and mutant to change within the various tissues, often with an increase in abnormal forms, and deterioration of symptoms over time. Over the last years, an increasing

G. F. Hoffmann et al. (eds.), *Inherited Metabolic Diseases*,
DOI: 10.1007/978-3-540-74723-9_D6, © Springer-Verlag Berlin Heidelberg 2010

Table D6.1 Important symptoms and findings in respiratory chain deficiency

Organ or tissue	Signs and symptoms
Brain	Seizures, stroke-like episodes, myoclonus, ataxia, Parkinsonism, migraine, dementia, leukoencephalopathy
Eye	Optic atrophy, pigmentary degeneration, cataract
Extraocular muscles	Ophthalmoplegia, ptosis
Ear	Deafness
Skeletal muscle	Myopathy, exercise intolerance
Bone marrow	Pancytopenia or failure of specific cell lines
Heart	Cardiomyopathy, conduction defects
Liver	Hepatic dysfunction, liver failure, cirrhosis, bile stasis
Intestine	Pseudo-obstruction
Testes and ovaries	Gonadal failure
Kidney	Tubulopathy, Fanconi syndrome
Pancreas	Diabetes mellitus, exocrine failure, pancreatitis
Endocrine organs (thyroid, parathyroid, adrenal, pituitary gland, and pancreatic β cells)	Failure of hormone secretion
Growth	Failure to thrive, wasting
Blood, CSF, and urine	Increased lactate or alanine

number of mutations in nuclear genes that affect mtDNA proliferation and stability and, if defective, that cause different diseases could be identified.

Despite the importance of mtDNA, most subunits of the five complexes of the mitochondrial respiratory chain are encoded by nuclear genes. The same is true for all transport proteins, proteins for mtDNA synthesis and maintenance, proteins required for transcription and translation, and assembly factors of the five complexes (Fig. D6.1). There are at least 1,000 nuclear genes involved in mitochondrial biogenesis, maintenance, and functioning. During the last years, mutations in nuclear genes coding for subunits of respiratory chain complexes (e.g., complex I) or assembly factors (e.g., complex IV) have been increasingly recognized, especially in mitochondrial disorders of infancy and childhood (see Table D6.2).

Mitochondrial disorders are among the most common metabolic disorder affecting ~ 1:5,000 already in childhood. They can involve any tissue at any age with any degree of severity. Table D6.1 lists some of the most

important symptoms associated with mitochondrial dysfunction. An otherwise unexplained combination of symptoms in different organ systems is the strongest indicator of a mitochondrial disease. Mitochondrial disorders may have prominent muscle involvement, although this presentation is rare in infancy and childhood. Other organs commonly affected include brain, retina, extraocular muscles, heart, liver, kidney, pancreas, gut, bone marrow, and the endocrine systems (Table D6.1). Physical growth may be impaired. Mild hypertrichosis is an unspecific sign of mitochondrial disorders as is thrombocytosis.

The consideration of mitochondrial disease proceeds along three axes – clinical symptoms, metabolic investigations, and functional assays. Molecular defects can be present in the mitochondrially encoded tRNAs, mitochondrial, and nuclear-encoded subunits of the oxidative phosphorylation complexes, and many other proteins. There are many areas of overlap – the same mutation can give rise to different syndromes, and the same syndrome can be caused by different functional impairments or mutations in different genes; so investigations are necessarily wide ranging, and it is difficult, even impossible, to provide guidelines which can by applied for all patients in all settings. Functional deficiencies of a single respiratory chain complex may be due to a mutation involving one of the subunits or assembly factors involved; mutations in genes involving translation usually give rise to multiple complex deficiency. The latter can also be found in nuclear gene defects impairing mtDNA maintenance or replication; however, respiratory chain activity can also be normal in some of these defects (see Table D6.2).

Clinically, there are some well-defined mitochondrial syndromes. Some of them can be heterogeneous, involving either several mitochondrial genes or several nuclear genes or even mitochondrial or nuclear genes such as Leigh syndrome. Table D6.3 gives an overview over the most important syndromes. Leigh syndrome is one of the most frequent manifestations of a mitochondrial disorder in infancy and childhood and illustrates the difficulties in the diagnosis of mitochondrial disorders. Affected patients present with developmental delay or a neurodegenerative course including extrapyramidal movement disorder, ataxia, strabismus, and swallowing difficulties. MRI reveals symmetric hyperintensities of basal ganglia, mesencephalon, and brain stem (Fig. D6.2). Additional symptoms as cardiomyopathy or renal insufficiency are possible and may help to pinpoint the genetic defect. Leigh syndrome is extremely heterogeneous and can be caused by mutations in the mtDNA, especially T8993G/C in *MTATP6* coding for

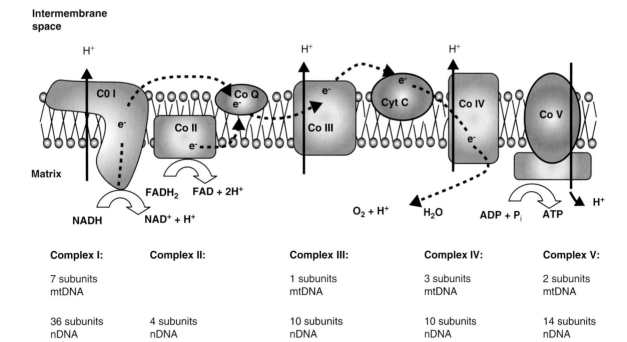

Fig. D6.1 Mitochondrial respiratory chain. Complex I (NADH:ubiquinone oxidoreductase), complex II (succinate:ubiquinone oxidoreductase), complex III (ubiquinol: cytochrome C oxidoreductase), complex IV (cytochrome c oxidase), and complex V (ATP synthase)

one of the complex V subunits, mutations in different nuclear genes, e.g., involving complex I subunits and assembly factors for complex IV and also mutations in the gene coding for the alpha subunit of pyruvate decarboxylase, the first of three enzymes in the pyruvate dehydrogenase complex (*PDHA1*). In the differential diagnosis of Leigh syndrome, muscle biopsy is necessary in order to narrow down the genetic investigations.

Over 100 pathogenic point mutations and 200 deletions, insertions, and rearrangements of mtDNA have been identified since the first mutations were described in 1988. The nuclear-encoded oxidative phosphorylation disorders and other mitochondrial syndromes are still difficult to elucidate although there has been great progress over the last few years. In infants and children, nuclear defects are much more common than mtDNA mutations that cause only 10–20% of respiratory chain disorders in this age group. As mostly the molecular basis of most nuclear defect is as yet unsolved, extended biochemical analysis in fresh muscle remains the gold standard for the diagnosis of many defects of the respiratory chain. This permits the determination of defects of regulation, posttranslational modification, signaling, import, quality control, folding, and assembly of the oxidative phosphorylation apparatus as a whole.

In daily clinical work, there are three different clinical scenarios where mitochondrial disorders are suspected (Fig. D6.3). First, clinical symptoms are so suggestive of a mitochondrial disease that subsequent investigations are warranted. Second, in the diagnostic work-up of a patient with more or less nonspecific symptoms results of either laboratory or other, e.g., neuroradiological investigations, point into the direction of a mitochondrial disorder. Third, in patients with unexplained symptoms and signs a mitochondrial disorder is considered as possible differential diagnosis, even without typical clinical or laboratory hallmarks supporting this idea. In the first scenario, it is possible to go directly to DNA analysis if the symptoms are typical of a certain syndrome as mitochondrial encephalomyopathy, lactic acidosis and stroke-like episodes (MELAS) or Alpers disease; if this turns out to be negative, muscle biopsy is necessary. In the second case, muscle biopsy is the first step, and depending on the results, tailored genetic investigations would follow (e.g., in complex I deficiency sequencing of genes coding for its subunits), perhaps also additional investigations as proteome analysis, candidate gene sequencing, etc. in a research setting. The third scenario is the most difficult one, as it is virtually impossible to exclude a mitochondrial disorder even with the most sophisticated work-up (save for

Table D6.2 Nuclear genes involved in mitochondrial disorders

Biochemical defect	Nuclear genes involved	Gene function	Other laboratory abnormalities
Deficiency of single enzymes			
Complex I deficiency	*NDUFA11, NDUFS1, NDUFS2, NDUFS3, NDUFS4, NDUFS6, NDUFS7, NDUFS8, NDUFV1, NDUFV2*	Structural subunits of complex I	
	B17.2L, C6ORF66, C20orf7, NDUFAF1	Assembly factors of complex I	
Complex II deficiency	*SDHA, SDHC, SDHD*	Structural subunits of complex II	Succinate elevated in cerebral ^{1}H-MRS
Complex III deficiency	*BCS1L*	Assembly factor of complex III	
Complex IV deficiency	*SURF1, COX15*	Assembly factor of complex IV	
	SCO1, SCO2	Copper incorporation	
	COX10	Heme synthesis	
	LRPPRC	Complex IV mRNA stabilization	
Complex V deficiency	*ATP12*	Complex V assembly gene	
Deficiency of multiple enzymes			
Impaired translation	*EFG1, TSFM, EFTu*	Mitochondrial translation elongation	
	MRPS16, MRPS22	Mitochondrial ribosomal proteins	
Impairment of coenzyme Q synthesis (decreased activity of complex I + III and II + III)	*PDSS1, PDSS2, COQ2, CABC1*	Coenzyme Q biosynthesis	Decreased ubiquinone content in muscle
Impaired intergenomic communication (activity of respiratory chain enzymes may be normal; depletion or multiple deletions of mitochondrial DNA (mtDNA) common)	*POLG1*	mtDNA replication (autosomal dominant and recessive mutations in several disorders)	
	TK2	Nucleotide salvage (mutated in mitochondrial mypoathy)	CK strongly elevated
	DGUOK	Nucleotide salvage (mutated in hepatocerebral mtDNA depletion)	
	MPV17	Mitochondrial inner membrane protein with unknown function	
	RRM2B	p53-Controlled ribonucleotide reductase subunit	Severe mtDNA depletion in muscle (1–2%); ragged red fibres
	SUCLA2	ADP-forming succinyl-CoA synthetase	Elevated excretion of methylmalonic acid
	SUCLG1	Succinate-coenzyme A ligase (fatal infantile lactic acidosis)	Elevated excretion of methylmalonate and methylcitrate
	C10ORF2	Twinkle, mtDNA replication	
	RARS2	Mitochondrial arginyl-tRNA synthetase (mutated in a type of pontocerebellar hypoplasia)	Only complex I may be abnormal

ANT1/SLC25A4	ADP/ATP translocator	
ECGF1	Thymidine phosphorylase (mutated in mitochondrial neurogastrointestinal encephalopathy)	Elevation of thymidine and deoxyuridine
PUS1	Pseudouridine synthase 1 (mutated in MLASA)	Sideroblastic anemia
Normal activity of respiratory chain complexes		
FXN	Frataxin, implied in iron homoestasis (mutated in Friedreich's ataxia)	
OPA1	mtDNA maintenance, mutated in patients with optic atrophy	
DDP1	Mitochondrial transport protein, mutated in x-linked dystonia deafness syndrome	
SPG7	Paraplegin (mutated in hereditary spastic sparaplegia type 7)	
ABCB7	Iron export (mutated in x-linked sideroblastic anemia with spinocerebellar ataxia)	Sideroblastic anemia
DARS2	Mitochondrial aspartyl-tRNA synthetase (mutated in LBSL)	Lactate elevated in ^{1}H-MRS, typical neuroimaging
DLP1	Dynamin-like protein, deficient fission of mitochondria and peroxisomes	Lactic acidosis and mild elevation of VLCFA
TAZ	Tafazzine (mutated in Barth syndrome)	Elevated excretion of 3-methylglutaconic acid

another firm diagnosis) and difficult to decide how far one should go with invasive and expensive diagnostic procedures as muscle biopsy.

Remember

In every patient diagnosed or suspected with a mitochondrial disorder, organs must be systematically screened for possible involvement. This includes cerebral MRI (and, if possible, ^{1}H-MRS to assess intracerebral lactate), CSF studies for lactate, alanine and protein, ECG and echocardiography to detect rhythm abnormalities and cardiomyopathy, urine studies to look for tubulopathies and pathological elevations of organic acids, liver function tests, assessment of retina, optic nerve, and hearing. Diabetes mellitus should be excluded. If these investigations remain normal and no other final diagnosis has been reached, they have to be repeated at regular intervals.

When muscle biopsy is performed, care must be taken that all necessary investigations are made. In adults, it is current practice to do only morphological studies, and the presence or absence of ragged red fibres is for some, enough to make or discard the diagnosis of a mitochondrial disorder (see Chap. D5). However, morphological studies are not enough! Every muscle biopsy in a patient with suspected mitochondrial disease has to be examined morphologically (if possible including electron microscopy to look at mitochondrial ultrastructure) as well as functionally. The latter investigation, the assessment of global respiratory chain function and activity of single complexes of the respiratory chain can be done wholly only in fresh muscle. Single complex activities can also be investigated in freshly frozen tissue, but its diagnostic yield is significantly inferior to the overall investigation of fresh tissue.

Table D6.3 Important mitochondrial syndromes

Syndrome	Genes involved	Inheritance	Important clinical features
LHON (Leber hereditary optic neuropathy)	Missense mutations in different mitochondrial DNA genes, especially complex I subunits	Mt, often be homoplasmic	Acute or subacute mid-life painless visual loss. Smoking as risk factor. Additional mild neurological symptoms possible, also preexcitation syndromes
MELAS (mitochondrial encephalomyopathy, lactic acidosis and stroke-like episodes)	Most common mutation A3243G in *MTTL1*; other mtDNA mutations	Mt	Stroke-like episodes, epilepsy, small stature, diabetes mellitus, deafness, cardiac conduction defects
MERFF (Mitochondrial encephalopathy with ragged red fibers and stroke-like episodes)	Most common mutation A8344G in *MTTK*; other mtDNA mutations	Mt	Progressive myoclonic epilepsy, ataxia, dementia
Kearns–Sayre syndrome (KSS)	Large mtDNA deletions (most common 4977 bp) of mtDNA	Mt (usually sporadic)	Progressive ataxia, dementia, cardiac conduction defect, deafness, elevated CSF protein and lactate, typical neuroimaging
Pearson marrow-pancreas syndrome	Large mtDNA deletions (identical to CPEO (chronic progressive external ophthalmoplegia) and KSS)	Mt, sporadic	Exocrine pancreas insufficiency and anemia, evolves into KSS
CPEO	Large mtDNA deletions; *POLG1, ANT1, POLG2, C10ORF2*	Mt (also sporadic); AD; AR	Progressive external ophthalmoplegia, additional myopathy possible
NARP (neuropathy, ataxia and retinitis pigmentosa)	T8993G/C in *MTATP6*	Mt	Neuropathy, ataxia, retinitis pigmentosa. If high rate of heteroplasmy → Leigh syndrome
Leigh syndrome	Many different genes, especially *SURF1* (nuclear DNA) and T8993G/C	Mt, AR, XL	Neurodegenerative disease with onset in infancy or early childhood: movement disorder, swallowing difficulties, strabismus. Additional symptoms possible. MRI with symmetric abnormalities in basal ganglia and brainstem
Alpers disease	*POLG1*, various mutations in mtDNA; other unknown nuclear genes	AR, mtDNA	Neurodegenerative disease with onset in childhood: status epilepticus, epilepsia partialis continua, liver failure (may be triggered by valproic acid), gastrointestinal dysmotility
Mitochondrial neurogastro-intestinal encephalopathy	*ECGF1* (coding for thymidine phosphorylase)	AR	Ptosis, CPEO, gastrointestinal dysmotility with pseudoobstruction, peripheral neuropathy, myopathy. MRI: diffuse leukoencephalopathy

AD Autosomal dominant; *AR* Autosomal recessive; *Mt* Mitochondrial; *XL* X-linked

Fig. D6.2 T2w axial images of a child with Leigh syndrome. Nucleus caudatus, pallidum, and the periaquaeductal area in the mesencephalon show elevated signal. Additionally, there are atrophy and white matter changes. ¹H-MRS of basal ganglia displays a strongly elevated lactate and decreased NAA. Courtesy of Dr. Inga Harting, Department of Neuroradiology, University Hospital Heidelberg

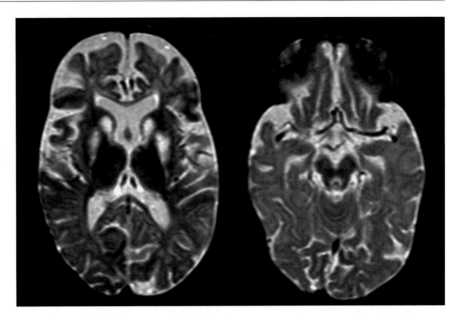

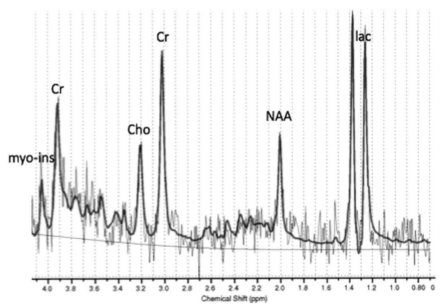

Remember

Muscle biopsy is necessary to confirm the diagnosis of a mitochondrial disorder and to help guiding further genetic investigations in most patients. Functional studies of respiratory chain function in fresh muscle tissue remain the gold standard in diagnosis. Morphological studies alone are not sufficient.

Prenatal diagnosis in mitochondrial disorders is straightforward if inheritance is Mendelian and the genetic defect is known. If Mendelian inheritance is suspected, e.g., autosomal–recessive inheritance in a consanguineous couple with an affected child, prenatal diagnosis is possible if a biochemical defect on the level of the respiratory chain has been proven in muscle and fibroblasts. For mtDNA mutations, prenatal diagnosis and assessment of disease severity in the offspring

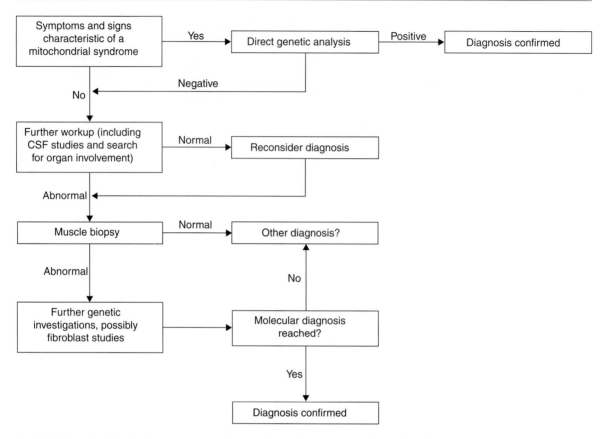

Fig. D6.3 Flowchart for the diagnostic approach in a patient with a suspected mitochondrial disorder

is difficult, even impossible, due to the random segregation of mtDNA, although there are efforts to assess levels of mutant DNA in oocytes, blastocysts, and chorionic villi. These investigations are performed only in a few highly specialized laboratories.

Remember

Prenatal diagnosis of mitochondrial disorders is straightforward if nuclear genes are affected and the mutation is known. In selected cases, biochemical assessment of respiratory chain function in chorionic villi is an option. With mtDNA mutations, prenatal diagnosis and risk assessment remain difficult.

There are many possible differential diagnoses for primary respiratory chain disorders. Metabolites in propionic and methylmalonic acidurias directly affect respiratory chain function and can thereby give rise to "mitochondrial" symptoms. The presentation of other inherited metabolic disorders, among others the group of congenital disorders of glycosylation, the glycogenoses or fatty acid oxidation defects, can mimic mitochondrial disorders very closely. Biotinidase deficiency causes lactic acidosis, deafness, and optic atrophy and has to be sought for in every child with elevated lactic acid, as it is treatable. Deficiency of the *PNPO* gene encoding pyridox(am)ine 5-phosphate oxidase may lead to greatly increased CSF lactate. Thiamine deficiency also results in severe lactic acidosis. Hypoxia, sepsis, and low cardiac output are systemic causes of lactate elevation. In several neurological disorders of childhood, lactate has been found to be intermittently increased in some patients, among them patients with Rett and Angelman syndromes. Even single enzyme deficiencies or decreased ATP production have been demonstrated in patients with variable other diagnoses. As correct diagnosis in these cases is important for prognosis and correct genetic counselling, clinical suspicion of other disorders must be high.

Remember

Besides respiratory chain disorders, there are many differential diagnoses for lactate elevation/lactic acidosis including nonmetabolic inherited and acquired disorders. The most common situation in which the concentration of lactic acid in blood is elevated is factitious, the result of improper technique, the use of a tourniquet, or difficulty in drawing the blood. Depending on the clinical setting, treatable disorders as biotinidase or PNPO deficiency or thiamine deficiency must be considered first.

Take Home Messages

> Respiratory chain disorders can present with a myriad of symptoms, at any age.
> Lactate (and alanine) elevation are common in respiratory chain disorders, but it can occur also in a variety of other inborn errors of metabolism, infection or circulatory failure or can be factitious.
> The gold standard for the diagnosis of a respiratory chain disorder is measurement of oxidation rates and single enzyme activities in fresh muscle tissue.
> Genetic investigations usually take the result of the muscle biopsy into account; if the clinical picture is very suggestive, the appropriate genetic test can be performed without a muscle biopsy.
> Secondary abnormalities of oxidation rates and single enzyme activities in muscle can be encountered in other genetic and acquired disorders.

Key References

Haas RH, Parikh S, Falk MJ et al (2007) Guidelines for the generalist on the diagnosis of mitochondrial disease. Pediatrics 120:1326–1333
The Mitochondrial Medicine Society's Committee on Diagnosis, Haas RH, Parikh S, Falk MJ et al (2008) The in-depth evaluation of suspected mitochondrial disease. Mol Gen Metab 94:16–37

Postmortem Investigations

D7

Piero Rinaldo

Key Facts

> All cases of sudden and unexpected death in childhood should be evaluated for a possible underlying metabolic disorder

> A history of "normal" newborn screening for metabolic disorders is not a sufficient reason to decline post-mortem evaluation

> Most important specimens to collect at autopsy are blood and bile, spotted on filter paper

The high mortality rate that is associated with acute episodes of metabolic decompensation has lead to a perceived association between sudden unexpected death in early life and several inborn errors of amino acid, organic acid, and energy metabolism (Dott et al. 2006). However, in most cases, these conditions do cause acute illness with obvious clinical symptoms that precede death by hours or days. The situation is significantly different when considering the large number of cases affected with a fatty acid oxidation (FAO) disorder who were diagnosed either postmortem or, retrospectively, after the identification of an affected sibling. The latter situation has become a relatively common event since the achievement of greater awareness

(Bennett and Rinaldo 2001) and, particularly, because of the broad implementation of expanded newborn screening for these disorders (Watson et al. 2006). Based on numerous observations, it has been postulated that without preventive intervention (i.e., newborn screening), FAO disorders might be responsible for up to 5% of children who die suddenly and unexpectedly from birth to 5 years of age, particularly among those with evidence of acute infection that routinely would not represent a life-threatening event (Boles et al. 1998).

Figure D7.1 shows a flowchart for the evaluation of sudden and unexpected death that is centered on the analysis of acylcarnitines in blood and bile spots (Rinaldo et al. 2002). Postmortem blood (Chace et al. 2001) and bile (Rashed et al. 1995) could be conveniently collected on a single filter paper card (Fig. D7.2), very similar to those used for newborn screening, which can be shipped at room temperature once properly dried. It is important to underscore the fact that both specimens should be collected in order to detect patients who may show mild or no apparent abnormalities in blood alone (Rinaldo et al. 2005). In cases with a higher level of suspicion, an effort should be made to collect a frozen specimen of liver (Boles et al. 1994) and a skin biopsy, which could be kept frozen to reduce cell culture workload (Gray et al. 1995). It has been possible to grow a viable line of cultured fibroblasts from a biopsy of the Achille's tendon collected as long as 72 h after death.

Although fatty infiltration of the liver and/or other organs (heart and kidneys) is a common observation in FAO disorders, the finding of macroscopic steatosis cannot be used as the only criterion in deciding whether to investigate a possible underlying FAO disorder during the postmortem evaluation of a case of sudden death (Boles et al. 1998; Dott et al. 2006).

P. Rinaldo
Biochemical Genetics Laboratory, Mayo Clinic College of Medicine, 200 First Street S. W., Rochester, MN 55905, USA
e-mail: rinaldo@mayo.edu

G. F. Hoffmann et al. (eds.), *Inherited Metabolic Diseases*,
DOI: 10.1007/978-3-540-74723-9_D7, © Springer-Verlag Berlin Heidelberg 2010

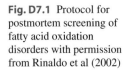

Fig. D7.1 Protocol for postmortem screening of fatty acid oxidation disorders with permission from Rinaldo et al (2002)

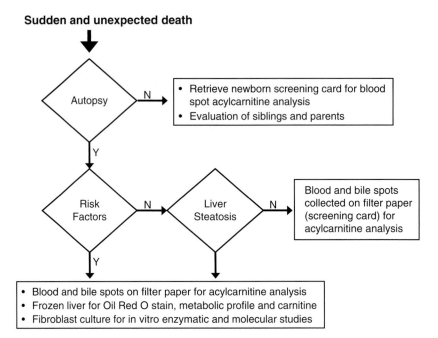

Fig. D7.2 Example of filter paper card for collection of postmortem blood and bile specimen

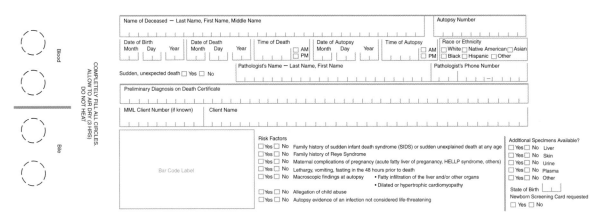

Special attention should be paid to the risk factors listed in Table D7.1, and allegations of child abuse should also be fully investigated, with the exception of obvious cases of trauma/physical harm. The frozen liver and skin biopsy could be discarded at a later time without further testing when a credible cause of death has been established, but could otherwise be crucial to reach a proper diagnosis and conclusive confirmation in vitro. If parental permission to perform an autopsy is not granted, it might be possible to retrieve leftover specimens collected during resuscitation efforts, which may still be available in the clinical laboratory. In cases when no autopsy is performed, retrieval of any unused portion of the blood spots collected for newborn screening could be arranged via a request submitted in writing to the local laboratory (for a template, see http://mayo-medicallaboratories.com/articles/communique/archive.html), as long as the period of storage, ranging from only a few weeks to indefinitely, had not expired already in the state where the patient was born (http://www2.uthscsa.edu/nnsis/)

Table D7.1 Factors which increase the risk of an undiagnosed fatty acid oxidation disorder

Birth at a location not yet providing expanded newborn screening by MS/MS
Family history of sudden infant death syndrome or other sudden, unexplained deaths at any age
Family history of Reye syndrome
Maternal complications of pregnancy (acute fatty liver of pregnancy, HELLP syndrome)
Lethargy, vomiting, fasting in the 48 h prior to death
Macroscopic findings at autopsy
Fatty infiltration of the liver and/or other organs
Dilated or hypertrophic cardiomyopathy
Allegation of child abuse (excluding obvious cases of trauma, physical harm)
Autopsy evidence of infection that routinely would not represent a life-threatening event

D7.1   Specimen Requirements

D7.1.1   Blood and Bile

Blood specimen collection is usually drawn into heparin-containing tubes from the proximal aorta or by intracardiac puncture. Bile collection is obtained by direct puncture of the gallbladder. These specimens are well preserved when spotted on a filter paper card. Two circles of the card are used for blood, two circles for bile (each 25 µL of volume). Blood and bile have to be dried before sending the filter paper card to the laboratory which performs the analysis. Relevant demographic patient information should be provided, together with a summary of relevant autopsy findings.

D7.1.2   Liver

A liver specimen of approximately 1–5 g should be collected and stored in all cases of sudden, unexpected death. The specimen should be frozen as soon as possible either at −70 °C, if feasible or at −20 °C. The liver should not be fixed or otherwise treated with a preservative. This specimen should be stored until the results of the postmortem screen on blood and bile, and the results from the original newborn screening card, are available.

D7.1.3   Skin/Tendon for Fibroblast Culturing

In cases with any risk factors, a 5 × 5-mm skin specimen should be collected and placed in culture media. If culture media is unavailable, the specimen can be placed in sterile saline. Although saline is not an optimal media for skin, it will be sufficient in most cases if the specimen is forwarded immediately for cell culturing. The skin specimen should be shipped at room temperature via overnight delivery.

D7.1.4   Urine

If urine is present, it should be collected and stored for all cases of sudden, unexpected death. Urine may be collected on a second filter paper card by swabbing the bladder. The specimen should be allowed to dry for 2–3 h. The urine specimen should be stored at room temperature until the results of the postmortem screen on blood and bile, and the results from the original newborn screening card are available.

Key References

Bennett MJ, Rinaldo P (2001) The metabolic autopsy comes of age. Clin Chem 47:1145–1146

Boles RG, Buck EA, Blitzer MG et al (1998) Retrospective biochemical screening of fatty acid oxidation disorders in postmortem liver of 418 cases of sudden unexpected death in the first year of life. J Pediatr 132:924–933

Boles RG, Martin SK, Blitzer MG et al (1994) Biochemical diagnosis of fatty acid oxidation disorders by metabolite analysis of post-mortem liver. Hum Pathol 25:735–741

Chace DH, DiPerna JC, Mitchell BL et al (2001) Electrospray tandem mass spectrometry for analysis of acylcarnitines in dried postmortem blood specimens collected at autopsy from infants with unexplained cause of death. Clin Chem 47:1166–1182

Dott M, Chace D, Fierro M et al (2006) Metabolic disorders detectable by tandem mass spectrometry and unexpected early childhood mortality: a population-based study. Am J Med Genet A 140:837–842

Gray RGF, Ryan D, Green A (1995) The cryopreservation of skin biopsies – a technique for reducing workload in a cell culture laboratory. Ann Clin Biochem 32:190–192

National Newborn Screening Report – 1997, National Newborn Screening and Genetics Resource Center (NNSGRC),

Austin, TX, pp. 31–32. http://www2.uthscsa.edu/nnsis/ Accessed May 2001

Rashed MS, Ozand PT, Bennett MJ et al (1995) Diagnosis of inborn errors of metabolism in sudden death cases by acyl-carnitine analysis of postmortem bile. Clin Chem 41: 1109–1114

Rinaldo P, Hahn SH, Matern D (2005) Inborn errors of amino acid, organic acid, and fatty acid metabolism. In: Burtis CA, Ashwood ER, Bruns DE (eds) Tietz textbook of clinical chemistry and molecular diagnostics, 4th edn. Elsevier Saunders, St. Louis, MO, pp 2207–2247

Rinaldo P, Matern D, Bennett MJ (2002) Fatty acid oxidation disorders. Ann Rev Physiol 64(16): 1–26

The metabolic autopsy: postmortem screening in cases of sudden, unexpected death. Mayo Reference Services Communiqué. *http://mayomedicallaboratories.com/articles/communique/ archive.html*. Accessed Sep 2003

Watson MS, Mann MY, Lloyd-Puryear MA, Rinaldo P, Howell RR, (eds) (2006) Newborn screening: toward a uniform screening panel and system (Executive summary). Genet Med 8(Supplement):1S–11S

Function Tests

D8

Johannes Zschocke

Key Facts

> The fasting test has been partly superseded by improved diagnostic methods such as acylcarnitine analysis. Remaining indications include the differentiation of disorders of gluconeogenesis from those with defective oxidation of pyruvate in patients with lactic academia; diagnostic work-up in patients with recurrent episodes of symptomatic ketonemia, recurrent cyclic vomiting, recurrent intermittent metabolic acidosis, or the suspicion of fluctuating neurometabolic disease; controlled determination of fasting tolerance to fine-tune the therapy of metabolic disorders; and the assessment of the duration of safe intervals between feedings, e g., in patients with mitochondrial disorders.

> The standardized determination of metabolic parameters before and after meals is particularly useful in the diagnosis of mitochondrial disorders, which typically show pathological postprandial increases of lactate, alanine, and other small amino acids.

> A controlled glucose challenge is useful to assess cellular respiration in patients with suspected disorders of energy metabolism, in whom lactate values have been repeatedly normal.

> The leucine challenge test examines the insulin reaction to food intake and the function of the blood sugar/insulin feedback mechanism and may be useful in patients with postprandial hypoglycemia or suspected hyperinsulinism–hyperammonemia syndrome.

> The phenylalanine challenge test may be useful for the identification of disorders of pterin metabolism in patients with unclear dystonic movement disorders, in particular when Segawa syndrome is suspected.

> The tetrahydrobiopterin (BH_4) test is intended to identify individuals with primary BH_4 deficiency or BH_4-sensitive phenylketonuria.

> The vitamin B_{12} test aims at identifying responsiveness to pharmacological doses of vitamin B_{12}, found in some defects of 5-deoxyadenosylcobalamin metabolism.

> The allopurinol test may be used for the diagnosis of heterozygous or mild ornithine transcarbamylase deficiency in cases of unclear transient or intermittent hyperammonemia, unclear comatose or encephalopathic episodes in both sexes, or stepwise regressing neurodegenerative disease in girls or women, especially those who show epilepsy and ataxia as prominent symptoms.

> The glucagon stimulation test is used as a provocative test for the diagnosis of glycogenosis type I (von Gierke disease).

> The major indication for the fructose tolerance test is a suspicion of hereditary fructose intolerance in patients in whom molecular analysis of the aldolase B gene failed to identify disease-causing mutations.

> The forearm ischemia test examines both anaerobic glycolysis and the purine nucleotide cycle through measurement of lactate and ammonia concentrations before and after anerobic exercise. It may be useful in patients with muscle cramps or other muscular symptoms on exertion.

J. Zschocke
Divisions of Human Genetics and Clinical Genetics, Medical University Innsbruck, Schöpfstr. 41,6020 Innsbruck, Austria
e-mail: johannes.zschocke@i-med.ac.at

G. F. Hoffmann et al. (eds.), *Inherited Metabolic Diseases*,
DOI: 10.1007/978-3-540-74723-9_D8, © Springer-Verlag Berlin Heidelberg 2010

D8.1 General Remarks

Many metabolic disorders show biochemical abnormalities only intermittently under metabolic stress, and normal findings in the interval may not reliably exclude a diagnosis in a particular patient. It is often possible to pinpoint the site or at least the area of a patient's metabolic abnormality by the use of a properly chosen challenge. A variety of in vivo function tests are used to create conditions that allow the assessment of metabolism in a controlled manner. Frequently, this entails ingestion of specific substances that give rise to diagnostic metabolites in certain disorders. Most tests are fairly safe; many are inconvenient, but some (including the frequently performed fasting test) can lead to potentially serious complications and should only be carried out by experienced pediatricians after other diagnostic options including mutation analysis of candidate genes have been exhausted. It is essential to carefully plan the collection of samples during the test and to prepare emergency measures in case complications occur.

Rapid advances in enzymatic, molecular, and other diagnostic techniques permit an increasing number of diagnoses to be obtained without tests of tolerance. However, functional studies may provide phenotypic information that more closely reflects the metabolic risk situation in the individual patient and will continue to have their place in the diagnostic work-up as well as in tailoring therapy.

D8.2 Tests of Fatty Acid Oxidation

D8.2.1 Monitored Prolonged Fast

Monitored fasting is a powerful tool in unraveling the nature of metabolic disorders of energy metabolism. It must, however, be emphasized that fasting is potentially dangerous, and should only be carried out after other, less risky investigations have been completed without a clear diagnosis. Fasting can cause life-threatening cardiac complications particularly in patients with long-chain fatty acid oxidation defects. Sudden cardiac arrest may occur even under controlled conditions in an intensive care unit and a fasting test

therefore is almost contraindicated in all patients with cardiomyopathy. Following a careful selection of patients and under careful observation it can be nevertheless carried out safely.

> **Remember**
>
> A fasting may cause life-threatening complications and should only be carried out with careful monitoring in a specialized hospital setting, and only after other, less risky investigations have been completed without a clear diagnosis.

Fasting results in a series of hormonal and metabolic responses to assure an endogenous supply of energy after cessation of exogenous intake. After each feeding, nutrients are supplied via gastrointestinal absorption. Depending on the amount and composition of the food, this absorption period can last for up to 6 h in adults. It is more often <4 h in infants and small children. With diminishing exogenous supply of glucose, plasma glucose concentrations fall and insulin levels decrease in parallel. The decrease of insulin and increase of counteracting hormones diminishes glucose consumption in muscle and peripheral tissues. The body begins to utilize glycogen reserves by glycogenolysis.

In principle, hypoglycemia may be the consequence of endocrine or metabolic disease. The whole picture can therefore only be obtained if insulin, cortisol, and growth hormone as well as metabolic parameters are measured simultaneously in patients who develop hypoglycemia. Patients with hyperinsulinism often have the shortest and sometimes variable fasting tolerance.

After 8–10 h of fasting, free fatty acids begin to substitute glucose as the primary energy source in muscle, while it often takes 17–24 h to deplete ordinary stores of glycogen. Two central metabolic adaptations to prolonged fasting are initiated in the liver. Glucose is synthesized via glyconeogenesis from alanine and from oxaloacetate derived from amino acids as well as from glycerol resulting from fatty acid oxidation; and most importantly, fatty acid oxidation funnels into ketone body production providing an alternative source of energy.

Infants and small children may have shorter tolerance of fasting. In prolonged fasting, the body finally draws selectively on its lipid resources to spare vitally needed proteins. Depending on the nutritional state, an adult with a defect in fatty acid oxidation may not become symptomatic until fasting has been prolonged for 36 h. In general, hypoglycemia following a short period of fasting signifies disordered carbohydrate metabolism; hypoglycemia that occurs only after prolonged fasting signifies disordered fatty acid oxidation or ketolysis. Some patients with electron transport defects follow the prolonged pattern, because fatty acid oxidation may be impaired secondarily.

Free fatty acids can be oxidized in most body tissues as an energy source. As they do not cross the blood-brain barrier; homeostasis of the brain energy supply depends on adequate production of ketone bodies. Defects of fatty acid oxidation, in which ketone production may be impaired and toxic intermediates are produced, may cause acute encephalopathy accompanied by hepatocelluar dysfunction, producing a Reye-like syndrome.

The fasting test has lost some importance with the advent of acylcarnitine analyses in dried blood spots and is now largely irrelevant if not contraindicated for the diagnosis of fatty acid oxidation defects. These disorders frequently show clinical symptoms only at times of fasting when there may be marked hypoketotic hypoglycemia and massive excretion of dicarboxylic acids without appropriate ketones in the urine. The single most important investigation is the determination of free fatty acids (elevated) and ketone bodies (no sufficient rise) in a serum or plasma sample at the time of symptomatic hypoglycemia. Diagnostic problems arise when the acute hypoglycemic illness is treated without prior collection of at least a serum sample for analyses, as biochemical abnormalities

may completely disappear with restoration of glucose homeostasis.

In fatty acid oxidation disorders, acylcarnitine profiles usually remain abnormal in the nonfasting state. Phenylpropionic acid (PPA) loading may confirm medium-chain acyl-CoA dehydrogenase (MCAD) deficiency or show an increased excretion of phenylhydracrylic acid as a marker of long-chain hydroxyacyl-CoA dehydrogenase (LCHAD) deficiency, but again this test has been largely superseded by acylcarnitine analysis. Analysis of fatty acid oxidation enzymes can be carried out in leukocytes or fibroblasts. The diagnosis of MCAD deficiency may be confirmed in most patients of European descent through the analysis of the common mutation K329E in the MCAD gene. Early analysis of the common LCHAD gene mutation E510Q is indicated if the clinical and biochemical symptoms are suggestive of LCHAD deficiency – progressive or episodic myopathy or cardiomyopathy and specific acylcarnitine pattern with or without bouts of hypoketotic hyoglycemia and hydroxydicarboxylic aciduria.

Determination of fasting tolerance through a monitored fast is indicated in patients with recurrent episodes of apparently fasting-related symptoms, such as episodes of decreased consciousness or especially recurrent documented hypoglycemia or Reye-like disease in whom other analyses (including acylcarnitines) were inconclusive. In particular, patients with a deficiency of mitochondrial 3-hydroxy-3-methylglutaryl-(HMG-) CoA synthase, an isolated disorder of ketogenesis, may show a normal acylcarnitine profile even during hypoglycemic episodes. A fasting test may reveal the typical, hypoketotic hypoglycemia and a unique spectrum of urinary organic acids. Primary mutation analysis is the method of choice to confirm the diagnosis.

A fasting test is also useful in patients with lactic acidemia to distinguish those with disorders of gluconeogenesis from those with defective oxidation of pyruvate (see Chap. B2.3). Other indications for controlled fasting include the following:

- Recurrent episodes of symptomatic ketonemia.
- Recurrent cyclic vomiting.
- Recurrent intermittent metabolic acidosis.
- Suspicion of fluctuating neurometabolic disease.
- Controlled determination of fasting tolerance not only to fine-tune the therapy of metabolic disorders, as in patients with glycogen storage diseases and nesidioblastosis, but also to judge the duration of safe intervals in between feedings, e.g., in patients with mitochondrial disorders.

D8.2.1.1 Preparations

A fasting test should be performed only if the patient is in a stable, steady-state condition. Caloric intake for the last 3 days should have been adequate for age. The test must be postponed in case of even minor intercurrent illness. What is especially important is a detailed history with respect to the individual fasting tolerance, and events and time courses of adverse reactions to previous fasting. With this information and that of the presumptive diagnoses, the timing of the fast can be optimally planned. The duration of the fasting period may be scheduled according to the age of the child (Table D8.1) unless a shorter period is indicated by the clinical history. In general, it is usually safe to allow fasting at night as long as the child usually goes without eating, but the period beyond should take place during the daytime. If hypoglycemia occurs, it should be at a time of optimal staffing.

A monitored fast should be undertaken only in settings in which the entire staff is experienced with the procedure, with close clinical supervision and well set out guidelines as to response to hypoglycemia or other adverse events. Necessary details must be explained to

Table D8.1 Suggested time periods for fasting in different age groups

Age	< 6 Mmonths	6–8 Mmonths	8–12 Months	1–7 years	> 7 years
Starting time	4 a.m.	Midnight	7 p.m.	5 p.m.	3 p.m.
Duration	8 h	15 h	20 h	24 h	24 h

everybody involved in advance. Special care must be taken to ensure complete collection of samples. It is advisable to fill out the forms and assemble and label all the tubes including day and timing of the samples prior to the start of the test.

The aim, nature, and possible adverse effects of the fasting test must be explained in detail to the patient and family to ensure optimal cooperation as well as early notification of symptoms. Informed consent must be obtained from the parents prior to the test.

An intravenous line must be established in order to provide immediate access for the treatment of hypoglycemia. It may be maintained with 0.9% NaCl or a heparin lock.

D8.2.1.2 Procedure

After baseline studies of plasma free fatty acids and ketone bodies (acetoacetate and 3-hydroxybutyrate) blood sugar and urinary organic acids, fasting is conducted with careful bedside monitoring of the concentrations of glucose in blood and ketones in urine. The patient is allowed to drink water and unsweetened tea, but no juices or soft drinks including "diet" beverages. Heart rate may be monitored by ECG.

An example of a fasting test of 24 h is given in Table D8.2. Under normal conditions, ketogenesis is brisk and especially after 15–17 h concentrations of acetoacetate and 3-hydroxybutyrate rise sharply, and gluconeogenesis occurs preserving normoglycemia. The fast is stopped at any time for the development of hypoglycemia, and with close monitoring it is usually possible to avoid symptoms of hypoglycemia.

Blood samples should be obtained at 15, 20, and 24 h and always at a time of hypoglycemia when the fast is stopped. The following basic laboratory parameters should be measured: blood sugar, free fatty acids and ketone bodies (acetoacetate, 3-hydroxybutyrate), lactate, electrolytes, blood gases, transaminases, and creatine kinase. In addition, dried blood spots must be obtained for the analysis of the acylcarnitine profile. Serum carnitine status and amino acids may be considered, and a spare serum sample should be obtained in case additional tests may be indicated. Hormone studies including insulin, glucagon, and growth hormone must be carried out during hypoglycemia. Urine is collected in 8 h aliquots for the quantitative determination of organic

Table D8.2 Twenty-four hour fast in a 6-year-old child[x]

Begin fast at time T = 0 h at 4 p.m.
T(ime) = 0 h (4 p.m.)
End of last meal with intake documented

T = 1 h (5 p.m.)
Serum *glucose*, electrolytes, creatine kinase. Blood gases. Lactate, pyruvate, *3-hydroxybutyrate*, acetoacetate from perchloric acid tube. *Plasma amino acids, free fatty acids, and carnitine.* Acylcarnitines.
Start collection of urine in 8 h aliquots. Monitor ketones in urine at the bedside

T = 1 h until T = 12h
Blood glucose concentration is monitored 3-hourly at the bedside.

From T = 12h (4 a.m.) onwards
Collect glucose levels hourly. Heart rate may be monitored by ECG.

T = 15 h (7 a.m.)
Serum glucose, electrolytes. Blood gases. Lactate, pyruvate, 3-hydroxybutyrate, acetoacetate. Plasma amino acids, free fatty acids

T = 20 h (noon)
Serum glucose, electrolytes. Blood gases. Lactate, pyruvate, 3-hydroxybutyrate, acetoacetate. Plasma amino acids, free fatty acids

T = 24 h (4 p.m.) or at the time of hypoglycemia
Serum *glucose*, electrolytes, creatine kinase. *Insulin, cortisol, growth hormone* and additional specimen for follow-up hormonal investigations. Blood gases. Lactate, pyruvate, *3-hydroxybutyrate*, acetoacetate. *Plasma amino acids, free fatty acids.* *Acylcarnitines*
Quantitative analysis of *organic acids* is performed on the first and last aliquots. The middle collection is to ensure a sample for analysis in a patient developing hypoglycemia during that period

[a]In this sample case, no adverse effect to overnight fasting was to be anticipated from the history
Parameters that are indispensible for evaluation and interpretation are highlighted in italics (see also Table D8.3)

acids. Hourly glucose determinations are made after the first missed feeding and are repeated more frequently if the blood sugar falls <50 mg/dL. All urine passed should be checked for ketones. Comprehensive investigation of intermediary metabolites and hormones in blood and urine are especially important at the scheduled end of the fast or at the time of developing hypoglycemia, when the fast is terminated.

In the investigation of lactic acidemia fasting is employed to distinguish disorders of gluconeogenesis from defects of oxidative phosphorylation (see Chap. B2.3). For this purpose, it is useful to give glucagon at 6 h into the fast (not in the evening or the night e.g. during a 24 hour fast). This may provide a presumptive diagnosis in a patient with glycogen storage disease type I. In addition, it depletes the liver of glycogen derived from exogenous glucose, and as the fast continues, gluconeogenesis is required to keep from hypoglycemia. A schedule is shown in Table 1 B2.3. If the suspicion for a defect of oxidative phosphorylation is especially high, it is possible to combine the fasting test with a glucose and/or protein load as the last feed.

D8.2.1.3 Treatment of Adverse Reactions

The fasting test must be terminated if the intravenous line is lost and cannot be immediately replaced or if the patient develops symptoms due to hypoglycemia or ketoacidosis, such as irritability, sweating, and drowsiness. It should also be discontinued at any sign of cardiac arrhythmia. The test is also terminated if hypoglycemia (blood glucose <40 mg/dL or 2.3 mmol/L) or significant metabolic acidosis (bicarbonate <15 mmol/L) is documented.

For treatment of hypoglycemia, 2 mL of 20% or 4 mL of 10% glucose/kg b.w. is given intravenously as a bolus followed by 3–5 mL 10% glucose/kg b.w./h until normoglycemia is restored and the patient retains oral food and fluid.

D8.2.1.4 Interpretation

If the patient develops hypoglycemia, the fasting test is abnormal. Accurate interpretation requires knowledge of age-dependant hormonal and metabolic responses

Table D8.3 Control ranges of metabolites of energy metabolism in response to controlled prolonged fasting

	Glucose mmol/L mg %	Ketones mmol/L	3-OH-BA mmol/L	3-OH-BA/ Acetoacetate	FFA mmol/L	FFA/ Ketones	FFA/3-OH-BA	Glucose × Ketones	Lactate	L/P
Infants										
15-h fasting	3.8–5.3 68–95	0.1–1.6	0.1–1.0	1.4–2.7	0.4–1.6	0.6–5.4	0.9–4.4	0.5–6	0.9–2.3	11–21
20-h fasting	3.5–4.7 63–85	0.6–3.5	0.4–2.5	1.7–3.1	0.6–1.4	0.3–1.7	0.5–2.1	3–12	0.8–2.0	12–19
24-h fasting	2.6–4.6 47–83	1.4–4.1	1.0–2.9	2.2–2.9	1.1–1.7	0.3–0.7	0.5–0.9	7–12	0.8–2.1	11–20
1–7 years										
15-h fasting	3.5–5.1 63–92	0.1–2.2	<0.1–1.0	1.2–3.2	0.6–1.8	0.6–4.0	0.9–11	0.7–8	0.6–1.7	12–18
20-h fasting	2.8–4.5 50–81	1.0–3.8	0.6–2.9	2.3–3.3	0.8–2.6	0.4–1.7	0.4–2.1	4–12	0.5–1.8	10–19
24-h fasting	2.8–3.9 50–70	2.1–6.1	1.5–3.4	2.5–3.5	1.0–2.9	0.4–0.9	0.4–1.3	8–13	0.6–1.8	10–18
7–18 years										
15-h fasting	3.8–5.3 68–95	< 0.1–0.8	<0.1–0.5	0.5–2.6	0.2–1.3	1.7–8	3.3–22	0.2–2.1	0.6–1.0	11–15
20-h fasting	3.5–4.7 63–85	0.1–1.5	<0.1–1.2	1.3–3.0	0.6–1.4	0.7–4.1	1.5–7.8	0.4–5.1	0.6–1.1	10–17
24-h fasting	2.6–4.6 47–83	0.7–4.1	0.5–1.6	1.5–3.1	0.9–1.8	0.5–2.0	1.1–2.4	2.4–8.1	0.4–1.0	8–18

FFA free fatty acids; *Ketones* sum of 3-hydroxybutyrate and acetoacetate; *L/P* lactate/pyruvate; *3-OH-BA* 3-hydroxybutyrate. Glucose concentration are converted from mg% into mmol/l by division by 18 and vice versa
The table has been modified from the work of Bonnefort et al. (1990) following the grouping of subjects and parameters considered and expanding the ranges from experiences with an additional 25 control subjects studied at the authors departments

to fasting as well as reference values from control individuals. Table D8.3 is based on experience with close to 100 control subjects from two published series and additional control subjects, which were selected after extensive metabolic investigations failed to give any indication of an inherited metabolic disease.

In older children and adults, ketone body production may not be maximal until the 2nd or 3rd day of fasting because of greater stores of glycogen and efficient gluconeogenesis. Prolonged fasting extended up to 36 or even 48 h may be justified in adults. Infants and small children have much lower glycogen stores and higher capacities to form and utilize ketone bodies. Significant ketone body production occurs before 24 h. Interestingly, infants show an intermediate response to fasting as compared to toddlers and older children. This can be explained by larger glycogen stores in infants because of high calorie meals at regular intervals. Ketone body production for children older than seven was variable and in some, only moderate even after 24 h (see Table D8.3). Metabolic defects of ketogenesis or ketolysis would still be expected to be diagnosed after 24-h fast.

Reliable quantification of acetoacetate and pyruvate is difficult. For the evaluation of the fasting response, ketone bodies (in particular 3-hydroxybutyrate) may be measured in a plasma or serum sample. However, the ratio of 3-hydroxybutyrate to acetoacetate is important in the work-up of a suspected defect of pyruvate metabolism or oxidative phosphorylation, and analysis should be carried out in deproteinized blood samples (perchloric acid extraction) if such a disorder is suspected. Additional clues to a defect of pyruvate carboxylase are bouts of hyperammonemia and elevated levels of citrulline and lysine on amino acid analysis.

A good indicator of blood pyruvate concentrations is the simultaneously determined level of alanine in plasma. An alanine level of 450 µmol/L corresponds to a blood pyruvate of 100 µmol/L, i.e., the upper limit of the normal range. Other amino acids to be evaluated at the end of a fasting test are the branched-chain amino acids isoleucine, leucine, and valine that are physiologically elevated during acute starvation. However, if the increase becomes excessive and allo-isoleucine detectable, a variant of maple syrup urine disease may

Table D8.4 Response to fasting in disorders of carbohydrate and energy metabolism

Presumptive diagnosis	Glucose	Blood ketones	3-OH-butyrate/ acetoacetate	FFA	FFA/ketones	Lactate	L/P
Glycogenosis I	↓↓	N – ↓	N	N	N – ↑	↑↑	N
Glycogenosis III, VI and 0	↓	↑	N	N	N	N	N
Defects of gluconeogenesis	↓↓	N – ↓	N	N	N – ↑	↑↑	N
Defects of fatty acid oxidation	↓↓	↓↓	N – ↓	N	↑↑	↑	N
Defects of ketolysis	↑ – N – ↓	↑↑	N	N	↓	N	N
Defects of pyruvate carboxylase	↓	↑	↓	N	N	↑↑	⇑
Defects of pyruvate dehydrogenase	↓	N – ↓	N	N	N	↑ – ↑↑	N
Defects of oxidative phosphylation	N – ↓	↑	↑ – ↑↑	N	N	N – ↑↑	↑ – ↑↑

FFA free fatty acids; *L/P* lactate/ pyruvate ratio; *N* normal values (see Table D8.3)
↑ pathologically elevated and ↓ decreased values
Parameters of specific diagnostic value are highlighted in bold and larger font

be the cause for recurrent episodes of hyperketotic hypoglycemia.

A diagnostic algorithm of differential metabolic responses to fasting in disorders of carbohydrate and energy metabolism is elaborated in Table D8.4. In general, a high level of free fatty acids and low levels of 3-hydroxybutyrate and acetoacetate indicate a disorder of fatty acid oxidation. In defects of ketolysis, an elevated product of blood glucose times ketones during fasting is the most suggestive parameter. A summary of metabolic and hormonal disorders in which pathological responses are elucidated by fasting is given in Table D8.5.

Congenital hyperinsulinism (previously described as nesidioblastosis or persistent hyperinsulinemia of infancy), the most common cause of persistent symptomatic hypoglycemia in neonates and small infants, leads to hypoketotic hypoglycemia with low levels of free fatty acids. This disorder can be due to defects of the sulfonylurea receptor. The same constellation of neonatal hypoglycemia and impaired lipolysis can be caused by hyperproinsulinemia. In such patients, insulin levels are low and proinsulin grossly elevated.

Diagnosis of hormonal disorders depends on the correct collection of specimens during fasting and interpretation in connection with the blood glucose concentrations. Diagnosis needs to be ascertained by repeated determinations of insulin or detailed studies of pituitary function and additional investigations in patients with insufficiency of one or more of the counteracting hormones. Single growth hormone determinations in response to hypoglycemia are of little value for the diagnosis of growth hormone deficiency, and different provocative tests should be employed if the diagnosis is clinically suspected. Catecholamine deficiency on the basis of dopamine-β-hydroxylase deficiency or tyrosine hydroxylase deficiency is an exceedingly rare condition with a tendency to hypoglycemia. It can be ascertained in patients primarily suffering from severe orthostatic hypotension by analysis of catecholamines in urine and biogenic amines in CSF.

A presumptive diagnosis of glycogen storage diseases is usually made before the diagnostic fast on the basis of significant hepatomegaly and repeated bouts of hypoglycemia. Fatty acid oxidation requires the coordinated action of at least 17 different enzymes and one additional transport protein. In each metabolic center, there are patients with definitive diagnoses of defective fatty acid oxidation, in whom the exact enzymatic defect could as yet not be determined. In addition, there are a number of enzymes involved in fatty acid oxidation and ketolysis for which no human defects have yet been discovered.

There are otherwise completely healthy children who can develop severe metabolic decompensation with excessive ketosis with or without hypoglycemia during intercurrent illnesses. In these children, similar reactions can be provoked by prolonged fasting. Although this is not a homogenous group of patients, an exaggerated uncoordinated production of ketone bodies and significant

Table D8.5 Differential diagnosis of pathological responses to fasting

Disorder	Response to fasting	Diagnostic markers (in addition to hypoglycemia)
Fatty acid oxidation disorders	Hypoketotic hypoglycemia	Free fatty acids/ketones >2 Carnitine deficiency, except for CPT I with elevated free carnitine. Dicarboxylic aciduria Variable elevations of lactate Acute illness – increased creatine kinase and uric acid
Glycogenoses I, III and VI	Hypoglycemia	Massive hepatomegaly. Variable elevations of lactate, urate, cholesterol, triglycerides, creatine kinase, and transaminases. Hypophosphatemia
Defects of gluconeogenesis	Hypoglycemia	Hepatomegaly. Elevations of lactate
Defects of ketolysis	Hyperketotic hypoglycemia	Persistently elevated free fatty acids and ketones[a]. Ketones × glucose >15 (fasting)
Mitochondrial disease	Hyperketotic hypoglycemia	Multisystem disease. Elevations of lactate and ketones as well as of L/P and 3-OH-BA/acetoacetate ratios
Maple syrup urine disease (intermittent variant)	Hyperketotic hypoglycemia	Maybe ataxia. Elevations of branched-chain amino acids including allo-isoleucine
Congenital hyperinsulinism (nesidioblastosis)	Hypoketotic hypoglycemia	Increased insulin levels >5 mU/L at glucose <30 mg% or >8 mU/L at glucose <40 mg%. Insulin (mU/L)/ glucose (mg%)/ >3. Low-free fatty acids and ketones
Hypocortisolism, growth hormone deficiency, panhypopituitarism	Hypoketotic hypoglycemia, but sometimes significant ketosis in patients with Addison disease	Cortisol <400 nmol/L. Deficiency of growth and/ or thyroid hormone
Catecholamine deficiency	Hypoketotic hypoglycemia	Decreased catecholamines
Cyclic vomiting (diminished glycogen and protein stores)	Hyperketotic hypoglycemia	No specific abnormalities

CPT I carnitine palmitoyl transferase I deficiency; Ketones sum of 3-hydroxybutyrate and acetoacetate; L/P lactate/ pyruvate; 3-OH-BA 3-hydroxybutyrate

[a]In normal fed children, the concentration of ketone bodies in the steady state are always <0.2 mmol/L

metabolic acidosis leading to nausea and protracted vomiting appears to be a common pathogenetic mechanism. The susceptibility to these reactions slowly diminishes with age but may persist into adolescence and young adulthood. True hypoglycemia is uncommon in these children, who appear to have a defect in ketone utilization. This condition is difficult to distinguish from abdominal migraine. Relatively low stores of fat and glycogen appear to be another common denominator for such exaggerated ketogenesis. Affected children are often slim and have relatively low muscle mass. Children with pathological muscular wasting, such as patients with spinal muscular atrophy, who have severely diminished glycogen and protein stores, are at especially high risk for metabolic decompensation during fasting. Similar metabolic constellations occur in milder forms of succinyl-CoA:3-oxoacid-CoA transferase deficiency.

D8.2.2 Phenylproprionic Acid Loading Test

PPA is a nontoxic substance that, through a single round of β-oxidation, is normally converted to hippuric acid, which is excreted in the urine. PPA oxidation is catabolized by enzymes that are specific for medium-chain acyl-CoA compounds, and the PPA loading test is traditionally performed to confirm MCAD deficiency. Like the other tests of β-oxidation function, the PPA loading test has now been largely superseded by acylcarnitine analysis in conjunction with enzyme studies or mutation analyses. Indeed, it has been shown that the PPA loading test can be normal in attenuated MCAD deficiency, which is still picked up by acylcarnitine analysis in dried blood spots.

D8.2.2.1 Procedure

The test is usually carried out in the morning (fasting)

- Obtain urine sample before PPA administration for organic acid analysis.
- PPA is given orally in a dose of 25 mg/kg. The substance is not licensed as a medical drug but may be obtained from metabolic laboratories. It has an unpleasant cinnamon taste and should be mixed, e.g., with jam or administered in 50–100 mL tea through a nasogastric tube. The child should be encouraged to drink plenty of water after ingestion of PPA and is allowed normal meals.
- Collect urine for 6 (–12) h after PPA administration for organic acid analysis.

D8.2.2.2 Interpretation

Normal activity of medium-chain β-oxidations is indicated by excessive excretion of hippuric and benzoic acids in urine, while marked excretion of phenylpropionylglycine and insufficient hippuric acid is indicative of MCAD deficiency. Increased excretion of phenylhydracrylic acid is another pathological response characteristic of LCHAD deficiency. However, the diagnostic sensitivity is far lower than in MCAD deficiency. Insufficient rise of hippuric acid without other abnormalities indicates insufficient PPA intake and thus makes the test results invalid.

D8.3   Tests of Energy Metabolism

D8.3.1   Preprandial/Postprandial Analyses (Protein/Glucose Challenge)

> **Remember**
>
> The standardized analysis of metabolic parameters in the preprandial and postprandial state may provide important functional clues for the diagnosis of metabolic disorders.

Many biochemical parameters show marked variation with food intake and should be routinely examined under preprandial conditions in order to determine baseline values. Reduced concentrations of amino acids or other metabolites may be diagnostically relevant but are sometimes only found in preprandial samples. On the other hand, some metabolic disorders that affect substrate utilization give rise to abnormal metabolite concentrations only in the postprandial state. In order to reliably detect relevant abnormalities it is often necessary to examine metabolic parameters before and after defined food intake. In practice, this may be a normal meal enriched with protein and carbohydrates, the exact composition of which is less important. This test is particularly useful in the diagnosis of mitochondrial disorders which typically show pathological postprandial increases of lactate, alanine, and other small amino acids. Alanine, in contrast to lactate, is not affected by cuffing or crying and when elevated is a more reliable indicator of disturbed energy metabolism. This test is also able to recognize amino acidemias and urea cycle defects but may trigger or aggravate acute neurological symptoms.

D8.3.1.1 Procedure

- Preprandial samples should reflect a neutral metabolic state (not a fasting reaction) and are best obtained 5–6 h (up to 8 h in older children) after the last meal. Measure blood gases, blood sugar, amino acids, lactate, and ammonia; obtain a deproteinized blood sample (perchloric acid extraction) for pyruvate and ketone bodies in case that lactate is elevated. In urine, check for ketones (ketostix) and measure lactate and/or organic acids and orotic acid if not previously normal.
- Give normal meal enriched with protein and sugar to attain a total amount of ≈1 g/kg b.w. each of protein and carbohydrate/sugar.
- Postprandial blood sample should be obtained 90 min after the meal; urine should be collected for 2 h. Measure the same parameters as in the preprandial samples.

D8.3.1.2 Interpretation

Blood lactate should not rise by >20% over baseline values and should not reach pathological values

(>2.1 mmol/L). When lactate is elevated, measure pyruvate, acetoacetate, and 3-hydroxybutyrate in the perchloric acid extract to determine the redox ratio. Acid–base status should remain normal. Most amino acids will be elevated in the postprandial sample, but the plasma concentration of alanine should stay under 600–700 µmol/L and the alanine/lysine ration should stay below three.

D8.3.2 Glucose Challenge

Remember

A controlled glucose challenge is useful to assess cellular respiration in patients with suspected disorders of energy metabolism in whom lactate values have been repeatedly normal.

For aerobic generation of energy, glucose is catabolized to pyruvate, transferred into the mitochondrion and fully oxidized via the Krebs cycle and the respiratory chain. High lactate (the reduced form of pyruvate) is the most valuable diagnostic marker of disturbed mitochondrial energy metabolism in respiratory chain defects and other disorders that affect cellular respiration. However, frequently lactate is elevated only after intake of glucose or glucogenic amino acids; single normal lactate values do not exclude a primary mitochondriopathy (see Chap. B2.3). A controlled glucose challenge is useful to assess cellular respiration in patients with suspected disorders of energy metabolism in whom lactate values have been repeatedly normal. It is relatively inexpensive as lactate can be measured in all general and pediatric hospitals but it requires frequent venipunctures and lactate concentrations may be affected by cuffing or crying of the child. The measurement of pyruvate is not necessary when lactate is normal, but deproteinized blood samples (perchloric acid extraction) should be obtained to determine the redox ration (lactate/pyruvate) when lactate is high. A glucose challenge should not be carried out when lactate has been consistently elevated or when a significant postprandial increase of lactate has already been demonstrated as it may cause acute metabolic decompensation. In such cases, appropriate enzyme studies (muscle biopsy) and possible molecular analyses should be undertaken immediately upon completion of the basic biochemical analyses. Other indications include unclear hypoglycemic episodes and suspected glycogen storage disease (see Chap. B2.3).

D8.3.2.1 Preparations

- Basic investigations including amino acids and organic acids should have been completed; blood lactate should have been normal in repeated measurements before and after meals at different times of the day.
- Glucose challenge should be carried out after overnight fasting in the morning, in younger infants at least 4–5 h after the last meal.
- Secure intravenous access.

D8.3.2.2 Procedure

- Measure baseline blood lactate, blood sugar, and acid–base status; obtain 10 mL urine for lactate and/or organic acids before test.
- Give glucose 2 g/kg (max. 50 g) as 10% oral solution. The solution may be administered through a nasogastric tube (flush with water) in small children; for administration in older children, the solution may be stored in the refrigerator as it is more pleasant to drink when cool.
- Measure blood lactate, blood sugar, and acid–base status 15, 30, 45, 60, 90, 120, and 180 min after the test; collect urine for 2 h for lactate and/or organic acids. Obtain deproteinized blood samples (perchloric acid extraction) for pyruvate and ketone bodies in case lactate is elevated.

D8.3.2.3 Interpretation

Blood sugar should be elevated after the test, but lactate should not rise by >20% over baseline values and should not reach pathological values (>2.1 mmol/L). Acid–base status and urine measurements should remain normal.

D8.4 Tests of Protein Metabolism

D8.4.1 Leucine Loading Test

Insulin secretion from the pancreas is controlled by a complex system involving several enzymes and transmembrane carriers. In some persons, inappropriate insulin release is triggered by food intake, and more specifically by the ingestion of large amounts of leucine (leucine-sensitive hypoglycemia). The leucine challenge test examines the insulin reaction to food intake and the function of the blood sugar/insulin feedback mechanism and may be useful in patients with postprandial hypoglycemia or suspected hyperinsulinism–hyperammonemia syndrome. It is important to appreciate, however, that some patients with hyperinsulinism syndrome may suffer severe, life-threatening hypoglycemia after quite small amounts of leucine, and appropriate emergency measures must be prepared before the test is started. A leucine challenge is not suitable for the diagnosis of maple syrup urine disease. In these circumstances allo-isoleucine would be used, which does not cause severe symptoms in affected patients.

D8.4.1.1 Procedure

The test is carried out in the morning after overnight fasting. Insert an intravenous cannula and prepare an intravenous 20% glucose solution for emergency application in case of severe hypoglycemia.

- Obtain blood samples for baseline measurements of blood sugar, insulin, and ammonia.
- Give L-leucine orally in a dose of 150 mg/kg or intravenously in a dose of 50 (75) mg/kg.
- Determine blood sugar, insulin, and ammonia 15, 30, 45, 60, and 90 min after leucine challenge.

D8.4.1.2 Interpretation

Patients with leucine-sensitive hyperinsulinism usually develop hypoglycemia caused by excessive insulin secretion (>3 mU/L at blood sugar <2.0 mmol/L) approximately half hour after leucine administration. Concomitant hyperammonemia is indicative of a defect of glutamate dehydrogenase.

D8.4.2 Phenylalanine Loading Test

The hydroxylation reactions of phenylalanine, tyrosine, and tryptophan require tetrahydrobiopterin (BH_4) as a cofactor. A deficiency in the biosynthesis or recycling of BH_4 may cause reduced synthesis of monoamine neurotransmitters. Frequently, this is not noticeable in plasma amino acid concentrations but can be demonstrated in the kinetics of phenylalanine hydroxylation after oral challenge. The phenylalanine challenge test may be useful for the identification of disorders of pterin metabolism in patients with unclear dystonic movement disorders, in particular when Segawa syndrome is suspected.

> **Remember**
>
> The phenylalanine challenge has little use in the diagnostic work-up of patients with phenylketonuria (PKU).

D8.4.2.1 Procedure

The phenylalanine challenge should be carried out at least 1 h after a light breakfast (minimal protein). No food is permitted until the end of the test. Obtain two separate samples of 1 mL EDTA blood for the determination of basal values of phenylalanine, tyrosine, and plasma pterins. For pterin analysis, it is important to immediately centrifuge the samples and freeze the plasma in two portions. Plasma should be stored at −70 °C or sent on dry ice to the metabolic laboratory.

- Give 100 mg/kg L-phenylalanine in orange juice, if necessary through a nasogastric tube. Do not use drinks containing protein or aspartame to mix. Phenylalanine does not dissolve well; therefore, stir the mix just before drinking, and rinse the residual phenylalanine with additional juice.
- Obtain blood samples 1, 2, 4, and 6 h after phenylalanine ingestion; again centrifuge and freeze plasma immediately in two portions for the analysis of phenylalanine/tyrosine and pterins.

D8.4.2.2 Interpretation

Plasma phenylalanine levels should rise sharply after ingestion with a maximum around 60 min and then decline continuously through conversion of phenylalanine into tyrosine. Biopterin concentrations should rise several fold above baseline (to >18 nmol/L). Plasma concentrations of phenylalanine should not exceed tyrosine more than fivefold after loading. A protracted rise and slow decrease of phenylalanine together with a delayed rise of tyrosine indicate a reduced hydroxylation capacity, which may be caused either by presence of a (heterozygous) mutation in the phenylalanine hydroxylase (PAH) gene or by reduced availability of BH_4. Further differentiation is possible by examination of pterins in blood, mutation analysis of the PAH gene, or repeating a modified phenylalanine challenge. This time BH_4 (20 mg/kg b.w.) is administered 1 h before or alternatively 3 h after phenylalanine (100 mg/kg b.w.). In case of reduced availability of BH_4, administration of BH_4 prior to phenylalanine results in a complete normalization of the test. If BH_4 is given after 3 h into the test, an immediate decrease of phenylalanine occurs together with a rise of tyrosine leading to normalization of metabolite levels (see later). In the latter setting, plasma amino acids are determined after another 1, 3, and 5 h, i.e., amino acids are determined prior to and 1, 2, 4, 6, and 8 h after phenylalanine loading.

D8.4.3 BH_4 Test

Neonatal screening in most Western countries includes the diagnosis of PKU, the severe deficiency of the hepatic enzyme PAH, which untreated causes highly elevated phenylalanine (Phe) concentrations in blood (hyperphenylalaninaemia) and mental retardation. More than 600 variants or mutations in the *PAH* gene with variable effect on enzyme function have been identified, and depending on dietary Phe tolerance, severe, moderate, and mild forms of PKU have been distinguished. The attenuated form of PAH deficiency that does not require treatment is denoted "mild hyperphenylalaninemia" (MHP). PAH requires BH_4 as a cofactor, and hyperphenylalaninemia is occasionally due to a primary deficiency of BH_4 biosynthesis. Oral administration of BH_4 does not significantly reduce plasma phenylalanine concentrations in newborns with

classical PKU but may rapidly normalize phenylalanine in patients with a primary defect of pterin synthesis or recycling. Also in many patients with mild or moderate PKU, oral administration of BH_4 enhances PAH activity and thus reduces plasma Phe concentrations. The BH_4 test is intended to identify individuals with either of these conditions, i.e., primary BH_4 deficiency or BH_4-sensitive PKU.

As responsiveness to BH_4 may be of immediate therapeutic relevance, a BH_4 test should be carried out prior to the introduction of a Phe-reduced diet in all the neonates with plasma phenylalanine concentration above 400 µmol/L (6.5 mg/dL). For the reliable exclusion of cofactor deficiency, it is also necessary to determine pterin concentrations in urine and to measure dihydropteridine reductase (DHPR) activity in a filter paper card (Guthrie card), which is usually sent together with the samples of the BH_4 test to the metabolic laboratory. The BH_4 test is not reliably performed when phenylalanine levels are <400 µmol/L as the therapeutic effect in cofactor deficiency is more difficult to recognize, and most MHP patients show BH_4 sensitivity, which, anyway, is not of therapeutic relevance due to the harmless nature of the condition.

Remember

A BH_4 test in conjunction with Phe loading is not recommended since interpretation is unreliable unless results are compared with the results of Phe loading without BH_4 administration.

D8.4.3.1 Procedure

- Collect 5–10 mL urine for pterin analysis, protect against light (urine may need to be collected in a dark bag) and freeze. Obtain 2 mL EDTA full blood, centrifuge, and freeze plasma for amino acid analysis. Collect a few drops of blood on a filter paper card (Guthrie card) for the analysis of Phe and tyrosine (Tyr) as well as DHPR activity. Plasma and urine samples should be sent on dry ice to the laboratory. Alternatively, urine may be oxidized with MnO_2 and sent at ambient temperature by express mail (for this purpose acidify 5 mL urine with 6 M HCl up to a pH of 1.0–1.5, add 100 mg MnO_2, shake for 5 min at ambient temperature, centrifuge for 5 min at 4,000 rpm, and mail supernatant protected against light in aluminum foil or in a dark container).

- Give 20 mg/kg BH_4 diluted in water 30 min before a normal meal. Beware of the photosensitivity of BH_4.
- Obtain dried blood spots or plasma samples 1, 4, 8, and 24 h after BH_4 administration for Phe and Tyr analysis. Collect urine 4–8 h after administration of BH_4 for pterin analysis (samples should be prepared in the same way as the baseline samples).

The infant or older patient may be fed or may eat regularly throughout the test.

D8.4.3.2 Interpretation

The BH_4 test is regarded as positive if Phe concentrations fall by at least 30%; this should usually correspond with a rise of Tyr concentrations. In primary BH_4 deficiency, Phe concentrations rapidly normalize within the first few hours after BH_4 administration. The differential diagnosis should be clarified through pterin analysis:

- GTP cyclohydrolase I deficiency: both neopterin and biopterin absent (or very low).
- 6-Pyruvoyl-tetrahydropterin synthase deficiency: elevated neopterin but absent (or very low) biopterin.
- Pterin-4a-carbinolamin dehydratase deficiency: elevated concentrations of various pterins, specifically primapterin.
- DHPR deficiency: markedly elevated biopterin, normal or mild elevation of neopterin, low DHPR activity.

Patients with (severe) PKU also show increased urinary excretion of biopterin and neopterin, with neopterin usually more markedly elevated than biopterin. A positive BH_4 test in PKU patients may indicate BH_4 sensitivity, but the therapeutic relevance of this phenomenon in the individual case has not yet been fully clarified.

D8.4.4 Vitamin B₁₂ Test

Friederike Hörster

Methylmalonic acidurias comprise a heterogenous group of diseases with accumulation of methylmalonic acid (MMA) in urine and other body fluids as the common denominator. They are caused by a defect of the mitochondrial enzyme methylmalonyl-CoA mutase (MCM, EC 5.4.99.2) or by one of the many defects in the uptake, transport, or synthesis of 5-deoxyadenosyl-cobalamin, the cofactor of MCM, the active metabolite of vitamin B_{12}. Primary deficiencies of MCM are further subdivided into defects without residual activity (mut^0) and defects with residual activity (mut^-), caused by mutations in the apomutase locus or in genes coding for the biosynthesis of cobalamin: *cblA*, *cblB*, *cblC*, *cblD*, *cblD* (variant 1 and 2), *cblE*, *cblF*, and *cblG*. MCM situated in the mitochondrium is part of the catabolic pathways of the amino acids isoleucine, valine, methionine, and threonine as well as of odd chain fatty acids, propionic acid coming from gut bacteria and cholesterol linking the degradation of these metabolites to the Krebs' cycle.

Some defects of 5-deoxyadenosylcobalamin metabolism respond to pharmacological doses of vitamin B_{12}. While *cblC* and *cblD* defects are routinely treated by vitamin B_{12}, only some patients with cblA and *cblB* or even with *mut⁻* disease will respond. Although response to vitamin B_{12} has been identified in many studies as an important prognostic factor and hallmark of therapy (Hörster et al. 2007), there is a large variation of practice at least in European centers. Therefore, Fowler et al. (2008) have proposed the following protocol to test the response to vitamin B_{12} in a standardized way.

D8.4.4.1 Procedure

- The patient should be clinically stable on the same treatment for at least 1 month. The intakes of protein and energy should be specified and recorded.
- If the patient is already receiving cobalamin, this should be stopped for at least 1 month before the test. If the patient appears to deteriorate, restart vitamin B_{12} and defer the test. Note a general rule that patients with MMA excretion >10,000 mmol/mol creatinine and those who are clinically unstable rarely respond to vitamin B_{12}.
- Baseline urine collections: at least three specimens should be collected on different days. Plasma concentrations may only be used if a sensitive assay (stable-isotope dilution assay) is available.
- Give hydroxocobalamin 1 mg intramuscularly on three consecutive days.
- After the cobalamin injection, collect urine (or plasma) specimens on alternate days for 10 days.

- The urine or plasma samples should be analyzed in the same run in a laboratory participating in a recognized quality control scheme for MMA using gas chromatography–mass spectrometry, in Europe ERNDIM EQA (http:// www.erndim.unibas.ch).

D8.4.4.2 Interpretation

A decrease of the mean urine and plasma MMA concentrations of >50% should be regarded as indicative of a beneficial response.

In parallel to this test, the enzymology including in vitro response to adenosylcobalamin and if possible the complementation group should be determined.

D8.4.5 Allopurinol Test

Various genetic disorders especially urea cycle defects show increased urinary excretion of the pyrimidine uridine or its precursor orotic acid. In the case of urea cycle defects, this is thought to be caused by mitochondrial accumulation of carbamoylphosphate, which is transferred into the cytosol and channeled into pyrimidine biosynthesis, thus bypassing the rate-limiting first step in that pathway catalyzed by the cytosolic enzyme carbamoylphopsphate synthase II (CPS II) (see Chap. B2.6 and Fig. B2.6.1). CPS II is different from the mitochondrial isoenzyme CPS I, which is required for the detoxification of ammonia. Orotic aciduria is a diagnostic feature particularly in ornithine transcarbamylase (OTC) deficiency which otherwise lacks specific amino acid changes. Nevertheless, orotic acid may be normal in the interval in mild forms of OTC deficiency and particularly in heterozygous carrier women. In these cases, it may be possible to demonstrate an increased throughput in pyrimidine biosynthesis through an excessive rise of orotic acid and its metabolite orotidine after allopurinol-mediated blockage of uridine monophosphate synthase, the enzyme that converts orotic acid to uridine monophosphate. The allopurinol test may be used for the diagnosis of heterozygous or mild OTC deficiency in cases of unclear transient or intermittent hyperammonemia, unclear comatose or encephalopathic episodes in both sexes, or stepwise regressing neurodegenerative disease in girls or women, especially those who show epilepsy and ataxia as prominent symptoms.

D8.4.5.1 Procedure and Interpretation

Avoid caffeine (decaffeinated coffee is acceptable), tea, coffee, cocoa, chocolate, chocolate biscuits, any cola drink, or benzoate-containing beverages 24 h before the test. Otherwise, there is no need for a special diet prior or through the test. Women should be 7–12 days after their last menstrual period if possible. The test is usually started in the morning.

- Collect 10 mL urine for baseline measurement of orotic acid and orotidine, which should be done by high-pressure liquid chromatography and not by a colorimetric method.
- Give allopurinol orally in a dose of 100 mg for preschool children, 200 mg for children between 6 and 10 years of age, or 300 mg for older children and adults.
- Collect urine over 24 h in four 6-h fractions (0–6 h, 7–12 h, 13–18 h, and 19–24 h); send 10 mL of each fraction. The samples should be sent together frozen or, after conservation with three drops of chloroform, at ambient temperature by express mail. It is important to label sample tubes accurately and to inform the laboratory of all medication taken during the test as well as on the preceding days.

Remember

Both false positive and false negative results of the allopurinol test have been reported.

Excessive rise of orotic acid and/or orotidine indicates increased throughput in pyrimidine synthesis as typically caused by mild (heterozygous) OTC deficiency. Positive tests can also be found in other genetic disorders including Rett syndrome, amino acid transport defects, creatine synthesis disorders, and mitochondrial disorders. A negative allopurinol test (or normal orotic acid after protein challenge) does not fully exclude heterozygous OTC deficiency as mosaicism in the liver (lyonization) may be skewed in favor of normal hepatocytes to a degree that renders the detection of metabolic effects impossible. OTC gene mutation analysis should be considered if OTC deficiency remains a possibility.

D8.5 Tests of Carbohydrate Metabolism

D8.5.1 Glucagon Stimulation

Glucagon is a counterregulatory hormone whose secretion is normally stimulated by hypoglycemia. It acts to stimulate hepatic glycogenolysis. It does this by stimulating phosphorylase, but *glucose-6-phosphatase* activity is required for release of free glucose into the blood. Thus, the glucagon stimulation test is an excellent provocative test for von Gierke disease, glycogenosis type I, in which the hepatic activity of this enzyme is in most patients absent or nearly absent (see also Chap. B3.3).

The test is usually done following a fast for at least 6 h. An overnight fast is usually employed in normal individuals. The duration of fasting in an infant with glycogenosis I depends on *tolerance* and may have to be 4 h or less. The dose of glucagon we generally employ is 0.5 mg intramuscular. Doses of 0.03–0.1 mg/kg have been used up to a maximum of 1 mg. We measure blood concentrations of glucose at time 0 and 15 min intervals after injection for 60 min, at 90 and 120 min. Lactate and alanine may also be measured in each sample in a patient of sufficient size. In a young infant, these determinations could be done on every other sample.

In control individuals, glucagon administration is followed by a prompt glycemic response, and the concentrations of lactate and alanine do not increase. In a patient with glycogenosis I, the curve for glucose may be flat or there may be a decline. In some patients, there may be a small elevation of glucose concentration in the blood, because 6–8% of the glucose residues of glycogen are released as free glucose by the debranching enzyme. However, the increase is usually not prompt and does not exceed 50% of the fasting level within 30 min. In glycogenosis type I, levels of lactate and alanine increase after glucagon. The level of lactate rises rapidly and may go very high, even over 15 mM.

In *glycogenosis type III* or debrancher deficiency, a presumptive diagnosis can be made by determining the response to glucagon in the fed and fasted state. Administration of glucagon after a 12–14 h fast is followed by little or no increase in blood glucose. The patient is then fed and the glucagon test repeated 2–6 h later at which time the glycemic response is normal. These patients do not have lactic acidemia, and concentrations of lactate do not increase following glucagon. Their concentrations of alanine are low.

In patients with *glycogen synthase deficiency*, glucagon administration in the fasting state is followed by no elevation of glucose, lactate, or alanine. In the fed state, glucagon is followed by a glycemic response. These patients can be distinguished from those with glycogenosis III by the elevation of lactate that occurs with a glucose tolerance test.

D8.5.2 Fructose Loading Test

Remember

Mutation analysis is the primary method of choice for the diagnosis of hereditary fructose intolerance.

The major indication for the fructose tolerance test is a suspicion of hereditary fructose intolerance in patients in whom molecular analysis of the aldolase B gene failed to identify disease-causing mutations. Evaluation of the response to fructose loading can also provide valuable diagnostic information for patients with suspected defects of gluconeogenesis, such as fructose-1,6-diphosphatase deficiency. It provides no additional information in patients with glycogen storage disease. It may be useful in guiding therapy in those patients with defects of oxidative phosphorylation in whom fructose administration leads to a major elevation of lactic acid. The test may cause potentially life-threatening hypoglycemia and should be performed with great care and only after other diagnostic options (including mutation analysis of the aldolase B gene) have been exhausted. Close clinical observation is essential, and resuscitation facilities must be available. The test may cause severe nausea and/or abdominal pain 15–90 min after oral fructose intake. Intravenous fructose challenge is preferable as nausea and vomiting are less common (15–50 min after intravenous administration), but intravenous fructose preparations are currently not available in most countries.

D8.5.2.1 Preparations

- Normal results of aldolase B gene mutation analysis.
- The child should have been on a fructose-free diet for at least 2 weeks and liver function tests should have normalized.

- Explain the potential risks (hypoglycemia, nausea, and vomiting) to the parents and obtain informed consent.
- Blood sugar before test should be in upper normal range to reduce the risk of life-threatening hypoglycemia.
- An intravenous line should be maintained with 0.9% NaCl to allow sampling of specimens and rapid infusion of glucose if necessary.
- Prepare intravenous glucose solution (20%) for emergency administration in case of hypoglycemia.

D8.5.2.2 Procedure – Oral Fructose Challenge

- Basal values: measure blood sugar, phosphate, magnesium, uric acid, and lactate; determine fructose if possible.
- Give oral fructose 1 g/kg as 20% solution over 5–7 min.
- Obtain blood samples after 15, 30, 45, 60, 90, and 120 min; measure the same parameters as in the basal sample.

D8.5.2.3 Procedure – Intravenous Fructose Challenge

- Basal values: measure blood sugar, phosphate, magnesium, uric acid, and lactate; determine fructose if possible.
- Give intravenous fructose 0.25 g/kg as 10% solution over 2–4 min.
- Obtain blood samples after 5, 10, 15, 30, 45, 60, and 90 min; measure the same parameters as in the basal sample.
- Optionally, measure sugars (including fructose) and amino acids in a baseline urine as well as urine collected over the 6–12 h after the load.

D8.5.2.4 Treatment of Adverse Reactions

In case of hypoglycemia (blood glucose <40 mg% or 2.3 mmol/L) or if the patient becomes symptomatic with irritability, sweating, and drowsiness, give 2 mL of 20% or 4 mL of 10% glucose/kg b.w. intravenously as a bolus, followed by 3–5 mL 10% glucose/kg b.w./h until normoglycemia is restored and the patient is able to take and retain oral food and fluid.

D8.5.2.5 Interpretation

In hereditary fructose intolerance, fructose loading leads to profound metabolic disturbances. The picture is dominated by progressive hypoglycemia. An even sharper fall of inorganic phosphate occurs within a few minutes. A sharp rise in fructose and uric acid is followed by a slight rise of magnesium. Levels of transaminases may increase, and there may be a slight fall in serum potassium. Lactate, pyruvate, alanine, free fatty acids, glycerol, ketone bodies, and growth hormone may also rise. Fructose may be found in the urine in amounts depending on the level of hyperfructosemia. The renal threshold is 20 mg/dL. Transitory renal tubular dysfunction may lead to mild aminoaciduria and proteinuria. The fall in glucose and phosphate along with the rise in urate are sufficient for an interpretation of hereditary fructose intolerance.

A hypoglycemic response to fructose administration is also observed in fructose-1,6-diphosphate deficiency. This disorder may be differentiated from fructose intolerance by a history of fasting hypoglycemia and lactic acidemia and an absence of aversion to fruits and sweets. Enzyme assay of biopsied liver provides the definitive diagnosis in both.

D8.6 Tests of Exercise Tolerance

D8.6.1 Forearm Ischemia Test

Adequate functioning of glycolysis is necessary for energy production during muscle exercise. With sufficient oxygen supply, glucose-6-phosphate is fully oxidized in the mitochondrion, while anaerobic glycolysis results in the production of lactate. Also required for adequate muscle function is the purine nucleotide cycle, which involves the deamination of adenosine monophosphate to inosine monophosphate and the release of ammonia. The forearm ischemia test examines both systems through measurement of lactate and ammonia concentrations before and after anaerobic exercise. It may be useful in patients with muscle cramps or other muscular symptoms on exertion. Normally, there is a marked increase in the concentration of both parameters after anaerobic exercise. Adequate rise of ammonia with absent rise of lactate indicates a deficiency in the breakdown of glycogen or in glycolysis as in glycogen storage disease types V (McArdle), III (Cori), or VII (Tauri). In contrast, absent rise of ammonia with normal lactate production indicates a deficiency in the purine nucleotide cycle such as muscle-AMP deaminase deficiency. The test is invalid if neither lactate nor ammonia is elevated as this implies insufficient muscle work. Significant increase of creatinine kinase after the test may indicate different metabolic disorders affecting the muscle, e.g., a long-chain fatty acid oxidation defect.

D8.6.1.1 Procedure

- Twenty to thirty minutes before the test, a urine sample should be obtained to determine myoglobin, and the patient should rest in bed.
- Just before the test, a large intravenous cannula is inserted into the cubital vein of the test arm, which should be the right arm in right-handed persons. A blood sample is taken for the measurement of lactate, ammonia, and creatinine kinase.
- An inflatable cuff for blood pressure measurements is attached to the upper test arm and pumped to a pressure of 250 or 20 mmHg above systolic blood pressure of the patient. The palmar arc may be blocked with a small cuff across the wrist. The patient is than asked to maximally exert the forearm and hand muscles. This may require strong encouragement and is difficult to achieve particularly in children, but insufficient exercise makes the test invalid. A standardized approach may involve a dynamometer which is best set at 80% maximum strength. Alternatively, a hand-powered torch may be used, which also gives feedback on muscle work (brightness of the light). Squeezing a firm roll such as a towel as hard as possible every 2 s does not usually cause a sufficient rise of lactate and ammonia and therefore is not a good alternative. After the end of muscle exercise the cuffs are released.
- Blood samples are obtained from the intravenous line immediately after muscle exercise and the following 1, 3, 5, and 7 min for the measurement of lactate, ammonia, and creatinine kinase. Myoglobin is determined in the first urine produced after muscle exercise.

D8.6.1.2 Interpretation

Normally, lactate should rise by >2 mmol/L and ammonia by >50 μmol/L above basal values. Insufficient rise of both lactate and ammonia indicates insufficient muscle activity and makes the test invalid. Insufficient rise only of lactate indicates deficient glyco(geno) lysis, while insufficient rise only of ammonia suggests muscle-AMP-deaminase deficiency. Elevations of creatinine kinase or myoglobin may reflect muscle cell damage which may be caused by metabolic disorders such as a long-chain fatty acid oxidation defect or electron chain disorders.

Key References

Bonham JR, Guthrie P, Downing M et al (1999) The allopurinal test lacks for primary urea cycle defects but may indicate unrecognized mitochondrial disease. J Inherit Metab Dis 22:174–184

Bonnefont JP, Specola NB, Vassault A et al (1990) The fasting test in paediatrics: application to the diagnosis of pathological hypo- and hyperketotic states. Eur J Pediatr 150:80–85

Cahill GF (1982) Starvation. Trans Am Clin Climatol Assoc 94:1–21

Fowler B, Leonard JV, Baumgartner MR (2008) Causes of and diagnostic approach to methylmalonic acidurias. J Inherit Metab Dis 31:350–360

Hörster F, Baumgartner MR, Viardot C, Suormala T, Burgard P, Fowler B, Hoffmann GF, Garbade SF, Kölker S, Baumgartner ER (2007) Long-term outcome in methylmalinic acidurias is influenced by the underlying defect (muto, mut-, cbIA, cbIB). Pediatr Res 62:225–30

Hyland K, Fryburg JS, Wilson WG et al (1997) Oral phenylalanine loading in dopa-responsive dystonia: a possible diagnostic test. Neurology 48:1290–1297

Morris AAM, Thekekara A, Wilks Z et al (1996) Evaluation of fasts for investigating hypoglycaemia or suspected metabolic disease. Arch Dis Child 75:115–119

Touatti G, Huber J, Saudubray JM (2006) Diagnostic procedures: function tests and postmortem protocol. In: Fernandes J, Saudubray JM, Van den Berghe G, Walter, J (eds) Inborn metabolic diseases, 4th edn. Springer, Berlin, pp 59–79

Family Issues, Carrier Tests, and Prenatal Diagnosis

D9

Johannes Zschocke

Key Facts

> Carrier tests should not be performed in asymptomatic children unless there is a medical consequence of the result for the tested individual in childhood.

> Standard invasive procedures required for prenatal analysis of inborn errors of metabolism have risk of abortion of 0.5–1%.

> Chorionic villus biopsy is the method of choice for DNA-based prenatal tests. It can usually be carried out from the 11th to the 12th week of pregnancy onward

> Preimplantation genetic diagnosis requires in vitro fertilisation and is illegal in many countries. An alternative is polar body analysis, which is more limited in its applications.

D9.1 General Remarks

Most inborn errors of metabolism are inherited as autosomal recessive traits. Diagnosis in a child thus implies a high recurrence risk for subsequent pregnancies in the family. Although clinicians caring for the child usually explain the genetic basis of the condition at an early stage (text box), many parents do not really appreciate all the implications, and formal genetic counselling including an explanatory letter to the parents is usually beneficial even in disorders with an apparently simple autosomal recessive inheritance. Genetic counselling also involves taking a standardised family tree and may help to identify other relatives with a high risk for an affected child, such as consanguineous partners in the same extended family. Genetic counselling should be recommended to these couples as well.

The human genome as a shelf of cook books

A simple way to explain the human genome and the molecular basis of inherited disorders to patients is a comparison with a kitchen shelf of books. The genetic information is stored in each cell in a collection of 46 books (chromosomes) that are comprised of a total of more than 23,000 recipes (protein coding genes). Each gene contains the information for a particular function that the cell may need to fulfil. Quite importantly, there are not 46 different books but 23 pairs of the same books with the same recipes, and each person thus has two copies of most recipes. The only exceptions are the sex chromosomes: females have two X chromosomes, but males have only one and an additional Y chromosome (which used to be an X chromosome many million years ago but over time has lost most of its genes, with the exception of a few genes that include some that trigger male sex development). When people have children, they pack one of the two copies of each book into the parcel for the child, which thus contains only 23 different exemplars. As a child gets a parcel from each parent, it again receives a total of 46 books. The text of the recipes consists of four letters ACGT, and one set of books has more than three billion letters. Because the books are copied by hand from generation to generation, they contain the occasional

J. Zschocke
Divisions of Human Genetics and Clinical Genetics, Medical University Innsbruck, Schöpfstr. 41,6020 Innsbruck, Austria
e-mail: johannes.zschocke@i-med.ac.at

G. F. Hoffmann et al. (eds.), *Inherited Metabolic Diseases*,
DOI: 10.1007/978-3-540-74723-9_D9, © Springer-Verlag Berlin Heidelberg 2010

spelling mistake or typing error, and there may be different variants (alleles) of the same recipes. Polymorphisms are variants that are quite common (>1% of gene copies in a population), while mutations are variants that change the information content and in consequence change or remove the normal function. It may be useful to point out that, for example, humans do not have two PAH genes (PAH codes for the enzyme phenylalanine hydroxylase deficient in phenylketonuria) but have two copies of the one PAH gene; just like having two copies of the same recipe for chocolate cake does not mean that one has two chocolate cake recipes. Any genetic abnormality may be explained with this example, from X-chromosome inactivation (only one book is used, the other exemplar is sealed) to genomic imprinting (a recipe can only be read on either the paternal or the maternal copy of the book, the other version is sealed) or balanced translocations (two books have fallen apart and have been wrongly glued together again).

D9.2 Carrier Tests

Once disease-causing mutations have been identified in a patient, it is easily possible to test other family members for the familial mutation(s). In autosomal recessive conditions, both the parents are normally carriers for the disease and mutation testing may not be necessary for confirmation. Sometimes, however, it is advisable to confirm the results in the child through carrier testing in both parents. In a child with homozygosity for a mutation, for example, it may be advisable to exclude the presence of a large deletion on one allele that may lead to PCR non-amplification on the other gene copy. When a child appears to be compound heterozygous for two mutations, it may be important to confirm that the two mutations are indeed in trans, i.e. on the two different chromosomal strands and not on the same chromosomal strand/in the same gene copy. In the latter case, the child is heterozygous for a double mutation, and the genotype does not confirm the disease. It should be kept in mind, however, that carrier tests in the parents may also lead to the identification of non-paternity which may be embarrassing (or worse) both for the couple involved and the doctor.

Carrier analyses in siblings of affected children or in more distant relatives may appear harmless on first sight. Nevertheless, there have been cases where the presence of mutations in completely healthy persons was misunderstood by the affected individual or others as a kind of disease and at worst had an adverse impact on insurance or employment. It is thus generally agreed that carrier tests should not be performed in underage siblings of patients with recessive disorders. This is true for all kinds of genetic tests. These should not be carried out in asymptomatic children unless there is a medical consequence of the result for the tested individual already in childhood. It is much wiser to let the child grow up to an age where she or he understands the implications and may request carrier testing in the course of genetic counselling. Growing up with the knowledge of the result may rob the child of the option to later actively work on this issue in the process of making a decision on testing.

D9.3 Prenatal Diagnosis

Many parents who experienced a severely debilitating or fatal inherited disease in a child and who have a high risk for the same disease in future pregnancies request prenatal diagnosis with the option of termination of pregnancy. The associated social and legal issues differ markedly between countries and are not discussed here. There is generally a window of opportunity between the 11th and 12th week of pregnancy when the placenta and foetus are sufficiently large for invasive testing, and the 22nd–23rd week when the foetus may survive outside the womb and termination of pregnancy is often regarded as much more problematic for ethical reasons. Termination of pregnancy in the second trimenon involves the induction of labour and delivery of a foetus which dies through the procedure, in contrast to the first trimenon when curettage is usually sufficient. After the 22nd–23rd week, the foetus is killed in the womb through injection of potassium into the heart (foeticide) in order to avoid that the child is born alive, a procedure that is emotionally and ethically very challenging or unacceptable for many parents and doctors. Parents should be offered genetic and/or psychosocial counselling when termination of pregnancy is considered. The decision for or against termination of pregnancy rests solely with the couple or the mother. Non-directive counselling is mandatory and is possible even when termination is requested by the parents but is rejected by the doctors or is deemed incompatible with legal regulations in the specific circumstances.

Prenatal diagnosis should be organised by a clinical geneticist in close contact with the gynaecologist who performs both the invasive procedure and possibly the termination. Parents should be advised to contact the geneticist as early as possible once a pregnancy has been confirmed. Traditionally, there are different approaches to prenatal diagnosis including metabolic analyses in amniotic fluid and enzyme tests in chorionic villus cells or amniocytes, but direct mutation analysis is now mostly regarded as the method of choice. Because of the enormous progress in the understanding of inherited disorders over the last years, it is now possible to test a foetus for almost all inborn error of metabolism once a disease has been recognised in a family.

Metabolic conditions are not usually recognised through abnormal ultrasound scans and invasive sampling of foetal cells or fluid is necessary for prenatal testing. There are three main approaches:

1. *Chorionic villus sampling* (CVS) is usually possible from the 11th week of pregnancy onwards. Small fragments of placental tissue are taken with a moderately large needle either through the abdomen or the cervix. Chorionic villi have both foetal and maternal components, and it is essential to carefully remove the latter after the sample has been taken. Cells may be either cultured, e.g. for chromosome analysis or enzyme studies, or may be used for DNA extraction. Chorionic cells are derived from the trophoblast and the extraembryonic mesoderm, and chromosomal abnormalities found in these cells (particularly when the abnormality is found only in a proportion of cells) do not necessarily reflect the chromosomal status of the foetus. For karyotype analysis, therefore, two different cell culture types are used. This is not necessary for molecular analyses, but it is mandatory to exclude maternal contamination when chorionic villi are used for genetic tests as presence of maternal cells may lead to false negative results. For this purpose, highly polymorphic microsatellite markers in DNA extracted from chorionic villi and maternal blood are compared; maternal contamination is excluded when only one of the two maternal alleles as well as one paternal allele are identified in the foetal sample. CVS has a risk for miscarriage of approximately 1%, i.e. 1 in 100 women loses a healthy child after the procedure. Because of the early availability of foetal DNA, CVS is the method of choice for prenatal diagnosis through mutation analysis.

2. *Amniocentesis* is usually possible from the 14th to 15th week of pregnancy onwards. Amniotic fluid contains foetal cells derived from the urinary tract or other sources and is obtained transabdominally with a long, relatively small needle. There is not usually sufficient cellular material for DNA extraction and amniocytes have to be cultured for 7–10 days both for chromosomal and molecular analyses. DNA is thus available for testing at least 4 weeks later than after CVS. In contrast to CVS, there is smaller risk of maternal contamination unless there is a significant amount of maternal blood in the amniotic fluid (which may be recognised, e.g. through a reddish colour). Compared with CVS, amniocentesis has a slightly lower risk for miscarriage of approximately 0.5%, although these figures also depend on the expertise of the gynaecologist who performs the procedure.

3. *Foetal blood sampling* is generally possible after the 20th week of pregnancy and has a risk of miscarriage of approximately 2%. Blood is taken transabdominally with a long needle from an umbilical vein at the insertion of the umbilicus into the placenta. As this foetal sampling approach becomes possible only relatively late in pregnancy, it is usually restricted to special indications.

D9.4 Preimplantation Genetic Diagnosis and Polar Body Analysis

As an alternative to prenatal diagnosis after several months of pregnancy, disease status may also be determined in the course of in vitro fertilisation (IVF) prior to implantation of the embryo into the womb. For preimplantation genetic diagnosis (PGD) one or two cells are taken from the embryo 2–3 days after fertilisation (in the four or eight cell stadium). PCR-based mutation analysis is performed after DNA extraction and amplification. This procedure requires a highly controlled laboratory setting and may have to be specifically established for the individual case. PGD is prohibited in several countries as discarding an embryo is deemed to violate its right to life when there is no conflicting interest of the mother (there is as yet no pregnancy), and there is a perceived risk of a "slippery slope" of easy selection of preferable characteristics in a child conceived through IVF. As an alternative to PGD in these countries, mutation status may be determined in DNA extracted from the polar bodies of an egg prior to fertilisation (polar body analysis). This method only allows testing for mutations carried by the mother and not the father, again may need to be specially established for the individual case and is offered by few specialised laboratories only. Both approaches require IVF, which may be stressful and carries additional risks, and is not necessarily covered by health insurances. However, they are options for parents who for religious or ethical reasons object to termination of pregnancy.

Key References

Besley GTN (2005) Prenatal diagnosis of inborn errors of metabolism. In: John M. Walker JM, Rapley R (eds) Medical biomethods handbook. Humana Press, Totowa, New Jersey

Sasi K, Sanderson D, Eydoux Cartier h, Scriver CR, Treacy E (1997) Prenatal diagnosis for inborn errors of metabolism and haemoglobinopathies: the Montreal Children's Hospital experience. Pren Diagn 17:681–685

Acidosis

Hyperchloremic diarrhea
Acrodermatitis, enteropathica
Infectious
Lactase deficiency
Sucrase deficiency
Renal tubular acidosis (RTA)
Cystinosis
Fanconi syndrome
Galactosemia
Glucose, galactose malabsorption
Hepatorenal tyrosinemia
Mitochondrial electron transport defect
Osteopetrosis and RTA
Topamax

Alopecia

An (hypo) hidrotic ectodermal dysplasia
Biotin deficiency
Cartilage hair hypoplasia
Conradi–Hünermann syndrome
Multiple carboxylase deficiency – holocarboxylase synthetase and biotinidase deficiencies
Trichorrhexis nodosa-argininosuccinic aciduria
Vitamin D-dependent rickets-receptor abnormalities

Angiokeratomas

Fabry disease
Fucosidosis
Galactosialidosis
GM_1 gangliosidosis
Sialidosis

Apparent Acute Encephalitis

Glutaric aciduria I
NARP
Propionic acidemia

Arthritis

Alkaptonuria
Farber disease
Gaucher type I
Gout-HPRT deficiency; PRPP overactivity
Homocystinuria
I cell disease
Lesch–Nyhan disease
Mucolipidosis III
Mucopolysaccharidosis IS; IIS

Bleeding Tendency

Abetalipoproteinemia
α-1-Antitrypsin deficiency
Congenital disorders of glycosylation (CDG)
Chediak–Higashi syndrome
Fructose intolerance
Gaucher disease
Glycogenoses types I and IV
Hermansky–Pudlak syndrome
Peroxisomal disorder
Tyrosinemia type 1

Calcification of Basal Ganglia

Albright syndrome
Bilateral striato-pallido-dentate calcinosis
Carbonic anhydrase II deficiency
Cockayne syndrome
Down syndrome
Fahr disease
Familial progressive encephalopathy with calcification of the basal ganglia (Aicardi–Goutieres syndrome)
GM1-gangliosidosis
Hallervorden–Spatz disease
Hypo-, hyper-parathyreoidism
Krabbe leukodystrophy
Lipoid proteinosis

G. F. Hoffmann et al. (eds.), *Inherited Metabolic Diseases*,
DOI: 10.1007/978-3-540-74723-9_E1, © Springer-Verlag Berlin Heidelberg 2010

Microcephaly and intracranial calcification
Mitochondrial cytopathies
Multiple endocrine neoplasia I
Neurofibromatosis
Pterin defects
    Dihydropteridine reductase deficiency
    GTP cyclohydrolase I deficiency
    6-pyruvoyletetrahydropterin synthase deficiency
    Sepiapterin reductase deficiency
    Spondyloepiphyseal dysplasia

Cardiomyopathy

Congenital muscular dystrophy
Danon disease
Disorders of fatty acid oxidation
Electron transport chain abnormalities
Fabry disease
Glycogenosis type III
Hemochromatosis
D-2-Hydroxyglutaric aciduria
3-Methylglutaconic aciduria II (Barth disease)
Mucopolysaccharidosis
Pompe disease

Cataracts – Lenticular Opacity

Delta1-pyrroline-5-synthase deficiency
Cerebrotendinous xanthomatosis
Electron transport chain disorders
Fabry disease
Galactokinase deficiency
Galactosemia
Homocystinuria
Hyperferritinemia-cataract syndrome
Hyperornithinemia (ornithine aminotransferase deficiency)
Lowe syndrome
Lysinuric protein intolerance
Mannosidosis
Mevalonic aciduria
Multiple sulfatase deficiency
Neonatal carnitine palmitoyl transferase (CPT II deficiency)
α'-Pyrroline-5-carboxylate synthase deficiency
Peroxisomal disorders

Cerebral Calcification

Abnormalities of folate metabolism
Adrenoleukodystrophy
Aicardi–Goutiere syndrome
Biopterin abnormalities

Biotinidase deficiency
Carnitine palmitoyltransferase II deficiency
Cockayne syndrome
GM2 gangliosidosis
L-2-hydroxyglutaric aciduria
Hypoparathyroidism
Kearns–Sayre syndrome
Krabbe disease
MELAS
Osteopetrosis and renal tubular acidosis (carbonic anhydrase II deficiency)
Mitochondrial disorders

Cerebral Vascular Disease

Fabry disease
Familial hypocholesterolemia
Homocystinuria
Menkes disease
5,10-Methylenetetrahydrofolatereductase deficiency
Myocardial infarction

Cerebrospinal Fluid Lymphocytosis

Aicardi–Goutieres syndrome

Cerebrospinal Fluid Protein Elevation

Congenital disorders of glycosylation CCDG
L-2-Hydroxyglutaric aciduria
Kearns–Sayre syndrome
Krabbe disease
MELAS – Mitochondrial encephalomyopathy, lactic acidemia, and stroke-like episodes
MERFF – Myoclonic epilepsy with ragged-red fibers
Metachromatic leukodystrophy
Multiple sulfatase deficiency
Neonatal adrenoleukodystrophy
Refsum disease

Cherry Red Macular Spots

Galactosialidosis
GM_1 gangliosidosis
Mucolipidosis I
Multiple sulfatase deficiency
Niemann–Pick disease
Sandhoff disease
Sialidosis
Tay–Sachs disease

Cholestatic Jaundice

Alagille syndrome
α-1-Antitrypsin deficiency
Byler disease
      (progressive familial intrahepatic cholestasis (PF1C1, BRIC1))
      PFIC2 (bile salt excretory pump (BSEP))
      PFIC 3 (MDR3)
Citrin deficiency
Cystic fibrosis
Dubin–Johnson syndrome
Fructose bisphosphate aldolase (B) deficiency (HNF-1B)
Hepatic nuclear factor 1β gene mutation
Hepatorenal tyrosinemia
LCHAD deficiency
Mevalonic aciduria
Niemann–Pick type C disease
Peroxisomal biogenesis disorders
Rotor syndrome
Tyrosinemia, hepatorenal

Chondrodysplasia Phenotypes

Conradi–Hünermann syndrome
Peroxisomal disorders
Warfarin embryopathy

Chronic Pancreatitis

Hereditary (dominant) (with or without lysinuria (cystinuria)): with or without pancreatic lithiasis or portal vein thrombosis
With hyperparathyroidism in multiple endocrine adenomatosus syndrome
MELAS
Organic acidemias
Pearson syndrome
Regional enteritis (Crohn)
Trauma – pseudocyst

Cirrhosis of the Liver

α-1-Antitrypsin deficiency
Citrin deficiency (citrullinemia)
Cystic fibrosis
Congenital disorders glycosylation
Defects of bile acid synthesis
Electron transport chain disorders
Galactosemia
Glycogen storage disease type IV
(Neonatal) Hemochromatosis

Peroxisomal disorder
Hepatorenal tyrosinemia
Niemann–Pick type C
Peroxisomal disorders
Pyruvate kinase deficiency
Transaldolase deficiency
Tyrosinemia type I
Wilson disease

Corneal Opacity

Cystinosis
Fabry
Fish eye disease (LCAT deficiency)
Galactosialidosis
GM_1 gangliosidosis
Hurler disease (MPS I)
I-cell disease
Mannosidosis
Mucolipidosis III
Multiple sulfatase deficiency

Corpus Callosum Agenesis

Adrenocorticotrophic hormone (ACTH) deficiency
Aicardi syndrome
Mitochondrial disorders (especially pyruvate dehydrogenase deficiency)
Nonketotic hyperglycinemia
Peroxisomal disorders

Creatine Kinase – Elevated

Aldolase A deficiency
Carnitine palmitoyl transferase II deficiency
Disorders of fatty acid oxidation
Drugs – Toxins, alcohol, statins
Glutaric acidemia (I)
Glycogenosis – III
Glycogenosis – V – McArdle
Glycogenosis – posphofructokinase
D-2-Hydroxyglutaric aciduria
Inflammatory myopathy – dermatomyositis, polymyositis
Infectious myositis
3-Oxothiolase deficiency
Mevalonic aciduria
Myoadenylate deaminase
Muscular dystrophy – Duchenne, Becker
3-Oxothiolase deficiency
Oxphos abnormalities
Traumatic muscle injury

Dermatosis

Acrodermatitic enteropathica
Biotinidase deficiency
Holocarboxylase synthetase deficiency

Diabetes Mellitus – Erroneous Diagnosis

Congenital disorders of glycosylation
Isovaleric acidemia
Methylmalonic acidemia
3-Oxothiolase deficiency
Propionic acidemia

Diarrhea

Abetalipoproteinemia
Congenital chloride diarrhea
Electron transport disorders
Enterokinase deficiency
Glucose galactose malabsorption
Johansson–Blizzard syndrome
Lactase deficiency
Lysinuric protein intolerance
Pearson syndrome
Schwachman syndrome
Sucrase deficiency
Wolman disease

Dysostosis Multiplex

Galactosialidosis
Generalized GM1 gangliosidosis
Hurler, Hurler–Scheie disease
Hunter disease
Maroteaux–Lamy disease
Mucolipidosis II, I-cell disease
Mucolipidosis III
Multiple sulfatase deficiency
Sanfilippo disease
Sly disease

Ectopia Lentis (dislocation of the lens)

Homocystinuria
Hyperlysinemia
Marfan syndrome
Molybdenum cofactor deficiency
Sulfite oxidase deficiency
Weiss–Marchesani syndrome

EEG Burst Suppression Pattern

Anesthesia-deep stages
Anoxia, cerebral hypoperfusion

B_6/pyridoxal-phosphate dependencies
Drug overdose (e.g., phenobarbital)
Molybdenum cofactor deficiency
Nonketotic hyperglycinemia
Organic acidemias (neonatal encephalopathy-propionic academia)
Purine metabolism defects

Exercise Intolerance

Defects of glycogenolysis
Disorders of fatty acid oxidation
3-Oxothiolase deficiency
Mitochondrial disorders
Myoadenylate deaminase deficiency

Fever Syndromes

Familial Mediterranean fever
Hyperimmunoglobulin D syndrome (mevalonic aciduria)
Muckle–Wells syndrome (neonatal onset multisystem inflammatory disease syndrome)
Tumor necrosis factor receptor-associated periodic syndrome

Glycosuria

Cystinosis
Diabetes mellitus
Hepatorenal tyrosinemia
Fanconi–Bickel syndrome – GLUT-2 mutations
Glycogen synthase deficiency
Pearson syndrome
Renal Fanconi syndrome
Wilson disease

Hair Abnormalities

Argininosuccinic aciduria
Kinky hair, photosensitivity, and mental retardation
Menkes disease (pili torti, trichorrhexis nodosa, monilethrix)
Pili torti: isolated, MIM 261900
Pili torti with deafness or with dental enamel hypoplasia MIM 262000 (Björnstad syndrome (complex 3))
Trichothiodystrophy: trichorrhexis nodosa, ichthyosis, and neurological abnormalities (Pollit syndrome) MIM 27550

HDL (lipoprotein) Low

Lecithin cholesterol acyltransferase (LCAT) deficiency
(fish eye disease)
Tangier disease
Hypoalphalipoproteinemia

Hemolytic Anemia

Defects of glycolysis
5-Oxoprolinuria
Purine and pyrimidine disorders
Wilson disease

Hemophagocytosis (Erythrophagocytosis)

Carnitine palmitoyl transferase I
Familial hemophagocytic lymphocytic histocytcosis
(perforin deficiency, PRF1)
Gaucher disease
Hemochromatosis
Lysinuric protein intolerance
Niemann–Pick disease
Propionic acidemia
Wolman disease

Hepatic Carcinoma

α-1-Antitrypsin deficiency
Galactosemia
Glycogen storage disease types I and IV
Hemochromatosis
Hepatorenal tyrosinemia
Progressive intrahepatic cholestasis
Thalassemia
Wilson disease

Hepatic Cirrhosis

α-1-Antitrypsin deficiency
Cholesteryl ester storage disease
Congenital disorder of glycosylation (CDG-X)
Cystic fibrosis
Coeliac disease
Electron transport disorders
Fructose intolerance
Galactosemia
Gaucher disease
Glycogenosis types I and IV
Hematochromatosis
Hepatorenal tyrosinemia
Hypermethioninemia
Mitochondrial DNA depletion
Niemann–Pick disease

Phosphoenolpyruvate carboxykinase deficiency
Progressive intrahepatic cholestasis
Thalassemia
Transaldolase deficiency
Urea cycle disorders
Wilson disease
Wolman disease

Hepatic Failure – Acute

α-1-Antitrypsin deficiency
Fatty acid oxidation disorders
Galactosemia
Hepatorenal tyrosinemia
Hereditary fructose intolerance
Mitochondrial depletion syndromes, esp. POLG1 and
MPV17 mutations
Neonatal hemochromatosis
Niemann–Pick types B and C
Urea cycle disorders
Wilson disease
Wolcott–Rallison syndrome

Hydrops Fetalis

Carnitine transporter deficiency
Congenital disorders of glycosylation
Farber disease (disseminated lipogranulomatosis)
Galactosialidosis
Glycogenosis type IV
GM1 gangliosidosis
Gaucher disease
Infantile free sialic acid storage disease (ISSD)
Mucolipidosis II – I-cell disease
Neonatal hemochromatosis
Niemann–Pick disease
Niemann–Pick disease type C
Pearson syndrome (anemia)
Siali inverted nipples dosis
Sly disease-β-glucuronidase deficiency
Wolman disease

3-Hydroxyglutaric Aciduria

Glutaryl-CoA dehydrogenase deficiency
Short-chain hydroxyacyl-CoA dehydrogenase
deficiency
Carnitine palmitoyltransferase I deficiency

Hyperammonemia

N-acetylglutamate synthetase deficiency
α-1-Antitrypsin deficiency

Argininemia
Argininosuccinic aciduria
Carbamoyl phosphate synthetase deficiency
Chemotherapy-induced hyperammonemia
Citrullinemia
Fatty acid oxidation disorders
HHH syndrome
HMG-CoA lyase deficiency
Isovaleric acidemia
Lysinuric protein intolerance
MCAD deficiency
Methylmalonic acidemia
Multiple carboxylase deficiency
Ornithine transcarbamylase deficiency
Pyruvate carboxylase deficiency
Pyruvate dehydrogenase complex deficiency
Propionic acidemia
Hyperthermia, malignant carnitine palmitoyl
transferase-II deficiency
Transient hyperammonemia of the newborn
Urinary tract infection – urea splitting bacteria
Valproate
Wilson disease

Hypertyrosinemia

Deficiency of 4-hydroxyphenylpyruvate dioxygenase
Drug – toxin
Hepatic infection
Hepatorenal tyrosinemia
Hyperthyroidism
Oculocutaneous tyrosinemia
Postprandial
Scurvy
Transient tyrosinemia of the newborn
Treatment with NTBC
Tyrosinemia type III

Hypoketotic Hypoglycemia

Carnitine transporter deficiency
CPT I deficiency
HMG-CoA lyase deficiency
LCAD
LCHAD/MTP
MCAD
VLCAD

Hypophosphatemia

Fanconi syndrome
Hyperparathyroidism
MELAS

Pearson
X-linked hypophosphatemic rickets

Hypouricemia

Fanconi syndrome, cystinosis, any proximal renal
tubular dysfunction
Isolated renal tubular defect (Dalmatian dog model)
Molybdenum cofactor deficiency
Phosphoribosyl pyrophosphate synthetase deficiency
Purine nucleoside phosphorylase deficiency
Wilson disease
Xanthine oxidase deficiency

Ichthyosis

CHILD syndrome (congenital hemidysplasia ichthyosis
and limb defects)
Congenital disorders of glycosylation (CDG) type 1f
Gaucher disease
Krabbe disease
Multiple sulfatase deficiency
Refsum disease
Sjogren–Larsson syndrome
X-linked ichthyosis – steroid sulfatase deficiency

Ichthyosis and Retinal Disease

Refsum syndrome
Sjogren–Larrson syndrome

Inverted Nipples

Biopterin synthesis disorders
Citrullinemia
Congenital disorders of glycosylation
Glycogenosis 1b
Hyperphenylalaninemia
Isolated – dominant (MIM163610)
Isovaleric acidemia
Menkes disease
Methylmalonic acidemia
Molybdenum cofactor deficiency
Niemann–Pick type C
SCAD deficiency
Propionic acidemia
Pyruvate carboxylase deficiency
VLCAD deficiency
Weaver syndrome

Isolated Deficiency of Speech as Presentation
in Metabolic Disease

Ethylmalonic aciduria
D-glyceric aciduria

Histidinemia
3-Methylglutaconyl-CoA hydratase

Lactic Acidemia

Electron transport chain
disorders
Fatty acid oxidation disorders
Lues, congenital
MELAS
MERRF
Organic acidemia, e.g., propionic
acidemia
Pyruvate carboxylase deficiency
Pyruvate dehydrogenase deficiency

Leigh Syndrome

Biotinidase deficiency
Electron transport chain disorders
Fumarase deficiency
3-Methylglutaconic aciduria
Pyruvate carboxylase deficiency
Pyruvate dehydrogenase complex
deficiency
Sulfite oxidase deficiency

Leukopenia with or without Thrombopenia and Anemia

Abnormalities of folate metabolism
Isovaleric acidemia
Johansson–Blizzard syndrome
Methylmalonic acidemia
3-Oxothiolase deficiency
Pearson syndrome
Propionic acidemia
Shwachman syndrome
Transcobalamin II deficiency

Macrocephaly

Bannayan–Ruvalcaba–Riley syndrome
Canavan disease
Glutaric aciduria type I
Hurler disease
4-Hydroxybutyric aciduria
L-2-hydroxyglutaric aciduria
3-Hydroxy-3-methylglutaric aciduria
Krabbe disease
Mannosidosis
Multiple acyl-CoA dehydrogenase deficiency
Multiple sulfatase deficiency
Neonatal adrenoleukodystrophy

Pyruvate carboxylase deficiency
Tay–Sachs disease

Megaloblastic Anemia

Cobalamin metabolic errors-methylmalonic acidemia
and homocystinuria-Cbl C and D
Folate metabolism, abnormalities of
B_{12} deficiency – vegan or breast-fed infant of vegan
mother
CblF cobalamin lysosomal transporter deficiency
Dietary folate deficiency
Folate malabsorption – hereditary – protein coupled
folate transport (PCFT) deficiency
Intestinal B_{12} transport deficiency – Imerslund–
Grasbeck-cubilin deficiency
Methylmalonic acidemia-homocystinuria-Cbl C + D
Mevalonic aciduria
Orotic aciduria
Pearson syndrome
Pernicious anemia – intrinsic factor
deficiency
Transcobalamin II deficiency

Metabolic Acidosis and Ketosis

Fabry disease
Familial hypocholesterolemia
Homocystinuria
Isovaleric academia
Menkes disease
Methylcrotonyl-CoA carboxylase deficiency
Methylmalonic/propionic acidemia
Multiple carboxylase deficiency
3-Oxothiolase deficiency

Methylmalonic aciduria

B_{12} deficiency, pernicious anemia, including
autoimmune
Cobalamin A
Cobalamin C, D
Imerslund–Gräsbeck – cobalamin enterocyte
malabsorption
Mut°, Mut⁻
Succinyl-CoA synthase deficiency
Transcobalamin II deficiency

Mongolian Spot – Extensive

GM_1 gangliosidosis
Hurler syndrome
Niemann–Pick disease

Myocardial infarction-cerebral vascular disease

Fabry disease
Familial hypercholesterolemia
Homocystinuria
Menkes disease
Oxothiolase deficiency
Propionic acidemia
SCHAD deficiency

Neonatal Hepatic Presentations in Metabolic Diseases

α-1-Antitrypsin deficiency
Cystic fibrosis
Fructose intolerance
Galactosemia
Glycosylation disorders, especially type Ib
Hemochromatosis
Hepatorenal tyrosinemia
Long-chain hydroxy-acyl-CoA dehydrogenase deficiency
Mitochondrial DNA depletion syndromes
Niemann–Pick type C disease
Wilson disease
Wolman disease
Sly disease

Odd or Unusual Odor

Dimethylglycinuria
Glutaric aciduria type II
Hepatorenal tyrosinemia
Isovaleric acidemia
Maple syrup urine disease
Phenylketonuria
Treatment of urea cycle disorder with phenylacetate
Trimethylaminuria

Optic Atrophy

ADP-ribosyl protein lyase deficiency
Adrenoleukodystrophy (ALD)
Biotinidase deficiency
Canavan disease
GM_1 gangliosidosis
Homocystinuria
Krabbe disease
Menkes disease
Methylmalonic acidemia
MERRF
Metachromatic leukodystrophy
3-Methylglutaconic aciduria, type III (Costeff)

Mevalonic aciduria
Mitochondrial energy metabolism, defects in – including
Leber hereditary optic neuropathy (LHON)
Multiple sulfatase deficiency
NARP
Neonatal adrenoleukodystrophy
Propionic acidemia
Sandhoff disease
Tay–Sachs disease

Orotic Aciduria

UMP synthase deficiency (hereditary orotic aciduria)
Urea cycle defects – ornithine transcarbamylase deficiency, citrullinemia, arginosuccinic aciduria, arginemia
Purine nucleoside phosphorylase (PNP) deficiency
Phosphoribosylpyrophosphate (PRPP) synthetase deficiency

Osteoporosis and Fractures

Adenosine deaminase deficiency
Gaucher disease
Glycogenesis I
Homocystinuria
I-cell disease
Infantile Refsum disease
Lysinuric protein intolerance
Menkes disease
Methylmalonic acidemia
Propionic acidemia

Pain and Elevated Erythrocyte Sedimentation Rate

Fabry disease
Familial hypercholesterolemia
Gaucher disease

Pancreatitis

Carnitine palmitoyltransferase II deficiency
Cytochrome c oxidase deficiency
Glycogenesis type I
Glycogenesis 1 plus apoE2 type III hypertriglyceridemia
Hereditary dominant, with or without lysinuria; with or without pancreatic lithiasis or portal vein thrombosis
Homocystinuria
Hydroxymethylglutaryl-CoA lyase deficiency
Hyperlipoproteinemia type IV
Isovaleric acidemia

Lipoprotein lipase deficiency, also type IV
Lysinuric protein intolerance
Maple syrup urine disease
MELAS
Methylmalonic acidemia
Ornithine transcarbamylase deficiency
Pearson syndrome
Propionic acidemia
Regional enteritis (Crohn)
Trauma – pseudocyst
With hyperparathyroidism in multiple endocrine adenomatosus syndrome

Paralysis of Upward Gaze

Leigh, Kearns–Sayre syndromes
Niemann–Pick type C
Peripheral neuropathy

Photophobia

Cystinosis
Oculocutaneous tyrosinemia

Polycystic Kidneys

Carnitine palmitoyl transferase II (CPT-II) deficiency
Congenital disorders of glycosylation
Glutaric aciduria type II, (multiple acyl-CoA dehydrogenase deficiency) (GA II)
Zellweger syndrome

Psychotic Behavior

Carbamoyl phosphate synthetase deficiency
Cbl disease
Ceroid lipofuscinoses
Citrullinemia
Hartnup disease
Homocystinuria
Hurler–Scheie, Scheie disease
Krabbe disease
Lysinuric protein
β-mannosidosis
Maple syrup urine disease
5,10-Methylenetetrahydrofolatereductase deficiency
Metachromatic leukodystrophy
Mitochondrial disease (MELAS)
Niemann–Pick type C disease
Ornithine transcarbamylase deficiency
Porphyria
Sanfilippo disease
Tay–Sachs, Sandhoff-late onset

Wilson disease

Ptosis

Dopamine deficiency syndromes
Kearn–Sayre syndrome
MNGIE (mitochondrial neurogastrointestinal encephalomyelopathy)

Ragged Red Fibers

Menkes disease
Mitochondrial DNA mutations

Red Urine

Beets
Hematuria
Hemoglobinuria
Myoglobinuria
Drugs: rifampicin, phenolphthalein, nitrofurantoin, ibuprofen, pyridium

Renal Calculi

APRT (adenosine phosphoribosyltransferase) deficiency
Cystinuria
HPRT deficiency-Lesch–Nyhan disease
Oxaluria
PRPP synthetase abnormalities
Wilson disease
Xanthine oxidase deficiency

Renal Fanconi Syndrome

Cystinosis
Electron transport defects
Galactosemia
Glycogenosis I and III
Hepatorenal tyrosinemia
Idiopathic
Lowe syndrome
Lysinuric protein intolerance
Wilson disease

Renal tubular acidosis (RTA)

Cystinosis
Fanconi syndrome
Galactosemia
Hepatorenal tyrosinemia
Mitochondrial electron transport defect
Osteopetrosis and RTA
Topamax

Retinitis Pigmentosa

Abetalipoproteinemia
Congenital disorder of glycosylation
Ceroid lipofuscinosis
Hunter disease
Kearns–Sayre syndrome
LCHAD deficiency
Mevalonic aciduria
NARP
Peroxisomal biosynthesis disorders
Primary retinitis pigmentosa
Refsum disease
Sjogren–Larsson syndrome (fatty alcohol oxidoreductase deficiency)

Reye Syndrome Presentation

Gluconeogenesis, disorders of Fatty acid oxidation disorders
Urea cycle disorders
Electron transport chain disorders
Fructose intolerance
Organic acidemia

Reynaud Syndrome

Fabry disease

Rhabdomyolysis

Aldolase A (fructose bisphosphate) deficiency
Disorders of fatty acid oxidation – LCHAD, CPTII
Drugs – methylenedioxymethylamphetamine (MDMA)
Glutaric acidemia I
Glycogenosis V-McArdle – myophosphorylase
VII – Tarui – phosphofructokinase
Glycolysis – phosphoglycerate kinase
– phosphoglyceromutase
Infection – myositis
Ischemic injury
Mitochondrial DNA deletions (multiple)
Mitochondrial point mutations (MELAS)
Oxphos defects – complex I, complex II
Quail ingestion – coturnism
Toxin-tetanus, snake venom, alcohol, cocaine, bee venom

Scoliosis

Congenital disorder of glycosylation
Homocystinuria

Self Injurous Behavior

Lesch–Nyhan disease
Neuroacanthocytosis

Sensorineural Deafness

Biotinidase deficiency
Canavan disease
Kearns–Sayre syndrome and other electron transport chain disorders
Peroxisomal disorders
PRPP synthetase abnormality
Refsum disease

Spastic Paraparesis

Argininemia
Biotinidase deficiency
HHH syndrome
Metachromatic leukodystrophy
Pyroglutamic aciduria
Sjögren–Larsson syndrome

Stroke-like Episodes

Carbamyl phosphate synthetase deficiency
Chediak–Higashi syndrome
Congenital disorders of glycosylation
Ethylmalonic encephalopathy
Fabry disease
Familial hypercholesterolemia
Glutaric aciduria type I
Homocystinuria
Hydroxymethylglutaryl-CoA lyase deficiency
Isovaleric acidemia
MELAS and other mitochondrial disorders
Menkes disease
Methylcrotonyl-CoA carboxylase deficiency
Methylmalonic acidemia
5,10-Methylenetetrahydrofolatereductase deficiency
Multiple acyl-CoA dehydrogenase deficiency
Ornithine transcarbamylase deficiency
Propionic acidemia
Phosphoglycerate kinase deficiency
Progeria
Pyruvate carboxylase deficiency
Pyruvate dehydrogenase deficiency
Respiratory chain disorders
Purine nucleoside phosphorylase deficiency
Sulfite oxidase deficiency

Subdural effusions

Glutaric aciduria I
D-2-Hydroxyglutaric aciduria
Menkes disease
Pyruvate carboxylase deficiency

Vomiting and Erroneous Diagnosis of Pyloric Stenosis

Ethylmalonic-adipic aciduria
Galactosemia
HMG-CoA lyase deficiency
4-Hydroxybutyric aciduria
D-2-Hydroxyglutaric aciduria

Isovaleric acidemia
Methylmalonic acidemia
3-Oxothiolase deficiency
Phenylketonuria
Propionic acidemia

Xanthomas

Cerebrotendinous xanthomatosis
Familial hypercholesterolemia
Lipoprotein lipase deficiency
Niemann–Pick disease
Sitosterolemia

Reference Books

E2

Blau N, Duran M, Blaskovics ME, Gibson KM (eds) (2003) Physician's guide to the laboratory diagnosis of metabolic diseases, 2nd edn. Springer, Berlin.

Detailed collation of clinical and laboratory findings in individual disorders. Very helpful for metabolic specialists and clinicians with experience of metabolic disorders but less well suited to clinicians who do not regularly see patients with inborn errors of metabolism.

Blau N, Duran M, Gibson KM (eds) (2008) Laboratory guide to the methods in biochemical genetics. Springer, Berlin.

A prime resource for metabolic specialists working in the laboratory that also provides excellent background information for clinicians interested in methodological background information.

Blau N, Hoffmann GF, Leonard J, Clarke JTR (eds) (2005) Physician's guide to the treatment and follow-up of metabolic diseases. Springer, Berlin.

The book gives detailed information with regard to the management of metabolic disorders. It is an intermediary between more general textbooks and dedicated original articles. A useful reference book for clinicians who see metabolic patients.

Bremer HJ, Duran M, Kamerling JP, Przyrembel H, Wadman SK (1981) Disturbances of amino acid metabolism: clinical chemistry and diagnosis. Baltimore-Munich, Urban & Schwarzenberg.

A unique, detailed source of information on amino acids and aminoacidopathies. Contains large tables of normal values in various body fluids. Somewhat outdated and unfortunately out of print, but worth an effort to get secondhand.

Clarke JTR (2006) A clinical guide to inherited metabolic diseases, 3rd edn. Cambridge University Press, Cambridge.

Hands-on description of five symptom-based presentations of metabolic diseases (CNS, heart or liver disease, the acutely ill neonate, and storage disorders) as well as other clinically relevant categories.

Fernandes J, Saudubray JM, van den Berghe G, Walter JH (eds) (2006) Inborn metabolic diseases – diagnosis and treatment, 4th edn. Springer, Berlin.

Accessible pathway-based approach to inborn errors of metabolism. Covers all the major groups of metabolic disorders and is particularly helpful for clinicians who seek basic information on diagnosis and treatment of individual defects. Individual chapters written by various authors and of variable quality.

Firth HV, Hurst JA (2005) Oxford desk reference clinical genetics. Oxford University Press, Oxford. A well-written, practical text. It is primarily aimed at clinical geneticist and does not have a specific focus on metabolic disorders but is an extremely valuable resource for all clinicians who encounter patient's genetic conditions.

Nyhan WL, Barshop BA, Ozand PT (2005) Atlas of metabolic diseases, 2nd edn. Hodder Arnold, London.

Detailed clinically oriented monographs of a wide range of individual metabolic disorders with excellent photographs.

Rimoin DL, Connor JM, Pyeritz RE, Korf BR (eds) (2006) Emery and Rimoin's principles and practice of medical genetics, 5th edn. Churchill Livingston, New York.

G. F. Hoffmann et al. (eds.), *Inherited Metabolic Diseases*,
DOI: 10.1007/978-3-540-74723-9_E2, © Springer-Verlag Berlin Heidelberg 2010

An excellent, comprehensive and mostly up-to-date textbook of clinical genetics. Chapters dealing with metabolic disorders are not always convincing. 3 Volumes, quite expensive.

Sarafoglu K, Hoffmann GF, Roth K (eds) (2009) Pediatric endocrinology and inborn errors of metabolism, McGraw Hill, New York.

Concise, comprehensive, and reasonably prized clinical textbook covering the whole field of metabolic as well as endocrine disorders. A must for every consultant pediatrician, not only endocrinologists and metabolic specialists.

Scriver CR, Beaudet AL, Sly WS, Valle D (eds) (2001) The metabolic and molecular bases of inherited disease, 7th edn. McGraw-Hill, New York.

The last printed version of the standard textbook on inborn errors of metabolism, extended to four volumes and nonmetabolic conditions. Special emphasis on molecular and pathophysiologal aspects of individual disorders. It has now turned into a huge online knowledgebase ("Online Metabolic and Molecular Bases of Inherited Disease") covering the widest possible range of inherited disorders but unfortunately requires an expensive annual subscription (www.ommbid.com).

Zschocke J, Hoffmann GF (2004) Vademecum metabolicum – manual of metabolic paediatrics, 2nd edn. Schattauer, Stuttgart.

A concise pocket book containing the essentials of metabolic pediatrics, with short descriptions of most inborn errors of metabolism.

Internet Resources

Society for the Study of Inborn Errors of Metabolism, SSIEM (www.ssiem.org)

Society for Inherited Metabolic Disorders (www.simd.org)

The homepages of the SSIEM (international, focus in Europe) and the SIEM (USA) provide excellent links to various internet resources concerned with inborn errors of metabolism, including learned societies, parent organisations, laboratory directories, etc.

National Center for Biotechnology Information, NCBI (www.ncbi.nlm.nih.gov)

The primary source for molecular biology information on the Internet. Home to Pubmed, OMIM, GenBank, and a vast range of other databases. May be difficult to navigate without some experience.

OMIM (http://www.ncbi.nlm.nih.gov/omim)

This is the online version of "Mendelian Inheritance in Man," the oldest collation of genetic disorders, originally edited by Victor A. McKusick. It is freely available from the NCBI. The database contains monographs of individual disorders and genes together with references and extensive links to other online resources. OMIM has an emphasis on molecular information, but there are also plenty of clinical data that are useful in daily practice. The number allocated to entries in the OMIM catalog is used in scientific publications worldwide for the exact identification of individual genetic disorders.

GeneTests (www.genetests.org)

A freely available medical genetics information resource, specifically for physicians and other health care providers, is funded by the National Institute of Health,

USA. Its "GeneReviews" are extremely useful monographs with detailed information on clinical presentation, diagnosis, differential diagnosis, management and genetic counseling, molecular genetics, etc., available now for a huge number of individual conditions. There are also directories of clinical centres and diagnostic laboratories particularly in the USA. GeneTests incorporates the previous GeneClinics Web site.

Orphanet (www.orpha.net) and EuroGentest (www.eurogentest.org)

Orphanet is an originally French database that developed into a major European portal for rare genetic diseases and orphan drugs. It was selected as the central database of EuroGentest, a more recent EU-funded Network of Excellence looking at various aspects of genetic testing, including quality management, information databases, and education. Together the websites provide a wealth of information on rare diseases and various resources particularly in Europe, including a laboratory directory, clinical centres, patient support groups, etc. The information is available in different languages; moreover, access to the site is free of charge.

European Directory of DNA Laboratories, EDDNAL (www.eddnal.com)

EDDNAL provides information on genetic services and molecular genetic laboratories in Europe. It was initiated by the European Molecular Genetics Quality Network (EMQN) initiative that provides quality assessment schemes for molecular tests. Access to the site is free of charge.

Human Genome Variation Society Website, HGVS (www.hgvs.org)

G. F. Hoffmann et al. (eds.), *Inherited Metabolic Diseases*,
DOI: 10.1007/978-3-540-74723-9_E3, © Springer-Verlag Berlin Heidelberg 2010

The HGVS aims to "foster discovery and characterization of genomic variations." The website provides links to a vast number of locus-specific mutation databases as well as standard recommendations for mutation nomenclature. An important resource for clinical molecular geneticists as well as clinicians and scientists trying to find additional mutation-related information.

Human Gene Mutation Database, HGMD (www.hgmd.cf.ac.uk)

This database on mutations causing human disorders, based in Cardiff, Wales, was originally established for the study of mutational mechanisms in human genes. Mutations were also identified by scanning published articles, a major effort. However, content freely available is not up-to-date, and the full "professional" version provided by a commercial partner is extremely expensive even for academic/nonprofit users.

GeneCards (www.genecards.org)

This is a concise, gene-oriented database that contains information on various functions of human genes including the respective proteins and associated disorders. There are copious links to other Internet databases. GeneCards are particularly useful for geneticists and researchers in the areas of functional genomics and proteomics.

Online Metabolic and Molecular Bases of Inherited Disease (www.ommbid.com)

It is the online successor of the standard textbook of inborn errors of metabolism, with detailed information on molecular and pathophysiological aspects of individual disorders. Though vastly expanded to cover the widest possible range of inherited disorders, it unfortunately requires an expensive annual subscription.

Index